EVOKED ELECTRICAL ACTIVITY IN THE AUDITORY NERVOUS SYSTEM

ACADEMIC PRESS RAPID MANUSCRIPT REPRODUCTION

The Proceedings of a Symposium held
at the University of Chicago, 1977

Evoked Electrical Activity in the Auditory Nervous System

Edited by
Ralph F. Naunton
Cesár Fernández

Department of Otolaryngology
University of Chicago
Chicago, Illinois

ACADEMIC PRESS New York San Francisco London 1978

A Subsidiary of Harcourt Brace Jovanovich, Publishers

ACADEMIC PRESS, INC.
111 Fifth Avenue, New York, New York 10003

United Kingdom Edition published by
ACADEMIC PRESS, INC. (LONDON) LTD.
24/28 Oval Road, London NW1 7DX

LIBRARY OF CONGRESS CATALOG CARD NUMBER: 78-19665

ISBN: 0-12-514960-3

PRINTED IN THE UNITED STATES OF AMERICA

CONTENTS

BRAINSTEM

Moderator: *Jerzy E. Rose*

BASIC AND CLINICAL ASPECTS OF BRAINSTEM RECORDING IN HUMANS

BRIEF FORMAL PRESENTATIONS AND ROUND TABLE DISCUSSION

Moderator: *Hallowell Davis*

BASIC AND CLINICAL ASPECTS OF BRAINSTEM RECORDING IN HUMANS

A ROUND TABLE DISCUSSION

Moderator: *Hallowell Davis*

CORTEX

Moderator: *Robert A. Butler*

SYMPOSIUM SUMMARY

CONTRIBUTORS

Numbers in parentheses indicate the pages on which authors' contributions begin.

J. Achor (443), University of California, Irvine
Francisco Antoli-Candela, Jr. (165), Centro Especial "Ramon y Cajal," Madrid
Jean-Marie Aran (239), Bordeaux II University
Jesper Barfod (525), Gentofte University Hospital, Copenhagen
H. A. Beagley (259), Royal National Throat, Nose and Ear Hospital
Michael V. L. Bennett (83), Albert Einstein College of Medicine
F. Owen Black (323), University of Pittsburgh
John F. Brugge (487), University of Wisconsin
Yves Cazals (239), Bordeaux II University
Manuel M. Cohen (551), Albert Einstein College of Medicine
Peter Dallos (141), Northwestern University
Hallowell Davis (575), Central Institute for the Deaf, St. Louis
Irving T. Diamond (463), Duke University
Josef J. Eggermont (209), University Hospital, Leiden
Donald H. Eldredge (69, 151), Central Institute for the Deaf, St. Louis
Robert Galambos (405), University of California, San Diego
George M. Gerken (409), University of Texas at Dallas
W. P. R. Gibson (259), Royal Throat, Nose, and Ear Hospital, London
William R. Goff (505), Yale University School of Medicine
John M. Harrison (353), Boston University
Raul Hinojosa (301), University of Chicago
Thomas Holton (91), Massachusetts Eye and Ear Infirmary, and Massachusetts Institute of Technology
Thomas J. Imig (487), University of Wisconsin
Eileen S. Kane (337), University of Massachusetts
Nelson Y. S. Kiang (165), Harvard Medical School
John R. Lindsay (301), University of Chicago
Alexander Ling, Jr. (91), Massachusetts Eye and Ear Infirmary, and Massachusetts Institute of Technology
Ralph F. Naunton (195, 221, 275), University of Chicago
P. Osterhammel (415), University Hospital, Copenhagen
William T. Peake (91), Massachusetts Eye and Ear Infirmary, and Massachusetts Institute of Technology
Isabelle Rapin (551), Albert Einstein College of Medicine
Ian J. Russell (113), University of Sussex
Gerhard Salomon (525), Gentofte University Hospital, Copenhagen

Peter M. Sellick (113), University of Sussex
Catherine A. Smith (3), University of Oregon
Heinrich Spoendlin (21), University Clinic, Innsbruck
Arnold Starr (443), University of California, Irvine
Knud Terkildosen (415), University Hospital, Copenhagen
A. Roger D. Thornton (429), Southampton University
Chiyeko Tsuchitani (373), University of Texas Health Science Center
W. Bruce Warr (43), The Boys Town Institute for Communication Disorders in Children, Omaha
Thomas F. Weiss (91), Massachusetts Eye and Ear Infirmary and Massachusetts Institute of Technology
F. Huis in 't Veld (415), University Hospital, Copenhagen
Stanley S. Zerlin (195, 221, 275), University of Chicago

PREFACE

Recognition of the recent growth of interest in the study of the human auditory nervous system by means of auditory evoked potentials prompted the decision to organize a symposium on this subject at the University of Chicago. The symposium, held October–November 1977, dealt with the anatomy, physiology, and clinical pathology of the end organ and first-order neuron, the brainstem, and the cortex; separate consideration was given to electrocochleography.

The contributors to this volume of the proceedings include basic scientists and clinicians from a variety of disciplines. The first section deals with the anatomy of the cochlear duct and the afferent and efferent innervation of the cochlea. The topic of the second section is the physiology of the end organ, with emphasis on hair cell physiology. This is followed by a third section on electrocochleography in animals and humans. Sections on the anatomy and physiology of the brainstem and cortex follow, each with subsections dealing with the clinical utility of electrical recordings from those areas. Finally, we present a review of the papers and discussions, and identification of promising avenues for further exploration.

One of the more valuable experiences provided by the symposium was the opportunity to see and hear clinicians and scientists interacting informally in open discussion; informal round table sessions were therefore included in the program and audience participation was encouraged. The resulting exchanges were recorded and are included in this volume.

R. F. NAUNTON AND C. FERNÁNDEZ

ANATOMY

Moderator: *Cesár Fernández*

Structure of the cochlear duct
Smith, Catherine A.

The afferent innervation of the cochlea
Spoendlin, Heinrich

The olivocochlear bundle: its origins and terminations in the cat
Warr, W. Bruce

Evoked Electrical Activity in the Auditory Nervous System

STRUCTURE OF THE COCHLEAR DUCT

Catherine A. Smith

University of Oregon

INTRODUCTION

There are a great many features of the structure of the cochlea that could be reviewed as a starting point for a discussion on electrical activity evoked by sound. It is not possible to consider all of them in an essay of this length, nor would it be desirable. I have chosen to summarize some of the more recent data. In particular the discussion will be centered about three topics:

1. In recent years a number of studies have been made in an effort to gain more information about ionic and molecular fluxes across the epithelium of the cochlear duct. Some of these investigations have made use of the passage of electron-dense tracers across or through the epithelial cells. Others were made by applying freeze-fracture techniques to the study of cell junctions.
2. It was postulated some years ago by Békésy (1953) and re-emphasized by Davis (1958) that the reticular lamina was a stiffened structure and that the hairs were moved across it by the tectorial membrane. Certainly by light and even electron microscopic examination the sub-surface apical cytoplasm of the Deiters and the hair cells is denser and more filamentous than that of the remainder of the cells. But do we have any definite morphological evidence that the surface of the organ of Corti is of unusual stiffness?
3. What is the present status of our knowledge regarding structure of the sensory cells?

The data presented here are the results of the efforts of many investigators working over the past twenty-five years, all of whom may not be named, but whose research has been basic and essential.

The membranous labyrinth is a closed epithelial tube. It begins in the embryo as an invagination of head ectoderm which moves inward and seals off to form a vesicle. The vesicle then expands and forms first the vestibular labyrinth and later the cochlea, each with its characteristic sensory and extra-sensory cell groups. Even though many specialized cells and structures evolve during matura-

ISBN 0-12-514960-3

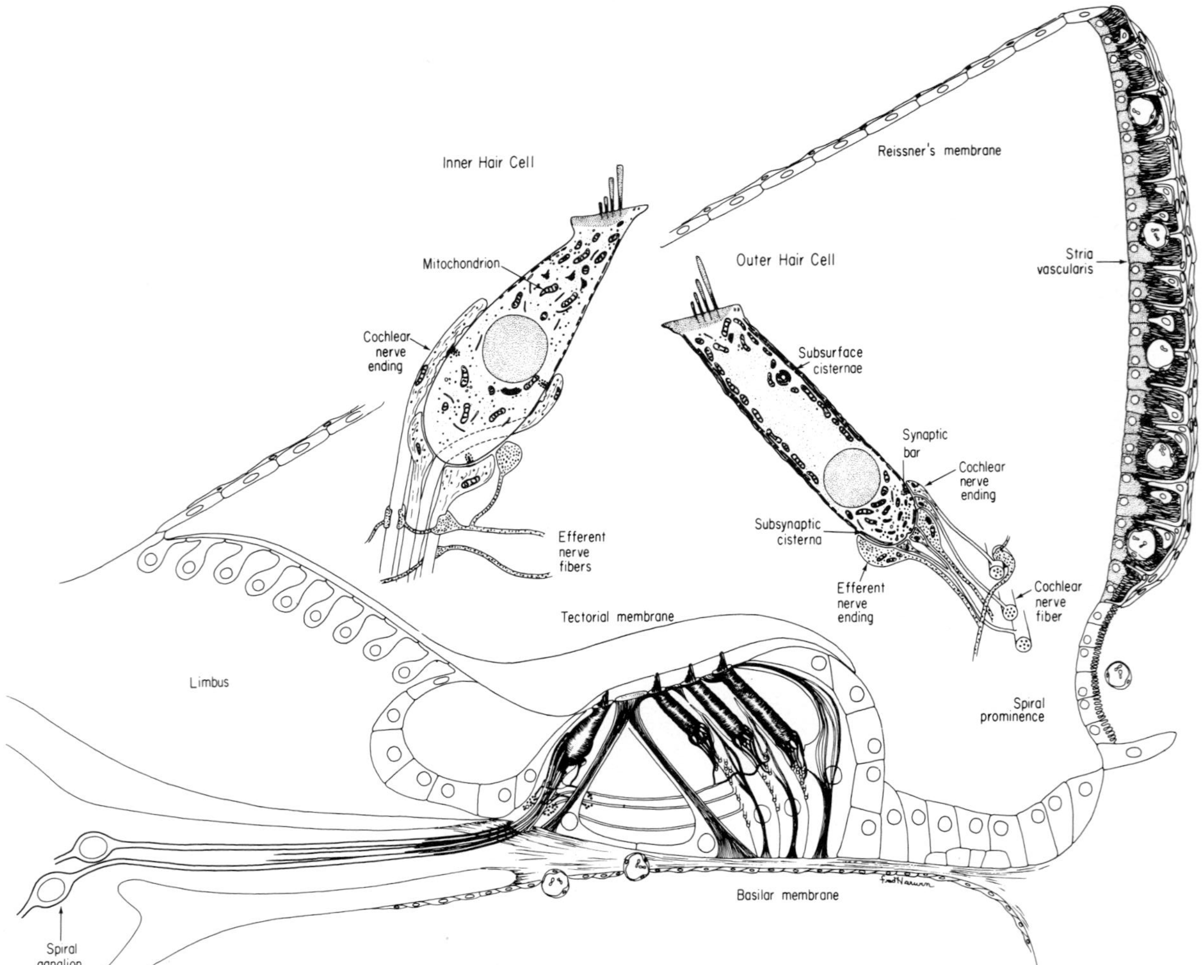

Inner Hair Cell
Reissner's membrane
Mitochondrion
Outer Hair Cell
Stria vascularis
Cochlear nerve ending
Subsurface cisternae
Synaptic bar
Cochlear nerve ending
Subsynaptic cisterna
Efferent nerve fibers
Efferent nerve ending
Cochlear nerve fiber
Tectorial membrane
Limbus
Spiral prominence
Basilar membrane
Spiral ganglion

Fig. 1. Drawing of the cochlear duct, second turn, guinea pig. (Reprinted from Smith, 1975 by permission from Raven Press).

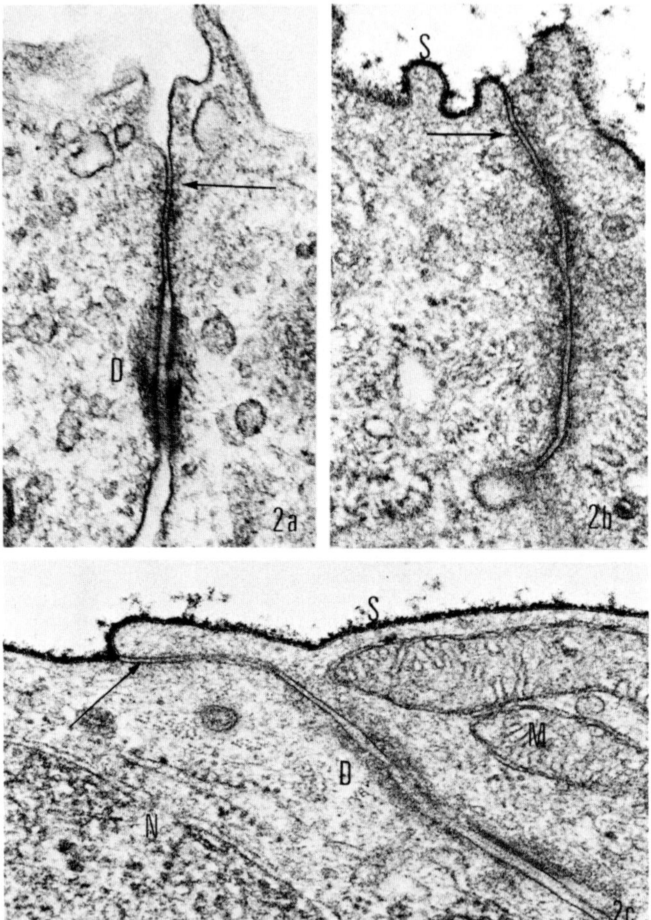
D
2a
S
2b
S
D
M
N
2c

tion, one thing remains unchanged, and that is the continuity of the epithelial layer (Fig. 1).

CELL JUNCTIONS

Junctions of the cochlear duct

The nature of the junctions between the epithelial cells that face the endolymph is of considerable importance because if the layer were leaky, the high potassium of endolymph would be difficult to maintain. Electron microscopists investigated this feature at an early date (Beagley, 1965; Iurato, 1965) and their micrographs revealed that there were tight junctions (as defined by Farquhar and Palade in 1963) between the apical ends of all the epithelial cells of the organ of Corti. It was also noticed by most investigators who studied the organ of Corti that there were long stretches of tight junctions between the basal parts of the Deiters cells.

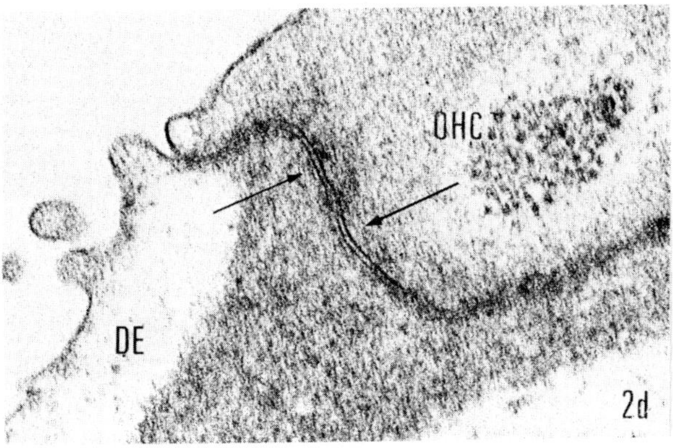

Fig. 2. Transmission electron micrographs (TEM) showing occluding junctions (arrows) at the apical ends of some of the epithelial cells lining the cochlear duct; a, Reissner's membrane; b, spiral prominence cells; c, marginal cells of stria vascularis; d, outer hair cell/Deiters' cell junctions. Mag.: a,b,c, 68,400 x; d, 53,900 x.

LABELS FOR THIS AND SUBSEQUENT FIGURES

BL, basal lamina
BM, basilar membrane
C, cochlear nerve ending
D, desmosome
DE, Deiters' cell
E, endolymph
EF, efferent nerve ending
ECS, extracellular space
M, mitochondrion
MT, microtubules
N, nucleus
OHC, outer hair cell
S, surface coat
Sc M, scala media
Sc T, scala tympani
Sc V, scala vestibuli
TR, tunnel rod cell

More recently, the use of tracers and freeze-fracture techniques have resulted in some re-definition of "tight" junctions, which are now divided into "gap" and "occluding" types. It has been re-confirmed that there are occluding junctions between all the cells which face the endolymph (Fig. 2a-d). This type of junction inhibits passage of most ions and molecules between cells, in this case from endolymph to perilymph (or interstitial fluid) or the reverse. Jahnke (1975b) and Gulley and Reese (1976) have used freeze-fracture methods to demonstrate occluding junctions between all cells at the reticular lamina (Fig. 2d) as well as in the inner and outer sulci in the guinea pig and chinchilla respectively. Franke et al. (1975) found narrow zonulae occludentes between the epithelial cells of Reissner's membrane (Fig. 2a). Reale et al., (1975) and Jahnke (1975a) have also described the occluding type of junctions between the marginal cells of the stria vascularis (Fig. 2c). There is therefore a complete system of occluding junctions between all the epithelial cells of the cochlear duct. Duvall and Sutherland (1972) injected horseradish peroxidase into the cisterna magna of the guinea pig's cerebrospinal fluid. Within 30 seconds, the peroxidase had passed into the cochlea (through the cochlear aqueduct), penetrated the basilar membrane and found its way into the intercellular spaces of the organ of Corti. Reaction product filled the intercellular spaces up to the zonulae occludentes, but was not present *between* these junctions. No reaction product was seen between or within the cells of the stria vascularis, only within the blood vessels in about one-half the animals. Hinojosa (1971, 1972) has shown that ferritin was carried *through* the epithelial cells of Reissner's membrane from perilymph to endolymph apparently by pinocytosis, and taken up by the marginal cells of the stria although not transported *across* the lateral wall within the time span of his experiments.

Reale et al., (1975) and Jahnke (1975a) found numerous zonulae occludentes between the basal cells of the stria vascularis. The occluding junctions between apical ends of marginal cells plus those between the basal cells make the stria a tightly sealed structure with the interstitial fluid of its interior separated from both endolymph and perilymph. The existence of this compartment is apparent after the administration of certain drugs such as diuretics which interfere with strial metabolism. A localized edema is produced only in the stria, which persists even after strial function, as shown by the endocochlear potential, has recovered to about three-fourths its normal activity (Brummett et al., 1977).

In summary, there is now ample evidence provided by the use of different kinds of tracers and techniques that the basilar membrane is fully permeable to at least small molecules in perilymph and that they penetrate rapidly to the sensory cells, but that the occluding junctions between all the epithelial cells facing the endolymph prevent ready ion diffusion between the two compartments containing endolymph or perilymph. The presence of a third compartment, in the stria vascularis, has been revealed: the apical surfaces of the marginal cells are bathed in endolymph, but the basal plasma membranes of the marginal cells, the capillaries, and the intermediate cells are sealed off from endolymph and perilymph by the basal cell layers (Fig. 3).

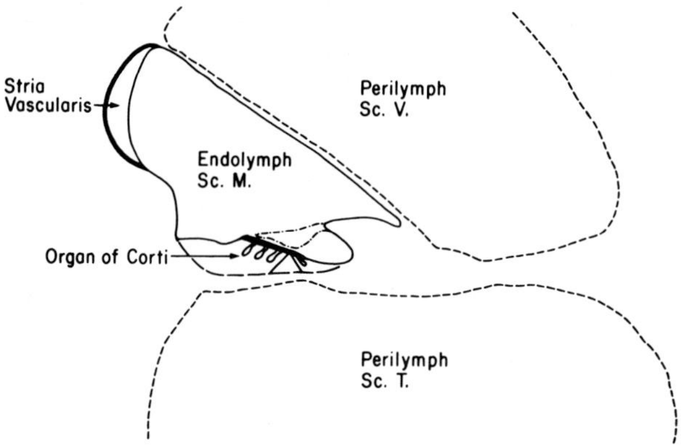

Fig. 3. Drawing illustrating compartments formed by occluding junctions. The thinner continuous line is the first compartment, filled by endolymph. The dashed line is the second compartment (perilymph). The thick line over the reticular lamina represents special junctions there. The thick line behind the stria vascularis represents special junctions between the basal cells which form the third compartment.

Junctions between the Deiters cells may also be of considerable physiological importance, but first, let us consider the reticular lamina.

The reticular lamina

The organ of Corti is composed of supporting and sensory cells (Fig. 1). The former extend from the basilar membrane to the reticular lamina, and hold the sensory cells in place. The outer supporting cells, the Deiters cells, are peculiar in that each has a thick basal column anchored on the basilar membrane. The upper part of this column forms a cup into which an outer hair cell with its nerve endings fits. The apical half of the Deiters cell is a slender process which arises from the cup and terminates in the reticular lamina. The lamina is a flat plate which is formed by the apical ends of the hair cells, the tunnel rods, the Deiters cells, and to some extent by the inner phalangeal cells. Only the hairs and small microvilli protrude from this flat surface which is continuous from basal to apical ends of the cochlea. If one views a section across the organ of Corti, large extracellular spaces are apparent between the tunnel rods and about the outer hair cells. Quite obviously the tunnel rods and Deiters' cells must have some intrinsic support otherwise they would never be able to hold the organ of Corti upright. The necessary stiffness is accomplished by means of bundles of microtubules. In the tunnel rods, the tubules spread out in the basal ends of the cells and have their origins very close to the plasma membrane (Fig. 4). They form a tight bundle in the slender central part of the cell, apparently being bound together by cross bonds, and spread out again at the apex in the reticular lamina. Hama and Saito (1976) have postulated that they may be inserted into the apical plasma membrane (the reticular lamina). The

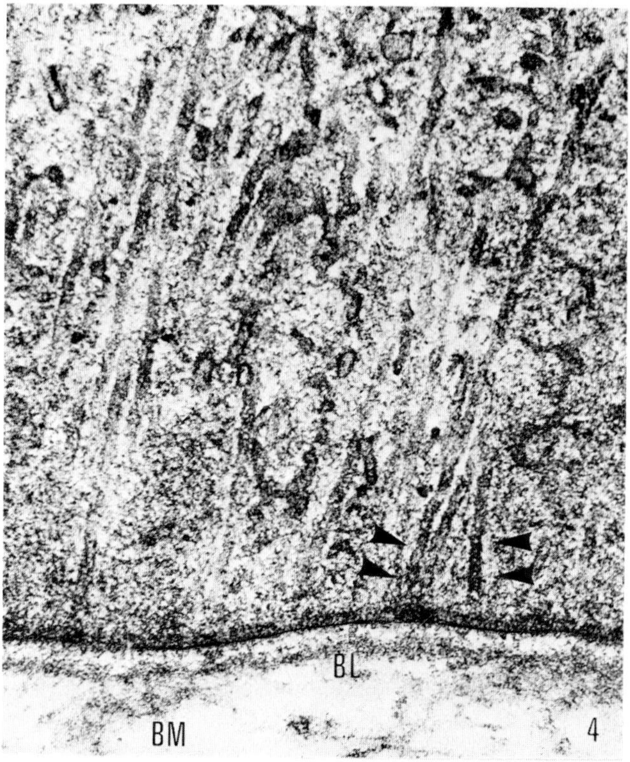

Fig. 4. TEM showing microtubules (arrowheads) which originate close to the plasma membrane of the tunnel rod cell. Mag.: 66,700 x, gerbil.

microtubules therefore apparently provide skeletal support for the organ of Corti and stiffness as well for the reticular lamina.

Freeze-fracture studies have shown that there is also a special junctional complex between the cells at the reticular lamina. All the cells of the reticular lamina are joined by a series of tight junctions which are of unusual depth and which encircle the apical end of each cell. These would lend stiffness to the lamina, as well as increase its resistance to stress. The function of the dense filamentous masses present within the sensory and supporting cell cytoplasm adjacent to the rings of occluding junctions is still unclear but they may also contribute to the overall stiffness of the lamina. It seems clear that we have good morphological evidence for stiffness in the organ of Corti, as well as at the reticular lamina.

The Deiters cells

The Deiters cells may have some function other than that of skeletal support. Electron microscopists have known for some time that there were long "tight"

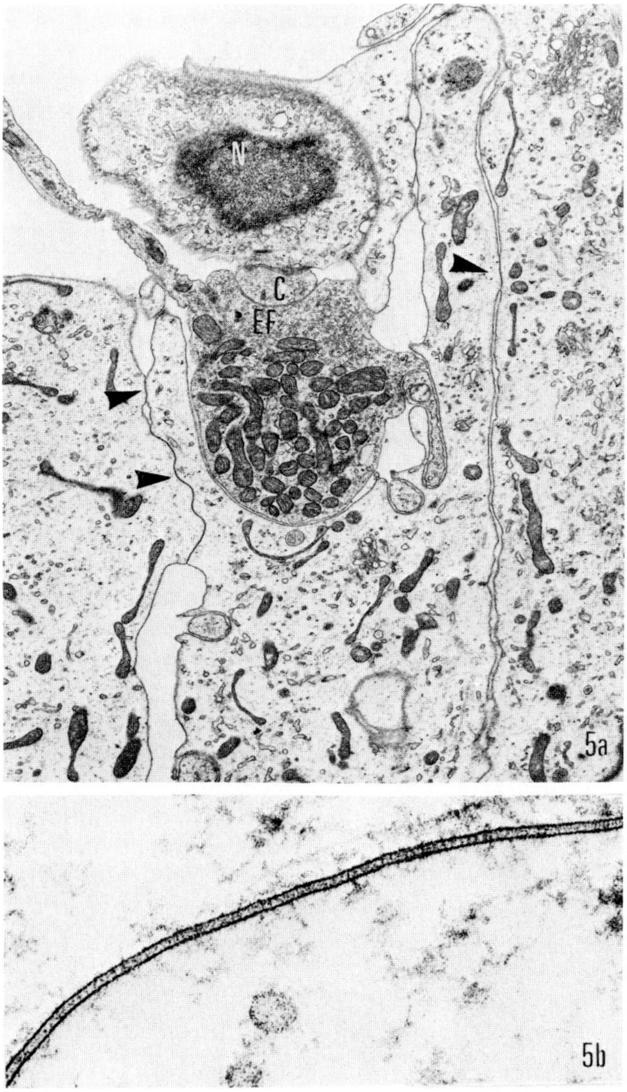

Fig. 5a. TEM of Deiters' cells with gap junctions between them in several places (arrowheads). The nucleus and basal tip of an outer hair cell is above, with cochlear and efferent nerve endings. Mag.: 11,120 x, gerbil.

b. Higher magnification (130,000 x) of a gap junction between Deiters' cells, guinea pig.

junctions between those cells (Fig. 5a,b). All investigators who have used the freeze-fracture techniques (Jahnke, 1975a, 1975b; Gulley and Reese, 1976; Hama and Saito, 1976, 1977) have found that these are gap junctions. This type of junction is characterized by a very narrow gap between the membranes (about 2-4nm.), with thin electron-dense bridges which span the gap (Fig. 5b). Globules on one face and complementary pits on the opposite face are revealed after freeze-fracturing (Hama and Saito, 1977). Gap junctions are the type of junction through which small ions (primarily K^+, N^+, $C1^-$) and some molecules pass from one cell to another. These cells are said to be ionically coupled.

There are some parallels between the glial cells of the brain and the Deiters cells. Both are interstitial cells surrounding other cells with excitatory properties; both are joined to adjacent cells of the same type by gap junctions. Recently Kuffler and Nichols (1976) have produced experimental evidence that the glial cells are very permeable to potassium ions and act like potassium electrodes. It has also been shown that glial cells are joined by gap junctions, so that ions can pass from one cell to another. Kuffler has advanced the theory that glial cells are important in regulating the ion environment of the neuronal population of the brain. It is possible that the Deiters cells perform a similar task for the hair cells and cochlear nerve dendrites. Hama and Saito (1977) have recently expressed a similar opinion.

Weiss et al. (1974) and Mulroy et al. (1974) recorded AC potentials from supporting cells as well as from sensory cells in the alligator lizard papilla. The magnitude of the potential in the two types of cells was similar, although the waveforms were different. Weiss et al. hypothesized that the sensory and supporting cells in the lizard papilla might be coupled by low resistance channels. There is no evidence that Deiters' cells are electronically coupled to the mammalian hair cells. Nor have such junctions been described between glial cells and neurons. There is some support for the proposal that Deiters' cells are susceptible to changes in their environment in the reaction of the Deiters cells to fixatives. Intravascular perfusion of very strong and hypertonic fixatives such as Heidehain-Susa fixative yield preparations in which the Deiters processes appear as slender rods. Osmium tetroxide sometimes produces the same result. Glutaraldehyde-formaldehyde fixatives often result in enlarged and irregular phalangeal processes (Fig. 6) which almost fill the extracellular spaces between hair cells. The tunnel rod cells do not usually react in this manner. Apparently under certain conditions, the Deiters cells readily take up water. It seems altogether probable that they have another function outside of physical support, and that is of maintaining a stable ion balance in the interstitial fluid around the outer hair cells and perhaps acting as miniature osmometers. It seems unlikely that the Deiters cells act in precisely the same manner as the glial cells. For, if their cell membranes as a whole were highly permeable to potassium, they would continually be absorbing potassium from endolymph. It is not inconceivable that their plasma membranes in the reticular lamina have different permeability properties from the remainder of the membrane.

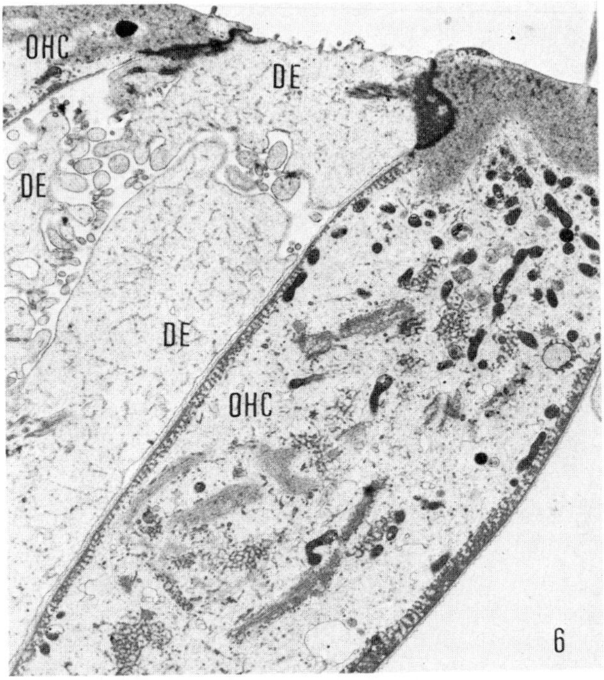

Fig. 6. TEM of Deiters' processes which are greatly enlarged between two outer hair cells. Mag.: 6,000 x, guinea pig.

Structure of the hair cells

All of the hair cells in the auditory system of vertebrates have some features in common: the cuticular plates with protruding bundles of hairs on their apical ends and sensory nerve endings about their basal ends. They all have a cuticular-free region on their apical ends where the kinocilia and/or the basal body resides in either the fetal or mature stage. Mammalian cochlear hair cells lose their kinocilia and possibly the basal bodies at maturity but most of the hair cells in reptiles and birds retain their kinocilia through adulthood. Beyond this, they vary considerably. The simplest hair cell form is that of a columnar or bottle-shaped cell, with a centrally placed nucleus, and organelles scattered throughout the cytoplasm. Cells of this type are found in the lateral line organ, and in reptilian and avian papillae. In the mammalian cochlea this cell-type is represented by the inner hair cell.

The inner hair cells are arranged as a single row of receptor cells that stretches from basal to apical ends of the cochlea. The hair bundle is composed of several rows of hairs which bisect the cuticular plate. The hairs on inner and outer hair cells are always arranged in stepwise length, the longest hairs being most lateral. Some of the nerve endings are long and finger-like and extend for almost 10 microns up the side of the cell; others terminate about the basal end. A single row

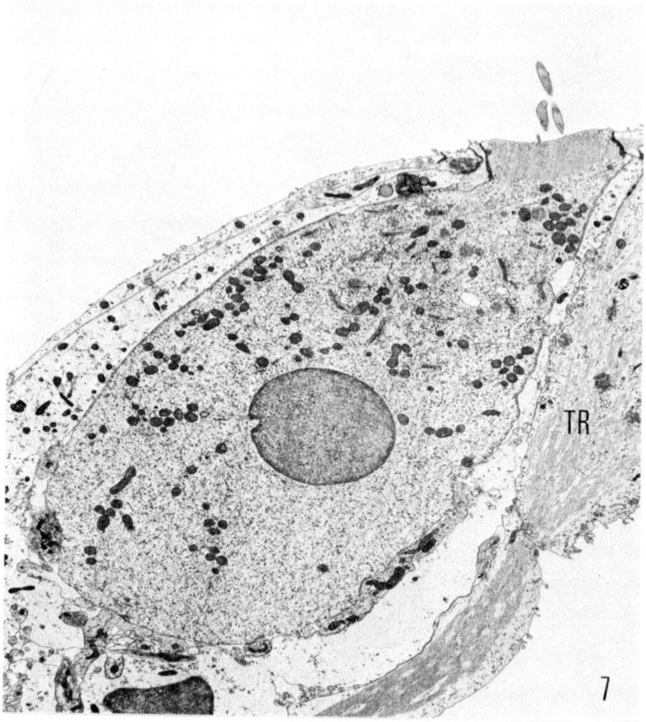

Fig. 7. TEM of inner hair cell with supporting cells. Mag.: 3,700 x, gerbil.

of cisternae or vesicles of endoplasmic reticulum is localized just beneath the plasmalemma (Fig. 7).

The outer hair cells are most highly specialized (Fig. 8) and are unique in the auditory or vestibular systems of vertebrates. The cells are polarized by their nuclei, and divided into large supra-nuclear portions and considerably smaller infra-nuclear parts (Smith, 1968). The apical portion has an organized system of smooth endoplasmic reticulum (ER) and mitochondria adjacent to the plasmalemma (Figs. 8,9). The plasmalemma of this part of the outer hair cell (but not the inner hair cell) is thick, irregular and less dense than usual (Smith and Dempsey, 1957). The ER forms multiple subsurface laminae in some mammals, but is restricted to a single layer in others. Whether the ER forms a single or multiple layer, mitochondria are always closely associated with it near the cell membrane. The outermost layer of ER is often seen as a long cisterna. The inner layers appear to be more vesicular and interconnected in a honeycomb form. Electron-dense bridges (Smith, 1975) appear to span the space between outer lamina and the plasmalemma (Fig. 9a-b). The bridges can be visualized in the outer hair cells of guinea pigs, gerbils and chinchillas, and even in squirrel monkeys which have only a single layer of ER. It is possible that some of the dense pin-points in Figure 9a may

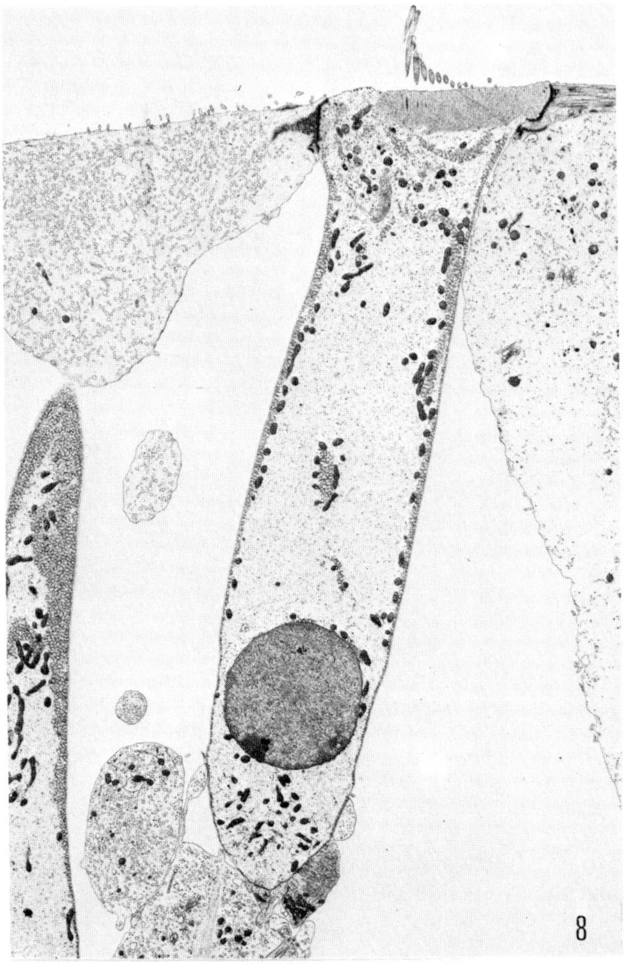

Fig. 8. TEM of outer hair cell. Mag.: 3,600 x, guinea pig.

actually be the terminals of inward dips of the plasma membrane. Whatever their nature, there is an unusually close relationship between plasma membrane and the sub-surface cisternae of ER. The significance of this unusual cell membrane/ER relationship is not clear.

It was originally proposed by Davis (1958) that there was a current flow across the cochlear duct with an important part of the circuit being through the hair cells and across the nerve endings. Johnstone and Sellick (1972) added to this another local flow which "short-circuited" across the apical part of the hair cell

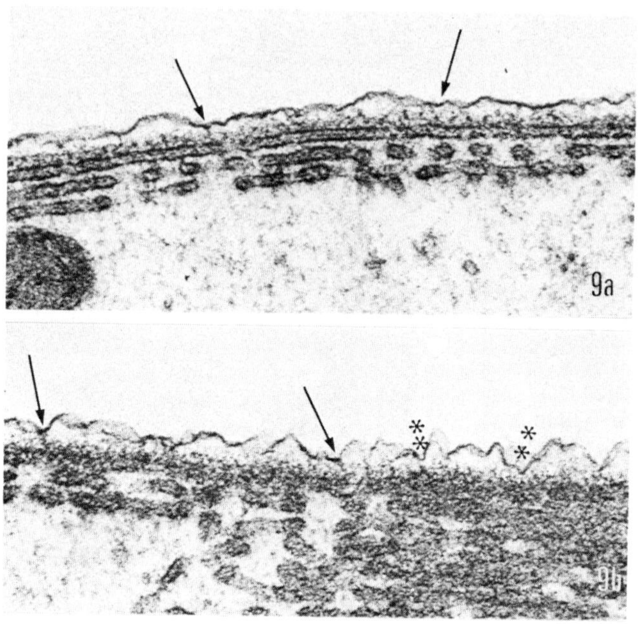

Fig. 9. TEM of peripheral cisternae of endoplasmic reticulum adjacent to the plasma membrane of an outer hair cell; 9a illustrates the dense material attached to the outermost cisterna and cross-bridges (arrows); 9b is cut tangential to the ER membranes and shows the manner in which the plasma membrane dips in toward the ER (asterisk); cross-bridges at arrows. Mag.: 59,000 x, guinea pig.

and then through the reticular lamina to endolymph. Dallos (1973) proposed a steady potassium flow from endolymph, in across the apical end of the hair cell and out through the hair cell membrane to the fluid in the spaces of Nuel. Johnstone's and Dallos' hypothetical circuits, with an outward flow across the upper part of the hair cell, could be fitted into its structure. Possibly this part of the outer hair cell membrane is more leaky than other tri-laminar membranes, and more so than the plasma membrane covering the lower half of the cell. Peters et al. (1966) noted that the contours of the axolemma at the node of Ranvier was irregular and that a layer of dense granular material was applied to the inner surface of the axolemma. There are some similarities between the node of Ranvier and hair cell membrane, but the two are not identical. However it would not be unreasonable to postulate rapid ion fluxes across the outer hair cell membrane. It is in searching for morphological correlates to complete a rapid circuit through the Deiters cells and across the reticular lamina that one runs into difficulties.

Another cell where there is a close relationship of ER to plasmalemma is the skeletal muscle cell. A triad is formed by close apposition of the invagination of the sarcolemma to the sarcoplasmic reticulum. It is believed that calcium is stored in the muscle ER cisternae. Perhaps the lamellar ER in the outer hair cells are ion storage sites and assist in maintaining the appropriate internal ion balance which might easily be upset by excessive activation of the sensory cells.

Finally, we come to the infra-nuclear parts of the hair cells where the nerve endings are located. The nucleus is large and almost completely fills the diameter of the cell. There is only a thin layer of cytoplasm between it and the plasma membrane. The nucleus might impede rapid ion or metabolite flow between the two parts of the cell. Alternatively it could act as a physical barrier to segregate the organelles which are relevant to production of the transmitter to the basal tip of the cell. The basal cytoplasm of the outer hair cells of some animals is packed with mitochondria and membranes (chinchilla and guinea pig), whereas in others, such as the gerbil, the cytoplasmic volume below the nucleus is so small that the few mitochondria present are pushed up into the nuclear membrane. It is suggested that the morphological polarization reflects a physiological compartmentalization and that the supra-nuclear part of the cell is specialized to produce the cochlear microphonics, but that the depolarization current may be impeded by some means from consistently spreading down to the infra-nuclear part of the cell to release the transmitter substance. The large and numerous efferent nerve endings may also play a part in preventing excessive depolarization of this region. It is hoped that these speculations will be thought-provoking and perhaps the sources of some experimental studies.

SUMMARY

1. There are occluding junctions between all of the epithelial cells of the cochlear duct so that we may assume that ion fluxes across this boundary are impeded.
2. The junctions between the apical ends of the cells of the organ of Corti are quite complex and contribute to the stiffness of the reticular lamina, as well as providing resistance to stress.
3. Another compartment is formed by the junctions between the basal cells of the stria vascularis and the occluding junctions at the apical ends of the marginal cells. This compartment encloses the basal ends of the marginal cells, the intermediate cells and the capillary network.
4. The Deiters cells may act as regulators of the ionic environment of the sensory cells.
5. The morphological polarization of the outer hair cells could reflect a dual function: production of an AC current flow and stimulation of the nerve endings.

These last two hypotheses need to be tested by physiological techniques.

REFERENCES

Beagley, H.A. Acoustic trauma in the guinea pig. II. Electron microscopy including the morphology of the cell junctions in the organ of Corti. *Acta Otolaryngol. 60:* 479-495, 1965.

Békésy, G.von, Description of some mechanical properties of the organ of Corti. *J. Acoust. Soc. Am. 25:* 770-785, 1953.

Brummett, R., Smith, C.A., Ueno, Y., Cameron, S. and Richter, R. The delayed effects of ethacrynic acid on the stria vascularis of the guinea pig. *Acta Otolaryngol. 83:* 98-112, 1977.

Dallos, P. *The Auditory Periphery. Biophysics and Physiology.* New York: Academic Press, 1973.

Davis, H. Transmission and transduction in the cochlea. *Laryngoscope 68:* 358-382, 1958.

Duvall, A.J. and Sutherland, C.R. Cochlear transport of horseradish peroxidase. *Ann. Otol. Rhinol. Laryngol. 81:* 705-714, 1972.

Farquhar, M.G. and Palade, G.E. Junctional complexes in various epithelia. *J. Cell Biol. 17:* 375-412, 1963.

Frank, K.D., Reale, E., Iurato, S., Luciano, L., Wermbter, G. and Pannese, E. Verbindungskomplexe an Zellen der Reissner-Membran in gefriergebrochenen Präparaten. *Acta Otolaryngol. 80:* 38-42, 1975.

Gulley, R.L. and Reese, T.S. Intercellular junctions in the reticular lamina of the organ of Corti. *J. Neurocyt. 5:* 479-507, 1976.

Hama, K. and Saito, K. Retangular arrays of intramembranous particles at the zonula adherens in the guinea pig organ of Corti. *J. Electron Micros. 25:* 299-302, 1976.

Hama, K. and Saito, K. Gap junctions between the supporting cells in some acoustico-vestibular receptors. *J. Neurocyt. 6:* 1-12, 1977.

Hinojosa, R. Transport of ferritin across Reissner's membrane. *Acta Otolaryngol.* Suppl. *292:* 1-27, 1971.

Hinojosa, R. Electron microscopic studies of the stria vascularis and spiral ligament after ferritin injection. *Acta Otolaryngol. 74:* 1-14, 1972.

Iurato, S. and Taidelli, G. Ultrastructure of the reticular membrane of the organ of Corti in rat. Est. da *Atti del V Cong. Ital. di Micros. Elettron.* Tipograf. de Seminario, Padua, 1965.

Jahnke, K. The fine structure of freeze-fractured intercellular junctions in the guinea pig inner ear. *Acta Otolaryngol.* Suppl. *336:* 1-40, 1975a.

Jahnke, K. Die Feinstructur gefriergeatzter Zell-membran-Haftstellen der Stria vascularis. *Anat. Embryol. 147:* 189-201, 1975b.

Johnstone, B.M. and Sellick, P.M. The peripheral auditory apparatus. *Quat. Rev. Biophys. 5:* 1-57, 1972.

Kuffler, S.W. and Nichols, J.G. *From Neuron to Brain. A Cellular Approach to the Function of the Nervous System.* Sunderland: Sinauer Assoc., 1976.

Mulroy, M.J., Altmann, D.W., Weiss, T.F. and Peake, W.T. Intracellular electric responses to sound in a vertebrate cochlea. *Nature 249:* 482-485, 1974.

Peters, A., Palay, S.L. and Webster, H. De F. *The Fine Structure of the Nervous System. The Cells and their Processes.* New York: Harper & Row, 1970.

Reale, E., Luciano, L., Franke, K., Pannes, E., Wermbter, G. and Iurato, S. Intercellular junctions in the vascular stria and spiral ligament. *J. Ultrastruct. Res. 53:* 284-297, 1975.

Smith, C.A. Electron microscopy of the inner ear. *Ann. Otol. Rhinol. Laryngol. 77:* 269-284, 1968.

Smith, C.A. The inner ear: it's embryological development and microstructure. In: *The Nervous System, Vol. 3: Human Communication and Its Disorders,* edited by D.B. Tower. New York: Raven Press, 1975, p. 1-18.

Smith, C.A. and Dempsey, E.W. Electron microscopy of the organ of Corti. *Am. J. Anat. 100:* 337-368, 1957.

Weiss, T.F., Mulroy, M.J. and Altmann, D.W. Intracellular response to acoustic clicks in the inner ear of the alligator lizard. *J. Acoust. Soc. Am. 55:* 606-619, 1974.

DISCUSSION

Galambos: There is reason to believe that at birth the human cochlea does not transduce tones above 3,000 or 4,000 Hz and that during the first few postnatal months the cochlea completes itself, so to speak, changing the youngster from one with a high frequency hearing loss into one with high frequency hearing. Do you have any information on that matter?

Smith: I assume you are talking about the human ear, because the human ear--

Galambos: I am talking about the human ear, but I suppose the situation would not be very different in other animals.

Smith: No, some animals are very immature when they are born. For example, the cat and the rat are very immature and the cochlea is not well developed at all. In the cat, for example, one would not find nerve fibers with their normal characteristics until about the second or third week after birth. But the human inner ear should be fully developed at birth, the sensory cells well differentiated and all neural connections within the cochlea complete. The guinea pig is born in a very mature state and its cochlea is functional at birth.

Galambos: My information comes from the effects of high pass noise on the brain stem responsivity of youngsters (Hecox, K. Electrophysiological correlates of human auditory development. In: *Infant Perception - From Sensation to Cognition,* Vol. II, edited by Cohen and Salapatek. New York: Academic Press, p. 151-191.) The best hypothesis is that the high frequency part of the cochlea is not yet functioning properly at birth.

Smith: There are some changes that occur in the human ear after birth, but these take place in the external and middle ear, according to all reports. For example, the configuration of the external ear canal changes.

It is probably within the external and middle ear, and more likely in brain stem pathways rather than in the cochlea itself that the changes occur which would be responsible for improvement in brain stem response.

THE AFFERENT INNERVATION OF THE COCHLEA

Heinrich Spoendlin

University Clinic, Innsbruck

ANATOMY

The afferent nerve supply of the cochlea consists of about 50,000 mainly bipolar neurons in the cat, 30,000 in man and 250,000 in whales (Hall, 1966) connecting the cochlear receptor to the cochlear nuclei. The ganglion cells are situated in the periphery, in Rosenthals canal. The central axons which are much longer than the peripheral, are remarkably uniform with diameters from 4-6μm and myelin sheaths of about 50 lammellae (Spoendlin, 1972; Hall et al., 1974). The peripheral axons, on the other hand, are much smaller with average diameters of 2-3μm but much great variability. Not only the axons but also most ganglion cells are provided with somewhat thinner myelin sheaths of 10-20 lammellae and a node of Ranvier on either side of the cell (Fig. 1). The peripheral axons take an essentially radial course through the osseous spiral lamina to reach the organ of Corti via the shortest route (Lorente de Nó, 1937), whereas the central axons are arranged according to the cochlear turns, the fibers from the cochlear apex being in the center and the fibers from the basal turn at the periphery of the nerve trunk (Sando, 1964). Unmyelinated nerve fibers are extremely rare in the cochlear nerve trunk (Spoendlin, 1972) but fairly numerous in the osseous spiral lamina (Paradisgarten et al., 1976).

Two main types of ganglion cells are found in the spiral ganglion (Spoendlin, 1971, 1973) (Fig. 1, 2A). About 95%, the type I cells, are large, myelinated and bipolar with a round nucleus, a prominent nucleolus and many ribosomes in the cytoplasm. The remaining 5% are of the quite different type II, about half the size, usually unmyelinated and pseudo-monopolar with a lobulated nucleus, a small nucleolus and a filamentous cytoplasm. The axons on the type II cells are unmyelinated in most cases and only rarely become thinly myelinated at a certain distance from the cell. Exceptionally, even type II ganglion cells are provided with a thin myelin sheath (Fig. 2A).

These type II ganglion cells are scattered through the spiral ganglion as single cells or in groups of two or three. We were never able to find structural evidence of synaptic contacts between different axons, ganglion cells and axons or ganglion

ISBN 0-12-514960-3

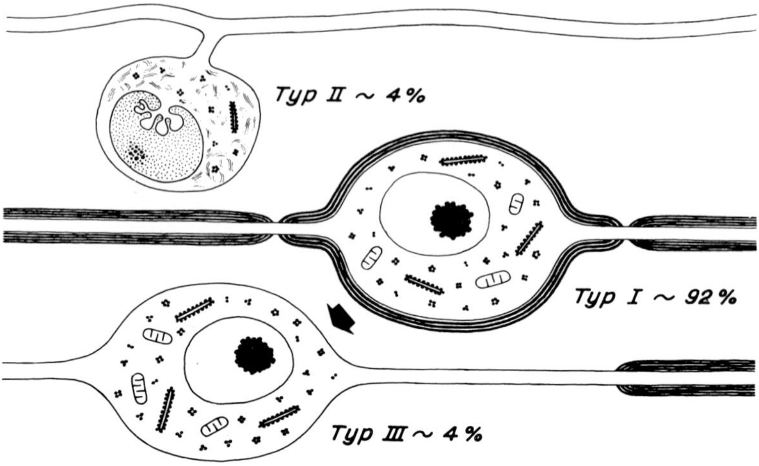

Fig. 1. Schematic drawing of the three types of ganglion cells found in the spiral ganglion of the cat. In normal animals there are only type I and type II cells whereas the type III cells are found after retrograde degeneration of the cochlear nerve.

cells. Although the unmyelinated axons of the type II cells are difficult to see in light microscopy, they can be followed over certain distances by interference contrast microscopy in very thick sections, by serial electronmicroscopic-sections or with the aid of methyline blue stain after degeneration of the type I neurons. They take a somewhat irregular but essentially radial course between the myelinated fibers of type I. We were unable to see them enter the intra ganglionic spiral bundle as suggested by Ross (1969) but they usually pass together with the other cochlear fibers into the osseous spiral lamina.

The innervation density of the organ of Corti with myelinated fibers varies considerably along the cochlear turns. The fiber density is highest in the basal turn with 400 fibers per 100μm which is more than twice the values of the lower and apical end of the cochlea (Fig. 3). The number of unmyelinated nerve fibers in the osseous spiral lamina is relatively constant throughout the cochlea, varying between 10% in the basal and middle turn and 35% of the myelinated fibers at the apex of the cochlea (Paradisgarten et al., 1976).

All fibers lose their myelin sheath before entering the organ of Corti through the habenular openings. Ten or 20 fibers pass together through one habenular opening. After having lost the myelin sheath all fibers passing through one habenular opening are individually surrounded by the extensions of one single special satellite cell, entirely separating the fibers from each other (Figs. 4,5). For each habenula opening there is one satellite cell with a rather light cytoplasm. Immediately beyond the habenula the fibers lose any sheathing and lie entirely bare adjacent to each other with no more than the usual intercellular gap of 200 Å between the axon membranes of the neighboring fibers (Fig. 6). There is however no mor-

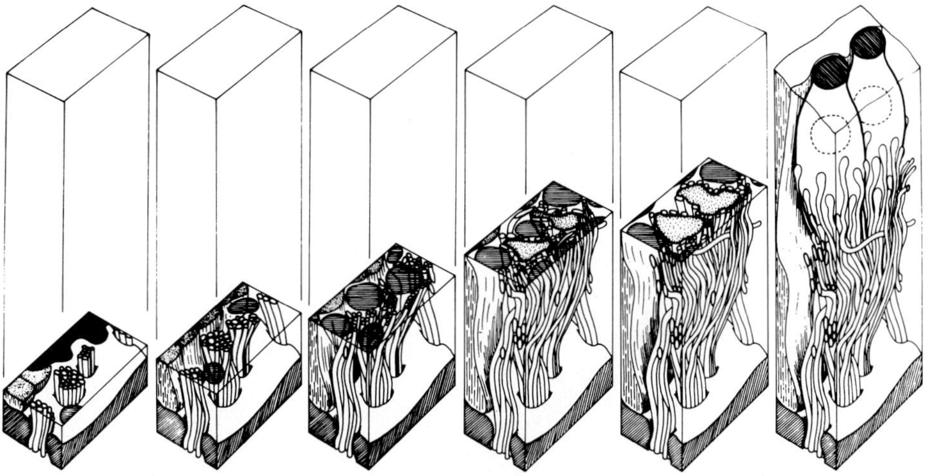

Fig. 7. Reconstruction of the area between habenula and two inner hair cells on the basis of serial EM sections. Most fibers entering the organ of Corti through the habenular opening lead directly to the nearest inner hair cell. Only about one out of 20 fibers turns outward to the outer hair cells.

The ultrastructural organization of the axoplasm varies to a certain extent between afferent fibers to outer and inner hair cells. The fibers for the outer hair cells contain mainly neurocanaliculi in their axoplasm whereas the fibers for the inner hair cells contain predominantly neuro fibrils. The endings at the inner hair cells usually form synaptic complexes with synaptic bars of varying sizes (Smith et al., 1961). The endings of the outer hair cells on the other hand have no synaptic ribbons in the cat and only relatively small ones in the guinea-pig (Rodriguez, 1967: Spoendlin, 1970; Dunn et al., 1975).

Fig. 6. Transverse section through a nerve bundle just after emerging from a habenular opening; the fibers are relatively large, contain many mitochondria at this level and are in close contact with each other. The fibers for the outer hair cells (of) tend to take a separate course immediately after the habenula. BM, basilar membrane.

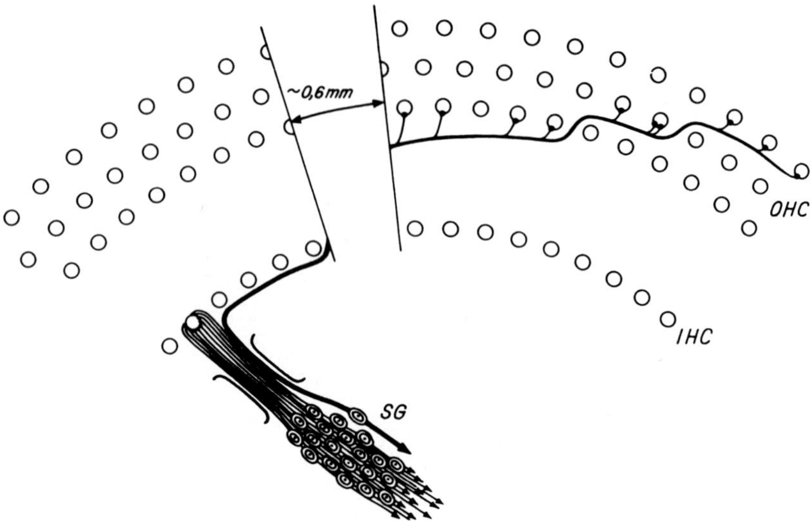

Fig. 8. Horizontal schema of the afferent innervation of the organ of Corti.

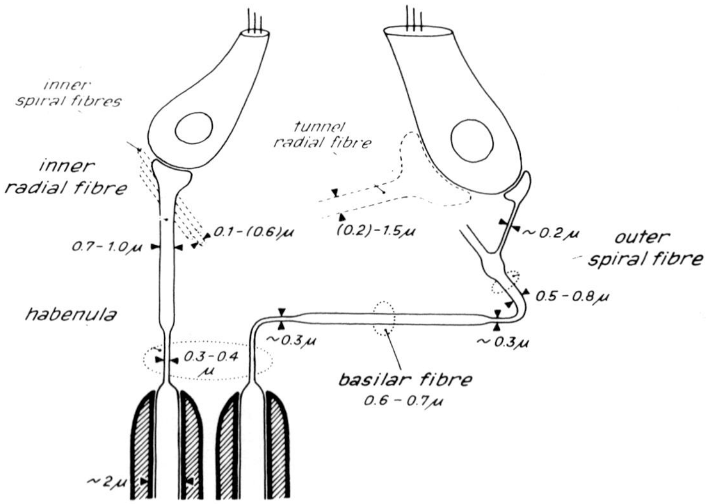

Fig. 9. Diameters of the nerve fibers within the organ of Corti.

The afferent innervation of the outer and inner hair cells shows a clearly distinguished pattern which can be summarized as follows (Fig. 8):

> The great majority of afferent neurons of the cochlear nerve (95% in the cat and 90% in the guinea pig (Spoendlin, 1972; Morrison et al. 1975) and in man (Nomura, 1976)) are associated with the inner hair cells and only a small minority (5% in the cat and 10% in the guinea pig) with the outer hair cells.
>
> The fibers associated with the inner hair cells are strictly radial whereas the fibers for the outer hair cells have a considerable spiral distribution.
>
> Each inner cell is innervated by about twenty unbranched individual afferent neurons and each outer hair cell is innervated by branches from several neurons, each of which participates in the innervation of about ten outer hair cells.
>
> The innervation mode is therefore basically different for the inner hair cell system with its great divergence (1:20) and for the outer hair cell system with its considerable convergence (10:1).
>
> The ultrastructural differences mainly of the synaptic contact with the hair cells indicate different functional mechanisms in the neurons of the outer and of the inner hair cell system.

BIOLOGICAL BEHAVIOR

The afferent neurons for the outer and inner hair cells differ not only in their anatomical distribution and structure but also in their biological behavior. The afferent fibers at the inner hair cells are very sensitive to metabolic disturbance such as anoxia or osmotic changes and react by a pronounced swelling of the axon, whereas the afferent fibers for the outer hair cells are resistent to such influences (Spoendlin, 1975). Also their degeneration behavior is different. After section of the cochlear nerve in the internal acoustic meatus of the cat, without disturbance of the cochlear blood supply, most cochlear neurons degenerate within 2 months but the organ of Corti remains intact (Fig. 10). This retrograde degeneration is a phenomenon peculiar to sensory bipolar neurons after division of one axon, as is well recognized in spiral ganglia (Ranson, 1905; Andres, 1961). Ganglion cell reactions to such lesions vary. Some cells respond only by loss of the myelin sheath and reduction of the endoplasmic reticulum but go on to survive; others undergo complete degeneration and disappear and still others remain unaffected. In the cochlea 90% to 95% of the spiral ganglion cells will disappear within six months following section of the cochlear nerve. The surviving ganglion cells are the type II cells, which seem to be unaffected by the retrograde degeneration after section of the cochlear nerve (Fig. 2B), and a small number of altered type I cells which have lost their myelin sheaths and which are referred to as type III cells. However, most axons of the bipolar type III cells remain myelinated (Fig. 1). As time of survival

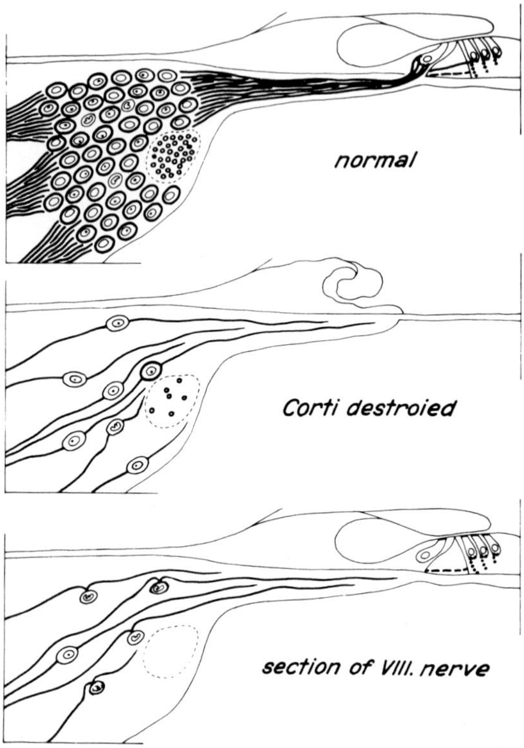

Fig. 10. Patterns of retrograde degeneration of the cochlear neurons. After destruction of the organ of Corti, mainly type III neurons survive; after section of the VIIIth nerve, mainly type II cells survive together with the complete afferent innervation of the outer hair cells.

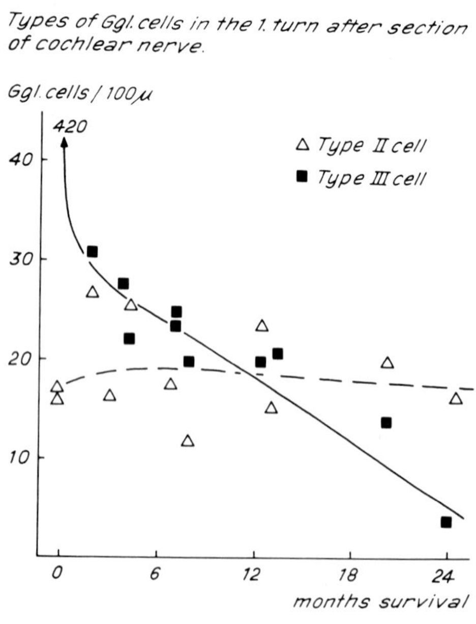

Fig. 11. Relative numbers of type II and III spiral ganglion cells after different survival times following section of the cochlear nerve. The number of the type III cells is gradually reduced whereas the number of the type II cells remains constant with increasing survival time.

lengthens, these type III cells have a tendency to be progressively reduced in number; after two years very few remain beside a normal population of type II cells (Spoendlin, 1976a, 1976b) (Fig. 11). In the organ of Corti most inner radial fibers associated with the inner hair cells disappear when the type I ganglion cells in the spiral ganglion degenerate. The afferent nerve supply of the outer hair cells, consisting of the basilar and outer spiral fibers with their endings at the bases of the outer hair cells, remain numerically and morphologically unchanged irrespective of the length of survival time. These surviving afferent neurons to the outer hair cells must therefore be related to the few surviving ganglion cells, particularly the type II cells, whose numbers are not reduced with increasing survival times. The area of the inner hair cells, however, is not totally devoid of nerve fibers after section of the VIIIth nerve. A small number of unusually large fibers is found in place of the normal radial fibers (Spoendlin, 1971). These giant fibers take their origin in the few surviving myelinated nerve fibers in the osseous spiral lamina (Fig. 13) and therefore probably belong to the surviving type III ganglion cells, which are the only remaining ganglion cells having myelinated axons (Spoendlin, 1976). The fibers penetrate the organ of Corti through every fifth to tenth habenular opening and divide into spirally expanding branches, making synaptic contacts with several inner hair cells (Fig. 12). When the efferent nerve supply is preserved in cases of selective section of the cochlear nerve, there are synaptic contacts between inner spiral efferent fibers and these giant fibers.

Three to eight months following section of the cochlear or VIIIth nerve these giant fibers are very few but after long survival their number increases surprisingly. Two years after the lesion, the area between habenula and inner hair cells is usually completely filled with spirally running nerve fibers of varying calibers despite the fact that only few ganglion cells and myelinated nerve fibers remain in the spiral ganglion and the osseous spiral lamina (Fig. 14) (Spoendlin, 1976). It must be assumed that the few neurons remaining after degeneration of the cochlear nerve undergo enormous ramification and proliferation to produce these neuroma-like agglomerations of spiral fibers in the area of the inner hair cells along the entire cochlea (Fig. 15).

A similar retrograde degeneration occurs following damage to the peripheral axons of the cochlear neurons by destruction of the organ of Corti. This type of retrograde degeneration has long been recognized but the organ of Corti changes inducing it are less certain (Bredberg, 1968; Schuknecht, 1953). Selective loss of outer hair cells has little effect on the cochlear neurons, while loss of inner hair cells, even when the supporting structures of the organ of Corti or the outer hair cells remain, is followed by massive retrograde degeneration of the cochlear neurons (Spoendlin, 1975). Although there is good correlation between the number of inner hair cells destroyed and the degree of retrograde degeneration (Johnsson, 1974) we observed degeneration in areas with inner hair cells present and areas with no degeneration despite extensive loss of inner hair cells (Fig. 17). The crucial factor for the initiation of retrograde degeneration is probably irreversible direct damage of the peripheral unmyelinated segments of the cochlear neurons associated with

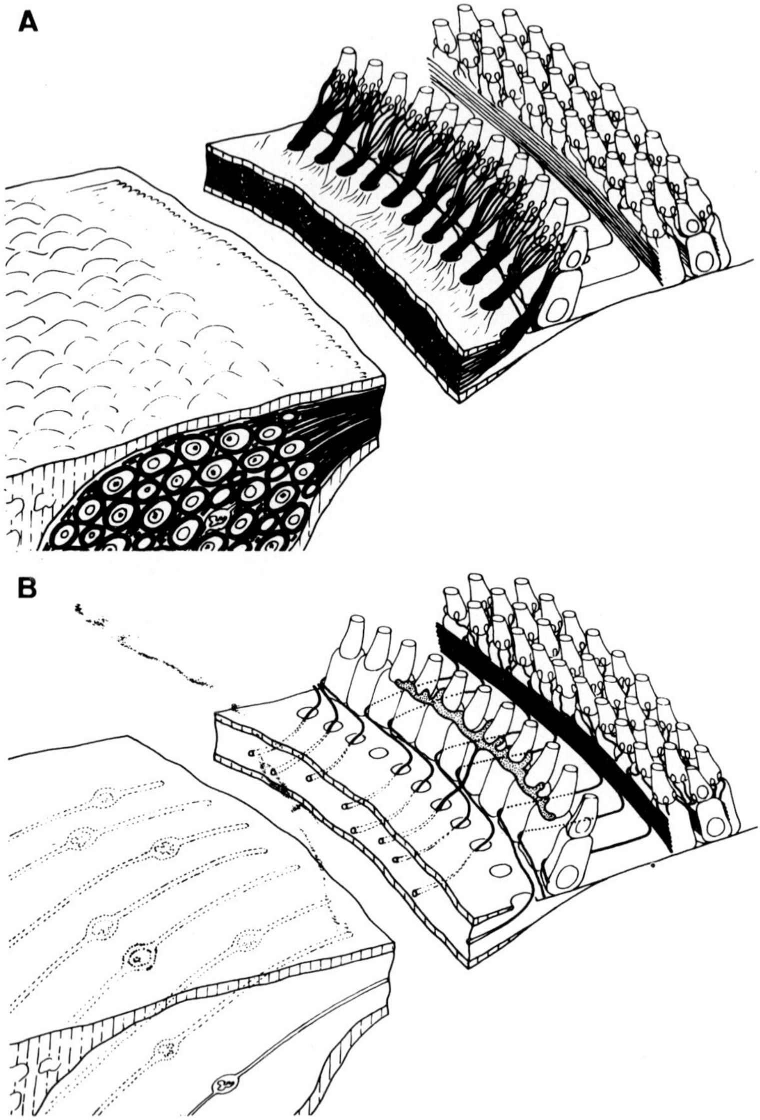

Fig. 12.

A. Afferent nerve supply of the organ of Corti in the normal animal.

B. Remaining afferent neurons after retrograde degeneration following section of the VIIIth nerve. The afferent nerve supply of the outer hair cell remains intact. At the level of the inner hair cells unusually large spirally-expanding giant neurons appear which normally are not present.

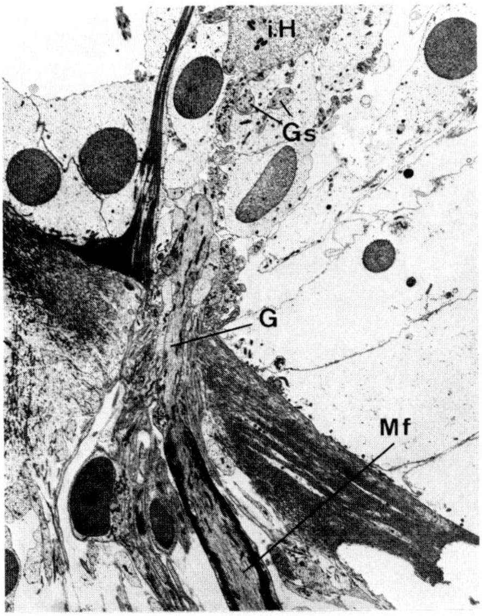

Fig. 13. Habenular area of a cat, eight months following section of the cochlear nerve. A giant nerve fiber (G) penetrates the habenula and evidently originates in a myelinated nerve fiber (Mf) from the osseous spiral lamina. Spirally running branches of giant nerve fibers (Gs) below the inner hair cell (iH).

the inner hair cells, a change occurring generally but not necessarily in conjunction with inner hair cell destruction.

After complete destruction of the organ of Corti by acoustic overstimulation, intoxication with ototoxic antibiotics or direct mechanical damage, retrograde degeneration never affects all neurons (Figs. 10, 17). About 10% are always spared provided the cochlear blood supply is not impaired. Up to 97% however, degenerate when the axons in the osseous spiral lamina are damaged close to the spiral ganglion. The degree of retrograde degeneration seems to be related to the distance of the axon damage from the ganglion cell bodies; the closer the damage is to the cell bodies the more complete the neuronal degeneration. Degeneration is always more pronounced in the basal turn and a greater percentage of neurons survives in the apical turns (Fig. 17). The process of retrograde degeneration following destruction of the organ of Corti is very slow, occupying several months. Most cells loose their myelin sheaths, the cytoplasmic organells are reduced and the nuclei frequently assume such irregular shapes that the cells are difficult to distinguish from type II ganglion cells. After survival times of a year or more the remaining cells, at least in the cat, are usually of type III (Fig. 2C, 10); ganglion cells with all the features of type II cells are extremely rare, in contrast to the situation following transection of the cochlear nerve where type II cells of normal appearance are found in normal numbers (Fig. 2B). The reasons for these differences in retrograde degeneration following section of the cochlear nerve and following destruction of the organ of Corti remain uncertain. It may be that the type II neurons send axons only to the organ

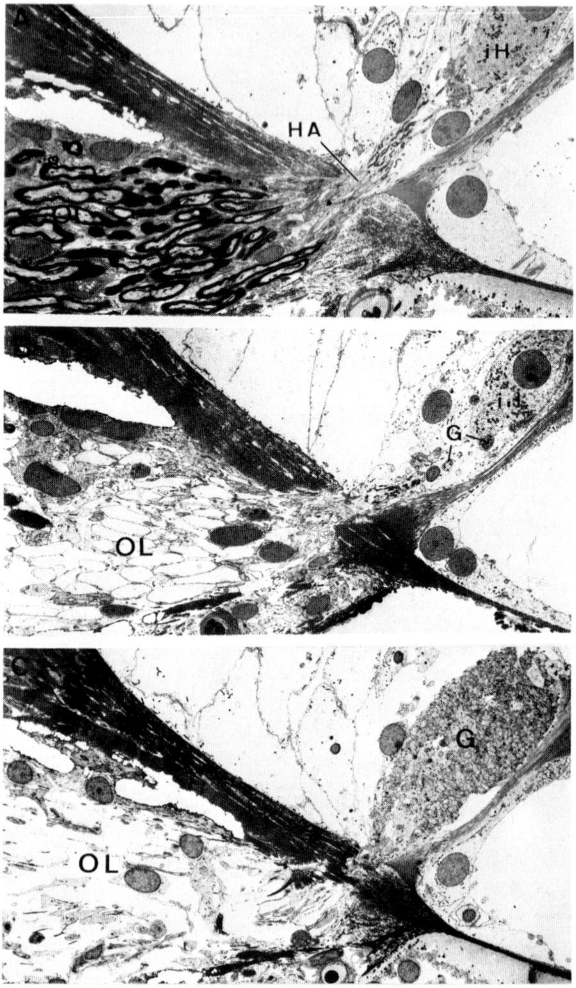

Fig. 14. Area of the habenula of a cat.

A. Normal situation. The osseous spiral lamina (OL) is filled with myelinated nerve fibers which penetrate the organ of Corti through the habenula opening (HA).

B. Situation eight months following section of the VIIIth nerve. The osseous spiral lamina (OL) is practically empty. In the area below the inner hair cell (IH) only a few giant fibers (G) remain.

C. Situation two years after section of the VIIIth nerve. The osseous spiral lamina (OL) is still practically empty. The area of the inner hair cell is filled with spirally-running nerve fibers of varying calibers (G) which represent an enormous proliferation of the peripheral branches of the few remaining neurons.

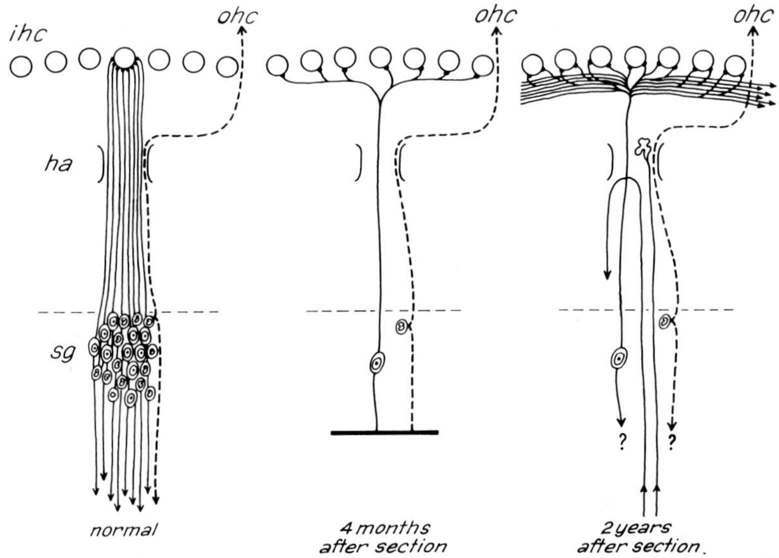

Fig. 15. Schematic representation of the degeneration and regeneration or proliferation behavior of the afferent cochlear neurons. Whereas the area of the inner hair cells contains only very few giant nerve fibers four months after section of the VIIIth nerve, the same area is filled with proliferating branches after longer survival times. Some other fibers ending in the habenula or turning back before the habenula can be found after long survival times. They may correspond to some type of regenerating fibers. The afferent fibers for the outer hair cells are not affected by these degenerative processes.

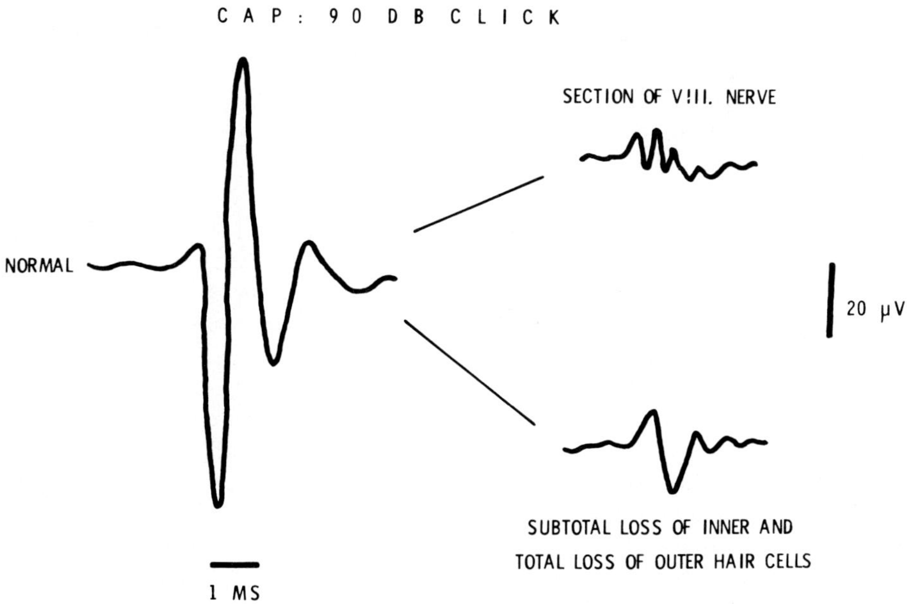

Fig. 16. Compound AP's in a normal cat, several months after section of the VIIIth nerve and after destruction of the organ of Corti.

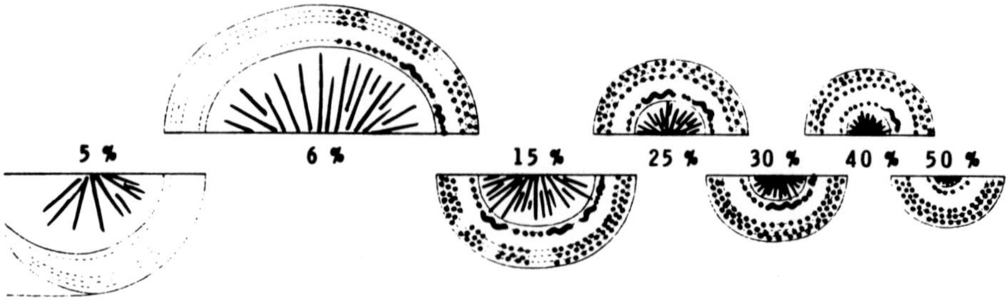

Fig. 17. Cochleographic reconstruction of a cat cochlea, one year following a single injection of 500mg Neomycin into the bulla. There is almost complete destruction of the organ of Corti with only very few severely altered inner hair cells remaining. (Small dots represent missing hair cells, wavy lines damaged hair cells and the numbers give the remaining nerve fibers in percentage of the normal nerve fiber population). The recording at the lower right of Figure 16 was made from this cochlea.

of Corti and are not connected to the central nervous system; thus lesions of the cochlear nerve in the inner acoustic meatus would not reach and affect them while destruction of the organ of Corti, in intimate contact with the outer hair cells, would affect them extensively. The fact that practically no unmyelinated nerve fibers are found in the cochlear nerve trunk could support this view, since the axons of type II cells are essentially unmyelinated. It could also explain why it has so far been impossible to demonstrate two distinct populations of neurons by single nerve recordings in the cochlear nerve trunk (Kiang, 1965).

On the other hand it is not clear how the outer hair cell system, which is associated with the type II neurons, could participate in cochlear function when there is practically no morphological evidence for synaptic contacts with the majority of type I cochlear neurons. Thus the question of the central connections of the type II neurons still remains open.

FUNCTIONAL CORRELATES

According to the innervation pattern, the outer hair cell system can work on a basis of spatial summation impossible for the inner hair cell system, which is quantitatively much more important and much better suited for tono-topical frequency perception and a greater dynamic range. Accordingly, one would assume that the outer hair cell system is of high sensitivity but small dynamic range; this would be in agreement with some electrocochleographic findings (Aran, 1971).

Other concepts of the outer hair cell system have been brought forward such as a monitoring action in the inner hair cell system (Lynn and Sayer, 1970). This, however, would presume a functional interaction between the fibers of outer and inner hair cells, a subject of much speculation (Evans, 1974; Zwislocki, 1974); unfortunately, no clear structural evidence and no direct functional evidence (Romahn et al., 1977) has been found. The only place where the fibers are close enough for possible functional interaction is in the habenular area, where they are surrounded by a common satellite cell. Whether such a satellite cell can mediate functional interaction between the different nerve fibers remains an open question. There is no structural evidence of synaptic contacts between satellite cell and the fibers; functional interaction, if it occurs, could only be on an electrical basis.

The diameters of the nerve fibers may have important functional implications in terms of conduction velocity, decrement of electronic excitation and possibly spike initiation at the initial segments, which might be determined by sudden changes of fiber diameter.

The degeneration and regeneration properties of the cochlear neurons are evidently of importance in considering the possibility of electrical stimulation of deaf ears. Even if all of these functional implications of structural organization appear logical, they are purely theoretical and may not correspond to actual effective mechanisms; these can only be elucidated by direct recordings from the different functional systems in the cochlea. In order to obtain objective information we produced typical damage patterns experimentally and measured cochlear function by electrocochleography. Section of the cochlear or VIIIth nerve had only a minor immediate effect on the compound action potentials of the cochlear nerve, -loss of the usually clearly visible P_1 waves in the high intensity stimulus range. However, four days after the lesion and in all subsequent recordings normal action-potentials disappeared, while cochlear microphonics remained normal (showing that the cochlear blood supply was not impaired). Instead of normal action-potentials, very strange stimulus-related electrical responses were recorded in all of these animals. Latencies were very short and did not change very much with stimulus intensities. They had maximum amplitudes between 10 and 20μV and were usually maintained over several milliseconds (Spoendlin, 1977) (Fig. 16).

This functional status must be correlated with the anatomical situation following section of the VIIIth nerve, with nearly complete loss of afferent neurons associated with the inner hair cells, an intact afferent nerve supply associated with the outer hair cells and mainly the 5% type II neurons left in the spiral ganglion. If the small unusual potentials prove to be real rather than artifactual, they are probably related to the afferent nerve supply of the outer hair cells. We must assume that the numerous nerve fibers in the organ of Corti which represent the afferent nerve supply to the outer hair cells produce some electrical activity upon stimulation. The complex and changing form of these recorded responses probably reflects highly dissociated and poorly synchronized activities; and the short latencies may indicate an origin peripheral to the initial segment of the neurons.

An entirely different picture results if secondary nerve degeneration is the result of destruction of the organ of Corti by locally applied ototoxic antibiotics or by direct mechanical damage.

A single 500mg dose of Neomycin injected into the bulla of the cat leads to complete loss of inner and outer hair cells except for a few remaining abnormal inner hair cells. After one year, 80-90% of the cochlear neurons have degenerated and disappeared (Fig. 17). Most of the surviving neurons are type III and a corresponding number of myelinated nerve fibers is found in the osseous spiral lamina. In contrast to the degeneration following transection of the VIIIth nerve, the afferent nerve supply of the outer hair cell disappears or is severely impaired.

In ECoG recordings the cochlear microphonics are entirely missing but weak yet typical compound action-potentials can still be recorded despite the total loss of outer hair cells and subtotal loss of inner hair cells (Fig. 16). Circumscribed mechanical destruction of the organ of Corti in the basal turn usually produces an almost complete loss of outer hair cells throughout the cochlea with a relatively good preservation of the inner hair cells. The functional consequence is a complete lack of cochlear microphonics, indicating that the outer hair cells are the main source of the cochlear microphonics which do not reflect activity of the inner hair cell. On the other hand, relatively typical AP's can still be recorded. The reduction of the AP is proportional to the reduction of myelinated cochlear nerve fibers (type I and III neurons) which frequently does not correspond with the loss of hair cells.

There is a major difference between secondary nerve degeneration following section of the VIIIth nerve and following damage to the organ of Corti. Following section of the VIIIth nerve, very few myelinated nerve fibers and an intact afferent nerve supply to the outer hair cells remain and no normal AP's can be recorded; following destruction of the organ of Corti a greater number of myelinated nerve fibers remains but the afferent nerve supply of the outer hair cells disappears or is highly impaired and some typical AP's can still be recorded in proportion to the remaining nerve fibers.

REFERENCES

Andres, K.H. Untersuchungen über morphologische Veränderungen in Spinalganglien währen der retrograden Degeneration. *Z. Zellforschung. 55:* 49-79, 1961.

Bredberg, G. Cellular pattern and nerve supply of the human organ of Corti. *Acta Otolaryngol.* Suppl. *236:* 1-135, 1968.

Dunn, R.A. and Morest, D.K. Receptor synapses without synaptic ribbons in the cochlea of the cat. *Proc. Nat. Acad. Sci. 72:* 3599-3603, 1975.

Evans, E.F. Auditory frequency selectivity and the cochlear nerve. In: *Facts and Models in Hearing,* edited by E. Zwicher and E. Terhardt. New York, Heidelberg, Berlin: Springer-Verlag, 1974, p. 118-129.

Johnsson, L.G. Sequence of degeneration of Corti's organ and its first-order neurons. *Ann. Otol. Rhinol. Laryngol. 83:* 249-303, 1974.

Hall, J.G. Hearing and primary auditory centers of the whales. *Acta Otolaryngol.* Suppl. *224:* 244-250, 1966.

Hall, J.G. An electron-microscopical analysis of the square areas and diameters of the cochlear nerve fibers in the cats. *Acta Otolaryngol. 77:* 305-310, 1974.

Lorente de Nó, R. Some unresolved problems concerning the cochlear nerve. *Ann. Otol. Rhinol. Laryngol.* Suppl. *40:* 1-28, 1976.

Lorente de Nó, R. Neural mechanisms of hearing: the sensory endings in the cochlea. *Laryngoscope 47:* 373-377, 1937.

Lorente de Nó, R. Anatomy of the eighth nerve. The central projections of the nerve endings of the internal ear. *Laryngoscope 43:* 1-38, 1933.

Morrison, D., Schindler, R.A. and Wersäll, J. A quantitative analysis of the afferent innervation of the organ of Corti in guinea pig. *Acta Otolaryngol. 79:* 11-23, 1975.

Nomura, Y. Nerve fibers in the human organ of Corti. *Acta Otolaryngol. 82:* 317-324, 1976.

Paradiesgarten, A. and Spoendlin, H. The unmyelinated nerve fibers of the cochlea. *Acta Otolaryngol. 82:* 157-164, 1976.

Ranson, S.W. Retrograde degeneration in the spinal nerves. *J. Comp. Neurol. 16:* 265-293, 1906.

Rodriquez-Echandía, E.L. An electron microscopic study on the cochlear innervation. I. The recepto-neural junctions at the outer hair cells. *Z. Zellforschung. 78:* 30-46, 1967.

Rohman, G. and Boerger, G. Filter function of the guinea pig cochlea after degeneration of outer hair cells. *Arch. Oto-Rhino-Laryngol. 215:* 223-229, 1977.

Sando, I. The anatomical interrelationships of the cochlear nerve fibers. *Acta Otolaryngol. 59:* 417-436, 1964.

Schuknecht, H.F., Igarashi, M. and Gacek, R.R. The pathological types of cochleo-saccular degeneration. *Acta Otolaryngol. 59:* 154-168, 1965.

Smith, C.A. Innervation of the cochlea of the guinea pig by use of the Golgi stain. *Ann. Otol. Rhinol. Laryngol. 84:* 443-458, 1975.

Smith, C.A. and Sjöstrand, F.S. A synaptic structure in the hair cells of the guinea pig cochlea. *J. Ultrastruct. Res. 5:* 184-192, 1961.

Spoendlin, H.H. *The Organ of the Cochlear Receptor.* Basel: Karger, 1966.

Spoendlin, H.H. Ultrastructure and peripheral innervation pattern of the receptor in relation to the first coding of the acoustic message. In: *Hearing Mechanisms in Vertebrates,* edited by A.V.S. de Reuck and J. Knight. London: Churchill, 1968, p. 89-119.

Spoendlin, H.H. Innervation patterns in the organ of Corti of the cat. *Acta Otolaryngol. 67:* 239-254, 1969.

Spoendlin, H.H. Structural basis of peripheral frequency analysis. In: *Frequency Analysis and Periodicity Detection in Hearing,* edited by R. Plomp and F.G. Smoorenburg. Leiden: Sijthoff, 1970, p. 2-36.

Spoendlin, H.H. Degeneration behavior of the cochlear nerve. *Arch. Klin. Exp. Ohren Nasen Kehlkoptheilkd. 200:* 275-291, 1971.

Spoendlin, H.H. Innervation densities of the cochlea. *Acta Otolaryngol. 73:* 235-248, 1972.

Spoendlin, H.H. The innervation of the cochlear receptor. In: *Basic Mechanisms in Hearing,* edited by A.R. Møller. New York: Academic Press, 1973, p. 185-234.

Spoendlin, H.H. Neuroanatomy of the cochlea. In: *Facts and Models in Hearing,* edited by E. Zwicker and E. Terhardt. New York, Heidelberg. Berlin: Springer-Verlag, 1974, p. 18-32.

Spoendlin, H.H. Neuroanatomical basis of the cochlear coding mechanisms. *Audiology 14:* 383-407, 1975.

Spoendlin, H.H. Retrograde degeneration of the cochlear nerve. *Acta Otolaryngol. 79:* 266-275, 1975.

Spoendlin, H.H. and Baumgartner, H. Electrocochleography and cochlear pathology. *Acta Otolaryngol. 83:* 130-135, 1977.

Spoendlin, H.H. and Suter, R. Regeneration in the VIII nerve. *Acta Otolaryngol. 81:* 228-236, 1976.

Zwislocki, J.J. and Sokolich, W.G. Neuro-mechanical frequency analysis in the cochlea. In: *Facts and Models in Hearing,* edited by E. Zwicker and E. Terhardt. New York, Heidelberg, Berlin: Springer-Verlag, 1974, p. 107-117.

DISCUSSION

Trahiotis: Would you discuss the data having to do with the efferent system in conjunction with what you have presented, in terms of apparently essentially all afferent units are affected by efferent stimulation? Mostly you have discussed what goes to the outer hair cells. You mentioned interaction, and I wondered if you had any thoughts about the data.

Spoendlin: I did not discuss the efferent innervation, since I was supposed to talk about the afferent system. It has always been intriguing that essentially all cochlear units are affected by efferent stimulation in spite of the enormous efferent innervation of the outer hair cells, which are only associated with a small minority of afferent neurons. The efferents to the outer hair cells influence directly and practically exclusively the sensory cells, whereas the efferents to the inner hair cell system have a direct influence on the afferent neurons. So far, all electrophysiologically recorded neurons probably belong to the inner hair cell system and we do not yet know the functional significance of the neurons associated with the outer hair cells.

Johnstone: Some three years ago I put forward a hypothesis that with very loud sounds it may be possible for the dendrites going to the inner hair cells to be directly mechanically stimulated, this possibly accounting for the long tails in the neural tuning curves. It would seem from your data here, where you can more or less wipe out lots of hair cells but still have some nerves and possibly dendrites left, that indeed this may be the case. Would you comment as to whether you think the possibility of a direct mechanical stimulation for loud sounds on the dendrites is a possibility and would fit in with your data?

Spoendlin: It is not possible to give an exclusive answer to this question. The fact is, however, that we still found typical but small AP in animals with total loss of outer hair cells and only very few heavily altered inner hair cells with a very odd shape and fused sensory hairs. Whether this means that the dendrites can be stimulated directly mechanically, cannot be concluded from this type of experiment. I would doubt it, however, because the mechanical events at this area below the inner hair cells are minimal.

Nadol: Is there a possibility that these regenerating fibers that you see, or giant fibers, are actually not cochlear neurons but are wandering vestibular or even facial neurons after section of the nerve?

Spoendlin: This is certainly a very interesting suggestion. I do not think this is the case because we can pretty much trace these giant fibers to the few remaining ganglion cells of the spiral ganglion. In the osseous spiral lamina their numbers decrease with survival time rather than increase as you would expect, if they were regenerating fibers. Only the peripheral ramifications within the organ of Corti show an enormous proliferation with longer survival times.

On the other hand, some regeneration of efferent or vestibular fibers does probably occur, because we regularly find after long survival times nerve fibers in the osseous spiral lamina which reach the habenula but then turn back again, as if they could not find their way through the habenular openings.

Zerlin: I have a question about the action potentials you showed at the end. When you said the smaller magnitude was related to the total number of cochlear nerves remaining, was that over the entire cochlea or just the basal section?

Spoendlin: Over the entire cochlea.

Zerlin: So that indicates that you are getting action potentials which are essentially summating over the entire cochlea rather than just the basal area?

Spoendlin: I would assume so, yes. I didn't say anything about threshold. This was a maximum response with high density.

McCormick: You showed swelling of nerve fibers with anoxia. Can you say how much anoxia can be tolerated for how long and still permit recovery of the fiber back to normal, with normal function?

Spoendlin: That is a very difficult question, because we have to kill the animal when we want to demonstrate it.

McCormick: Yes, but you let it live for different lengths of time after the anoxia.

Spoendlin: That's right. We produced anoxias for different lengths of time. After anoxic periods of less than 30 minutes, we found morphological recovery of the dendrites but after anoxia of thirty minutes and more the dendrites burst and the neurons degenerated. These experiments gave no information on the time course of recovery after anoxic damage.

Smith: What happens to the adrenergic nerve fibers after you have cut the cochlear fibers? You mentioned that some of the fibers go up to the habenula and turn back. Some might be coming in with the blood vessels.

Spoendlin: Some of these fibers which turn back at the habenula might well be autonomic fibers. However we never find them in normal cats and must therefore assume that they are some sort of regenerating fibers from the autonomic or efferent system or from the vestibular nerve.

Davis: Regarding those small surviving action potentials that Dr. Zerlin inquired about, was the latency of these potentials normal? What was it? I hope there was a latency.

Spoendlin: Yes, there was one. It was slightly increased. I think you have seen it in Stockholm where I have shown cochleograms of such animals.

Thornton: Again on the residual nerve fibers, you showed a stable Type II population, but the Type III population got smaller and smaller over a two-year period with sectioning of the nerve. The population that remains after ototoxic damage you said was predominantly Type III. Does it show the same degeneration with time, or is that more stable?

Spoendlin: I can't give you this answer yet. I have to wait for longer survival times. The longest survival time after ototoxic damage was one and a half years. Up to this moment I still had about 10% surviving Type III neurons.

Fernandez: Your suggestion is that the Type II neuron may be considered as an interneuron. Where is the terminal of the central axon?

Spoendlin: I was never able to follow the central axon of the type II neurons further than the bony channels connecting Rosenthals Canal with the modiolus, where they seem to fade away. It might well be that this type II neurons have no central connections at all. They do not necessarily have to go to the central nervous system; this is the case with the interneurons in the retina. As I said, some evidence speaks for such an assumption and some speaks against it; so that the question for the time being is still open.

THE OLIVOCOCHLEAR BUNDLE: ITS ORIGINS AND TERMINATIONS IN THE CAT

W. Bruce Warr

The Boys Town Institute for Communication Disorders in Children, Omaha.

INTRODUCTION

The purpose of the experiments to be described here was to identify the cells of origin of the olivocochlear bundle (OCB) and to study the projections of these cells to the organ of Corti in the cat using axonal transport techniques. These two problems, namely the origins and terminations of the OCB, have been difficult ones for the neuronanatomist because until very recently, the methods available for their study were either too insensitive, or too cumbersome to provide a satisfactory resolution. Regarding the identity of olivocochlear neurons, the best available evidence, though largely circumstantial, was that some of the acetylcholinesterase-containing neurons in the superior olivary complex of the brain stem project to the cochlea by way of the crossed OCB. The basis for this belief was as follows: Rasmussen (1946) found that the lesions most effective in producing degeneration in the crossed OCB were ones located within or dorsal to the medial nucleus of the trapezoid body of the cat. Osen and Roth (1969), using a histochemical technique which localizes acetylcholinesterase (AChE), identified large stellate neurons in this general area and also recognized AChE-containing axons traveling dorsally from the medial nucleus of the trapezoid body toward the decussation of the OCB in the floor of the fourth ventricle. Because ten years earlier, Schuknecht et al. (1959), had shown that sectioning the crossed OCB resulted in a substantial loss of AChE activity in the organ of Corti, it was obviously tempting to conclude that the origins of the crossed OCB were at last known, at least in a general way. Attempts to demonstrate these neurons by experimental means, specifically by the technique of retrograde cell changes following axotomy had been largely unsuccessful or incomplete (Papez, 1930, Rasmussen, 1946; Luk et al., 1974).

Rasmussen (1960, 1964, 1967) later described an uncrossed component of the OCB which he ultimately concluded took origin from neurons dorsal to the lateral superior olivary nucleus. He believed this ipsilateral component contained only about 100 axons or one quarter the number estimated to travel in the crossed

ISBN 0-12-514960-3

OCB. There was little basis for supposing that this component also arose from AChE-stained neurons because Schuknecht's experiments had shown such a dramatic loss of AChE activity in the cochlea supposedly after cutting only the crossed OCB. Moreover, AChE-stained axons were clearly visible traveling dorsally only from the region of the medial nucleus of the trapezoid body. Such was not the case for the region of the lateral superior olivary nucleus, although the presence of small fusiform cells, heavily stained for AChE, was reported by Osen and Roth (1969).

Paradoxically, the terminations of the OCB are somewhat better known than are its origins. In fact, even before experimental approaches were brought to bear on the projections of the OCB, several investigators had correctly identified the efferent nature of certain presynaptic structures on outer haircells (Engstrom, 1958) and on afferent dendrites beneath the inner hair cells (Smith, 1961). This was done purely by analogy with the characteristic fine structure of synaptic endings found elsewhere in the nervous system. Later application of the electron microscope-antergrade degeneration method has fully confirmed these observations (Kimura and Wersall, 1962; Smith and Rasmussen, 1963; Spoendlin 1966, 1970; Nakai and Igarashi, 1974).

Of particular interest in the present context is the question of the differential terminations of the crossed and uncrossed components of the OCB. This problem has received no satisfactory solution to date because the selective destruction of the uncrossed OCB could not be undertaken and verified in experimental animals until its origins and intramedullary course had been more completely described. No such problem attends the selective destruction of the *crossed* component, and for this reason a number of studies in a variety of animal species have been done on its terminations. There is unanimous agreement that the major synaptic consequence of this latter maneuver is the degeneration and disappearance of up to 90% of the large, vesicle-containing presynaptic structures on the outer hair cells. Moreover, in the cat and monkey, associated with this extensive loss of large vesicle-containing endings, there is axonal degeneration of: 1) most of the outer spiral fibers in the space of Nuel, 2) most of the upper tunnel radial fibers in the tunnel of Corti, 3) a variable portion of the tunnel spiral bundle adjacent to the inner pillars, and 4) a variable portion (up to 50% in some specimens) of the inner spiral bundle beneath the inner hair cells (Spoendlin, 1970; Nakai and Igarashi, 1974). Only when both the crossed and uncrossed components are severed do virtually all of these elements degenerate (Smith and Rasmussen, 1963); and, most importantly, does one observe the unequivocal loss of the axo-dendritic synapses between the inner spiral fibers and the dendrites and terminal varicosities of spiral ganglion peripheral process beneath and adjacent to the inner hair cells.

In the studies to be reported here, I have made exclusive use of light microscopic methods to identify axonally transported tracer substances. By such means I located the OCB cells (retrograde transport of HRP) and determined their projections (anterograde transport of radioactively labelled protein). The findings, although still in need of confirmation, suggest that the current mode of dealing with olivocochlear projections in terms of crossed and uncrossed components may require modification. The findings appear to reveal the existence of two different cell types of origin of the OCB and two different sites of termination for these cells, but neither type is exclusively crossed or uncrossed.

METHODS

Experimental Series 1 Retrograde Axonal Transport of Horseradish Peroxidase (HRP)

Thirty-six kittens ranging in age from newborn to three weeks were anesthetized and the round window of one side was exposed and injected with 1-20 microliters of aqueus 10% HRP (Sigma Type VI). After 24 hours, the animals were re-anesthetized and perfused transcardially with cacodylate buffered (pH 7.2) fixative containing 5% glutaraldehyde and 4% paraformaldehyde. The brains were removed and soaked overnight at 4° C in a mixture of fixative in 30% sucrose. Frozen sections of the brain stem were cut at 40μm and incubated in 0-dianisidine for the demonstration of HRP according to the procedure of Graham and Karnovsky (1966). Some of these same sections were further incubated for the demonstration of acetylcholinesterase according to the method of El-Badawi and Schenk (1966). Sections were mounted on slides and lightly counterstained with cresyl violet, and coverslipped in the usual manner.

Experimental Series 2 Anterograde Axonal Transport of Radioactively Labelled Protein *(In collaboration with Dr. John J. Guinan, Jr., Eaton-Peabody Laboratory of Auditory Physiology, Massachusetts Eye and Ear Infirmary, Boston, Mass.).*

Six adult cats were anesthetized with Dial-Urethane and prepared for bilateral acoustic stimulation. A gross recording electrode was advanced through the superior olivary complex via a ventral approach through the basioccipital bone (Guinan et al., 1972). Using evoked auditory responses as landmarks, the depths of various nuclei of the olivary complex were charted. The gross electrode was then withdrawn and an injection pipet affixed to a microliter syringe was inserted to an appropriate depth. An injection of 0.5 - 12μCi of ^{35}S Methionine (New England Nuclear Corp.) was delivered continuously in a volume of 20-60 nanoliters of distilled water at a constant rate of 0.7 nanoliters per minute. The animal was maintained on anesthesia and kept at 37°C for 24 hours. Fixation was by transcardial perfusion with phosphate buffered (pH 7.4, 0.1M) 0.5% Paraformaldeyde and 2% Glutaraldehyde. The brain was removed and sectioned at 30μm on a freezing microtome. Every 10th section was mounted defatted in Xylene and dried. The cochleas were also removed, decalcified for 48 hours in Decal and embedded in Araldite plastic to which 8% by volume of dibutylphthalate had been added as a softener. Sections were cut on a rotary microtome at 4μm or 10μm (depending on the animal) in the plane of the modiolus. Three consecutive 4μ

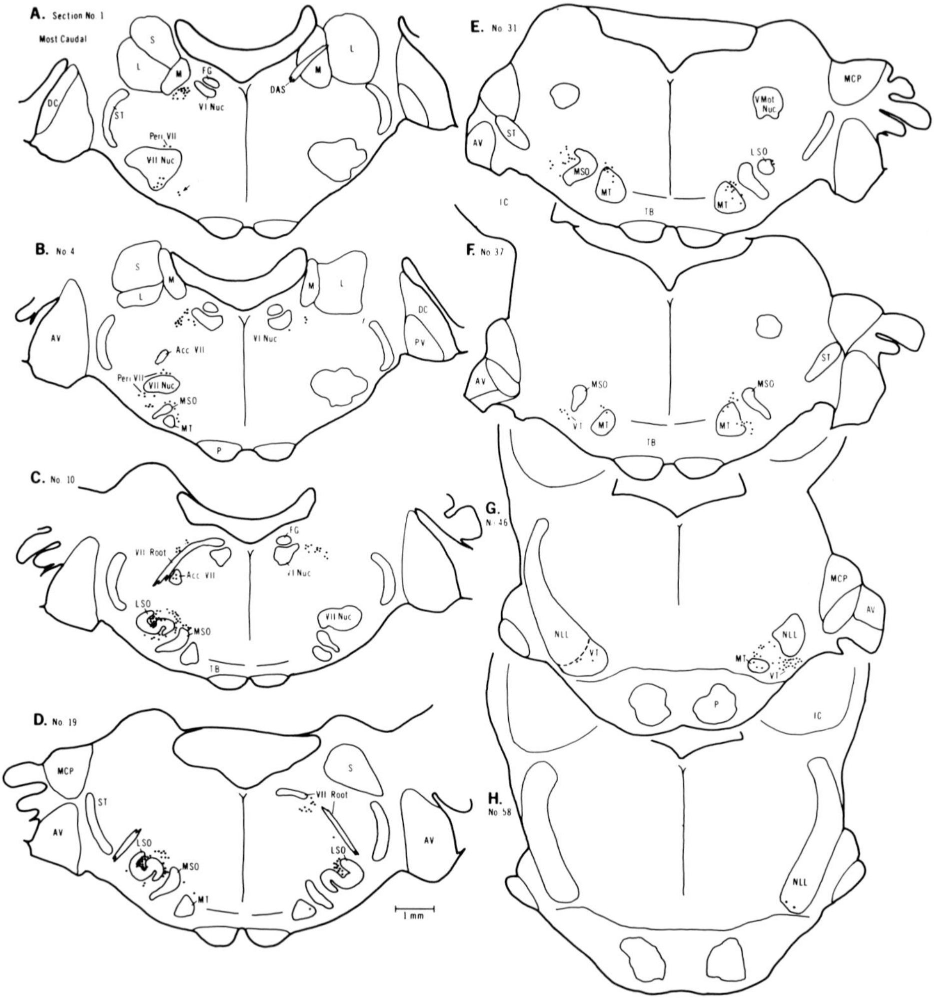
A. Section No 1
Most Caudal
B. No 4
C. No 10
D. No 19
E. No 31
F. No 37
G. No 46
H. No 58
1 mm

sections were saved and mounted every 50μm. All the 10μm sections were saved and mounted. All slides were processed for autoradiography (AR) in Kodak NTB-2 or NTB-3 liquid emulsion, boxed with dessicant and stored at 4°C until developed (Cowan et al., 1972). Exposure times for the brain sections ranged from 7 to 42 days, and for the cochleas, from 14 to 90 days. Following development, slides were usually counterstained with either neutral red (brain) or toluidine blue (cochleas), dehydrated, and covered in Permount. In assessing the autoradiographs of the cochleas, we set criteria that ensured that silver grains were significantly above local background levels before being considered an autoradiographically (AR) positive finding. These criteria were set in order to reduce to a minimum the chance that randomly scattered "background" silver grains would be mistaken for grains caused by the disintegration of ^{35}S.

RESULTS

Experimental Series 1

In Figure 1 I have mapped the location of all neurons labelled with HRP following an injection into the left labyrinth of a 1 day old kitten. I shall focus here only upon those cells located within the superior olivary complex, since these are presumably the principal, if not the exclusive source of the olivocochlear bundle. A more detailed report of the other findings has appeared elsewhere (Warr, 1975).

Perhaps the most striking feature illustrated in Figure 1 is the wide bilateral distribution of labelled cells. There appears to be little tendency toward clustering of these neurons into discrete nuclear groups. None are located directly in the two principal olivary nuclei. A comparison of the two sides with regard to loci containing labelled neurons suggests a modest degree of symmetry; that is, homonymous cell groups of both sides tend to contain labelled neurons. For example, the dorsal hilus of the lateral superior olivary nuclei, and the medial nuclei of the trapezoid body, exhibit labelled cells in essential identical regions.

Fig. 1. Plot of labelled neurons at eight levels of the brain stem in Kitten 21. Each dot represents one labelled neuron, except in the dorsal hilus of the ipsilateral LSO where there were more labelled neurons than could be indicated. The cochlea on the left side was injected with HRP. The most caudal section in the figure was assigned the number "1" and each successive 40 μ section was numbered rostrally through 58 (H). Arrow, labelled neurons in lateral paragigantocellular nucleus. Abbreviations: Acc. VII, accessory facial nucleus; AV, anteroventral cochlear nucleus; DAS, dorsal acoustic stria; DC, dorsal cochlear nucleus; FG, facial genui; IC, inferior colliculus; L, lateral vestibular nucleus; LSO, lateral superior olivary nucleus; M, medial vestibular nucleus; MCP, middle cerebellar peduncle; MSO, medial superior olivary nucleus; MT, medial nucleus of the trapezoid body; NLL, nucleus of the lateral lemniscus; P, pyramidal tract; Peri VII, neurons surrounding the facial nucleus; PV, posteroventral cochlear nucleus; S, superior vestibular nucleus; ST, spinal tract of the trigeminal nerve; TB, trapezoid body; VT, ventral nucleus of the trapezoid body; V Mot. Nuc., motor nucleus of trigeminal nerve; VI Nuc., abducens nucleus; VII Nuc., facial nucleus.

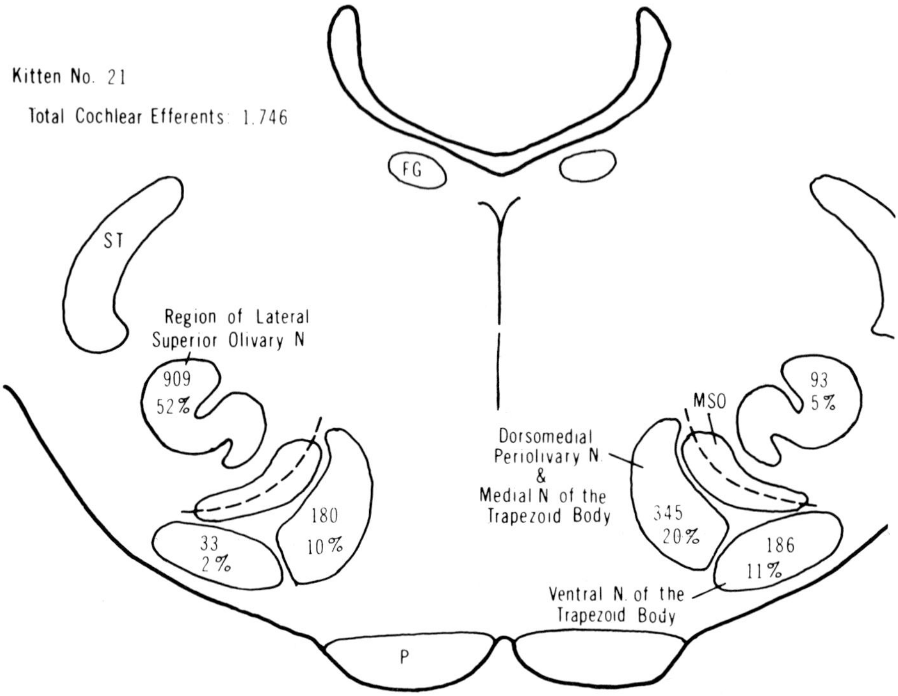

Fig. 2. Summary of counts of cochlear efferent neurons in Kitten No. 21 in which HRP had access to only one labyrinth. Injected side is on the left. Broken line passing through the medial superior olivary nucleus indicates the line of demarcation between the region of the lateral superior olivary nucleus and the regions of the dorsomedial periolivary and medial nuclei of the trapezoid body. Percentages are based upon the total number of olivocochlear efferent neurons. Abbreviations: FG, Facial Genu; MSO, Medial Superior Olivary Nucleus; P, Pyramidal Tract; ST, Spinal Tract of the Trigeminal Nerve.

A major assymetry visible in Figure 1 however, is the *number* of cells in homonymous loci. Thus there are far more labelled cells in the vicinity of the lateral superior olivary nucleus on the injection side than on the opposite side. The reverse is true of the medial nucleus of the trapezoid body and its dorsally and ventrally neighboring cell groups, the dorsomedial periolivary and ventral nucleus of the trapezoid body. I have quantified these observations in this animal (Figure 2) which presents the number of labelled cells counted bilaterally in three regions of the superior olivary complex, together with the percent of total of olivocochlear efferents that each represents.

The size and shape of labelled cells show distinct differences depending on their location. Those in the area surrounding the lateral superior olivary nucleus (Figure 3) were noticeably smaller and more fusiform than those in the medial or ventral nuclei of the trapezoid body (Figure 4), or in the dorsomedial periolivary nucleus. Although I found virtually no small neurons in these latter loci, a few fairly large cells were usually observed on the margins of the lateral superior olive.

Finally, I studied sections which had been incubated both for peroxidase and for acetylcholinesterase (AChE) and found that virtually all of the neurons which contained HRP also were positively stained for AChE as well. Unfortunately, the combined HRP-AChE incubations were carried out on several animals in which only one cochlea was injected and in which, furthermore, the number of HRP-labelled neurons totaled, for unknown reasons, only about 500 - 600. Therefore there were many AChE stained cells which lacked HRP in their cytoplasm. Thus, it is still not possible to conclude that *all* of the AChE-positive neurons in the superior olivary complex contribute to the olivocochlear bundle, although there is nothing in these data which would preclude this.

In the second series of experiments to be described below, I collaborated with Dr. John J. Guinan, Jr. at the Eaton-Peabody Lab of the Massachussetts Eye and Ear Infirmary in an effort to determine the projections of the different cells that contribute to the olivocochlear bundle. In particular, we concentrated our efforts on the issue of whether the small cells in the vicinity of the lateral superior olivary nucleus had different projections to the cochlea than the large cells scattered in the area of the medial and ventral nuclei of the trapezoid body.

Experimental Series 2

The upper panel of Figure 5 shows an injection site centered in the left medial nucleus of the trapezoid body. A total of 0.5 microcuries of ^{35}S Methionine in 20 nanoliters of distilled water was injected. The two lower panels present reconstructions of the cochleas of this animal, together with the sites of silver grain clusters which met or exceeded criterion, represented here as "filled" symbols. The exposure time was 90 days, or approximately one "half life" of ^{35}S. In both cochleas, the region around the bases of outer hair cells is virtually the only place where silver grains were sufficiently clustered to meet criterion, and here the criterion was generally massively exceeded, particularly in the right cochlea (Fig. 6). Only rarely were there any silver grains associated with the inner hair cells, or perhaps more precisely, with the subadjacent zone which contains the inner spiral bundle. These instances, two in the upper basal turn of the right cochlea and one in the apical turn of the left cochlea, barely met criterion. The number of silver grains in association with the bases of outer hair cells in the right cochlea was consistantly greater than in the left cochlea. Dr. Guinan and I have more recently extended some of these findings to the ventral nucleus of the trapezoid body, a region which the experiments with HRP indicate is rich in *large* neurons which project almost exclusively to the opposite cochlea (Fig. 1). As would be expected, an injection of ^{35}S Methionine into this nucleus resulted in AR positive findings in the opposite cochlea in association with the outer hair cells. The ipsilateral cochlea has not yet been evaluated.

In the next case, shown in Figure 7, an injection of 12μCi^{35}S Methionine in

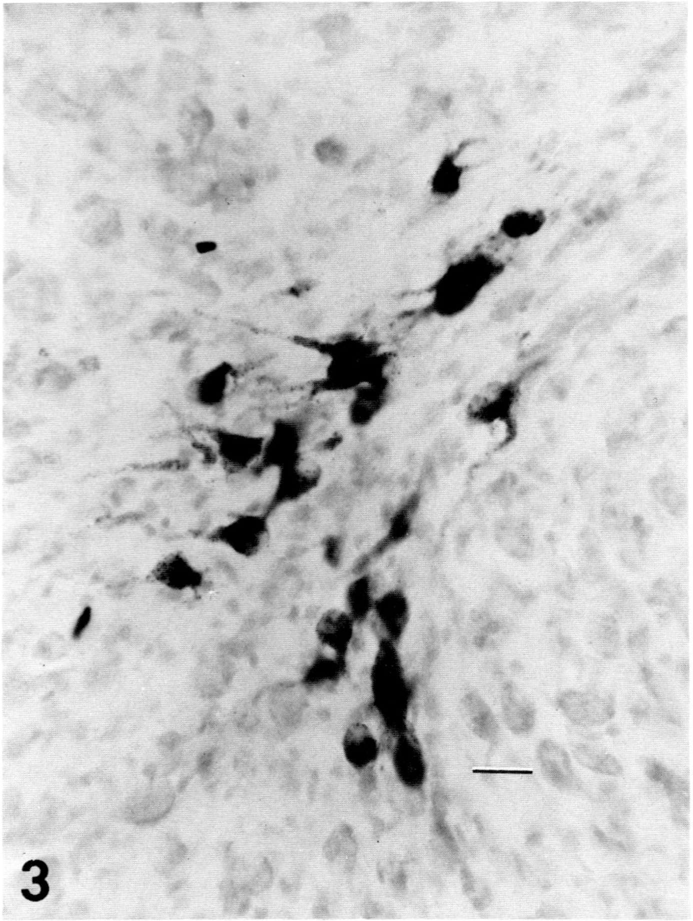

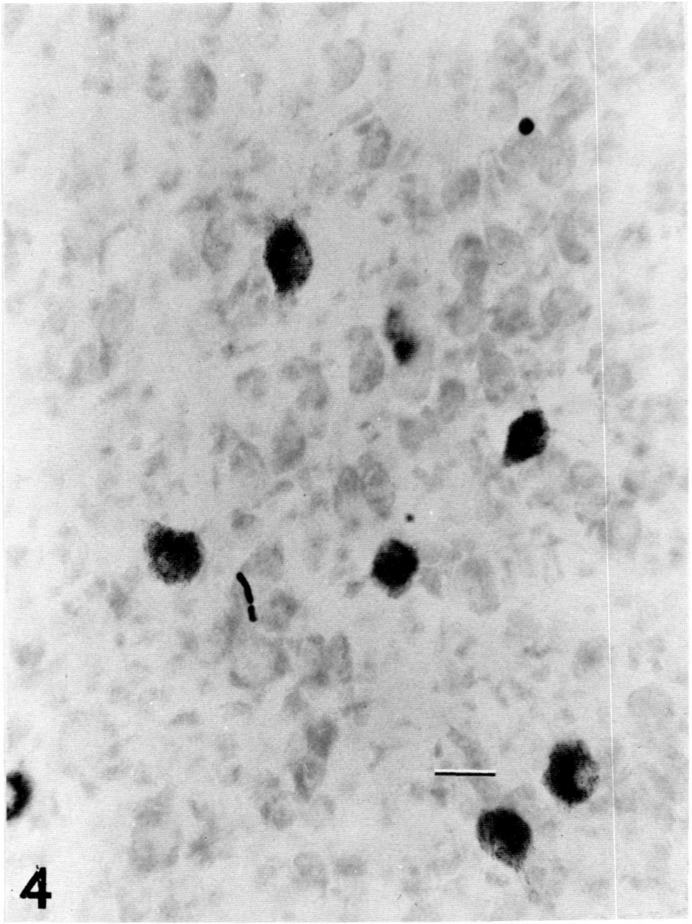

Fig. 3. Small, fusiform olivocochlear neurons in the dorsal hilus of the lateral superior olivary nucleus are labeled with HRP after an injection into the ipsilateral cochlea. Bar at lower right: 20 microns.

Fig. 4. Large olivocochlear neurons spanning the territories of the contralateral medial nucleus of the trapezoid body and the dorsally adjacent dorsomedial periolivary nucleus. Same kitten as in Fig. 3. Bar at lower right: 20 microns.

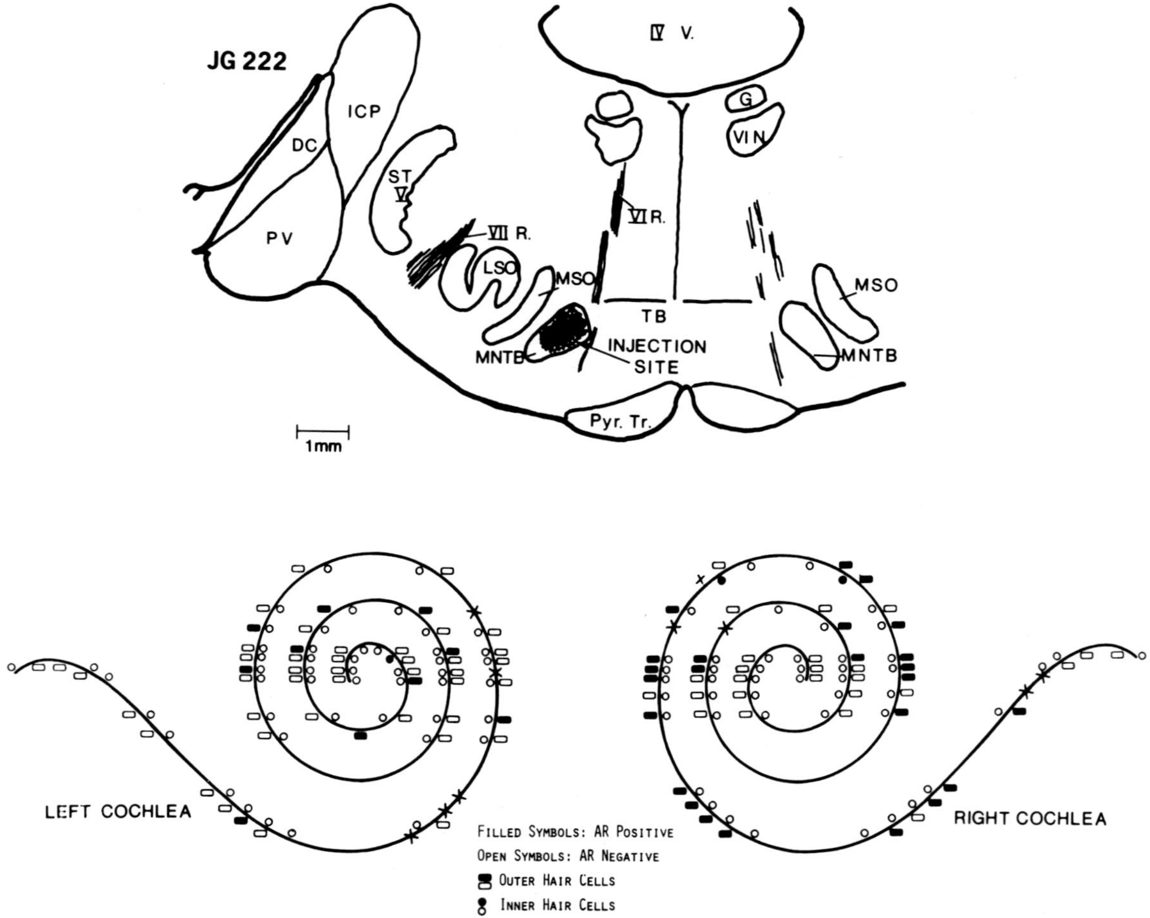
JG 222
IV V.
G
VI N
ICP
DC
PV
ST
V
VII R.
VI R.
LSO
MSO
MNTB
TB
INJECTION SITE
MSO
MNTB
Pyr. Tr.
1mm
LEFT COCHLEA
RIGHT COCHLEA
Filled Symbols: AR Positive
Open Symbols: AR Negative
Outer Hair Cells
Inner Hair Cells

Fig. 5. Summary of autoradiographic observations in cat JG-222. In the upper portion of the figure is shown the center of the injection site located in the left medial nucleus of the trapezoid body (MNTB) where large olivocochlear neurons are distributed. The lower two panels of the figure show the sites of silver grains (filled symbols) within the organ of Corti in the reconstructed cochleas. Crosses on the cochlear spirals indicate that this portion of the organ of Corti could not be reliably evaluated owing to the presence of either histological or autoradiographic artefacts. Abbreviations: DC, Dorsal Cochlear Nucleus; G, Genu of Facial Nerve; ICP, Inferior Cerebellar Peduncle; LSO, Lateral Superior Olivary Nucleus; MNTB, Medial Nucleus of the Trapezoid Body; MSO, Medial Superior Olivary Nucleus; PV, Posteroventral Cochlear Nucleus; Pyr. Tr, Pyramidal Tract; STV, Spinal Tract of Trigeminal Nerve; TB, Trapezoid Body; IV V, Fourth Ventricle; VI N, Abducens Nerve; VI R, Abducens Root; VII R, Facial Root.

60 nanoliters of distilled water was made into the dorsal hilus of the lateral superior olivary nucleus. The exposure time for the brain stem section was 7 days and that for the cochleas was 90 days. Within the organ of Corti of both sides, silver grains meeting criterion were almost entirely confined to the zone beneath the inner hair cells. On the ipsilateral (left) side, heavy accumulations of silver grains were found throughout the length of the cochlea, always in association with the inner hair cells (Fig. 8). In the opposite (right) cochlea, areas containing silver grains meeting criterion were fewer than in the ipsilateral cochlea and were, moreover, characterized by containing relatively fewer silver grains per unit area. Furthermore, the zones that did meet criterion tended to be located under the inner hair cells of only the more apical two turns of the cochlea. The right cochlea also presented two instances in which clusters of silver grains which barely met our criterion were found under the outer hair cells.

DISCUSSION

Origins of the OCB

The finding that emerged repeatedly in the series of experiments with HRP was that not only were there far more olivocochlear neurons than previously believed, but that the majority of these project to the cochlea of the same side, not to that of the opposite side as I expected. A likely source of this discrepancy, both in terms of the total number of efferent neurons and as regards the principal side of origin, may be that previous counts were performed on myelin-stained preparations which would have failed to reveal any unmyelinated axons which were present. That unmyelinated axons may be present in the cat is suggested by the observations in guinea pigs of Terayama and Yamamoto (1972) and by some unpublished counts made by R.S. Kimura (personal communication) who found that in the guinea pig 42% of the OCB axons in the vestibulo-cochlear anastomosis were unmyelinated. The data which show the ipsilateral side to be the major source of OCB axons would be accounted for if this ipsilateral component were largely unmyelinated. I have no experimental evidence to suggest that this is in fact the case, but it may be significant that the principal source of the ipsilateral component consists of rather small neurons, and that the AChE method and light microscope fail to resolve these axons (Osen and Roth, 1969). Thus, the small cells may possess fine diameter axons which are lightly myelinated or may even lack a myelin sheath entirely.

Another somewhat surprising result was that most regions of the superior olivary complex where OCB cells are found appear to contain, in reality, a dual population of efferent neurons. One population sends its axons to one cochlea, and the second population sends its axons to the cochlea of the opposite side. Although an alternate explanation of these data would be that some "special neurons" within each locus possess axons which bifurcate within the brain stem, one branch going to one cochlea and another branch to the opposite cochlea, this notion would appear to be without precedent and is less probable than the interpretation first proposed.

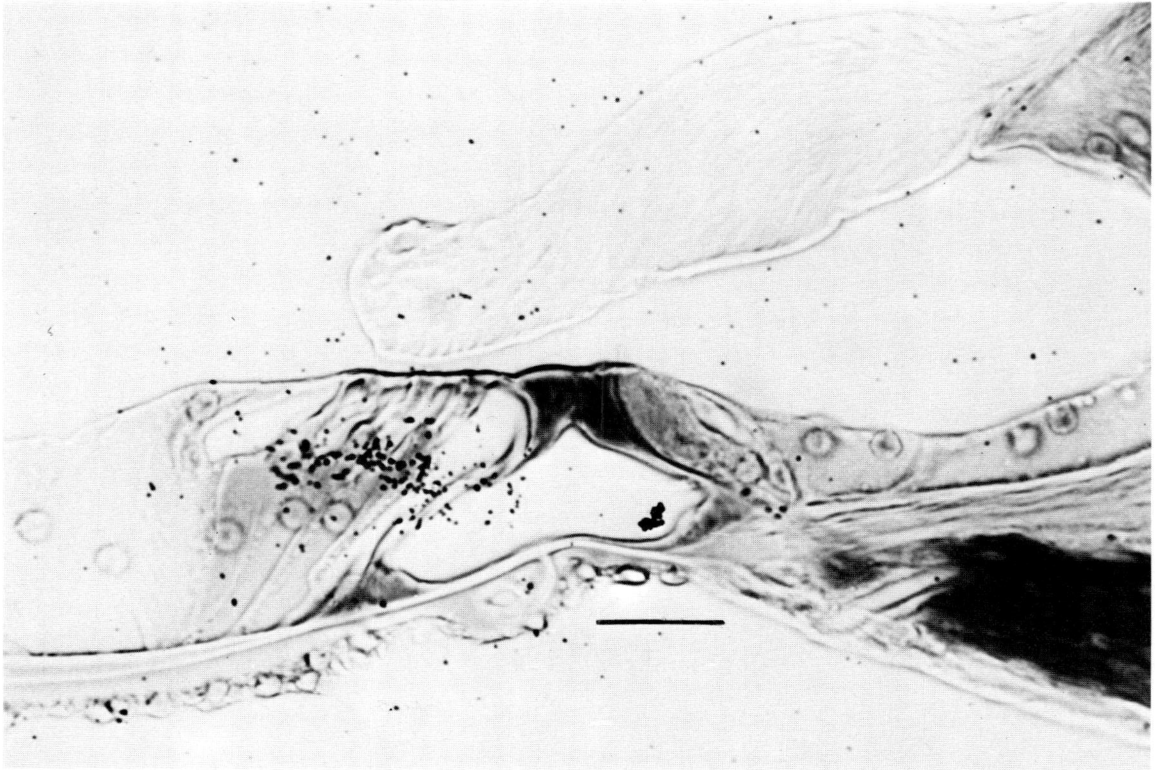

Fig. 6. Autoradiograph of the basal turn of the cochlea on the side opposite an injection in the medial nucleus of the trapezoid body. Bar equals 20μ.

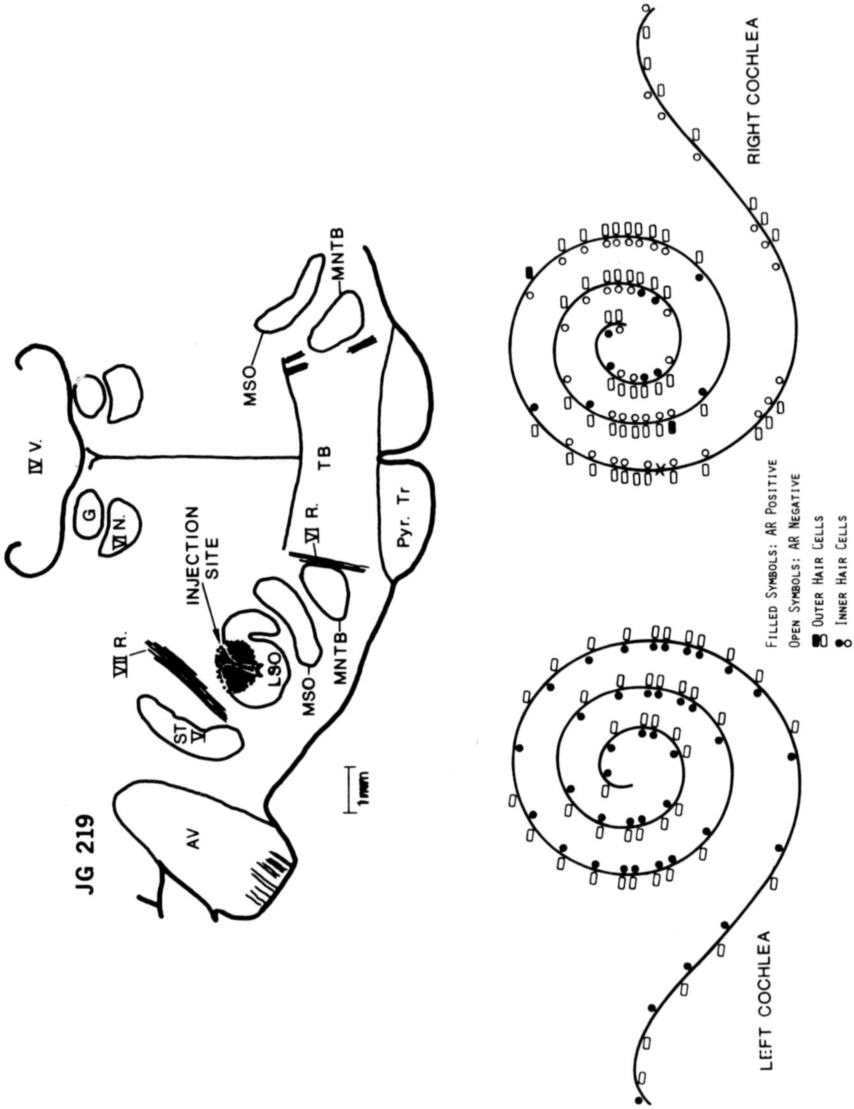

The regions of the superior olivary complex which were here demonstrated to contain olivocochlear neurons coincide precisely with the location of AChE-stained neurons previously mapped by Osen and Roth (1969). In fact, we have observed a close correspondance not only in the distribution of these cells, but also in regard to the morphological features of the individual neurons. Thus the perikarya and dendrites of neurons containing AChE match perfectly with the features of HRP labelled neurons in our experimental cases. Finally, that these neurons, namely

Fig. 7. Summary of autoradiographic observations in cat JG-219. In the upper portion of the figure is shown the center of the injection site located directly in the dorsal hilus of the left lateral superior olivary nucleus (LSO) where Experiment Series 1 had revealed the presence of a particularly heavy concentration of small olivocochlear neurons (see Figure 3). The lower two panels of the figure show the sites of silver grain clusters (filled symbols) located on reconstructions of the organ of Corti. Crosses on the cochlear spirals indicate sites where the organ of Corti could not be reliably evaluated owing to the presence of either histological or autoradiographic artifacts. Abbreviations same as Figure 5.

those reactive for AChE and those labelled with HRP, are perhaps identical, is suggested by the demonstration, following dual incubation for the two enzymes HRP and AChE, that neurons which contain the former virtually always contained the latter (Warr, 1975).

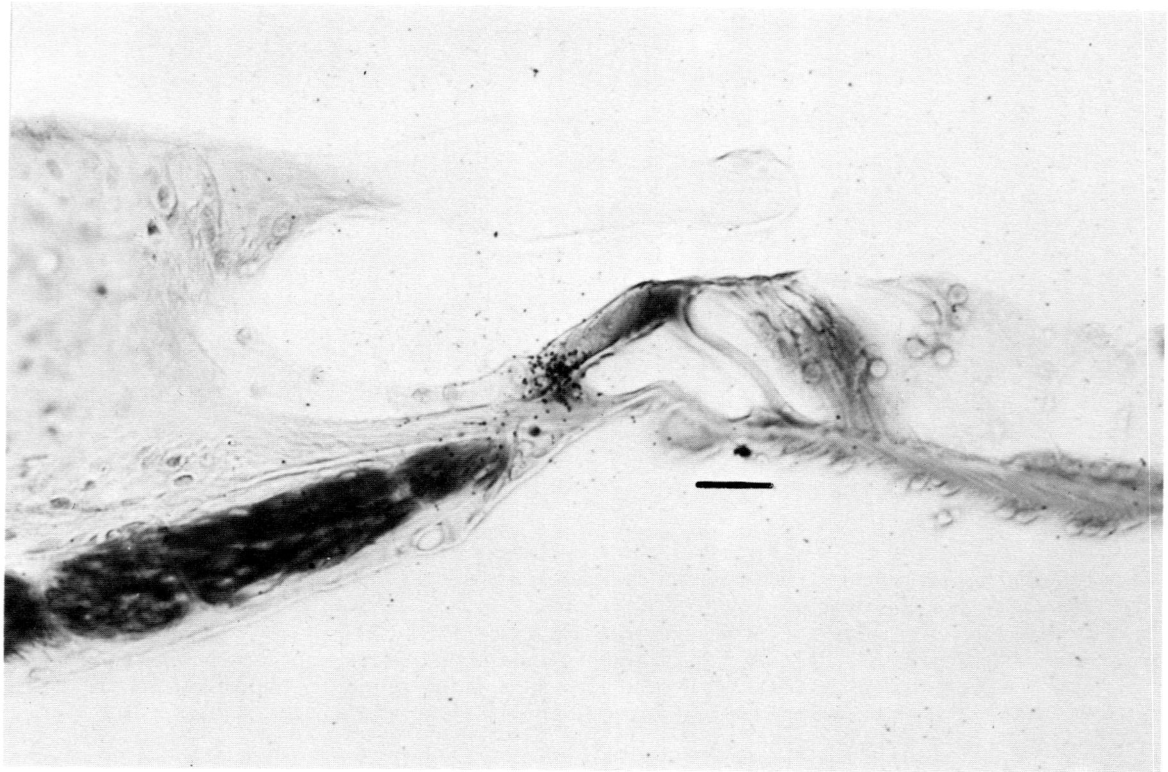

Fig. 8. Autoradiograph of the basal turn of the cochlea on the same side as an injection in the lateral superior olivary nucleus. Bar equals 20μ.

Differential Projections of Small and Large OCB Neurons

The preliminary evidence presented here suggests that olivocochlear neurons differ markedly in their projections to the organ of Corti. The large neurons in the area of the medial and ventral nuclei of the trapezoid body have as their synaptic destination the outer hair cells. A majority of these neurons project to the cochlea on the side opposite their origin, but according to my data a sufficient number to produce a recognizable autoradiographic signal also project from the medial nucleus of the trapezoid body to the cochlea of the same side. The finding of a projection predominantly to outer hair cells of the opposite cochlea is in perfect agreement with the many experimental studies cited in the introduction to this paper, where section of the crossed OCB results in substantial loss of large vesicle-containing synaptic structures on the bases of the outer hair cells (for review see Klinke and Galley, 1974; Guth et al., 1976). The existence of a smaller projection to the outer hair cells of the ipsilateral cochlea is also perhaps not unexpected because sectioning the crossed OCB does not produce a total loss of large endings on the outer hair cells, but rather a loss of at most 90% in the basal turn and a lesser proportion more apically in the monkey (Nakai and Igarashi, 1974). Similar detailed studies of the cat are unfortunately lacking.

The small neurons in the region of the lateral superior olivary nucleus project predominantly to the cochlea of the same side. This is entirely consistent with the results obtained with the HRP method, but also with the EM degeneration study of Smith and Rasmussen (1963). More importantly, these small neurons appear to be limited in their synaptic relations to the zone underlying the inner hair cells. This zone, containing the inner spiral bundle, has been beautifully analyzed by Smith (1961) in reconstructions of serial electron micrographs. She demonstrated that axons of the inner spiral bundle exhibit varicosities along their course which are in reality en passant presynaptic specializations which have as their virtually exclusive post-synaptic member an afferent axon (or peripheral preterminal process of a spiral ganglion cell) destined to terminate on an inner hair cell. Thus, some of the axons of the inner spiral bundle are engaged in axoaxonic synapses with the peripheral process of spiral ganglion cells. Furthermore, the location of these synapses requires that they be regarded as exerting their physiological influence at a post-synaptic level, or in other words, at a point along the axon which is temporally subsequent to the influence of the inner hair cell itself. This is in sharp contrast to the synaptic relations of large vesicle-containing structures in direct contact with outer hair cells.

The injections of the radio-labelled precurser amino acid, ^{35}S Methionine in the lateral superior olivary nucleus and in the medial nucleus of the trapezoid body in the two animals presented here were so situated as to provide labelling of neurons which differed maximally in terms of their morphology. The results show that the synaptic destinations of axons arising from these cells, while to some degree sharing the same cochlea as their target, exhibit virtually no commonality as regards their specific site of synaptic influence, at least as could be determined with

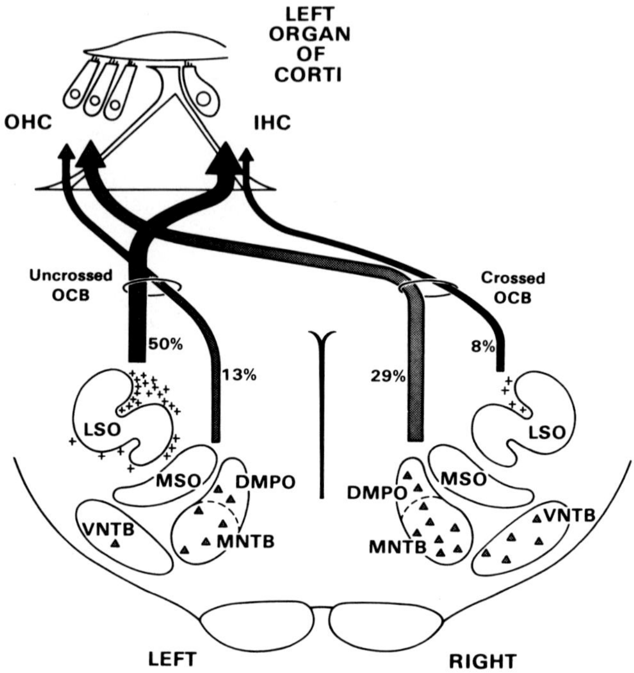

Fig. 9. A schema of the origins and terminations of the olivocochlear bundle in the cat, based upon HRP injections (origins and numerical estimates) and upon ^{35}S Methionine injections into the superior olivary complex (Zones of termination). Crosses represent small OCB neurons; triangles represent large OCB neurons. The number of symbols of each kind and the widths of the lines originating from each region are proportional to neuronal contribution. It can be seen that a majority of OCB neurons to one cochlea originates on the ipsilateral side. Furthermore, the majority of OCB neurons are small, originate bilaterally, and do not innervate outer hair cells. Abbreviations: DMPO, dorsomedial periolivary nucleus; IHC, inner hair cells; LSO, lateral superior olivary nucleus; MNTB, medial nucleus of the trapezoid body; MSO, medial superior olivary nucleus; OCB, olivocochlear bundle; OHC, outer hair cells; VNTB, ventral nucleus of the trapezoid body.

the light microscopic methods employed. Efforts are now underway to confirm these inchoate observations both at the light and electron microscopic levels using the autoradiographic technique.

It is tempting to provide a tentative synthesis of the results of the two series of experiments, the one using HRP, and the second using the labelled amino acid. Such an attempt is shown in Figure 9, where the numerical data relating to the various sources of the olivocochlear bundle is based exclusively upon the HRP experiments (see Warr, 1975, Figure 2F), and the data concerning the terminations of these cell groups is based exclusively upon injections of amino acids. I have assumed that the large cells of the *ventral* nucleus of the trapezoid body have projections similar to the large cells of the *medial* nucleus of the trapezoid body. The

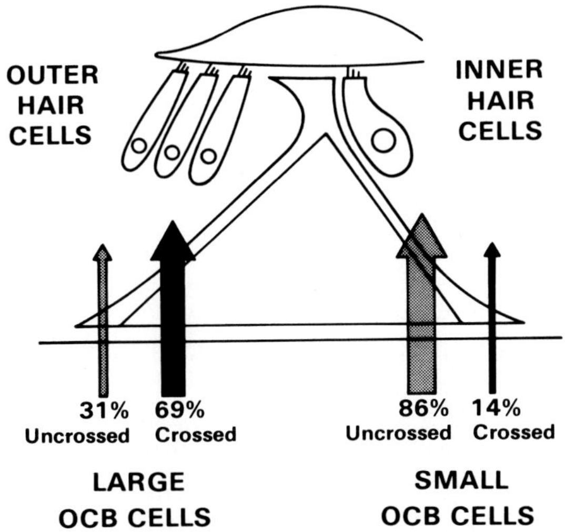

Fig. 10. The relative proportions of crossed and uncrossed olivocochlear neurons contributing to each of the two efferent synaptic fields within the organ of Corti. Calculations were based upon the same data base as Figure 9.

number of symbols (crosses and triangles) indicating small and large cells respectively is proportional to the actual cell counts in each region seen with the HRP method and the line widths also further reflect the proportional contribution of each cell group to the combined OCB to one cochlea.

Figure 10 presents these same data in a different way. Here I wish to emphasize the proportion of crossed vs. uncrossed innervation to outer hair cells on the one hand (left) and to the peripheral processes of spiral ganglion cells on the other (right).

In conclusion, it may be permissible to speculate that the existence within the OCB of two kinds of axons with distinct origins within the brain stem and separate terminations in the organ of Corti suggest that there may be two distinct physiological mechanisms by which the central nervous system may influence the peripheral auditory receptor. It would seem that sufficient anatomical data are now in hand to permit the selective manipulation of these two efferent pathways for the purpose of determining their contributions to the hearing process.

SUMMARY

The origins and terminations of the olivocochlear bundle (OCB) were studied by means of axonal transport methods in the cat. The cells of origin of the OCB were localized by injecting horseradish peroxidase unilaterally into the cochleas of kittens where it was taken up by synaptic endings in the organ of Corti and transported intra-axonally to neurons in the superior olivary complex of the brain stem.

In the kitten, approximately 1800 efferent neurons project to one cochlea, of which more than half are located ipsilaterally. The single largest contingent originates from small fusiform neurons located near the lateral superior olivary nucleus (LSO) of the same side. The next largest contingent, comprising about a third of the total, arises contralaterally from large stellate neurons located medial and ventral to the medial superior olivary nucleus (MSO). Although each group of olivocochlear neurons projects preferentially to either the same or opposite side, neither group can be said to have exclusively crossed or uncrossed projections to the cochlea.

In a second series of experiments on adult cats, the distribution within the cochlea of synaptic terminals and preterminal axons belonging to the efferent neurons was studied by the method of anterograde intra-axonal transport of radioactively labelled protein, and subsequent autoradiography on histological sections of the cochleas. Injection of ^{35}S-methionine, were made into the region of the LSO (small OCB neurons) and into the medial and ventral nuclei of the trapezoid body (large OCB neurons). In the former cases, a heavy accumulation of autoradiographic silver grains is localized beneath the inner hair cells of the ipsilateral cochlea, and a slight accumulation of silver grains is observed under inner hair cells of the opposite cochlea. On the other hand, injections into the mediolateral trapezoid nuclei produces a heavy accumulation of silver grains at the bases of outer hair cells on the side opposite the injections, and a slight accumulation at the bases of outer hair cells in the cochlea of the same side.

These findings suggest that the OCB in the cat may be comprised of two distinct neuronal pathways. The first consists of small laterally located OCB neurons which presumably synapse on the peripheral processes of spiral ganglion cells beneath the inner hair cells. The second pathway consists of larger, medially located OCB neurons which terminate predominantly in association with outer hair cells. The large cell pathway is mostly crossed and the small cell pathway is mostly uncrossed, but significant contingents of each pathway do not follow this rule.

Acknowledgement

This work supported by USPHS grant # NS07720.

REFERENCES

Cowan, W.M., Gottleib, D.I., Hendrickson, A.E., Price, J.L. and Woolsey, T.A. The autoradiographic demonstration of axonal connections in the central nervous system. *Brain Res. 37:* 21-51, 1972.

El-Badawi, A., and Schenk, E.A. Dual innervation of the mammalian urinary bladder. *Am. J. Anat. 119:* 405-428, 1966.

Engström, H. On the double innervation of the sensory epithelia of the inner ear. *Acta Otolaryngol. 49:* 109-118, 1958.

Graham, R.C. Jr. and Karnovsky, M.J. The early stages of absorption of injected horseradish peroxidase in the proximal tubules of mouse kidney: ultrastructural cytochemistry by a new technique. *J. Histochem. Cytochem. 14:* 291-302, 1966.

Guinan, J.J. Jr., Guinan, S.S. and Norris, B.E. Single auditory units in the superior olivary complex. *Intern. J. Neurosci. 4:* 101-120, 1972.

Guth, P.S., Norris, C.H., and Bobbin, R.P. The pharmacology of transmission in the peripheral auditory system. *Pharm. Rev. 28:* 95-125, 1976.

Kimura, R.S. and Wersäll, J. Termination of the olivocochlear bundle in relation to the outer hair cells of the organ of Corti in guinea pig. *Acta Otolaryngol. 55:* 11-32, 1962.

Klinke, R. and Galley, N. Efferent innervation of vestibular and auditory receptors. *Physiol. Rev. 54:* 316-357, 1974.

Luk, G.D., Morest, D.K. and McKenna, N.M. Origins of the crossed olivocochlear bundle shown by an acid phosphatase method. *Ann. Otol. Rhinol. Laryngol. 83:* 382-392, 1974.

Nakai, Y. and Igarashi, M. Distribution of the crossed olivocochlear bundle terminals in the squirrel monkey cochlea. *Acta Otolaryngol. 77:* 393-404, 1974.

Osen, K.K. and Roth, K. Histochemical localization of cholinesterases in the cochlear nuclei of the cat, with notes on the origin of acetylcholinesterase-positive afferents and the superior olive. *Brain Res. 16:* 165-185, 1969.

Papez, J.W. The superior olivary nucleus: its fiber connections. *Arch. Neur. Psychiat. 24:* 1-20, 1930.

Rasmussen, G.L. The olivary peduncle and other fiber projections of the superior olivary complex. *J. Comp. Neurol. 84:* 141-219, 1946.

Rasmussen, G.L. Efferent fibers of the cochlear nerve and cochlear nucleus. In: *Neural Mechanisms of the Auditory and Vestibular Systems,* edited by G.L. Rasmussen and W.F. Windle. Springfield, Ill.: Charles C Thomas, 1960, p. 105-115.

Rasmussen, G.L. Anatomic relationships of the ascending and descending auditory systems. In: *Neurological Aspects of Auditory and Vestibular Disorders,* edited by W.S. Fields and B.R. Alford. Springfield, Ill.: Charles C Thomas, 1964, p. 5-19.

Rasmussen, G.L. Efferent connection in the cochlear nucleus. In: *Sensorineural Hearing Processes and Disorders,* edited by A.B. Graham. London: Churchill, 1967, p. 61-75.

Schuknecht, H.F., Churchill, J.A. and Doran, R. The localization of acetylcholinesterase in the cochlea. *Arch. Otolaryngol. 69:* 549-559, 1959.

Smith, C.A. Innervation pattern of the cochlea. The internal hair cell. *Ann. Otol. Rhinol. Laryngol. 70:* 504-527, 1961.

Smith, C.A. and Rasmussen, G.L. Recent observations on the olivocochlear bundle. *Ann. Otol. Rhinol. Laryngol. 72:* 489-505, 1963.

Spoendlin, H. *The Organization of the Cochlear Receptor. Adv. Oto-Rhino-Laryngol. 13.* New York: S. Karger, 1966.

Spoendlin, H. Structural basis of peripheral frequency analysis. In: *Frequency Analysis and Periodicity Detection in Hearing,* edited by R. Plomp and G.F. Smoorenburg. Leiden: Sitjhoff, 1970, p. 2-40.

Terayama, Y. and Yamamoto, K. Olivo-cochlear bundle in the guinea pig after central transsection of the crossed bundle. *Acta Otolaryngol. 72:* 385-396, 1971.

Warr, W.B. Olivocochlear and vestibular efferent neurons of the feline brain stem: their location, morphology and number determined by retrograde axonal transport and acetylcholinesterase histochemistry. *J. Comp. Neur. 161:* 159-182, 1975.

DISCUSSION

Galambos: You have emphasized that your data are for the cat. If I remember rightly, the rodent has a third origin for OCB cells, somewhere in the midline. What is that all about?

Warr: I don't know what that is all about, Bob. I think that data is based largely on acetylcholinesterase stain. I don't believe those cells have been positively identified as really having projections to the cochlea itself. My own opinion is that the only way to do that is perhaps to use horseradish peroxidase or perhaps even the antegrade transport technique with autoradiography. So, how general these findings are is a very valid question. It ought to be done on the monkey and guinea pig, and I am sure it will be done ultimately.

Spoendlin: Does horseradish peroxidase also go into the afferent neurons when applied to the round window or only when it is applied to the efferents? I am very pleased to hear your results, because on the basis of degeneration behavior I always had the impression that the efferent population for the inner hair cells is different from that of the outer hair cells. The efferents of the outer hair cells degenerate very early, within 12 hours, whereas the efferents of the inner hair cell area take several days.

Warr: Yes. Others have observed that too, Heinrich, and a lot of facts seem to militate in favor of the notion that there are separate origins, if not terminations, for the efferent system.

With regard to the first question, do the afferents take up horseradish peroxidase, the answer is that we often saw horseradish peroxidase in the axons of the eighth nerve. I don't recall carefully studying the ganglion itself to find out whether peroxidase was in the ganglion cells. We did some sections of the cochlea, but we were primarily interested in other matters. We wanted to be sure the horseradish peroxidase had reached all the turns. We were not concerned with conduction or transport by afferents. It occurs, though. I am not sure why we didn't see it more prominently or more often.

Bodian: Does the trapezoid body show a cholinesterase reaction?

Warr: The ones that projected the cochlea are stained with cholinesterase techniques, both in the nucleus of the trapezoid body and those around the lateral olive as well. I didn't go into the data, but we actually were able to demonstrate in a number of preparations that horseradish peroxidase was inside the very same cells as were stained with cholinesterase. So, we know it is the cholinesterase group of cells that is projecting to the cochlea, and nothing else.

Bodian: And that applies to the trapezoid nuclei as well?

Warr: Precisely.

Bodian: In the monkey, at least, there are conspicuously more granular vesicles in the efferent synaptic terminals, on the afferent dendrites to the inner hair cells, than one finds in the efferent endings on the outer hair cells. I just wonder whether we are dealing with the same transmitter system.

Warr: Well, there seems to be widespread evidence that all these efferent fibers can be stained with the usual Karnovsky cholinesterase methods. The only efferent supply to the cochlea which is not, is apparently the adrenergic innervation which presumably comes from the superior sympathetic ganglion. However, those that originate in the central nervous system do seem to be cholinergic.

Smith: In some studies that Dr. Eldredge, Dr. Iurato and I were doing in the chinchilla in which the crossed tract was cut in the floor of the fourth ventricle, we found differences in degeneration of the large nerve endings on the outer hair cells along the basilar membrane. There was no degeneration of large efferent endings in the round window portion of the cochlear duct, very little in the first turn, and then more degeneration in the second turn of the chinchilla. I wonder if when you injected your tagged amino acids you found any differences in different places along the basilar membrane.

Warr: Of course we did, but whether it is significant at all at this point is not clear, because that would depend a great deal on precisely where our injection was made within the olivary complex. For example, we may have labeled preferentially cells with a higher frequency representation than certain others. So, what I am saying is that until we sample systematically all the zones of origin, perhaps using four or five different animals, we will not be able to come out and say there is a zonal projection, a limited projection, from any one region of the brain stem to any one region of the cochlea.

There are some subtleties in this data that are suggestive, and they are the kind of thing I will be glad to talk over with you; but we need the pictures in front of us.

At the present stage I don't believe I can say anything about limited projections. What is remarkable, though, is that projection from the lateral superior olive is extremely intense throughout the extent of the cochlear duct, whereas there did seem to be more limited projections from our injections in the medial nucleus of the trapezoid body. Of course, because of the different density of clustering of the cells in the two regions we would have labeled ten times more neurons after injection in the lateral olive than in the medial nucleus of the trapezoid body. So, we have to be very careful about drawing any conclusions yet. But ultimately I think we will make some progress with this method.

PHYSIOLOGY

Moderator: *Jay M. Goldberg*

Electrical equivalents of the Békésy traveling wave in the mammalian cochlea
Eldredge, Donald H.

Mechanisms of afferent discharge from electroreceptors: implication for acoustic reception
Bennett, Michael V. L.

Which structures determine frequency selectivity and tonotopic organization of vertebrate nerve fibers? Evidence from the alligator lizard
Weiss, Thomas F., Peake, William T., Ling, Alexander, Jr., and Holton, Thomas

Intracellular studies of cochlear hair cells: filling the gap between basilar membrane mechanics and neural excitation
Sellick, Peter and Russell, Ian J.

Cochlear electrophysiology
Dallos, Peter

Interpretation of evoked neural responses: facts and illusions related to the methods for recording whole-nerve action potentials
Eldredge, Donald H.

Unit activity underlying the N_1 potential
Antoli-Candela, Francisco, Jr. and Kiang, Nelson, Y. S.

ELECTRICAL EQUIVALENTS OF THE BÉKÉSY TRAVELING WAVE IN THE MAMMALIAN COCHLEA

Donald H. Eldredge

Central Institute for the Deaf, St. Louis

INTRODUCTION

The earliest stages in the process of hearing are acoustical and mechanical. The amplitudes and phases of the mechanical motion at the stapes footplate are relatively simple transformations of those of the sound pressures at the tympanic membrane. Békésy (1943, 1947, 1949) first described for us the complex patterns of motion along the basilar membrane that follow simple sinusoidal motion at the stapes. Using direct observations under the microscope with stroboscopic illumination, he was able to see waves travel and grow along the basilar membrane to a place of maximum amplitude and then decay abruptly to amplitudes too small to be seen. From his collected studies (Békésy, 1960) we know that the graded properties of stiffness of the cochlear partition from base to apex can account for the orderly pattern of delays in the responses along the basilar membrane that give this appearance of a traveling wave.

In recent years it has been possible to confirm in principle many of Békésy's observations. Johnstone and Boyle (1967), Johnstone et al., (1970), Rhode (1971), Rhode and Robles (1974) and Robles et al., (1976) have employed the Mössbauer technique to measure amplitudes and phases as functions of frequency at a few places in the cochleas of guinea pig and squirrel monkey. Kohllöffel (1972a, 1972b, 1972c) employed interference patterns under laser illumination to measure amplitudes and phases over a distance of several miilimeters in the basal turn of the guinea pig. Wilson and Johnstone (1975) measured amplitude and phases as functions of frequency in the basal turn of the guinea pig with a subminiature capacitative probe.

Each of the above studies is limited to a restricted place or set of places in only one area of the basilar membrane and, although giving results quite consistent with Békésy's findings, do not show in detail the spatially distributed traveling wave. Earlier Tasaki et al., (1952) had shown that the cochlear microphonic (CM) measured from several turns in the cochlea of guinea pig could be used to sample amplitude and phase as functions of frequency at these several widely separated

ISBN 0-12-514960-3

places. Then Teas et al., (1962) devised a method for interpolation of CM values between each of the measurement stations in order to produce longitudinal spatial voltage gradients. From photographs of a series of such gradients it was possible to make a motion picture of the electrical traveling wave. In 1969 Benitez, and Templer, then working in my laboratory, undertook to learn these procedures and to apply them to the CM responses to several different acoustic signals. This exercise did not provide any really new scientific information, but it yielded the longitudinal voltage gradients that, either as a set of static gradients or projected as a motion picture, help the observer better to appreciate the nature of the Békésy traveling wave. The movie has been presented on several formal occasions (Eldredge et al., 1971a, 1971b, 1973) and is repeated here.

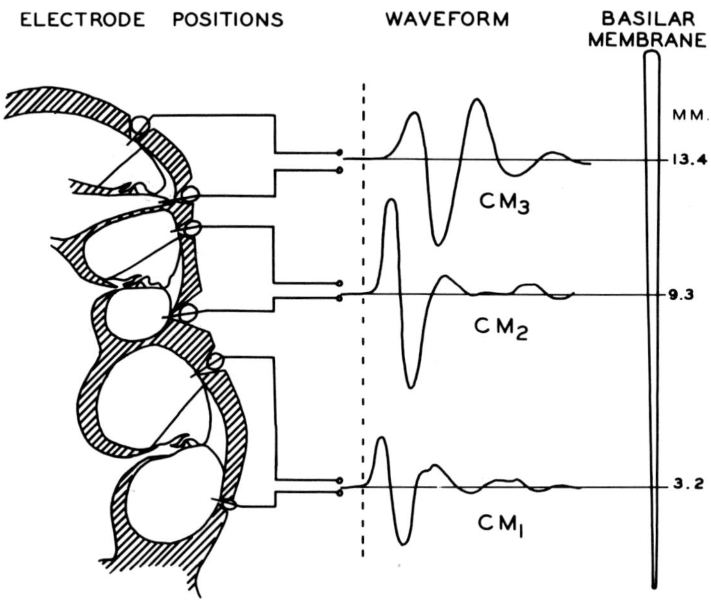

Fig. 1. Diagrams relating placements of three pairs of differential cochlear electrodes in chinchilla (left) to the different CM waveforms recorded from each of the three cochlear turns (center) and to position along the basilar membrane in millimeters from the round window end (right).

METHODS

After the method of Tasaki et al., (1952) CM was measured differentially with pairs of electrodes across the cochlear partition in each of the three cochlear turns of chinchilla. This orientation of electrode pairs, indicated on the diagram at the left in Figure 1, discriminates against evoked neural or whole-nerve action potential responses and favors recording of CM generated within a few millimeters of the electrodes over that generated more remotely. In the middle of Figure 1 are shown the electrical waveforms in time for CM_1, CM_2 and CM_3 in response to a 650-Hz low-pass transient or thump. Békésy (1951) showed that CM is proportional to displacement at the basilar membrane. Since it is not likely that the constants of proportionality are exactly the same in the different turns, the longitudinal voltage gradients to be reported are only similar to the actual mechanical traveling waves. The places of the electrodes, as indicated on the right in Figure 1, were reconstructed from measurements on every fifth section of several cochleas.

Each CM function in time contains several distinctive and recognizable features. These include an onset, a first positive peak, a zero crossing, a first negative peak, a second zero crossing, a second positive peak, etc. Also the CM functions in time show characteristic delays between turns. Note that we can measure the peak voltages at each place and we can measure the time required for each dis-

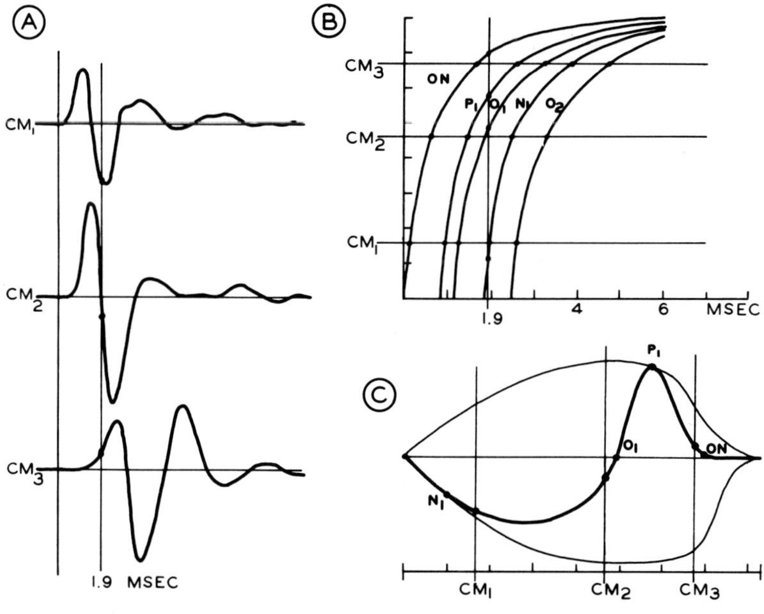

Fig. 2. Diagrams showing the methods used to infer a voltage gradient along the basilar membrane from the CM responses measured at three places. A: CM waveforms as measured in three turns with values 1.9 msec after onset marked. B: Plot of measured interturn delays for onset, first positive peak, and second zero crossing with smoothed interpolations and extrapolations basally and apically. Locations of onset, first positive peak at 1.9 msec after onset are marked. C: CM voltages as functions of place along the basilar membrane. The light line above is the envelope of first positive peaks smoothly interpolated from zero at each end through the peak values measured in each turn. The light line below is the corresponding envelope for the first negative peaks. The heavy line is interpolated through the values appropriate to 1.9 msec after onset. See text for details.

tinctive feature to travel between turns. In order to make a longitudinal voltage gradient, it is necessary to interpolate values appropriate to intermediate places.

The first step in this interpolation is to erect on the abscissas corresponding to the places of measurement along the basilar membrane ordinates that are proportional to the measured peak voltages at each place. Then, as in Figure 2c, values for intermediate places are assumed to follow a spatial envelope that smoothly changes from zero at each end through the measured values. A separate envelope is drawn for each positive and negative peak. Only one of each is shown in Figure 2c.

For the second step in the interpolation the ordinates for place of measurement are related to the delays between distinctive features as shown in Figure 2b. The measured points are connected by functions with smoothly decelerating slopes and extrapolated both basally and apically. Zero time is set as the extrapolation of the onset back to zero distance along the basilar membrane.

Now it is possible at a single moment in time to learn many values for voltage along the basilar membrane. In the example shown in Figure 2 at 1.9 msec there are three measured values for each turn as shown in Figure 2a and these values are replotted at the appropriate places in Figure 2c. In Figure 2b we see that the onset has traveled apical to the place for CM_3, the first positive peak is about half way between the second and third turns, the first zero crossing is just apical to the electrodes in the second turn and the first negative peak is still basal to the electrodes in the first turn. The onset and zero crossing are given values of zero at the corresponding places in Figure 2c and the positive and negative peaks are assigned the values of their interpolated spatial envelopes at the corresponding places. Finally a spatial voltage gradient is interpolated from zero at each end through each of the seven values. Superficially it appears that there is too much freedom of choice for this last interpolation. But, if we maintain the criterion that all points along the interpolated voltage gradients move smoothly as functions of space and time, then there turns out in practice to be very little freedom of choice and the interpolated values and the spatial gradients cannot actually be very different from those to be shown. Incorrect choices for spatial voltage gradients are quickly revealed when pauses, jumps, or reversals become necessary in order to be consistent with measured values.

RESULTS

In Figure 3 are shown the CM functions in time for the acoustic thump generated when a 0.7 msec rectangular electrical pulse, band-passed 20-650 Hz, was led to a PDR-10 earphone sealed to a speculum sewed into the ear canal of a chinchilla. The sound pressure was only 50 dB SPL (peak equivalent) and 20 responses were averaged to achieve a better ratio of signal to noise. The CM_1 waveform approximates the sound pressure waveform at the tympanic membrane, but is more nearly proportional to the instantaneous stapes velocity than to stapes displacement. The CM_2 waveform is very similar but larger and slightly delayed. The CM_3 waveform is further delayed and shows both lengthening of its periodicity

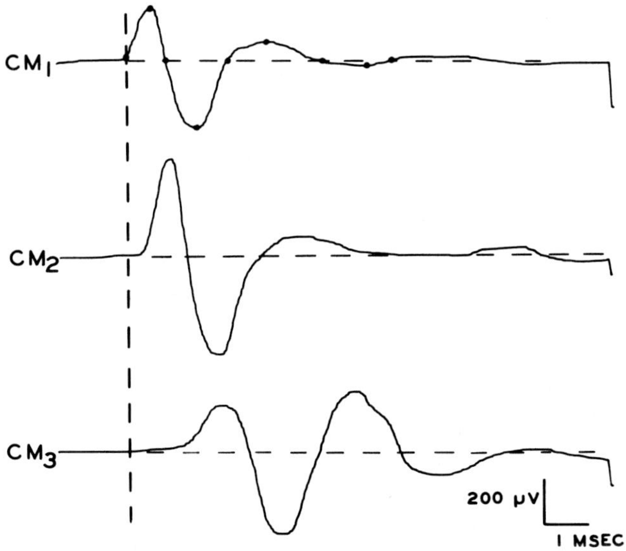

Fig. 3. First, second and third turn CM responses to 650-Hz, low-pass acoustic thump at 50 dB SPL, peak equivalent.

and an increase in the relative magnitude of the second positive peak. These features reflect additional low-pass filtering by the basilar membrane at this place where the best frequency is about 300 Hz.

The corresponding CM functions in space are shown in Figure 4. The sequence of gradients begins with the thinnest line above and progresses to the thickest, then jumps to the thinnest line below and continues to the thickest line below. The first gradient is at 0.6 msec after onset and successive gradients are at 0.4 msec intervals through 4.8 msec after onset. On close examination of the gradients several interesting features are apparent. Starting at the base CM amplitude is significant even in the relative absence of acoustic energy at high frequencies. Over relatively long distances the CM is nearly in phase and local voltages are changing in the same direction. Note also that, as they travel along the basilar membrane the first and second positive peaks grow and decay through different spatial envelopes.

In Figure 5 are shown the CM waveforms in time for a wide-band acoustic click produced by applying a 0.1 msec rectangular pulse to the PDR-10 earphone and speculum system. Except for a broad resonance between 2.5 kHz and 5.0 kHz with a peak of 12 dB at 3.6 kHz, the acoustic response at the tympanic membrane was flat within ±5 dB from 50 Hz to 8 kHz. Again the sound pressure was 50 dB SPL, peak equivalent, and 20 responses were averaged to improve the ratio of signal to noise. These CM responses show different periodicities that reflect the respective corner or best frequencies for each place. The relatively large first negative peak in the CM_2 response is characteristic at low signal levels. With increasing level, the first positive peak grows more rapidly and eventually becomes relatively larger than the negative peak. CM_3 is relatively smaller at all signal levels. Note that the three waveforms are distinctively different. When electrode placements are poor, it is easy to see electrical crosstalk and it is appropriate then to infer that the waveforms reflect responses from distant as well as local sources.

The CM functions in space for the wide-band click are shown in Figure 6. Again the sequences for the traces proceed from light to heavy traces and from upper to lower groups of traces. The first gradient is for 0.1 msec after the onset and subsequent gradients are at intervals of 0.1 msec through 1.8 msec after onset. In the upper set of six, note that the onset initially moves apically very rapidly. By the fourth trace in the upper set there are two quite clear positive peaks along the membrane and the pattern of a second peak closely chasing the first along the membrane persists clearly through the fourth trace in the second set. Unlike the sequence for the thump, here there are large phase differences at different places.

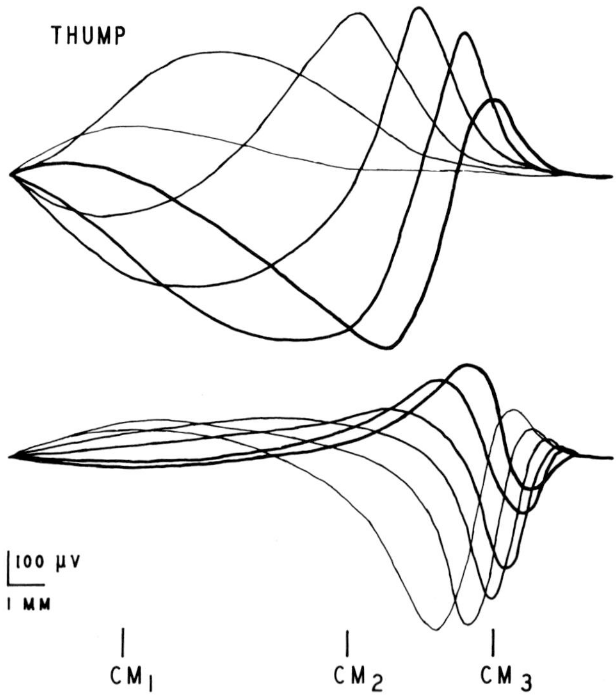

Fig. 4. Longitudinal CM voltage gradients for CM responses to the 650-Hz low-pass acoustic thump. The first gradient at 0.6 msec after onset is the lightest trace in the upper group. Subsequent traces proceed at intervals of 0.4 msec. The thinnest line in the group below follows the thickest line above.

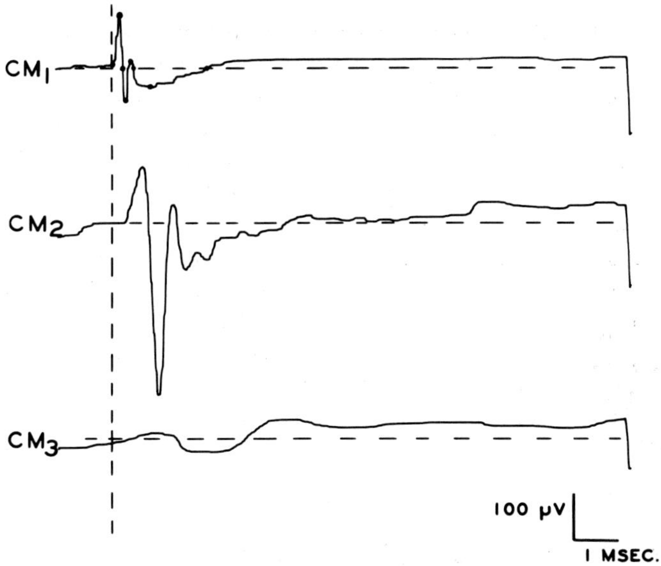

Fig. 5. First, second and third turn CM responses to wide-band click at 50 dB SPL, peak equivalent.

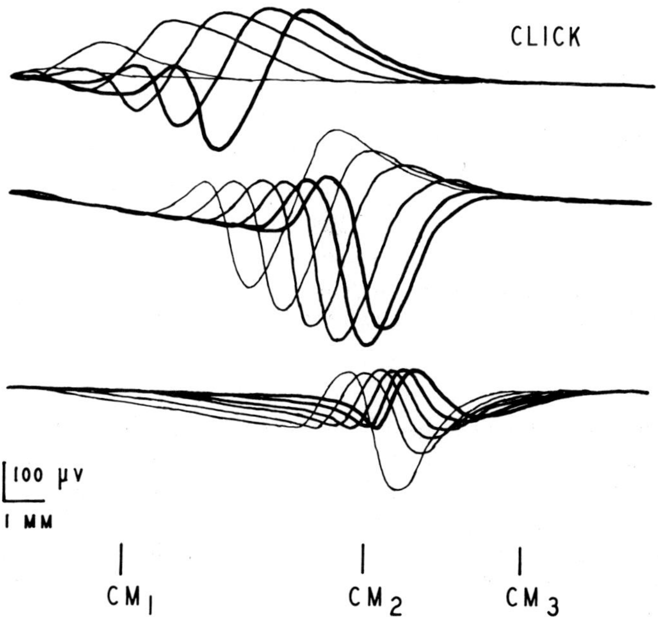

Fig. 6. Longitudinal voltage gradients for CM responses to wide-band click. The first gradient at 0.1 msec after onset is the thinnest line in the upper group of traces. Subsequent traces are at intervals of 0.1 msec. Within groups heavier lines follow lighter lines and the overall sequence proceeds from the upper to the middle and then to the lower group of traces.

Also, something like this regular growth of the first negative peak to a place just apical to the electrodes in the second turn and then a relatively abrupt decay in amplitude is clearly required by the CM waveforms in time shown in Figure 5.

When the signals were pure tones, the CM responses in chinchilla closely followed the relations reported for guinea pig by Tasaki et al., (1952). The three CM responses in time to a brief gated tone of 150 Hz at 55 dB SPL are shown in Figure 7. Again 20 responses were averaged to improve the ratio of signal to noise. The voltages grow systematically with distance from the base and are largest in the third turn. The response in the second turn is in phase with that from the basal turn and the response in the third turn shows a delay of less than 1 msec which is less than 0.3 π radians at this frequency. The successive additions to the duration of the response as it moves from the basal turn to the third turn were also present at higher levels and presumably reflect some resonant ringing along the basilar membrane.

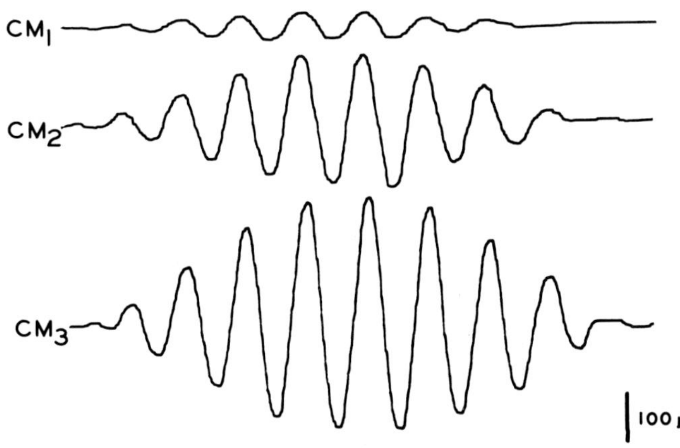

Fig. 7. First, second and third turn CM responses to tone pip of 150 Hz at 55 dB SPL. Calibration for time should be inferred from the period of 6.67 msec.

The three CM responses to a brief gated tone of 500 Hz at 45 dB SPL are shown in Figure 8. At this frequency the voltages in the second turn are the largest. The CM_3 response does not change linearly with level as the signal is gated on and off. Furthermore, the 500 Hz component of the response is riding on a slow wave with a period roughly corresponding to the envelope of the gated onset. From base to third turn the delays of the traveling wave are clearly apparent. CM_3 lags CM_1 by slightly more than one cycle or 2 msec.

The three CM responses to a brief tone of 2000 Hz at 41 dB SPL are shown in Figure 9. At this frequency the largest voltages are found in the basal turn. The smaller response recorded from the second turn is delayed by about 0.6 msec or

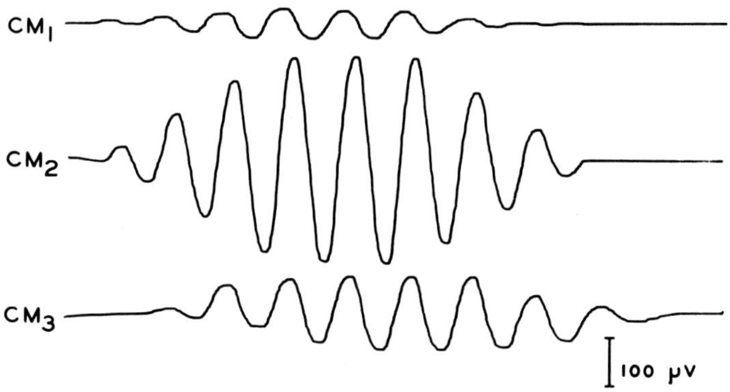

Fig. 8. First, second and third turn CM responses to tone pip of 500 Hz at 45 dB SPL. Calibration for time should be inferred from the period of 2.0 msec.

slightly more than one period, does not change linearly with level as the tone is gated on and off, and is superimposed on a slow wave. In the third turn the 2000 Hz component of the response is entirely gone and only the slow wave remains. The onset of this slow wave in the third turn follows the onset of the 2000 Hz component in the basal turn by about 2 msec. It appears that the acoustic energy in the envelope of the tone pulse has been detected more basally and then traveled apically as an independent mechanical event.

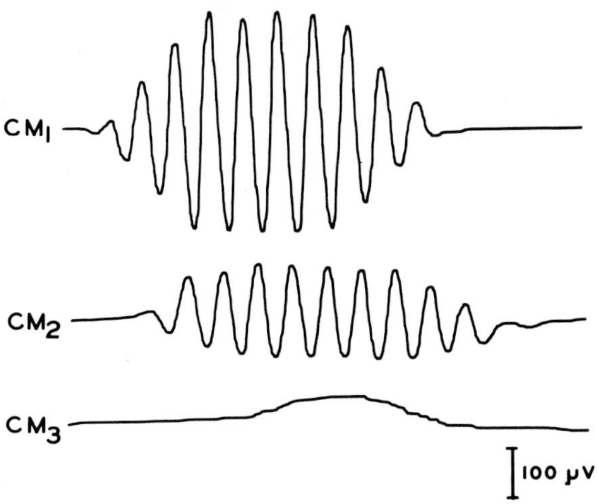

Fig. 9. First, second and third turn CM responses to tone pip of 2000 Hz at 41 dB SPL. Calibration for time should be inferred from the period of 0.5 msec.

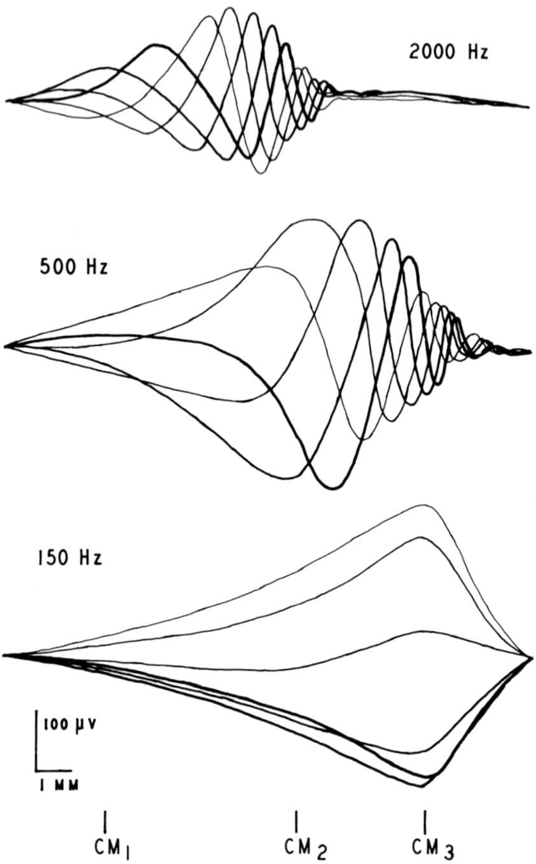

Fig. 10. Longitudinal voltage gradients for CM responses to tones at 150 Hz, 500 Hz and 2000 Hz. In each set the sequence of gradients starts with the lightest trace and continues to the darkest trace. For 500 Hz and 2000 Hz the sequence then returns again from the darkest trace to the lightest trace. The intervals between gradients are 0.8 msec at 150 Hz, 0.4 msec at 500 Hz, and 0.1 msec at 2000 Hz.

The longitudinal voltage gradients for these three tones are shown in Figure 10. These were constructed using the same methods as for the click and the thump from a cycle during the maximum responses. At 150 Hz the six gradients are plotted for intervals of 0.8 msec and span a total time of only 4 msec out of a full period of 6.67 msec. The lack of significant phase change leads to simple patterns for the voltage gradients. It is as if the basilar membrane were swinging as a gate with only a slight lag or "whipping" at the end.

At 500 Hz the five longitudinal voltage gradients plotted at intervals of 0.4 msec are sufficient to show one full period of 2 msec. These voltage gradients in sequence from the lightest to the darkest line clearly show the travel or progression described by Békésy. An entirely similar pattern confined to the basal half of the basilar membrane appears for the gradients at 2000 Hz. Here five longitudinal voltage gradients at intervals of 0.1 msec suffice to show one full period of 0.5 msec.

DISCUSSION

Appreciation of the mechanical events in the cochlea in response to sounds can be greatly enhanced by comparisons of the voltage waveforms in time at different places, both to each other and to the voltage gradients in space along the cochlear partition. It is even better to see a series of the longitudinal gradients projected in time as in a motion picture. Dr. von Békésy wrote to me that the motion picture we have prepared in this way showed many details of movement that are impossible to describe in a paper but that these were exactly as he had remembered seeing them. It is also important to have established so securely by these methods that the traveling wave is not just a response characteristic to high signal levels, but appears intact at the low levels used here.

Nevertheless, some caveats are in order. As noted earlier, we do not know that the ratios of CM to displacement are the same at different places. To the extent that they are not, the quantitative relations shown in these illustrations should be altered. Also the choice of zero voltage at each end of the longitudinal voltage gradients is quite arbitrary and possibly wrong. The spatial distributions of currents and voltages in the cochlear tissues and fluids are complex and not well understood. Unexpected complexities can easily appear in the sequence of transformations from displacements to local currents at hair cells and again to CM voltages as measured by these gross electrodes. We may just be fortunate that these records correspond to the mechanical events as closely as they appear to do.

Acknowledgements

Most of the measurements for the figures were performed by Luis D. Benitez, M.D. and Jerry W. Templer, M.D. in 1969 while in postdoctoral training in the Research Department of Central Institute for the Deaf.

Preparation of this manuscript was supported by Grant No. NS-03856 from the National Institute of Neurological and Communicative Disorders and Stroke to Central Institute for the Deaf.

REFERENCES

Békésy, G.von, Über die Resonanzkurve und die Abklingzeit der verschiedenen Stellen der Schneckentrennwand. *Akust. Zeits. 8:* 66-76, 1943.

Békésy, G.von, The variation of phase along the basilar membrane with sinusoidal vibrations. *J. Acoust. Soc. Am. 19:* 452-460, 1947.

Békésy, G.von, Microphonics produced by touching the cochlear partition with a vibrating electrode. *J. Acoust. Soc. Am. 23:* 29-35, 1951.

Békésy, G.von, *Experiments in Hearing,* edited and translated by E.G. Wever. New York: McGraw-Hill, 1960.

Eldredge, D.H., Benitez, L.D. and Templer, J.W. Electrical traveling waves in the cochlea of chinchilla. *Proceedings of the International Union of Physiological Sciences, Vol. VIII,* XXV International Congress, Munich, 1971a, p. 33-34.

Eldredge, D.H., Benitez, L.D. and Templer, J.W., Templer Electrical traveling waves in the cochlea of the chinchilla. In: *Physiology of the Auditory System, A Workshop,* edited by M.B. Sachs. Baltimore: National Educational Consultants, Inc., 1971b, p. 51-54.

Eldredge, D.H., Benitez, L.D. and Templer, J.W. Electrical traveling waves in the cochlea of the chinchilla. In: *Physiology of the Auditory System, A Workshop,* edited by M.B. Sachs. Baltimore: National Educational Consultants, Inc., 1971b. p. 51-54.

Johnstone, B.M. and Boyle, A.J.F. Basilar membrane vibration examined with the Mössbauer technique. *Science 158:* 389-390, 1967.

Johnstone, B.M., Taylor, K.J. and Boyle, A.J. Mechanics of the guinea pig cochlea. *J. Acoust. Soc. Am. 47:* 504-509, 1970.

Kohllöffel, L.U.E. A study of basilar membrane vibrations. I. Fuzziness-detection: a new method for the analysis of microvibrations with laser light. *Acustica 27:* 49-65, 1972a.

Kohllöffel, L.U.E. A study of basilar membrane vibrations. II. The vibratory amplitude and phase pattern along the basilar membrane (Post-mortem). *Acustica 27:* 66-81, 1972b.

Kohllöffel, L.U.E. A study of basilar membrane vibrations. III. The basilar membrane frequency response curve in the living guinea pig. *Acustica 27:* 82-89, 1972c.

Rhode, W.S. Observations of the vibrations of the basilar membrane in squirrel monkeys using the Mössbauer technique. *J. Acoust. Soc. Am. 49:* 1218-1231, 1971.

Rhode, W.S. and Robles, L. Evidence from Mössbauer experiments for nonlinear vibration in the cochlea. *J. Acoust. Soc. Am. 55:* 588-596, 1974.

Robles, L., Rhode, W.S. and Geisler, C.D. Transient response of the basilar membrane measured in squirrel monkeys using the Mössbauer effect. *J. Acoust. Soc. Am. 59:* 926-939, 1976.

Tasaki, I., Davis, H. and Leguouix, J.-P. The space-time pattern of the cochlear microphonics (guinea pig) as recorded by differential electrodes. *J. Acoust. Soc. Am. 24:* 502-519, 1952.

Teas, D.C., Eldredge, D.H. and Davis, H. Cochlear responses to acoustic transients: an interpretation of whole-nerve action potentials. *J. Acoust. Soc. Am. 34:* 1438-1459, 1962.

Wilson, J.P. and Johnstone, J.R. Basilar membrane and middle-ear vibration in guinea pig measured by capacitative probe. *J. Acoust. Soc. Am. 57:* 705-723, 1975.

DISCUSSION

Witter: I am wondering if you have done any of this work on noise-damaged ears to see if there are any changes in the impedance of the basilar membrane as a result of scarring.

Eldredge: We haven't done these reconstructions. Too much work goes into making the reconstructions of the longitudinal voltage gradients. However, in noise-damaged ears with "wipeouts" or complete absence of the organ of Corti of 6 or 8 mm in the basal turn of the cochlea and many missing cells apically the CM delays and waveforms are essentially normal, albeit greatly reduced, in the second and third turns. This observation has important implications bearing on the choice of a powerful hearing aid over a prosthesis with direct electrical stimulation.

If you have any hair cells left that could be excited by a powerful hearing aid, you probably would get more normal distribution of an input traveling wave pattern to whatever remaining neurons there are by using such an aid than you could ever get by going to an artificial electrical stimulation. In the foreseeable future electrical prostheses will not be able to reproduce the pattern in space and time of the traveling wave. However, even in badly damaged ears the pattern is preserved with minimal qualitative changes wherever there is some residual function.

MECHANISM OF AFFERENT DISCHARGE FROM ELECTRORECEPTORS: IMPLICATIONS FOR ACOUSTIC RECEPTION

Michael V. L. Bennett

Albert Einstein College of Medicine

The acoustico-lateralis receptors are those organs innervated by the VIIIth cranial nerve. Most are mechanoreceptors and include in higher vertebrates cochlear receptors and labyrinthine receptors, and in fish and amphibia, lateral line receptors and in fish only, the specialized lateral line organs, electroreceptors (cf. Bennett, 1971a, b; 1976; Bennett and Clusin, 1978; Fessard, 1974). The weakly electric fishes have electric organs which set up a field around the animal; distortions in this field are detected by the electroreceptors distributed variously over the body surface. The receptors can also detect the discharges of other electric fishes of the same or different species. Some non-electric fishes also have electroreceptors. A typical electroreceptor has a canal leading to the outside and sensory epithelium with receptor cells that synapse on afferent fibers. The receptors are situated so as to sense the potential difference between the lumen, which is continuous with the outside via the canal, and the inside of the body. The receptor cells contain many vesicles and presynaptic dense bodies which are typical of all acoustico-lateralis receptors and also vertebrate photoreceptors and retinal bipolar cell synapses. There are tight junctions between the receptor cells and the supporting epithelial cells which prevent leakage of current between the cells. When a potential is applied across the epithelium that is lumen-positive, current flows through the inner face; thus such a voltage gradient tends to depolarize the membrane of the inner face. Study of synaptic transmission in the electroreceptors may be relevant to other acoustico-lateralis receptors, since their receptor cells are in a sense "bald" hair cells without kinocilia in which the stimulus for synaptic transmission is provided by the external field rather than mechanoelectric transduction.

One class of electroreceptor is the tonic, low frequency, or DC receptor, which has a tonic discharge frequency in the absence of any stimulus. When the outside is made positive, depolarizing the presynaptic membrane, there is

ISBN 0-12-514960-3

an increase in the frequency of the nerve discharge; conversely, a stimulus of opposite polarity hyperpolarizes the presynaptic membrane and causes a decrease in discharge frequency. Several observations suggest that transmission at the synapse is chemically mediated; it is a Ca dependent and blocked by high Mg and there is a synaptic delay. Transmission is believed to involve release from vesicles, partly on morphological grounds and partly by analogy with the saccular fibers of the goldfish where there is direct evidence for quantal release (Ishii et al., 1971); the variability of intervals between impulses in the afferent nerve fibers also suggest quantal release. The transmitter is suspected to be glutamate, since application of 10^{-6}M L-glutamate causes restoration of firing after depression of synaptic release with high Mg. Asparate, D-glutamate, and cholinergic or adrenergic agents have little or no effect. It remains to be shown that release of glutamate can be evoked by stimulation, and that iontophoretic application of glutamate involves the same permeability changes in the postsynaptic cell as those produced by the physiologically-released transmitter.

The receptor cells themselves are not electrically excitable, in that they show no detectable electrical response to a stimulus adequate to cause a pronounced change in the afferent nerve discharge. However, since Ca apparently is involved in transmitter release, there are presumably voltage-dependent Ca channels in the secretory membrane. The response is extremely sensitive; depolarizing the presynaptic face by a millivolt causes a dramatic increase in the amount of transmitter release, as judged from increased impulse frequency in the nerve, and a similarly small hyperpolarization turns the nerve discharge off altogether. There appears to be a tonic release of a single transmitter which is modulated up and down; the input-output relation (stimulus voltage versus impulse frequency) is linear through zero voltage, and it is hard to imagine this being the result of a continuous nerve discharge accelerated by an excitatory transmitter and decelerated by an inhibitory transmitter released by depolarization, and hyperpolarization, respectively. There are two important differences between the receptor synapse and the classical squid giant synapse: there is a shift along the voltage axis such that transmitter is being released in the absence of external stimuli, and the sensitivity is considerably increased.

What factors might be involved in this increased sensitivity? The sensitivity is unlikely to be in the relation between transmitter concentration and PSP amplitude or in the relation between PSP amplitude and impulse frequency, since the postsynaptic membrane apparently is noticeably affected by the contents of a single presynaptic vesicle, as is true of many other synapses. Thus, the mechanism controlling the release of vesicles is a more likely candidate. The tonic receptor is electrically linear; that is, there is no voltage amplification at the membrane with respect to the applied stimulus voltage. There are no data on two other possibilities, namely the relation of voltage change to Ca influx and the relation of Ca influx to release of transmitter.

In another class of receptors, the phasic, high frequency, or AC receptors, the responses are very different from those seen in the tonic receptors. There is either no spontaneous activity in the afferent fiber or only irregular activity; but when stimulated, there are regenerative oscillations recorded external to the receptor at the onset and termination of stimuli. These oscillations can be accompanied by afferent discharges, but the impulses are poorly correlated with them. The oscillations are generated by the receptor cells themselves, for they can persist after denervation. Again, transmission to the afferent fiber is in most cases chemically mediated as indicated by the lack of correlation between responses of the receptor cells and the afferent discharge, the sensitivity of the afferent discharge to high Mg, and the presence of a significant synaptic delay. A striking correlation across species is that the oscillations recorded outside the receptors have a frequency that is close to the main frequency present in the electric organ discharges. Also the afferent discharges are maximally sensitive at these frequencies (Hopkins, 1976). The suggestion is that these receptors are acting as tuned amplifiers or active filters for the signals that the animal is putting out or picking up from conspecifics.

One kind of phasic receptor exhibits a very good all-or-nothing action potential which carries regenerative responsiveness to its extreme. This is the most sensitive of the phasic receptors, and it responds to stimuli of a few tenths of a millivolt. It is specialized in that the resting potential and threshold are held very close together and, perhaps as a consequence, it exhibits considerable spontaneous activity.

The origin of the electrical responsiveness of the receptor cells might be any kind of voltage-sensitive channel; however, the observation that these voltage-sensitive channels are tetrodotoxin (TTX) insensitive while all the Na channels of nerve and muscle in the electric fishes are sensitive to TTX suggests that Ca channels may be involved. (Direct evidence for Ca channels is available from marine fishes, see below). During the course of evolution, the receptor cell may have increased the number of Ca channels present in the presynaptic face, and thereby developed an electrically excitable response. As Ca channels show little inactivation in many systems, they may allow a cell to remain poised near threshold without accommodating.

The presence of an all-or-none response gives the fish a different option for mode of transmission. In the case noted above, transmission to the afferent fiber appears to be electrically mediated, as indicated by the lack of effect of high Mg solutions, a transmission delay of less than 0.3 msec as opposed to 1 msec for chemical synaptic delay, and bidirectional transmission across the synapse. In a different receptor apparently serving the same function, Srivastava (1972) has described gap junctions. Electrical amplification, by means of which the excitable membrane of the receptor cell provides the energy to excite the postsynaptic nerve fibers, may be relevant to some of our own acoustico-lateralis receptors. Our Type I vestibular receptors have gap junctions (Hamilton, 1968) and the spontaneous discharges recorded in the afferent fibers (Goldberg and Fernandez, 1971) show the same kind of pattern as seen in this class of electroreceptor. A similar mechanism may be involved, but one which detects potentials produced by stimulation of the mechano-receptor hairs rather than potentials from an external source.

The electroreceptors of marine fishes are extraordinarily sensitive, responding to signals in the 1 to 10 μ V range. This greater sensitivity may relate to the presence of less electrical noise in the marine environment as contrasted to the freshwater environment (cf. Hopkins, 1973). Seawater is much more conductive and voltages caused by atmospheric disturbances and perhaps other physical phenomena are likely to be much weaker than in freshwater where they commonly exceed the threshold of the electroreceptors. The receptors (in elasmobranchs and the marine catfish Plotosus) have a tonic discharge in the afferent nerve fibers which is accelerated by excitatory stimuli, but the receptors themselves can also generate action potentials. These responses are clearly Ca dependent, and involve a Ca permeability change (Akutsu and Obara, 1974; Clusin and Bennett, 1977a,b).

In the skate it is the lumenal membrane that generates the action potential. Perfusing the lumen with EGTA or Co solution blocks the response; there is considerable recovery after washout. The responses are TTX insensitive. Voltage clamp of the receptors reveals an initial inward current followed by an outward current as in a typical action potential. The Ca equilibrium potential is given by the intersection of the leakage current line with the linear region of the early current. Injection of EGTA into the canal, which lowers the Ca concentration, causes an appropriate shift in the Ca equilibrium potential and a reduction in the Ca current.

In contrast to records from squid axon, the late outward current decreases and finally stops as the Ca equilibrium potential is approached. This observation, which still holds when the Ca equilibrium potential is changed by changing the Ca concentration, suggests that this is a Ca-activated current, i.e., the current is turned on by Ca at the inner surface of the membrane, not by depolarization. In this preparation, where there are no voltage-sensitive Na or K conductance changes, one can be confident that this is a separate conductance mechanism, not just an effect of Ca on a voltage-sensitive channel. Although there are no direct data yet, comparative considerations suggest that this is a Ca-activated K channel (cf. Meech and Standen, 1975).

An interesting property of the receptor in the marine catfish Plotosus is that when it is electrically isolated, the excitable receptor membrane becomes hyperpolarized and the nerve is virtually silent (Obara, 1974, 1976). No discharge is produced in the nerve until a depolarizing stimulus reaches the point where the Ca conductance begins to be turned on. In the short-circuited preparation, as the receptor is in situ, the excitable membrane is depolarized into the region where there is some Ca activation. Correspondingly, there is a spontaneous discharge in the nerve that is accelerated by a small stimulus that increases Ca activation and decelerated by a small stimulus that decreases Ca activation. Thus, we have direct evidence for an ongoing Ca activation producing the ongoing release of transmitter and resultant nerve discharge. A similar but more complicated situation obtains in the skate receptor (Clusin and Bennett, 1978). The in situ receptors oscillate asynchronously, and stimulation modulates this activity to modulate the release of transmitter.

There remains the problem of the extreme sensitivity of the electroreceptors in the marine fishes. Cole and colleagues (1970) have introduced the notion of the gain of an action potential mechanism; an ideal impulse-generating mechanism sitting at threshold has an infinite gain, for an infinitesimally small depolarization will cause a finite action potential. A repetitively firing cell may also be very sensitive if it spends enough of the activity cycle near threshold. A difficulty in realizing such a mechanism is to adjust the membrane potential close to threshold, without too much accommodation or spontaneous firing for a stimulus to produce a detectable change. Since some degree of spontaneous discharge is a common feature of sensitive receptors, one would expect that the best compromise is to allow some spontaneous activity, and also a spontaneous discharge could reset any accommodative processes. A further aspect of spontaneous activity is that it allows signalling of inhibitory stimuli as in tonic receptors. The sensitivity of the electroreceptors of the skate indicates that they have achieved an excellent balance between spontaneous activity and sensitivity. One mechanism whereby this balance is achieved may involve the Ca-activated outward current demonstrated for these cells. If a receptor cell is inactive, it will have a very low cytoplasmic Ca concentration, the Ca-activated outward current channels will be turned off and (presumably) the cell will depolarize and become active. Conversely, if the cell is very active, enough Ca will enter to turn on the outward current and thus reduce the activity. The Ca-activated mechanism may provide the cell with a way of integrating its activity over a number of oscillations better than the conventional Na and K activation and inactivation mechanisms. In other words, Ca-activated mechanisms may give the cell a better "short-term memory" of its previous activity, with respect to which it adjusts its threshold.

Another aspect of the process whereby threshold and activity level are adjusted is the accommodation that the skate receptors exhibit. In the presence of a maintained stimulus of moderate strength the response level and incremental sensitivity gradually return to near the resting level, a change equivalent to readjustment of threshold. This accommodation is very different from light adaptation in photoreceptors where sensitivity to changes in absolute intensity greatly decrease as background illumination increases. Accommodation to maintained shifts in level without increase of incremental threshold may be of importance for any receptor (or presynaptic membrane) that must respond to very small voltages. This is likely because relatively large changes in membrane potentials generated by the cells, as well as changes in DC signals from a variety of outside sources (such as the stria vascularis in the cochlea), would be expected to occur during changes in physiological state of the animal or even during aging.

The properties of the electroreceptors have a number of implications for acoustico-lateralis receptors in general. There can be chemical transmission from the receptor cells to afferent fibers, and glutamate is a likely candidate transmitter. Transmitter release is Ca-dependent as at other synapses, but may occur in the absence of external stimulation and be modulated toward either increase or decrease. Transmission can also be electrical. There is Ca activation in the phasic receptors and in the very sensitive receptors of marine fishes that provides voltage amplification. In the skate at least there is a Ca-activated outward current that is likely to function in accommodation and adjusting incremental threshold to its optimal value. Hair cells of lower vertebrates have intracellular microphonics of a fraction of a millivolt, which is well within the range of electroreceptor sensitivity (Harris et al., 1970; Hudspeth and Corey, 1977; Weiss et al., 1974). In mammalian inner hair cells receptor potentials are larger, but are at most a few millivolts near threshold for hearing (Russell and Sellick, 1977 and this volume). It is thus reasonable that these phylogenetically similar receptor cells may use the same mechanisms that have been demonstrated in the electroreceptors.

Acknowledgments

This paper is a modification and updating of a Brain Information Service summary of a lecture given to the Society of Neuroscience in 1976. More complete discussions will be found in Bennett and Clusin (1978) and Clusin and Bennett (1978). Supported in part by NIH grants HD-04248, NS-07412 and NS-12627 and BNS75-19120 from the National Science Foundation.

REFERENCES

Akutsu, Y. and Obara, S. Calcium dependent receptor potential of the electroreceptor of marine catfish. *Proc. Japan. Acad. 50:* 247-251, 1974.

Bennett, M.V.L. Electroreception. In: *Fish Physiology, Vol. V,* edited by W.S. Hoar and D.S. Randall. New York: Academic Press, 1971a, p. 493-573.

Bennett, M.V.L. Electrolocation in fish. *Ann. N.Y. Acad. Sci. 188:* 242-269, 1971b.

Bennett, M.V.L. Transmission at receptor synapses. In: *Mechanisms in Transmission of Signals for Conscious Behavior,* edited by T. Desiraju. Amsterdam: Elsevier, 1976, p. 345-366.

Bennett, M.V.L. and Clusin, W.T. Transduction at electroreceptors: origins of sensitivity. In: *Membrane Transduction Mechanisms,* edited by R.A. Cone and J.E. Dowling. New York: Raven Press. *Symp. Soc. Gen. Physiol. 33,* 1978 (In press).

Clusin, W.T. and Bennett, M.V.L. Calcium activated conductance in skate electroreceptors: current clamp experiments. *J. Gen. Physiol. 69:* 121-143, 1977.

Clusin, W.T. and Bennett, M.V.L. Calcium activated conductance in skate electroreceptors: voltage clamp experiments. *J. Gen. Physiol. 69:* 145-182, 1977.

Clusin, W.T. and Bennett, M.V.L. The ionic basis of oscillatory responses of skate electroreceptors. To be submitted to *J. Gen. Physiol.* 1978.

Cole, K.S., Guttman, R. and Bezanilla, F. Nerve membrane excitation without threshold. *Proc. Nat. Acad. Sci. 65:* 884-891, 1970.

Fessard, A. (Ed.) *Handbook of Sensory Physiology, III/3. Electroreceptors and Other Specialized Receptors in Lower Vertebrates.* New York: Springer-Verlag, 1974.

Goldberg, J.M. and Fernández, C. Physiology of peripheral neurons innervating semicircular canals of the squirrel monkey. III. Variations among units in their discharge properties. *J. Neurophysiol. 34:* 676-684, 1971.

Hamilton, D.W. The calyceal synapse of Type I vestibular hair cells. *J. Ultrastruct. Res. 23:* 98-114, 1968.

Harris, G.G., Frishkopf, L.S. and Flock, Å. Receptor potentials from hair cells of the lateral line. *Science 167:* 76-79, 1970.

Hopkins, C.D. Lighting as background noise for communication among electric fish. *Nature 242:* 268-270, 1973.

Hopkins, C.D. Stimulus filtering and electroreception: tuberous electroreceptors in three species of gymnotid fish. *J. Comp. Physiol. 111:* 171-207, 1976.

Hudspeth, A.S. and Corey, D.P. Sensitivity, polarity and conductance change in the response of vertebrate hair cells to controlled mechanical stimuli. *Proc. Nat. Acad. Sci. 74:* 2407-2411, 1977.

Ishii, Y., Matsuura, S. and Furukawa, T. Quantal nature of transmission at the synapse between hair cells and eighth nerve fibers. *Japan J. Physiol. 21:* 79-89, 1971.

Meech, R.W. and Standen, N.B. Potassium activation in *Helix aspersa* neurones under voltage clamp: a component mediated by calcium influx. *J. Physiol. London 249:* 211-239, 1975.

Obara, S. Receptor cell activity at 'rest' with respect to the tonic operation of a specialized lateralis receptor. *Proc. Japan. Acad. 50:* 386-391, 1974.

Obara, S. Mechanisms of electroreception in ampullae of Lorenzini of the marine catfish, *Plotosus.* In: *Electrobiology of Nerve, Synapse and Muscle,* edited by J.P. Reuben, D.P. Purpura, M.V.L. Bennett and E.R. Kandel. New York: Raven Press, 1976, p. 129-147.

Russell, I.S. and Sellick, P.M. Tuning properties of cochlear hair cells. *Nature 267:* 858-860, 1977.

Srivastava, C.B.L. Morphological evidence for electrical synapses of 'gap' junction type in another vertebrate receptor. *Experientia 28:* 1029-1030, 1972.

Weiss, T.F., Mulroy, M.J. and Altmann, D.W. Intracellular responses to acoustic clicks in the inner ear of the alligator lizard. *J. Acoust. Soc. Am. 55:* 606-619, 1974.

WHICH STRUCTURES DETERMINE FREQUENCY SELECTIVITY AND TONOTOPIC ORGANIZATION OF VERTEBRATE NERVE FIBERS? EVIDENCE FROM THE ALLIGATOR LIZARD

Thomas F. Weiss, William T. Peake, Alexander Ling, Jr. and Thomas Holton

Massachusetts Eye and Ear Infirmary and

Massachusetts Institute of Technology

INTRODUCTION

At each anatomical level in the vertebrate inner ear and auditory nervous system, responses to acoustic stimuli show frequency selectivity. Usually, maximal sensitivity of the response to tones occurs at a particular frequency, the characteristic frequency or CF. In addition, an orderly mapping or tonotopic organization relates frequency-selective properties, such as CF, to location at each level. These notions are cornerstones of our current understanding of the organization of the auditory system.

Tonotopic organization originates in the inner ear. Measurements of basilar membrane motion in mammals (Békésy, 1960; Johnstone and Boyle, 1967; Rhode, 1971; Kohllöffel, 1972; Wilson and Johnstone, 1975) show there is a systematic mapping of CF to longitudinal position in the cochlea, i.e. a mechanical tonotopic organization. In Békésy's view, the spatial variation in the mechanical stiffness of the basilar membrane (resulting from the gradual increase in its width from the basal to the apical end of the cochlea) is the structural basis of mechanical tonotopic organization. In the cochlear nerve, tonotopic organization (Sando, 1965; Kiang et al., 1965) is similar to that of the basilar membrane in that at both levels CF varies monotonically from a low value at the apex to a high value at the base. However, the frequency selectivity of cochlear nerve fibers has been reported to be sharper than that of the basilar membrane motion (Geisler, Rhode, and Kennedy, 1974; Evans, 1975; Evans and Wilson, 1975); this view is contraversial (see eg. Helfenstein, 1973; Kim and Molnar, 1975). These observations would imply that the relation of basilar membrane motion to cochlear nerve-fiber responses is frequency-dependent; several possibilities have been suggested for processes that might be involved (eg. Billone and Raynor, 1973; Steele, 1973; Hall, 1977; Allen, 1977; and papers and comments in Zwicker and Terhardt, 1974).

ISBN 0-12-514960-3

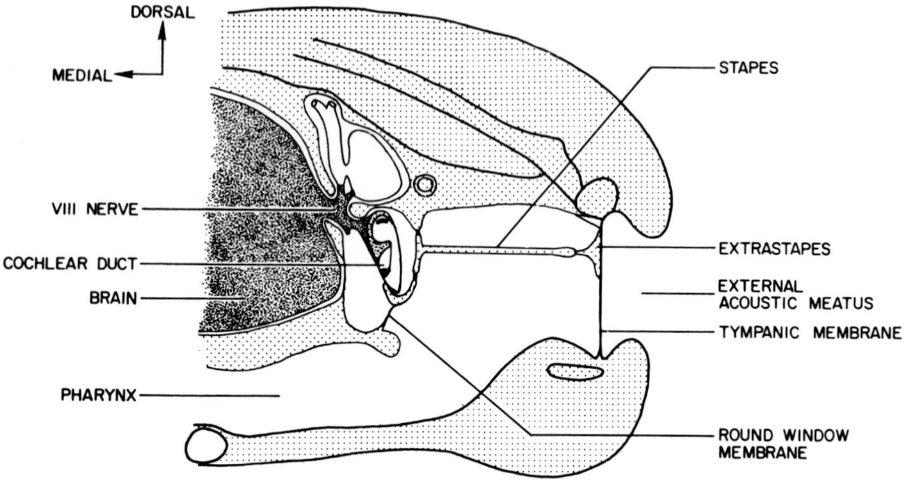

Fig. 1. Diagram of a section of the head of the alligator lizard showing the external, middle, and inner ear (not to scale). In experiments reported here acoustic stimuli were generated by an earphone in a cavity sealed to the external meatus. A calibrated probe microphone was used to measure sound pressure near the entrance to the meatus. Adapted from Weiss, *et al* (1974).

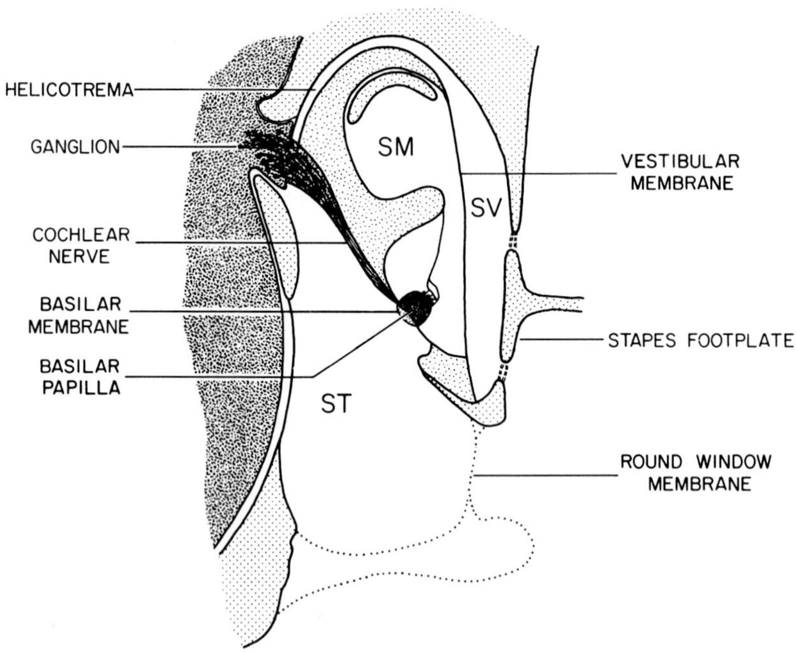

Fig. 2. Enlargement of inner ear portion of Figure 1. SV, SM, and ST are scala vestibuli, media, and tympani. Dotted lines indicate structures that are surgically removed to expose the basilar papilla and cochlear nerve. Adapted from Weiss, *et al.*

This paper describes results from the inner ear of the alligator lizard, Gerrhonotus multicarinatus. Because this inner ear is anatomically similar to the mammalian ear in some respects but different in others, investigation of its physiology may provide clues to the structural bases of frequency selectivity and tonotopic organization in vertebrates. Since the auditory receptor organ in the alligator lizard is relatively flat and accessible, it is possible to measure basilar membrane motion, intracellular potentials in the receptor organ, and spike discharges of cochlear nerve fibers over the entire organ. Our results indicate that frequency selectivity and tonotopic organization of cochlear nerve fibers are not determined by the motion of the basilar membrane in the alligator lizard cochlea. We suggest other structures that may be important in determining frequency-selective properties.

STRUCTURE OF THE PERIPHERAL AUDITORY SYSTEM

The structure of the peripheral auditory system of the alligator lizard has been described by Wever (1965); Miller (1966, 1973); Mulroy (1968, 1974); Weiss et al. (1976), and is briefly summarized here. The external ear consists of a short external acoustic meatus terminated by a tympanic membrane (Fig. 1). The cartilaginous extrastapes and the bony stapes connect the tympanic membrane with the oval window which opens into scala vestibuli (Fig. 2). Scala tympani communicates with scala vestibuli via the helicotrema. The cochlear duct is a sac protruding from the saccule. The lumen of the duct, scala media, is separated from scala vestibuli by the vestibular (Reissner's) membrane and from scala tympani by the basilar membrane and limbus.

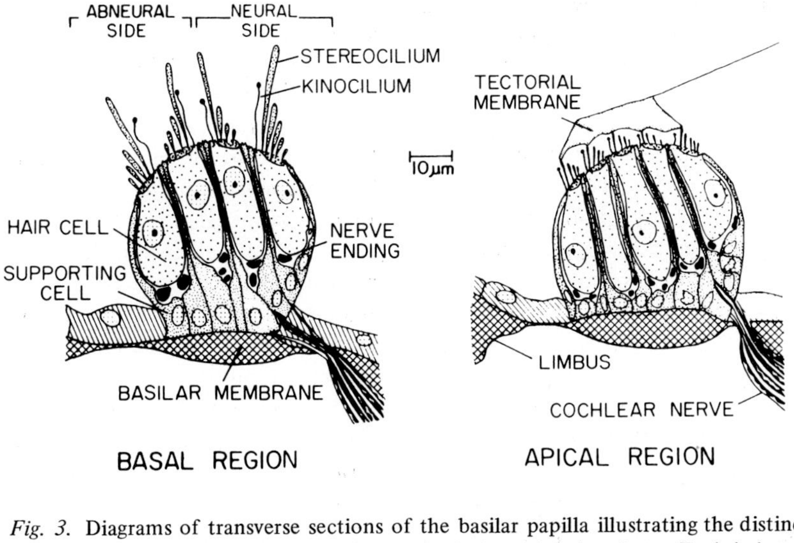

Fig. 3. Diagrams of transverse sections of the basilar papilla illustrating the distinct differences in ciliary and tectorial structures in the apical and basal regions. Each hair cell has about 60 stereocilia and one eccentrically located kinocilium; the direction of morphological polarization is defined as pointing from the stereocilia toward the kinocilium. Adapted from Mulroy (1974).

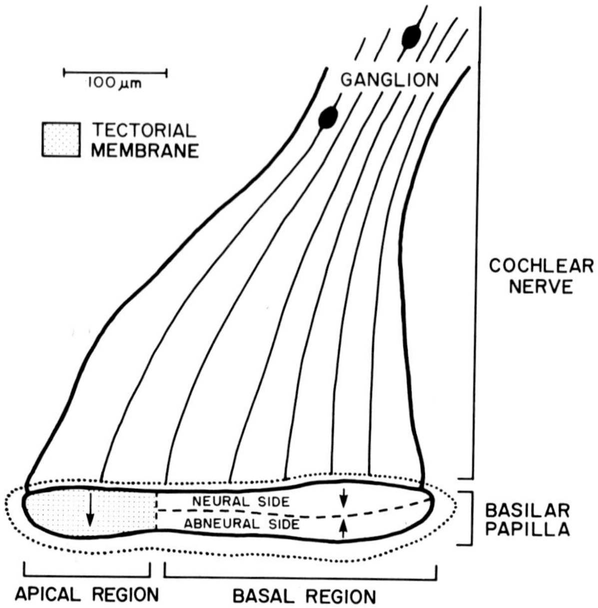

Fig. 4. Schematic view of the basilar papilla and cochlear nerve as seen from scala tympani. A solid line outlines the basilar papilla. A dotted line outlines the boundary between the basilar membrane and the surrounding limbus. The width and thickness of the basilar membrane vary by less than 30% along its length. The basilar papilla is divided (by dashed lines) into three regions. Arrows indicate the direction of morphological polarization of hair cells in each region. The stippled area indicates the region of the basilar papilla covered by a tectorial membrane. Six of the nerve fibers are shown schematically along with two of the biopolar cell bodies. Nerve fibers are arranged in parallel fascicles near the papilla, in the region where spikes were recorded from single fibers. The more central course of these fibers (in the region where the nerve forms a compact bundle) is not known and is indicated schematically in this diagram.

The basilar papilla, which rests on the basilar membrane, is generally considered to be the reptilian homolog of the mammalian organ of Corti (Wever, 1974). The basilar papilla is a short strip of neuroepithelium (approximately 400 μm long, 50μm wide, and 60μm high), containing hair cells, supporting cells, and unmyelinated terminal portions of cochlear nerve fibers. There are two morphologically distinct regions of the basilar papilla (Figs. 3 and 4). In the apical region (containing about 50 hair cells), the stereocilia on the hair cells are short (the longest cilia are roughly 7μm), and all the hair cells are morphologically polarized in the same direction; a tectorial membrane (which appears to contact the longer cilia in each ciliary tuft) is present, and vesiculated nerve terminals (whose ultrastructural features are those of efferent presynaptic terminals) are present on the bases of hair cells. In the basal region (containing about 100 hair cells), the stereocilia on the hair cells are longer (the longest cilia range from 12 to 31μm), and hair cells are morphologically polarized in either of two directions; no tectorial membrane is present, and no vesiculated nerve terminals are found at the bases of hair cells.

The cochlear nerve consists of about 600 myelinated nerve fibers (with an average axis-cylinder diameter of 1μm) which fan out from a compact bundle near the ganglion to a thin sheet of fibers organized in parallel fascicles near the basilar papilla (Fig. 4). The fibers become unmyelinated as they penetrate the basilar membrane. The branching pattern of the fibers in the papilla is not known.

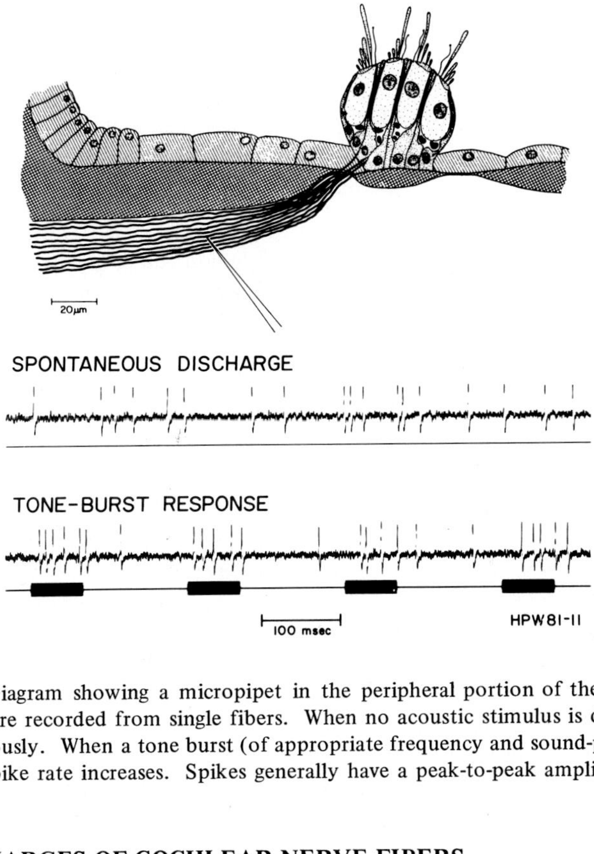

Fig. 5. Diagram showing a micropipet in the peripheral portion of the cochlear nerve where spikes were recorded from single fibers. When no acoustic stimulus is delivered, spikes occur spontaneously. When a tone burst (of appropriate frequency and sound-pressure level) is delivered, the spike rate increases. Spikes generally have a peak-to-peak amplitude of roughly 1 mV.

SPIKE DISCHARGES OF COCHLEAR NERVE FIBERS

Spike discharges of single fibers were recorded with micropipets in the cochlear nerve (Fig. 5). The frequency selectivity of a fiber was characterized by the "neural tuning curve," which gives the tone level and frequency required to obtain a fixed increment in spike rate above the spontaneous rate. Tuning curves of lizard fibers (Fig. 6) are roughly similar to those of other vertebrate cochlear nerve fibers (Weiss et al., 1976). The frequency of maximal sensitivity, corresponding to the tip of the tuning curve, is the neural characteristic frequency or CF_N. The sound-pressure level at the tip of the tuning curve is called the "threshold." In alligator lizards, CF_N's range from 0.2 to 4.0 kHz (Fig. 7A).

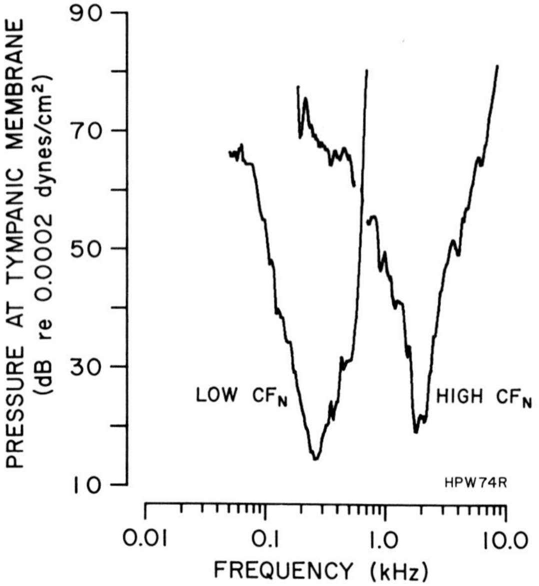

Fig. 6. Tuning curves of two cochlear nerve fibers: one an apical fiber (CF_N = 0.26kHz), and the other a basal fiber (CF_N = 1.88 kHz). Tuning curves were measured automatically using tone-burst stimuli (duration, 50 msec; repetition rate, 10 bursts/sec). A computer system set the frequency of the tone bursts and determined the sound-pressure level required to evoke a constant spike rate from the fiber. Measurements were made at 32 points per octave of frequency.

The distribution of CF_N has two disjoint ranges that correspond to the two anatomically distinct regions of the basilar papilla (Weiss, et al., 1976). Fibers projecting to the apical region have lower CF_N (0.2 - 0.8 kHz) than do fibers projecting to the basal region (CF_N: 0.9 - 4.0 kHz). We refer to this correspondence between CF_N and region of the papilla as "dichotomous tonotopic organization." Apical and basal fibers show physiological differences in addition to differences in CF_N: tuning curves of apical fibers have much higher slopes for frequencies above CF_N than do those of basal fibers; in this sense, apical fibers are more sharply tuned than basal fibers. Apical fibers tend to have lower spontaneous discharge rates than do basal fibers (Frezza, Holton, and Weiss, in preparation). Apical fibers exhibit two-tone rate suppression whereas basal fibers do not (Holton and Weiss, 1977); by definition two-tone rate suppression occurs when the average discharge rate of a fiber to an excitatory tone (one that evokes an increased discharge rate when presented alone) is reduced by the addition of a second tone.

In basal fibers there is a systematic relation between the CF_N of a fiber and its position in the nerve (Fig. 8): CF_N increases toward the basal end. We refer to this relation as "graded tonotopic organization." In the apical portion of the nerve, maps of CF_N versus position have given variable results perhaps because access to the apical portion of the nerve close to the basilar papilla is often limited and the geometry of the nerve changes from a thin sheet of fibers near the papilla to a thicker bundle at more central locations. Hence, it is possible that a graded tonotopic organization may also exist in apical fibers.

We conclude that there is a dichotomous tonotopic organization in the nerve; apical fibers have low CF_N whereas basal fibers have high CF_N. In addition, basal fibers exhibit a graded tonotopic organization. In contrast to the mammalian

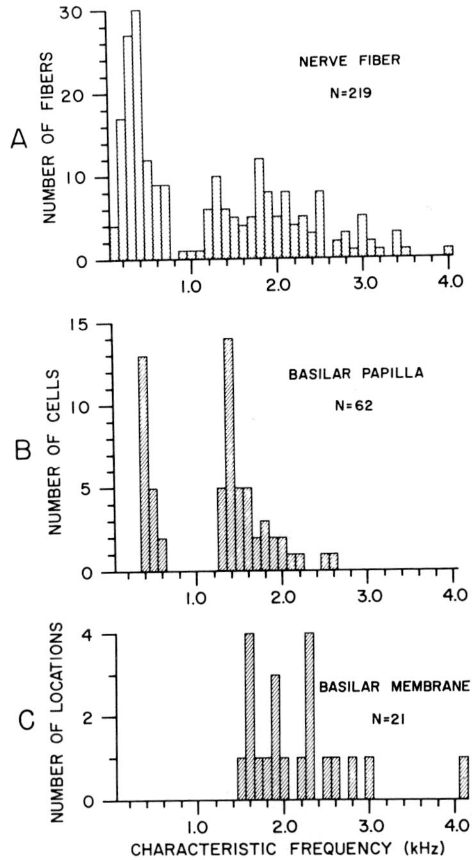

Fig. 7. Comparison of histograms of characteristic frequencies of cochlear nerve fiber discharges, basilar papilla intracellular potential responses, and basilar membrane velocities.

A. Histogram of characteristic frequency (CF_N) from tuning curves of 219 nerve fibers (Weiss, *et al,* 1976).

B. Histogram of characteristic frequency (CF_P) of intracellular potential response from Fourier-analyzed click responses of 62 cells in the basilar papilla (Weiss, *et al,* 1974).

C. Histogram of characteristic frequency (CF_M) of basilar membrane velocity from mechanical tuning curves for 21 different locations in 16 lizards. Because the mechanical tuning curves often had broad minima, the following method was used to measure CF_M: The mechanical tuning curve was first smoothed by a 3-point triangular window function, and the minimum SPL of the smoothed mechanical tuning curve was determined. A line was drawn at a level 5 dB above this minimum. The CF_M was defined as the geometric mean of the frequencies of the two points of intersection of this line with the smoothed mechanical tuning curve.

cochlea, basilar membrane dimensions in the alligator lizard do not appear to vary appreciably with location along the membrane. Thus, spatial variations in the dimensions of the basilar membrane are an unlikely source of either kind of tonotopic organization.

INTRACELLULAR POTENTIAL RESPONSE IN HAIR CELLS AND SUPPORTING CELLS

Intracellular potentials were recorded with micropipets in the basilar papilla. When an acoustic stimulus is applied to the ear, the intracellular potential changes from its resting value (Fig. 9). We call this change the intracellular potential response; the intracellular response recorded in a hair cell is often called the receptor potential. Intracellular potential responses have been recorded in hair cells and supporting cells (Mulroy et al., 1974; Weiss et al., 1974). It is likely that responses recorded from supporting cells result from mechano-electric transduction in hair cells and electric coupling of hair cells to supporting cells by low-resistance electric pathways. Gap junction, which are thought to mediate electrical connec-

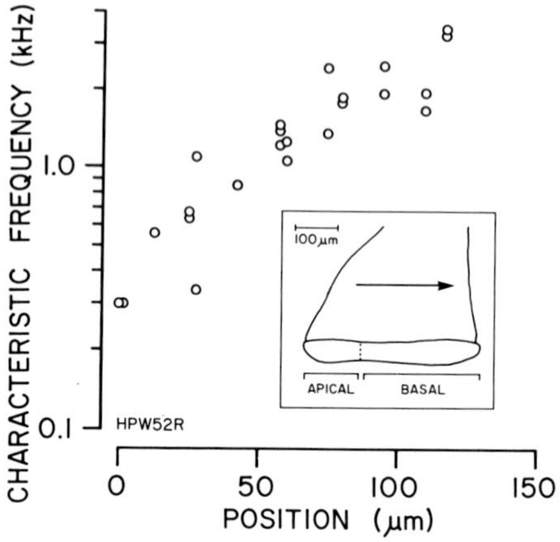

Fig. 8. Map of characteristic frequency of a fiber (CF_N) versus position of the fiber in the nerve. A single micropipet was used to record tuning curves of 23 fibers located along a path parallel to the long axis of the basilar papilla (as indicated schematically by the arrow in the inset). The path was traversed twice: once from basal to apical directions and once from apical to basal directions. The position of the micropipet in the nerve (the abscissa) was measured relative to the most apically located fiber from which a tuning curve was obtained. Fibers with $CF_N \leqslant 0.8$ kHz were found more apically than fibers with $CF_N \geqslant 0.9$ kHz, reflecting the dichotomous tonotopic organization in the nerve. For basal fibers ($CF_N \geqslant 0.9$ kHz) there is a tendency for CF_N to increase with increasingly basal positions. This graded tonotopic organization of basal fibers has been consistently seen in 9 such maps. For apical fibers ($CF_N \leqslant 0.8$ kHz) there is a suggestion of a trend of increasing CF_N with increasing position in this map, but this trend has not been consistently seen in all maps.

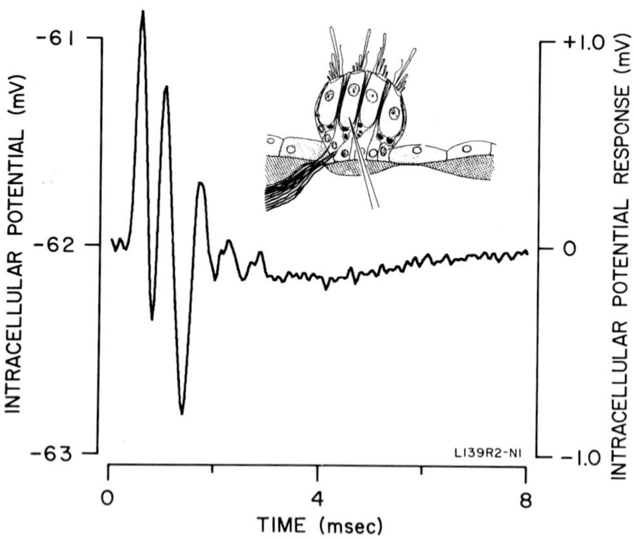

Fig. 9. Schematic diagram showing a micropipet recording intracellularly from a hair cell. The trace shows an averaged response to acoustic clicks recorded from a hair cell whose resting potential was −62 mV. After recording this click response, dye was injected into the cell which was later identified histologically.

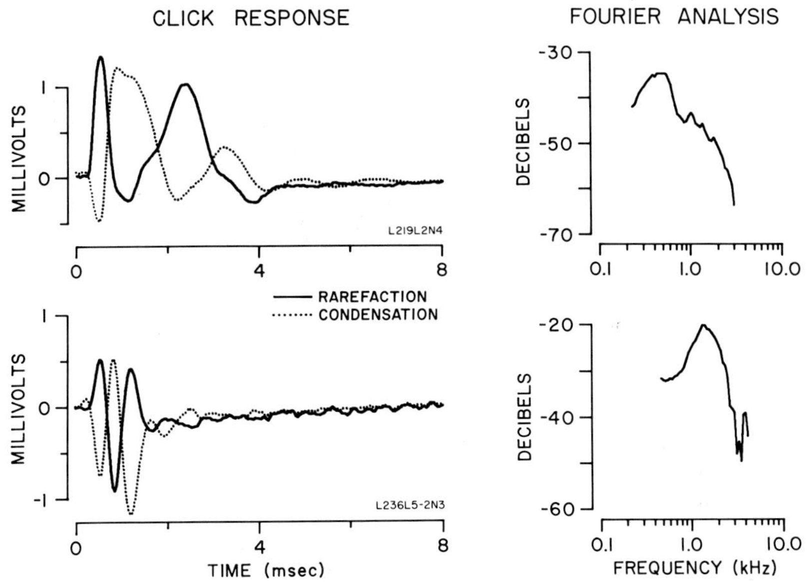

Fig. 10. Averaged click responses of two cells showing predominantly oscillatory responses to clicks (left). The peaks and valleys of the oscillations in response to rarefaction and condensation clicks interleave. The time between peaks is relatively long in one cell (upper) and short in the other (lower). Fourier analysis of the averaged click responses was used to estimate a characteristic frequency (CF_p) for each cell (see Weiss, *et al*, 1974 for details). A transfer ratio of intracellular potential to tympanic membrane pressure was computed for both click polarities and the two transfer ratios averaged. The averaged ratio is plotted (right) over the frequency range for which the angles of the two transfer ratios are within ±60° of each other. CF_p is determined from the frequencies of the maxima. One cell (upper) has a CF_p = 0.48 kHz, the other cell (lower) has a CF_p = 1.3 kHz. The reference level for the ordinate scale (right) is 1 $\mu V/0.0002$ dynes/cm^2.

tions between cells (Bennett, 1973), occur between hair cells and supporting cells in the basilar papilla of the alligator lizard (Nadol et al., 1976). Waveforms of intracellular responses to acoustic clicks vary in the different cell types, but most waveforms contain an oscillatory component (Fig. 10). The frequency of this oscillatory component varies from one cell to another indicating that different cells are selectively tuned to different frequency ranges. Estimates of the characteristic frequency associated with the intracellular potential response, CF_p, were obtained by Fourier analysis of click responses (Fig. 10). The distribution of CF_p is disjoint (Fig. 7B) with a low CF_p range (0.35-0.8 kHz) and a high CF_p range (1.3-2.6 kHz). Preliminary results with tonal stimuli indicate that CF_p's of the ac components of intracellular responses have a disjoint distribution similar to that obtained from Fourier analysis of click responses.

The relation of CF_p to position in the basilar papilla has not been definitively determined. However, there are indications (Weiss, et al., 1974) that hair cells that

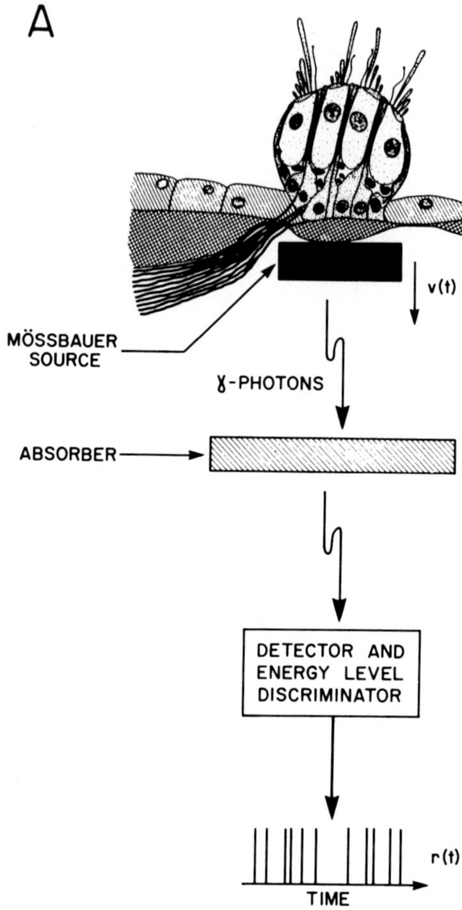

Fig. 11. Basic features of the Mössbauer method used to measure velocity of the basilar membrane.

A. Perilymph is aspirated from scala tympani and a radioactive Mössbauer source is advanced to the basilar membrane on the tip of a pipet held in a micromanipulator. The source tends to stick to the basilar membrane on contact. While perilymph refills scala tympani, the pipet holds the source on the basilar membrane. The pipet is then removed and the source stays in place. A typical Mössbauer source (Co^{57} electroplated onto a palladium foil) has dimensions of 40 × 40 × 12 μm and a mass of 0.2 μgrams. Photons (γ-rays) are emitted by the source, passed through a resonant absorber (stainless steel enriched with Fe^{57}) and detected with a gas-tube proportional counter. The energy-level discriminator was adjusted to select photons of the energy level (14.4 keV) which exhibit the Mössbauer effect.

B. Relation between photon rate, r, and source velocity, v. Because of the Doppler shift in the energy of the photons, the number of photons passing through the absorber depends on the source velocity. The large solid curve shows the theoretical relation between r and v. Two examples are shown in which this curve is used to predict the rate waveform which results from sinusoidal velocity waveforms. For small velocity amplitude, V, r(t) varies sinusoidally (small solid traces). For large values of V (dotted traces), r(t) is quite distorted and the mean rate, $\overline{r(t)}$, is increased (dashed line). In our experiments, source velocity waveforms were obtained by measuring r(t) and the relation between r and v was used

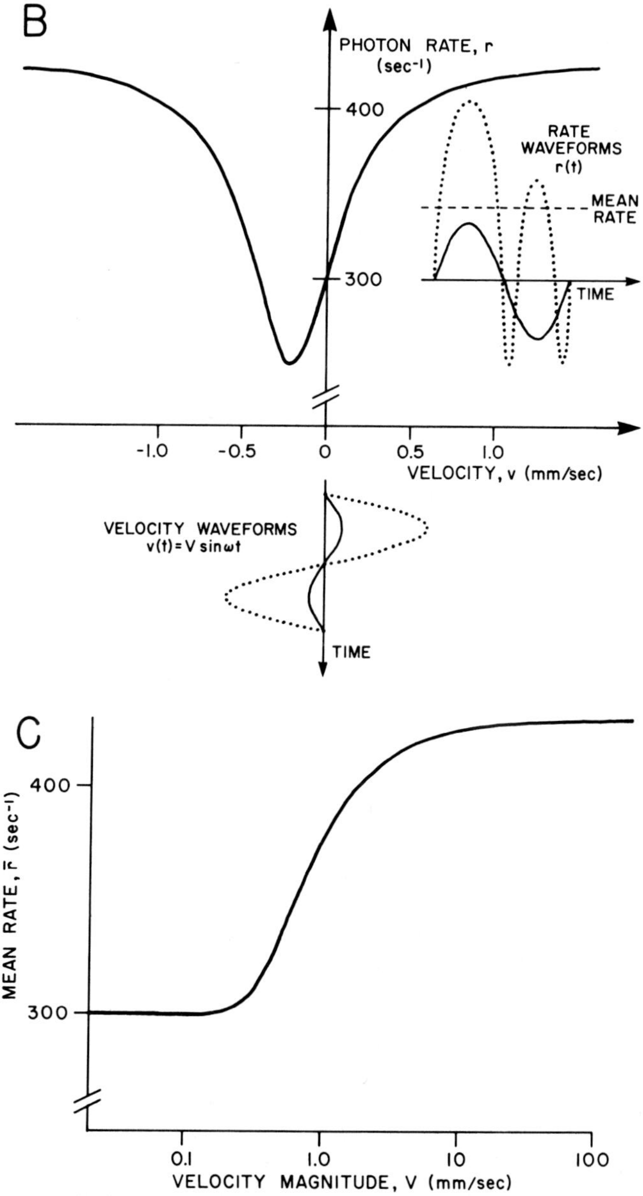

to compute v(t). This method was used for $V < 0.2$ mm/sec (Fig. 16). About 10 minutes of data were required to determine a velocity waveform when $V \approx 0.1$ mm/sec.
C. Theoretical dependence of mean photon, $\overline{r(t)}$, on V for a sinusoidal velocity, $v(t) = V \sin 2\pi ft$. Mechanical tuning curves were measured with a computer controlled system in which the acoustic stimulus level is adjusted at each frequency to produce a constant value of $\overline{r(t)}$ and, hence, of V. These mechanical tuning curves were obtained with $V \approx 0.8$ mm/sec. [This velocity corresponds to a displacement of about 1 μm at 100 Hz and 0.1 μm at 1 kHz.] Such constant velocity curves could be measured at 10 to 15 frequencies in about 10 minutes.

have click responses with low CF_p are located in the apical region, whereas those with high CF_p are in the basal region of the basilar papilla.

We conclude that the distributions of CF_p of cells in the papilla and of CF_N of cochlear nerve fibers are similar. The dichotomous tonotopic organization observed in cochlear nerve fibers appears to be present in receptor potentials of hair cells.

BASILAR MEMBRANE MOTION

Basilar membrane velocity was measured with the Mössbauer method (Gilad et al., 1967; Johnstone and Boyle, 1967; Rhode, 1971). In this method, a small radioactive source is placed on the basilar membrane (Fig. 11A). When the basilar membrane vibrates, the source moves, and the rate of the detected photons depends upon the source velocity (Fig. 11B and C).

Two important questions arise in interpreting Mössbauer measurements of basilar membrane velocity:

1. Does the placement or presence of the Mössbauer source on the basilar membrane alter responses of the inner ear? Measurements (with a gross electrode) of cochlear potential responses to clicks and tones demonstrated that sources could be placed on the basilar membrane without producing large changes in these potentials. In

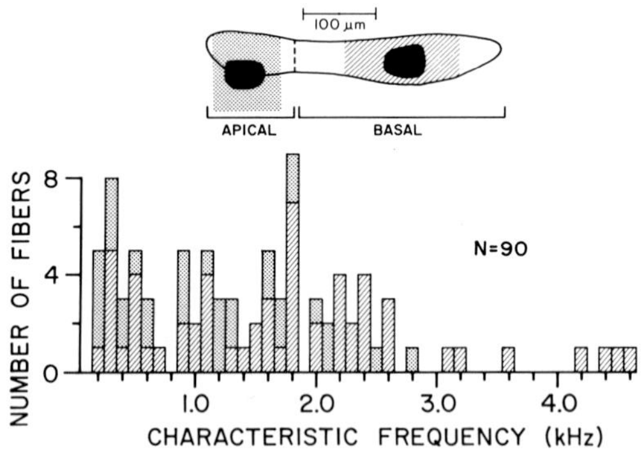

Fig. 12. Histogram of CF_N from all cochlear nerve fibers studied in the two ears in which a Mössbauer source was in place on the basilar membrane while nerve fiber responses were recorded. During the experiment, the location of the source on the basilar papilla was observed through a dissecting microscope. In one of these cases, the source was also located on the dissected cochlear duct with a compound microscope. The shaded areas on the sketch of the basilar papilla indicate the approximate location of the source (whose size is shown in black). As indicated in Fig. 4, the thin part of the basilar membrane extends somewhat beyond the outline of the basilar papilla. The type of shading also relates histogram entries to source location.

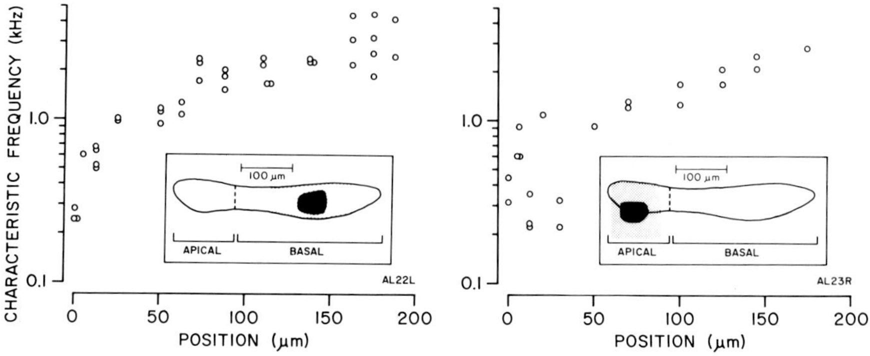

Fig. 13. Maps of CF_N versus position of the fiber in the nerve for the two ears in which the Mössbauer source was in place on the basilar membrane while nerve fiber measurements were made. The inset sketches indicate the size of the Mössbauer source (solid) in its approximate location for each ear (see Fig. 12). Each map was constructed as indicated in Fig. 8. Fiber positions which were approximately opposite the center of the source are 110 μm (left) and 50 μm (right).

two experiments, neural tuning curves of 90 fibers were measured with a source in place on the basilar membrane, once in the apical region and once in the basal region. In both ears, apical and basal fibers had CF_N's (Fig. 12) and thresholds in the normal range. In addition, tonotopic organization (Fig. 13), and tuning curve shapes (Fig. 14) were normal. Thus the placement and presence of the radioactive source on the basilar membrane apparently did not alter either the tonotopic organization or the frequency selectivity of cochlear nerve fibers.

2. Does the Mössbauer source adhere well enough to the basilar membrane to make the measured source velocity equal to the basilar membrane velocity? To examine this, we attached a lizard's head to a vibrator and determined that over the frequency range 0.1-4.0 kHz the velocity of a source on the basilar membrane was roughly equal to that of a large source firmly attached to the skull; the difference in estimated velocities of the two sources was 2.9 ± 1.8 dB (mean ± standard deviation) over the whole frequency range; results showed that variations in estimates of absolute velocity were in range ± 3 dB. Hence, if we assume that the velocity of the skull and basilar membrane are approximately equal in this experiment, then we can conclude that the source and basilar membrane velocities are also approximately equal. Thus the source adhered to the basilar membrane in this control experiment, and we assume that it also does when the ear is stimulated acoustically.

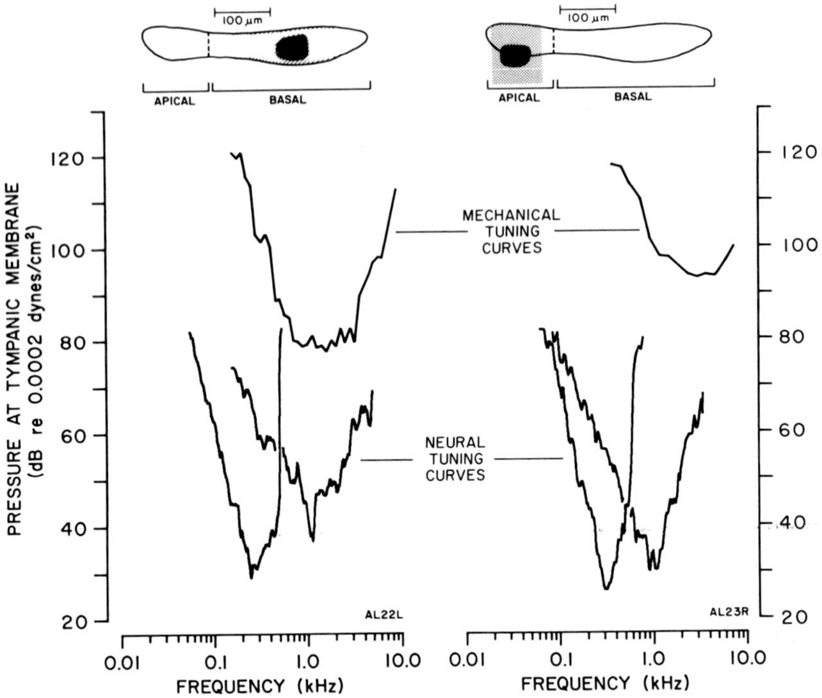

Fig. 14. Mechanical tuning curves of the basilar membrane (measured at constant velocity, V = 0.8 mm/sec) and examples of neural tuning curves from the two cochleas in which neural measurements were made while Mössbauer sources were in place on the basilar membrane. Typical low and high CF_N tuning curves are shown for each ear. Frequency resolution: Mechanical tuning curves, 20 points per decade (left) and 10 points per decade (right); neural tuning curves, 32 points per octave.

Apparently the basilar membrane moves relative to the surrounding tissue, since with the Mössbauer source on the limbus or nerve (adjacent to the basilar membrane), the acoustic stimulus level had to be increased by about 20 dB to obtain the same source velocity.

Mechanical tuning curves are measures of frequency selectivity of basilar membrane motion. They are relatively broad (Fig. 14 - 16) with most sensitive or mechanical characteristic frequencies, CF_M's, in the range 1.5-4.1 kHz (Fig. 7C). A key finding is that mechanical tuning curves do not appear to change appreciably with source location along the basilar membrane (Fig. 15). In particular, CF_M's obtained from sources placed on the apical end did not differ significantly from those obtained from the basal end. Neither was there a significant difference in CF_M between the apical and basal halves of the basal region. The contrast between the properties of mechanical and neural tuning curves is clearly seen in the two experiments in which both curves were measured in the same ear (Fig. 14). Whereas mechanical tuning curves from apical and basal locations both have CF_M

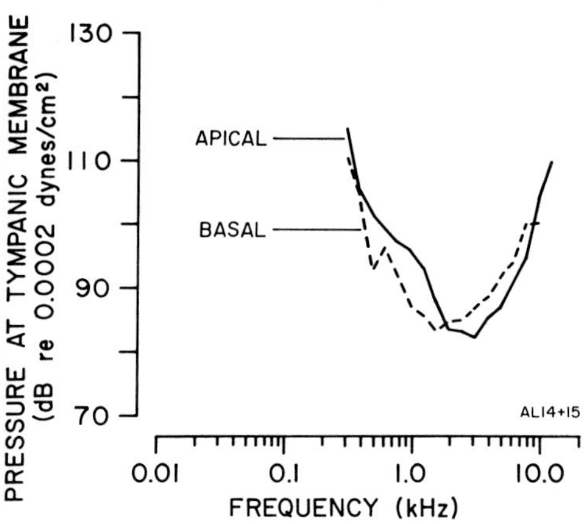

Fig. 15. Typical mechanical tuning curves from two ears. The Mössbauer source was placed on the apical end of the basilar membrane in one ear and on the basal end in the other. The velocity amplitude V was 0.5 mm/sec for the apical location and 0.8 mm/sec for the basal location. [The value of V was determined after measurements were made at constant values of $\bar{r}$.] These two curves are typical of measurements from 21 source placements on the basilar membrane: CF_M was 2.2 ± 0.6 kHz; threshold (sound-pressure level at the minimum of the mechanical tuning curve) was 82 ± 5 dB SPL (mean ± standard deviation). The values of V for these 21 curves were estimated to be in the range 0.5 - 1.1 mm/sec.

above 1.5 kHz, neural tuning curves span the range 0.22-4.6 kHz (Fig. 12) and are organized tonotopically in the nerve (Fig. 13).

Figure 14 demonstrates two other points. Mechanical tuning curves are broader than neural tuning curves. Also, sound-pressure levels required to measure mechanical tuning curves (for $V \approx 0.8$ mm/sec) were much higher than those used for neural tuning curves. If the mechanical system were non-linear, constant velocity curves taken at lower velocities might have a different frequency dependence (as reported for squirrel monkeys by Rhode, 1971; Rhode and Robles, 1974). We have made a few measurements at lower levels. For example, in Figure 16 two constant-velocity curves with velocity levels 16 dB apart have approximately the same frequency dependence, and they are separated by about 16 dB. These results do not exhibit any large non-linear effects.

The motions of the extrastapes and basilar membrane have a similar frequency dependence (Fig. 17), although the basilar membrane sensitivity falls off somewhat faster at low frequencies. Perhaps at these low frequencies ($\lesssim$ 0.4 kHz) there is significant volume flow through the helicotrema which reduces the relative motion of the basilar membrane. CF's determined from mechanical tuning curves of extrastapes motion were highly correlated with CF's of basilar membrane motion. Therefore, a portion of the variation in CF_M seen in Figure 7C results from differences in middle ear transmission in different preparations.

We conclude that measurements of the velocity of the basilar membrane in apical and basal regions do not exhibit the dichotomous tonotopic organization seen in hair cell and nerve fiber responses. Also the continuous gradation of CF which occurs in nerve fiber responses from the basal end of the basilar papilla is not evident in measurements of basilar membrane motion. The frequency-dependence of basilar membrane motion appears to be strongly influenced by the characteristics of the middle ear.

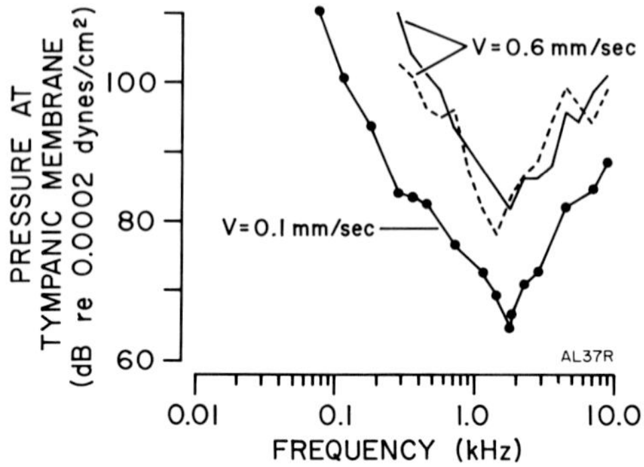

Fig. 16. Dependence of mechanical tuning curves on velocity level. The upper curves (solid and dashed) were obtained by determining the sound pressure necessary to maintain the velocity V = 0.6 mm/sec (at 10 points per decade of frequency) according to the method described in Figure 11C; 3 minutes were required to measure each of these curves. The lower curve was obtained from velocity and sound-pressure waveforms at each frequency according to the method described in Figure 11B; about 6 hours were required to obtain these data. The actual peak values of the fundamental component of the velocity waveforms ranged from 0.06 to 0.16 mm/sec with an average of 0.1 mm/sec; all points have been normalized to the same velocity magnitude (V = 0.1 mm/sec) assuming linearity. The 2nd and 3rd harmonics of the velocity waveforms were at least 13 dB below the fundamental except for the point below 100 Hz for which the second harmonic was 5 dB less than the fundamental.

DISCUSSION

Structure-Function Correlation in the Alligator Lizard Cochlea

Dichotomous Tonotopic Organization

The dichotomy in CF of cochlear nerve fibers appears to correspond to the anatomical division of the receptor organ into apical and basal regions. A dichotomy in CF is also observed in responses of cells in the receptor organ, but not in the motion of the basilar membrane (Fig. 7). Which steps leading to the generation of the receptor potential might be responsible for dichotomous tonotopic organization? Presumably motion of the stapes results in motion of the cilia of the hair cells. Displacements of cilia produce conductance changes of the hair cell membrane (Hudspeth and Corey, 1977) which result in current flow that causes the receptor potential. Any structures that affect ciliary motion differently in apical and basal regions could produce dichotomous tonotopic organization even though the motion of the basilar membrane is the same in these two regions. We suggest that the striking difference in morphology of tectorial and ciliary structures between the apical and basal regions is the basis of difference in ciliary motion.

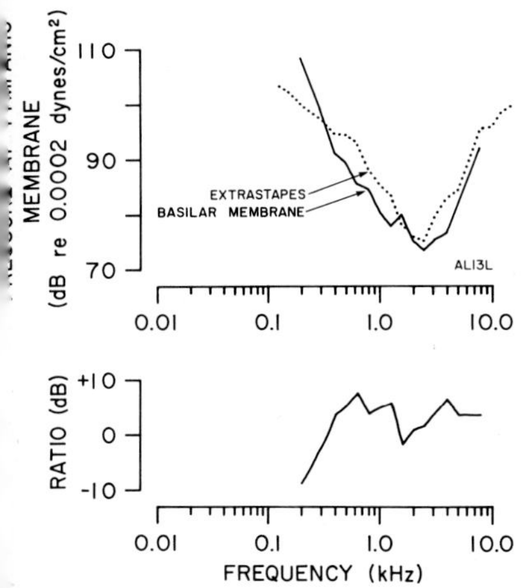

Fig. 17. Comparison of basilar membrane and extrastapes motion. Results are representative of data from 9 ears. Upper: Constant velocity characteristics obtained with Mössbauer sources on the basilar membrane (basal region near apical-basal border) and on the tympanic membrane over the extrastapes. V = 0.4 mm/sec. Lower: The ratio (difference in dB) of the two curves shown above.

Graded Tonotopic Organization

Basal cochlear nerve fibers exhibit a graded tonotopic organization as shown by the regular mapping between the CF_N of a fiber and its location in the nerve (Fig. 8 and 13). Measurements of basilar membrane velocity show no evidence of a graded tonotopic mapping of CF_M to position along the basilar membrane. What structures are responsible for this finer level of tonotopic organization? Presumably some structures in the basal region of the basilar papilla vary systematically along the longitudinal direction. The lengths of ciliary tufts of hair cells in the basal region vary continuously from 12μm in the basal end to 31μm near the basal-apical border (Mulroy, 1974). We suggest that this gradual variation in ciliary length may be the anatomical basis of the graded tonotopic organization of basal cochlear nerve fibers.

Implications for Acoustic Receptors in Vertebrates

Apparently factors other than basilar membrane motion are involved in determining frequency selectivity and tonotopic organization of cochlear nerve fibers in alligator lizards. Let us consider this conclusion in the context of results obtained from a broad range of vertebrates. From available anatomical (eg., Baird, 1974; Wever, 1974) and physiological knowledge, we can group acoustic receptors of vertebrates into three categories:

1. Acoustic receptors not located on a basilar membrane. In fish and amphibians, the receptor organs are located on structures that (on anatomical bases) are thought not to vibrate significantly. Yet VIIIth nerve fibers that innervate these organs exhibit frequency selectivity that varies from fiber to fiber (Enger, 1963; Furukawa

and Ishii, 1967; Capranica, 1976). Differences in frequency selectivity may well result from differences in tectorial and ciliary structures observed in these organs (Lewis and Li, 1975; Popper, 1976; Lewis, 1977; Platt, 1977; Dale, 1977).

2. Acoustic receptors located on a short basilar membrane. In certain reptiles, the receptor organs are located on a relatively short basilar membrane. In the alligator lizard, the basilar membrane's dimensions vary little over the length of the organ, and its motion exhibits no tonotopic organization. In contrast, cochlear nerve fibers are tonotopically organized. Furthermore, neural frequency selectivity is sharper than mechanical frequency selectivity.
3. Acoustic receptors located on a long basilar membrane. In crocodylians and birds, the basilar membrane and receptor organ are elongated. In mammals, the basilar membrane is even longer, and its dimensions vary systematically from base to apex. Mechanical tonotopic organization, which has been demonstrated in mammalian and avian cochleas (Békésy, 1960), is presumed to be a major determinant of neural tonotopic organization in these animals. However, as indicated in the INTRODUCTION, neural frequency selectivity has been reported to be sharper than mechanical frequency selectivity in mammals. Since the frequency selectivity of receptor potentials of cochlear inner hair cells appears to be about as sharp as that of cochlear nerve fibers (Russell and Sellick, 1977), some process whose frequency selectivity is sharper than that of the basilar membrane displacement must occur prior to the generation of the receptor potential in mammals. This process may well involve motion of ciliary and tectorial structures, whose dimensions are known to vary in the mammalian cochlea (Iurato, 1967).

Evidence from a number of species suggests that frequency selectivity and tonotopic organization of nerve fibers depend upon processes in addition to basilar membrane motion. We conclude that processes such as the ones we have suggested for the alligator lizard may well be important in other species including mammals.

Acknowledgements

This research was supported by U.S. Public Health Service Grants 1 PO1 NS 13126 and 5 KO4 NS 00113. A number of people contributed to this work. We especially appreciate the contribution of D.G. Beil who helped with surgery and histology and drafted all the figures. K.E. Michel, S.A. Nelson, B.E. Norris, J.D. Pusey, and G.S. Roberts were helpful in many ways. K. Baden-Kristensen and D.W. Altman participated in some experiments reported here. T.J. Lynch, III, provided several components of Figure 11. Helpful comments on the manuscript were obtained from: K. Baden-Kristensen, L.S. Frishkopf, J.J. Guinan, Jr., N.Y.S. Kiang, M.C. Liberman, and W.M. Siebert.

REFERENCES

Allen, J.B. Cochlear micromechanics - a mechanism for transforming mechanical to neural tuning within the cochlea. *J. Acoust. Soc. Am. 62:* 930-939, 1977.

Baird, I.L. Anatomical features of the inner ear in submammalian vertebrates. In: *Handbook of Sensory Physiology. V/1. Auditory System: Anatomy, Physiology (Ear),* edited by W.D. Keidel and W.D. Neff. Berlin, Heidelberg, New York: Springer-Verlag, 1974, p. 159-212.

Békésy, G.von, Experiments in Hearing, edited by E.G. Wever. New York: McGraw-Hill, 1960.

Bennett, M.V.L. Permeability and structure of electrotonic junctions and intercellular movements of tracers. In: *Intracellular Staining in Neurobiology,* edited by S.B. Kater and C. Nicholson. New York: Springer-Verlag, 1973, p. 115-134.

Billone, M. and Raynor, S. Transmission of radial shear forces to cochlear hair cells, *J. Acoust. Soc. Am. 54:* 1143-1156, 1973.

Capranica, R.R. Morphology and physiology of the auditory system. In: *Frog Neurobiology,* edited by R. Llinás and W. Precht. New York: Springer-Verlag, 1976, p. 551-575.

Dale, T. The labyrinthine mechanoreceptor organs of the cod *Gadus morhua L.* (Teleostei: Gadidae). A scanning electron microscopical study, with special reference to the morphological polarization of the macular sensory cells. *Norw. J. Zool. 24:* 85-128, 1976.

Enger, P.S. Single unit activity in the peripheral auditory system of a teleost fish. *Acta Physiol. Scand.* 59: 1-48, 1963.

Evans, E.F. The sharpening of cochlear frequency selectivity in the normal and abnormal cochlea. *Audiology 14:* 419-442, 1975.

Evans, E.F. and Wilson, J.P. Cochlear tuning properties: concurrent basilar membrane and single nerve fiber measurements. *Science 190:* 1218-1221, 1975.

Furukawa, T. and Ishii, Y. Neurophysiological studies on hearing in goldfish. *J. Neurophysiol. 30:* 1377-1403, 1967.

Geisler, C.D., Rhode, W.S., and Kennedy, D.T. Responses to tonal stimuli of single auditory nerve fibers and their relationship to basilar membrane motion in the squirrel monkey. *J. Neurophysiol. 37:* 1156-1172, 1974.

Gilad, P., Shtrikman, S., Hillman, P., Rubinstein, J. and Eviatar, A. Application of the Mössbauer method to ear vibrations. *J. Acoust. Soc. Am. 41:* 1232-1236, 1967.

Hall, J.L. Spatial differentiation as an auditory "Second Filter": assessment on a nonlinear model of the basilar membrane. *J. Acoust. Soc. Am. 61:* 520-524, 1977.

Helfenstein, W.M. Beitrag Zur Messung der Akustisch Bedingten Bewegungen und Identifikation des Mechanischen Teils des Innenohrs der Katze, Thesis, Eidgenössischen Technischen Hochschule Zürich, Switzerland, 1973.

Holton, T. and Weiss, T.F. Two-Tone rate suppression in lizard cochlear-nerve fibers: relation to auditory receptor morphology. *J. Acoust. Soc. Am. 62:* S45, 1977.

Hudspeth, A.J. and Corey, D.P. Sensitivity, polarity, and conductance change in the response of vertebrate hair cells to controlled mechanical stimuli. *Proc. Natl. Acad. Sci. 74:* 2407-2411, 1977.

Iurato, S. *Submicroscopic Structure of the Inner Ear.* New York: Pergamon, 1967.

Johnstone, B.M. and Boyle, A.J.F. Basilar membrane vibration examined with Mössbauer technique. *Science 158:* 389-390, 1967.

Kiang, N.Y.S., Watanabe, T., Thomas, E.C. and Clark, L.F. Discharge patterns of single fibers in the cat's auditory nerve. Cambridge: MIT Press, 1965.

Kim, D.O. and Molnar, C.E. Cochlear mechanics: measurements and models. In: *The Nervous System. 3: Human Communication and Its Disorders,* edited by D.B. Tower. New York: Raven Press, 1975, p. 57-68.

Köhlloffel, L.U.E. A study of basilar membrane vibrations. III. The basilar membrane frequency response curve in the living guinea pig. *Acustica 27:* 82-89, 1972.

Lewis, E.R. Structural correlates of function in the anuran amphibian papilla. In: *Scanning Electron Microscopy. II: Biological Applications of SEM,* edited by O. Johari and R.P. Becker. Chicago: IIT Research Institute, 1977, p. 429-435.

Lewis, E.R. and Li, C.W. Hair types and distributions in the otolithic and auditory organs of the bullfrog. *Brain Res. 83:* 35-50, 1975.

Miller, M.R. The cochlear duct of lizards. *Proc. Cal. Acad. Sci. 33:* 255-359, 1966.

Miller, M.R. Scanning electron microscope studies of some lizard basilar papillae. *Am. J. Anat. 138:* 301-330, 1973.

Mulroy, M.J. Ultrastructure of the basilar papilla of reptiles. Ph.D. Diss. Dept. Anat., University of California, San Francisco, 1968.

Mulroy, M.J. Cochlear anatomy of the alligator lizard. *Brain Behav. Evol. 10:* 69-87, 1974.

Mulroy, M.J., Altmann, D.W., Weiss, T.F. and Peake, W.T. Intracellular electric response to sound in a vertebrate cochlea. *Nature 249:* 482-485, 1974.

Nadol, J.B., Mulroy, M.J., Goodenough, D.A. and Weiss, T.F. Tight and gap junctions in a vertebrate inner ear. *Am. J. Anat. 147:* 281-301, 1976.

Platt, C. Hair cell distribution and orientation in goldfish otolith organs. *J. Comp. Neurol. 172:* 283-297, 1977.

Popper, A.N. Ultrastructure of the auditory regions in the inner ear of the lake whitefish. *Science 192:* 1020-1023, 1976.

Rhode, W.S. Observations of the vibration of the basilar membrane in squirrel monkeys using the Mössbauer technique. *J. Acoust. Soc. Am. 49:* 1218-1231, 1971.

Rhode, W.S. and Robles, L. Evidence from Mössbauer experiments for nonlinear vibration in the cochlea. *J. Acoust. Soc. Am. 55:* 588-596, 1974.

Russell, I.J. and Sellick, P.M. Tuning properties of cochlear hair cells. *Nature 267:* 858-860, 1977.

Sando, I. The anatomical interrelationships of the cochlear nerve fibers. *Acta Otolaryngol. 59:* 417-436, 1965.

Steele, C.R. A possibility for sub-tectorial membrane fluid motion. In: *Basic Mechanisms in Hearing,* edited by A.R. Møller. New York: Academic Press, 1973, p. 69-90.

Weiss, T.F., Mulroy, M.J. and Altmann, D.W. Intracellular responses to acoustic clicks in the inner ear of the alligator lizard. *J. Acoust. Soc. Am. 55:* 606-619, 1974.

Weiss, T.F., Mulroy, M.J., Turner, R.G. and Pike, C.L. Tuning of single fibers in the cochlear nerve of the alligator lizard: relation to receptor morphology. *Brain Res. 115:* 71-90, 1976.

Wever, E.G. Structure and function of the lizard ear. *J. Aud. Res. 5:* 331-371, 1965.

Wever, E.G. The evolution of vertebrate hearing. In: *Handbook of Sensory Physiology. V/1. Auditory System: Anatomy, Physiology (Ear),* edited by W.D. Keidel and W.D. Neff. Berlin, New York, Heidelberg: Springer-Verlag, 1974, p. 423-454.

Wilson, J.P. and Johnstone, J.R. Basilar membrane and middle-ear vibration in guinea pig measured by capacitive probe. *J. Acoust. Soc. Am. 57:* 705-723, 1975.

Zwicker, E. and Terhardt, E. *Facts and Models in Hearing.* New York: Springer-Verlag, 1974.

DISCUSSION

Spoendlin: I have a question about the coupling of your Mössbauer source on the basilar membrane. I wonder whether the wide mechanical tuning curve and the lack of tonotopical behavior could also be the consequence of poor coupling.

Weiss: To definitively determine the coupling of the source to the basilar membrane, one needs to independently measure both the motion of the basilar membrane and the motion of the source. This has not been done. However, the experiment described in our paper, in which the lizard's head is vibrated, suggests that motion of the source does not differ appreciably from that of the membrane.

Gerken: Is there any correlation between the lizard's life style in its environment and the dichotomous tuning curve function? Secondly, how do you know that there is not some kind of movement artifact?

Weiss: In response to your first question, I don't know of any behavioral correlate of dichotomous tonotopic organization. If I understand the second question correctly, you asked, is the intracellular electric response to sound stimulation that we record, generated by the hair cell or by the micropipette? In other words are these potentials of physiological origin or are they artifacts? Experiments in which sodium pentobarbital placed in scala tympani resulted in reduction of intracellular responses without changes in basilar membrane motion suggest that the measured potentials do not arise from mechanical vibration of the micropipet tip (Mulroy et al., *Nature 249:* 482-485, 1974).

Durrant: I have a two-part question. Have you looked at the ability of these neurons to lock onto the phase of the stimulus? If so, do you see any dichotomy there between the two apparent populations? Secondly, can I assume that the spontaneous rate of discharge represents a random rate for both populations, or is there any background frequency such as in vestibular fibers?

Weiss: Lizard fibers do show synchronized responses to low frequency tones. However, we have not looked systematically at the synchrony of the response to tones as a function of stimulus parameters. Both apical and basal fibers have similar spontaneous discharges resembling those found in mammalian auditory nerve fibers. However, the distribution of average discharge rate of the population of apical fibers differs from that of the population of basal fibers.

Platt: In fishes at least there do not appear to be bulbed cilia, but I know in lizards and amphibians there are. Could you make a statement on frequency of the bulbs on the cilia?

Weiss: Bulbs are seen on kinocilia in Gerrhonotus multicarinatus (see Miller, *Am. J. Anat., 138:* 301-329, 1973). I don't have any quantitative information on the frequency of occurrence.

Goldberg: I have a question or two. There is a notion which is nicely exemplified here, a concept that emerged over the last four or five years, of a second filter. You have to invoke a second filter. It seems to me the mechanical curves are so distant from the frequency tuning curves that you would need a hell of a filter to explain a unit tuned at 200 Hz with your mechanical tuning curves up around .002. Do you have any insight as to what class of mechanism would give you such a sharp second filter used solely in a descriptive way.

Weiss: Not really. But let me comment on your use of the term "second filter". If a second filter is defined to exist when there is a difference in the shapes of mechanical (as measured on the basilar membrane) and neural tuning curves, then indeed a second filter is required in the alligator lizard cochlea. However, this second filter need not be viewed as coming *after* a filter representing the basilar membrane hydrodynamics. In other words, the mechanical input to a hair cell, which we might regard as the motion of the cilia, need not be uniquely determined by the motion of the basilar membrane.

Goldberg: When you talk about discrepancy in mammals you are talking about a substantial discrepancy. Just viewing the slides qualitatively this would seem a greater discrepancy. I wouldn't care to define how I would measure that.

Weiss: The differences between mechanical and neural tuning curves is certainly larger in the alligator lizard than it is in mammals.

Goldberg: A second question. One of the arguments for the existence of a second filter in mammalian cochlea has been that you can manipulate the shapes of the tuning curves by a variety of techniques which usually are injurious to the cochlea. Do you have any kind of similar observations in your preparation?

Weiss: We have not examined this systematically.

INTRACELLULAR STUDIES OF COCHLEAR HAIR CELLS: FILLING THE GAP BETWEEN BASILAR MEMBRANE MECHANICS AND NEURAL EXCITATION

Peter M. Sellick and Ian J. Russell

University of Sussex

INTRODUCTION

Mechanical measurements of basilar membrane vibration to pure tones show that the amplitude of vibration varies along the length of the basilar membrane depending in a graded way upon the frequency of the tone (Békésy, 1960; Johnstone and Boyle, 1967; Rhode, 1971; Wilson and Johnstone, 1975). It has been found that the vertical vibration of the basilar membrane is more broadly tuned, ie. less frequency selective, than the response of the auditory nerve fibers that innervate the hair cells in the organ of Corti (Evans, 1972). This discrepancy exists because there is no obvious reason why the hair cells and hence the afferent fibers should not have the same frequency response as the basilar membrane. Hence it is necessary to propose a mechanism to explain neural sharpening. In the absence of experimental data concerning the transduction of mechanical movement to hair cell receptor potential and subsequent initiation of impulses in the auditory nerve, a large number of models have been put forward to explain the discrepancy between basilar membrane and neural frequency selectivity. These models all start with the broad tuning of the basilar membrane and propose some sharpening mechanism to produce the tuning properties of the auditory nerve. They may be divided into three classes. Firstly, there are mechanical models that propose that the vertical or measured motion of the basilar membrane is not directly responsible for stimulating the hair cells but that this motion undergoes some transformation at the top of the hair cells to produce sharpening (Tonndorf, 1960; Duifhuis, 1976; Steele, 1973). Secondly, neural models which propose that neural interaction occurs within the organ of Corti to produce sharpening of the response of the auditory nerve or hair cell (Nieder, 1971; Zwislocki, 1974). Thirdly, electrical interaction models which propose that receptor potentials from adjacent hair cells interact electrotonically (Manley, 1977).

The existence of so many different models emphasizes how little we know about the processes occurring between the basilar membrane motion and neural

ISBN 0-12-514960-3

excitation. An obvious first step towards understanding these processes is to record the frequency response of the hair cells themselves. However, in the past measurements of the cochlear microphonic and summating potential have been made extracellularly with single ended electrodes on the round window (Adrian, 1931) or in scala media (Honrubia and Ward, 1968) or differentially across the cochlear partition (Dallos, 1973). These methods suffer from the disadvantage that the potentials are smeared out by the cable properties of the cochlear partition making it difficult to determine the response of an individual hair cell and hence compare it with that of the basilar membrane or auditory nerve. In this paper we describe the results of intracellular measurements from inner hair cells in the first turn of the guinea pig cochlea in an attempt to bridge the gap between basilar membrane mechanics and neural excitation.

METHODS

The experimental details have been described in detail elsewhere (Russell and Sellick, 1978) and only a brief description of special methods used in these experiments will be given here.

The cochlea of the anesthetized guinea pig was exposed by displacing the mandible and opening the bulla ventro-laterally. The first turn of the cochlea was illuminated from behind, on the scala vestibuli side, by placing a 1 mm diameter fiber optic light source against it. This permitted a view of blood vessels in the bone of the first turn during exposure of the basilar membrane and facilitated the positioning of the microelectrode. The cochlea was opened by thinning the bone over the scala tympani at the first turn thus exposing the basilar membrane in the 15-23 kHz region. The threshold (within 10 dB) of the compound action potential (AP) evoked by a pure tone burst of 2 msec duration was monitored during exposure of the basilar membrane by a fine Teflon-insulated silver wire positioned close to the round window and secured to the skull with cyanoacrylic cement. It was possible to expose the basilar membrane in this way while preserving the original AP threshold.

The microelectrodes used in these experiments had initial resistances of about 700 MΩ and 200 MΩ when filled with 6% aqueous solution of Procion yellow and 4M potassium acetate respectively. Their resistances were reduced to half these values by bevelling the electrode tips on a grinding wheel to facilitate penetration of the basilar membrane (Brown and Flaming, 1975). A hydraulic microdrive was used to advance the electrode through the basilar membrane. A Bioelectric P1 probe equipped with capacitance compensation was used to measure intracellular receptor potentials. Optimal compensation of the probe produced an amplification of signals between 1 kHz and 20 kHz of 5-6 times depending on the degree of capacitance compensation and the electrode resistance. The magnitude of CM is, therefore, subject to a small unsystematic error.

The AC component of the receptor potential was measured with potassium acetate electrodes and two Brookdeal 9503SC lock-in amplifiers in quadrature. The modulus of the signal was obtained from a Brookdeal Omniphase and stored on an FM tape recorder for future analysis.

Resistance measurements were made from hair cells during sound stimulation and simultaneous recording of the DC component of the receptor potential. The measurements were made according to the method of Pinto and Pak (1974). Sinusoidal currents (1.5×10^{-11} A) with frequencies of either 40, 100 or 150 kHz were passed through the recording electrode via a bridge circuit into the impaled hair cell. Voltage changes due to the electrode's intrinsic impedance were balanced out with the amplifier bridge circuit and voltage changes due to changes in the resistance of the hair cell were measured with the lock-in amplifiers, one set in phase and one 90° out of phase. Thus the real and imaginary impedances of the hair cell could be observed and the time constant of the hair cell calculated. Measurements of the real and imaginary impedance changes at different frequencies indicated that the changes in impedance were due to pure resistance changes.

RESULTS

Amplitude and Frequency Response of the Receptor Potentials

Large, 5-23mV depolarizing receptor potentials, which follow the envelope of a tone burst and therefore correspond to extracellularly recorded summating potentials, have been recorded intracellularly from morphologically identified inner hair cells in the organ of Corti (Russell and Sellick, 1977a, 1977b, 1978) (Fig. 1). We have termed this potential the DC component of the receptor potential. When we were convinced that we could successfully aim our electrode towards inner hair cells, and that these were the cells which responded with a large DC potential to tone bursts, we abandoned the Procion dye-filled electrodes which were essential for morphologically identifying the inner hair cells, for potassium acetate-filled microelectrodes which had lower resistances, and consequently higher frequency responses. When intracellularly recorded receptor potentials were measured from inner hair cells with these microelectrodes it was found that the DC component was modulated by a smaller potential corresponding to the extracellularly-recorded cochlear microphonic potential, and we have named it the AC component of the receptor potential.

The DC and AC components of the receptor potential recorded from an inner hair cell in response to 80 msec tone bursts of varying frequency and 10 dB SPL intervals is illustrated in Figure 1. The DC component has a maximum magnitude of about 12mV at CF and has a broad frequency response at high SPLs. As the SPL is reduced the response bandwidth decreases until the receptor potential is reduced to noise level. These data may be compared with the isointensity-rate response of the auditory nerve which has similar characteristics. The AC component on the other hand is smaller, maximally about 0.6mV at CF and shows slightly different characteristics at high SPLs in that the response is largest for low frequencies, declines, and has a peak around the characteristic frequency of the cell. As the SPL

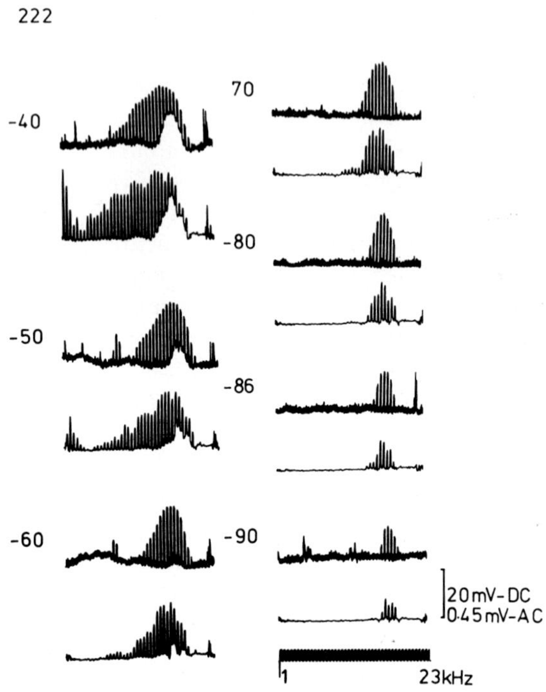

Fig. 1. DC (upper trace) and AC (lower trace) receptor potentials to 80msec tone bursts from a presumed inner hair cell. In each pair of traces the upper trace is the output from the probe amplifier and the lower trace is the modulus output from the lock-in amplifiers. The numbers by the side of each pair of traces indicate dB attenuation of the sound system. The notches in the traces for -40 and -50dB attenuation is due to leakage through the electronic switch. The lower right hand trace shows the trigger pulses for individual tone bursts at 500 Hz intervals—the frequency scale is linear from 1 to 23 kHz.

is reduced the low frequency response disappears to leave a response similar to that of the DC component.

A plot of the ratio of the DC and AC components vs frequency shows that the AC component falls off at a rate of 6-9 dB/octave with respect to the DC component (Fig. 2). This frequency-dependent attenuation of the AC component is probably due to the low pass characteristics of the hair cell membrane rather than to some frequency dependency of the mechano-electric transduction process, because the extracellularly recorded AC component is not attenuated at high frequency (Russell and Sellick, 1978). This proposal is further supported by measurements of the hair cell time constant which was found to be between 0.31 and 0.76 msec in the 7 cells in which it was measured. Thus for a cell with a time constant of 0.7 msec the cutoff frequency is 210 Hz and the intracellular AC component will fall

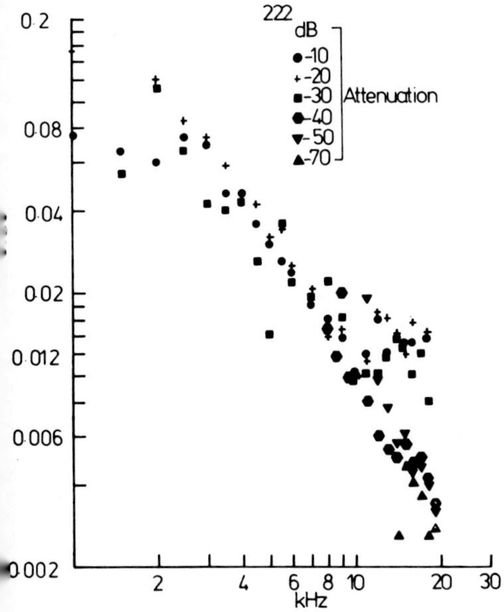

Fig. 2. The ratio of the AC and DC components of the receptor potential vs frequency showing the fall off from 69dB/octave of the AC component with respect to the DC component.

off at a rate of 6 dB/octave above this frequency, if it is assumed that the hair cell behaves as a simple RC network and the space constant of the hair cell is large compared to the cell's dimension.

The release of chemical transmitter and hence neural excitation occurs during the depolarization phase of the hair cell receptor potential (Sand et al., 1975). The importance of the AC component of the receptor potential in this process and hence the occurrence of phase locking in the auditory nerve will depend on its relative size with respect to the DC component. The fact that the AC component falls at a rate of 6 dB/octave from about 200 Hz with respect to the DC component might indicate that it is this which limits phase locking. However there are other factors that could also be limiting, eg. the frequency response of transmitter release and the temporal resolution of excitatory postsynaptic potentials. It is, therefore, premature to implicate the magnitude of the AC component in the reduction in phase locking with increasing frequency found by Rose et al. (1967). One thing is certain, however, at frequencies about 5 kHz, where phase locking to the stimulus is not observed and the AC component is small, the DC component of the receptor potential must be entirely responsible for neural excitation.

Intensity Functions for the DC and AC Component of the Receptor Potential

It is evident from the raw data in Figure 1 that the receptor potentials behave nonlinearly throughout the frequency range. Simply, the low frequency responses are reduced more rapidly with decreasing SPL than the responses around the CF of

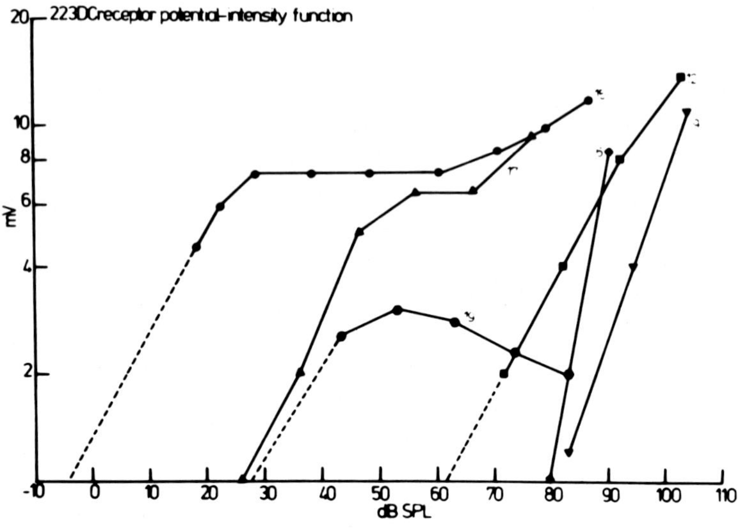

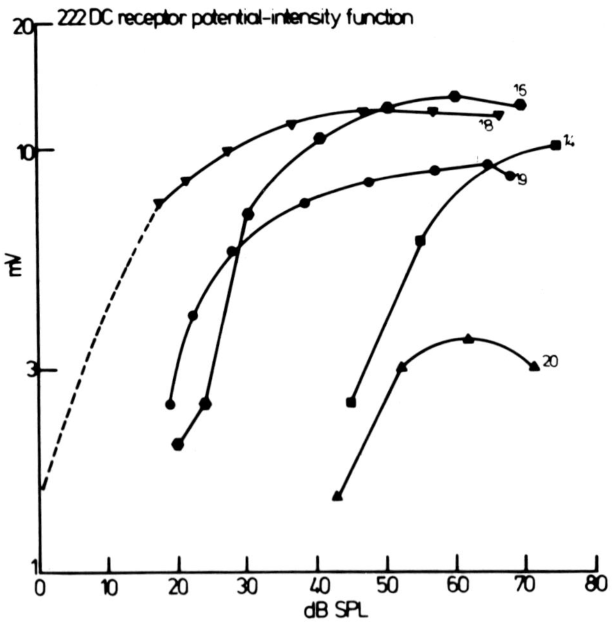

Fig. 3. Intensity functions for the DC and AC components of the receptor potential. The numbers by the side of each intensity function denote frequency.

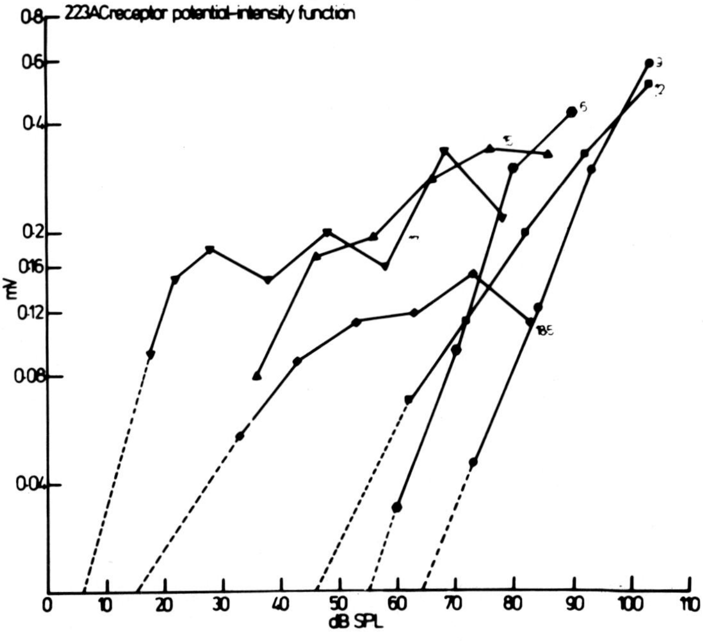
223AC receptor potential-intensity function
mV
dB SPL

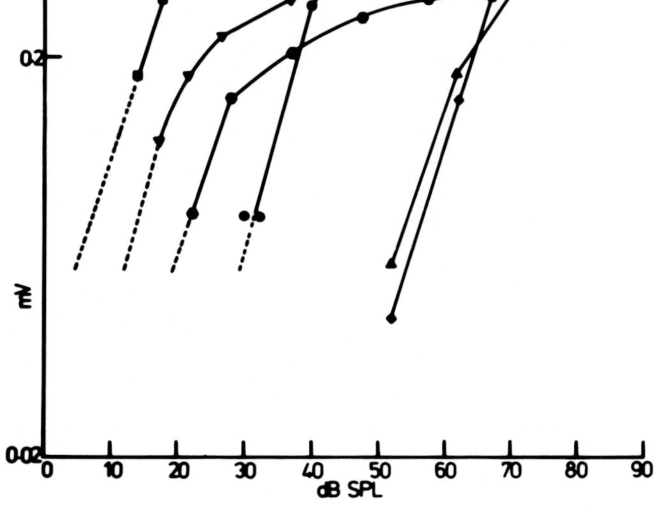
222AC receptor potential-intensity function
mV
dB SPL

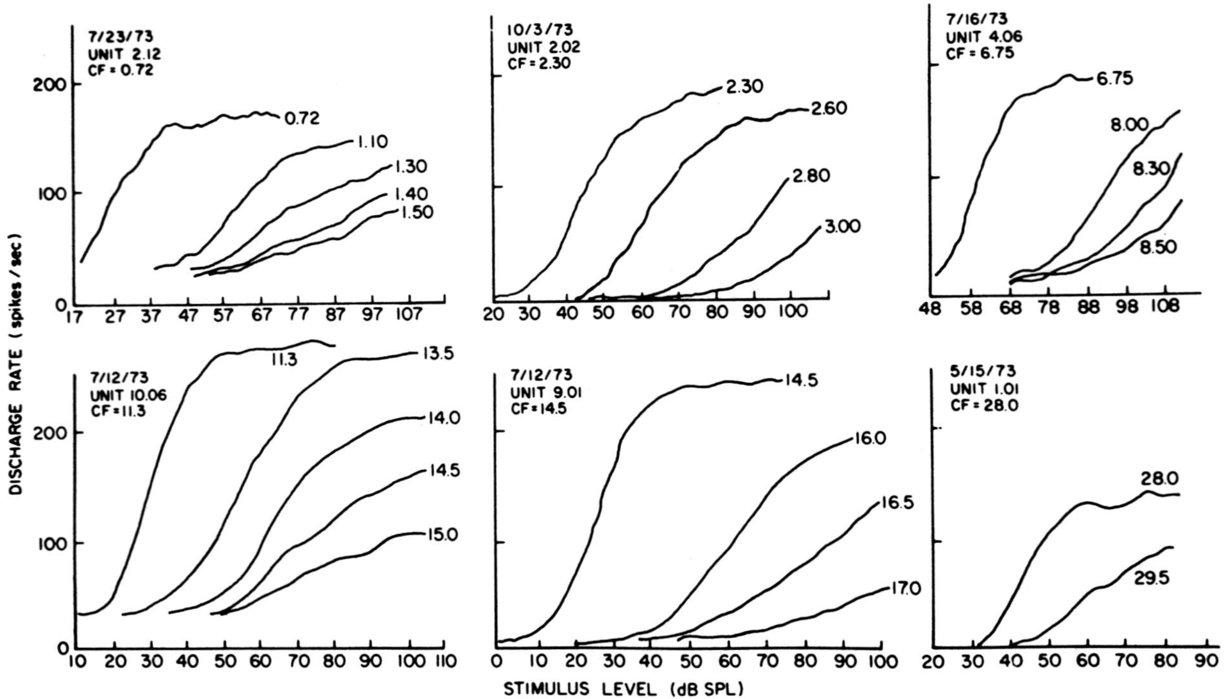

Fig. 4. Rate-versus-level functions for tones at CF and higher frequencies from the cat auditory nerve. Frequency of the tone corresponding to each curve is given in kilohertz. From Sachs and Abbas *J. Acoust. Soc. Amer. 56,* 1835-1847, by permission of the authors.

the cell. This behavior is more easily examined from the relationship between amplitude of receptor potential vs stimulus intensity at fixed frequencies (intensity functions) in Figure 3. The DC component at frequencies substantially below the CF rise linearly from the noise level and do not reach saturation within the SPLs used. However as the CF is approached the potentials saturate at low amplitudes and this trend continues through and above CF. A similar trend is observed for the AC component except that the amplitude at the low frequency end is higher with respect to CF due to the low-pass characteristics of the cell. The curves are also moved toward lower SPLs as the CF is approached and back to higher SPLs at frequencies above CF.

The rate functions of the auditory nerve will reflect the intensity functions of the receptor potential though possibly distorted by the several transformations which occur between the production of a receptor potential in a hair cell and the generation of impulses in the afferent fiber innervating it. The release of chemical transmitter from the hair cell, the depolarization of the postsynaptic membrane and the initiation of impulses in the nerve are all rate limited functions whose characteristics have not been measured in the peripheral auditory system and are likely to account for differences between hair cell intensity functions and neural rate functions. However, the two relationships are in fact rather similar as is seen from the rate functions for single fibers in the cat auditory nerve from Sachs and Abbas (1974) Figure 4. One obvious difference between neural rate functions and the hair cell intensity functions is that the former is sigmoidal while the latter rises linearly from the noise level before saturating. The hair cell intensity function may also be sigmoidal but with the lower inflexion masked by the noise level. However, the lower inflexion of the neural rate function is more likely to be caused by the limitations of the synaptic and spike generating mechanism, as predicted by the model of Schroeder and Hall (1974) for mechanical to neural transduction. This may explain the differences at frequencies above CF where the receptor potential saturates at very low amplitudes and the neural responses appear to rise very slowly from threshold. The important similarity between hair cell intensity functions and neural rate functions is that the level at which saturation occurs declines progressively with increasing frequency through and above CF. From a comparison between Figures 3 and 4, it is clear that at CF both sets of curves saturate over a similar range of SPL, ie. 30 dB. Thus saturation of neural rate function occurs not because of saturation of the synaptic mechanism or the refractory period of the nerve fiber but because the receptor potential itself saturates. It is unlikely that this saturating nonlinearity is a property of the hair cell since it is frequency-dependent, but has its origin in the basilar membrane mechanics as predicted by Kim et al. (1973).

Isoamplitude Curves for Intracellular Receptor Potentials

Our primary aim in these experiments was to make a comparison between the tuning properties of hair cells and auditory nerve fibers. The frequency response of single fibers in the auditory nerve has been described in terms of isothreshold or isorate contours which are referred to as neural frequency tuning curves (FTC). They are derived by measuring the threshold for an arbitrarily determined increase

TABLE I

Expt. No.	CF kHz	Resting Potential mV	AP Threshold SPL dB	DC FTC[1]					AC FTC				
				Q_{10dB}	Threshold dB SPL	HF slope dB/oct.	LF slope dB/oct.	Tip-Shoulder dB SPL	Q_{10dB}	Threshold dB SPL	HF slope dB/oct.	LF slope dB/oct.	Tip-Shoulder dB SPL
105	23	35	15	7.7	21.5	500	253	26					
222	17.5	30	0	6.0	-2	475	136	66	9	5	800	190	65[2]
223	17	20	0	8.5	8	340	104	79	7.4	12.5	400	135	59[3]
225	17	30	0	8.7	5	460	162	67					
211	18	43	20	5.3	50	400	45	35	4.9	43	300	75	42[4]
210	15	35	30	6.0	42	650	98	29					
218	17	40	10	9.4	7	425	130	69	8.5	8	460	144	62[5]
197	17	30	10	11.3	6	350	170	67					

1 Based on 2mV FTC
2 Based on 0.2mV FTC
3 Based on 0.4mV FTC
4 Based on 0.06mV FTC
5 Based on 0.04mV FTC

in firing rate of the nerve fiber at different frequencies of sound stimulation. Hair cell FTCs are isoamplitude contours derived from the isointensity functions and minor extrapolation and interpolation of these are made when necessary to fill gaps in the data. Therefore, before any comparison can be made between neural and hair cell FTCs, it is essential to discover the amplitude of receptor potential which corresponds to a just-noticeable increase in the background activity in an auditory nerve. This may be estimated from the threshold to pure tones of the compound action potential of the cochlear nerve (AP) measured at the round window, which Johnstone (1977) has shown to approximate the threshold of the spiral ganglion cells (cell bodies of the auditory nerve fibers). Our data (Table 1) suggests that AP threshold corresponds to about 2mV for the DC component and about 0.01mV for the AC component at a CF of 17 kHz.

The shapes of neural FTCs are defined by four main characteristics, namely the Q_{10dB} defined as the characteristic frequency divided by the bandwidth measured 10 dB from the tip as a measure of frequency selectivity and three related characteristics, namely the high and low frequency slopes in dB/octave and the difference between tip and low frequency tail in dB.

The receptor potential and neural FTCs resemble each other in several respects (Figs. 6 and 8). The high and low frequency slopes of the hair cell FTCs measured within 5 and 25 dB of the tip fall within the ranges of 100 and 600 dB/octave, and 100 and 300 dB/octave respectively, which are similar to the values measured by Evans (1972) for the corresponding slopes of neural tuning curves in the guinea pig. The sharpness of neural and hair cell FTCs expressed as Q_{10dB} fall within the same range of 6-11 and the difference between the low frequency tail and tip of the FTC is comparable to those of neural FTCs. Furthermore the tuning

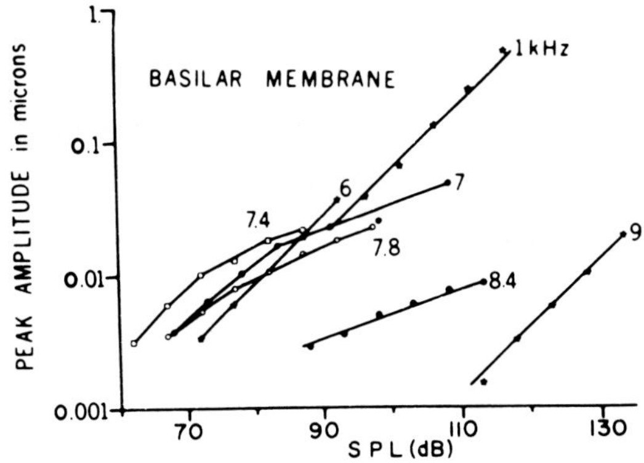

(a)

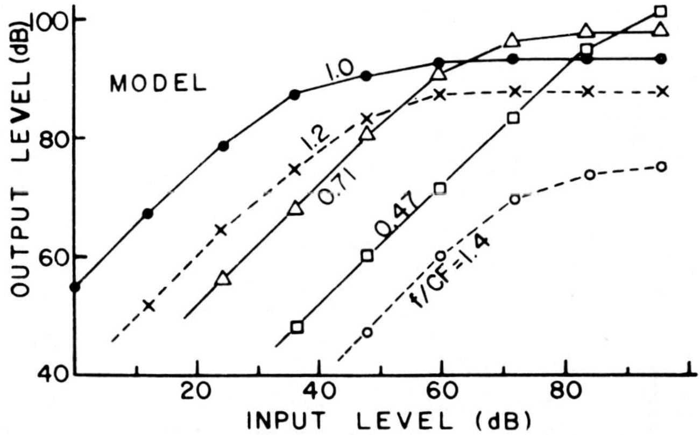

Fig. 5a. Peak amplitude of displacement of a point on the basilar membrane versus sound pressure level for several frequencies of sinusoidal inputs (from Rhode, 1971).

b. Output level (peak-to-peak) of the model of Kim et al versus input level for several frequencies of sinusoidal inputs. The reference of the input and the output levels of the model is an arbitrary constant. Note the decreasing level of saturation of the output with frequency and the crossover of the intensity functions at high input level which result in a reduction of the CF. From Kim et al (1973) *J. Acoust. Soc. Amer. 54,* 1517-1529, by permission of the authors.

properties of hair cells and nerve fibers exhibit a similar independence of SPL (Geisler et al., 1974) (Fig. 9) ie. the characteristics of the receptor potential and neural FTCs are largely independent of the amplitude of receptor potential and threshold criterion selected to derive FTCs except for the high frequency slope of the FTC which behaves nonlinearly. It is obvious from the receptor potential intensity functions in Figure 3 that this would be the case, since the amplitude at which the receptor potentials saturate decreases rapidly after CF and the high frequency

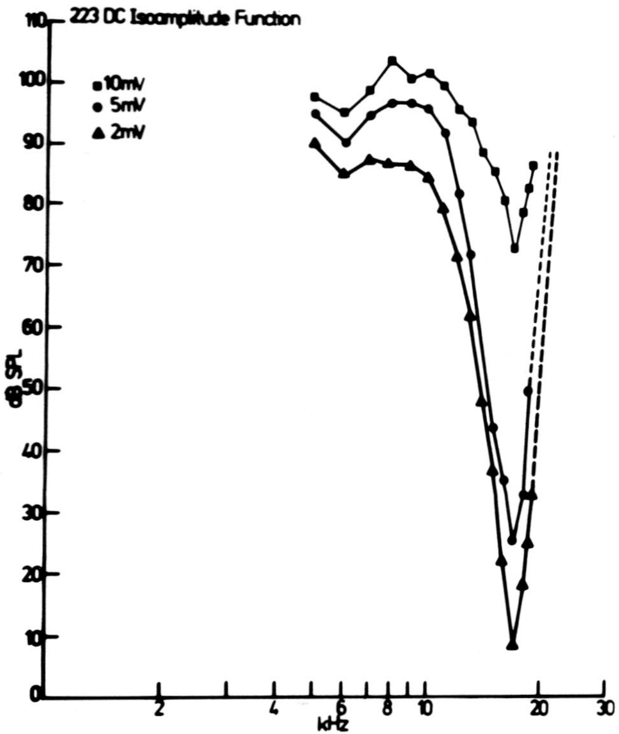
223 DC Isoamplitude Function
10mV
5mV
2mV
dB SPL
kHz

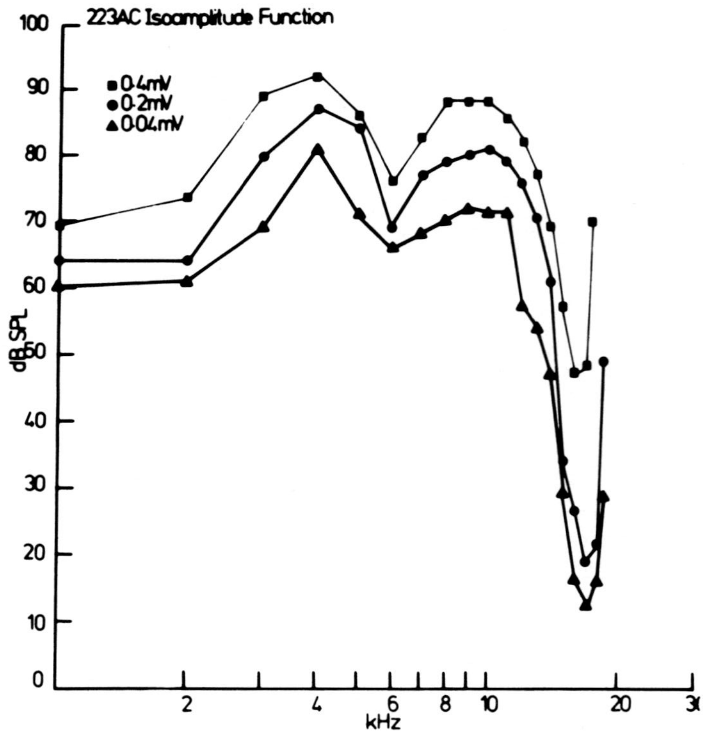
223AC Isoamplitude Function
0·4mV
0·2mV
0·04mV
dB SPL
kHz

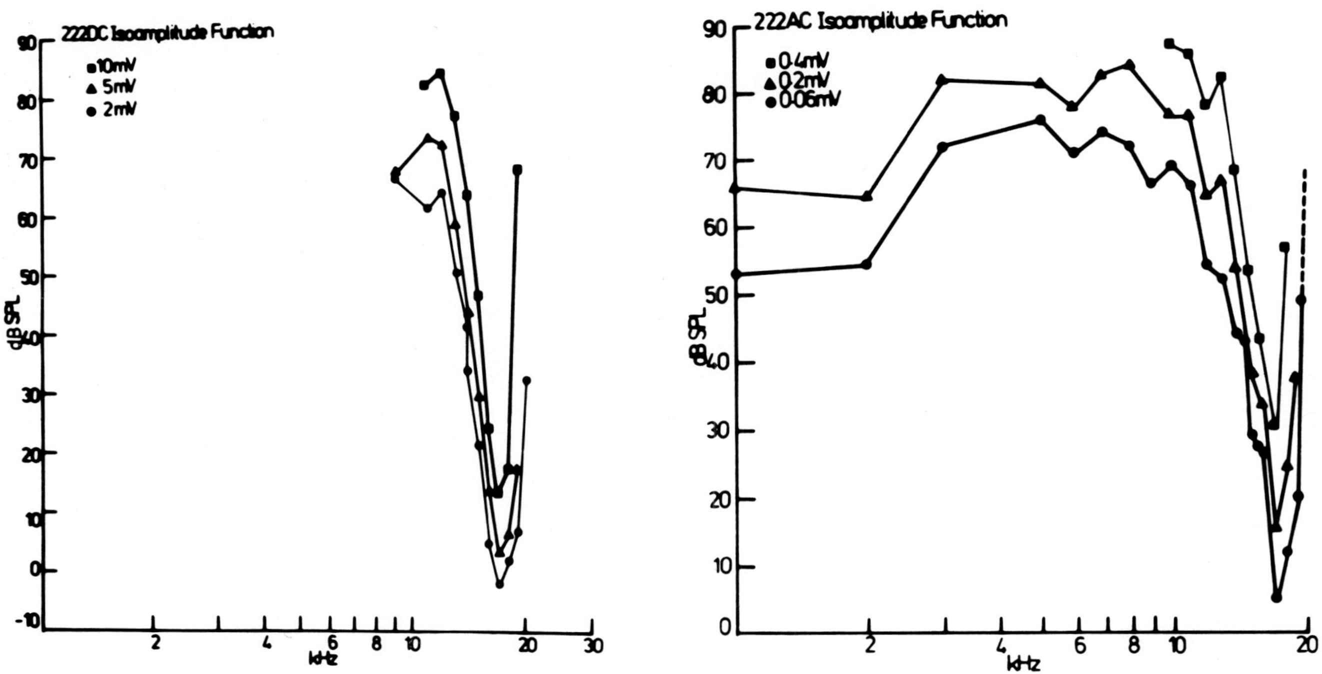

Fig. 6. Isoamplitude curves for the DC and AC component for two cells.

slope for the FTCs must have been derived from a very nonlinear region of the intensity function. As the amplitude criterion of the FTC is increased into the nonlinear range of the CF intensity function, the FTC changes shape markedly, the tip moves up and the Q_{10dB} is decreased. There may also be a shift of CF towards low frequencies due to the cross over of the intensity functions at high SPL. This finding corresponds to the behavior of neural FTCs in response to loud sound (Evans, 1977). We conclude that the shapes of the neural tuning curves are determined by the frequency-intensity characteristics of individual inner hair cells.

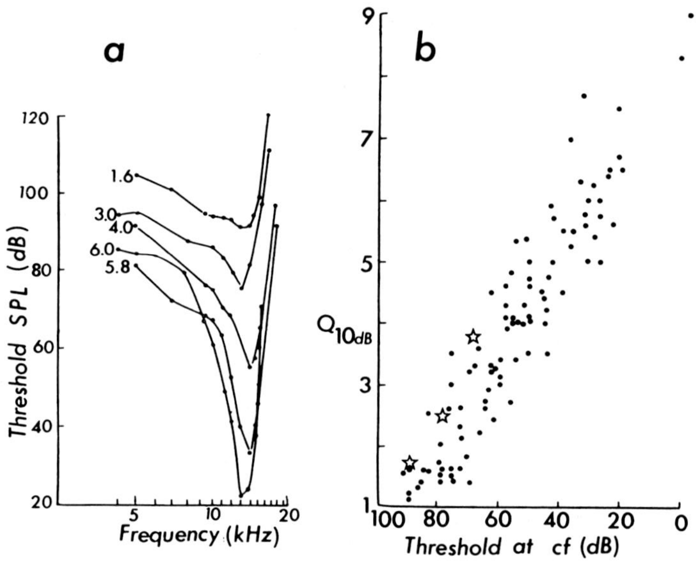

Fig. 7a. Representative tuning curves each from a different animal showing the gradation in sensitivity and sharpness of the tuning curves. FTCs were obtained from the spiral ganglion of the guinea pig.

b. Pooled data from 94 cells showing the close relationship between Q_{10dB} and the threshold at the CF. The range of CFs included is 12-19 kHz; closed circles are the neural data from the spiral ganglion. Stars are the Q_{10dB} values from Rhode (1971) of the basilar membrane vibration at the 8 kHz point in the squirrel monkey. From Robertson and Manley (1974) *J. Comp. Physiol. 91*, 363-375, by permission of the authors.

Resistance Changes in Hair Cells During Sound Stimulation

Davis (1957) postulated that displacement of the cilia on the apical surface of the hair cells altered the resistance across the top of the cell and thus modulated the driving voltage between scala media and hair cell to produce the receptor potential.

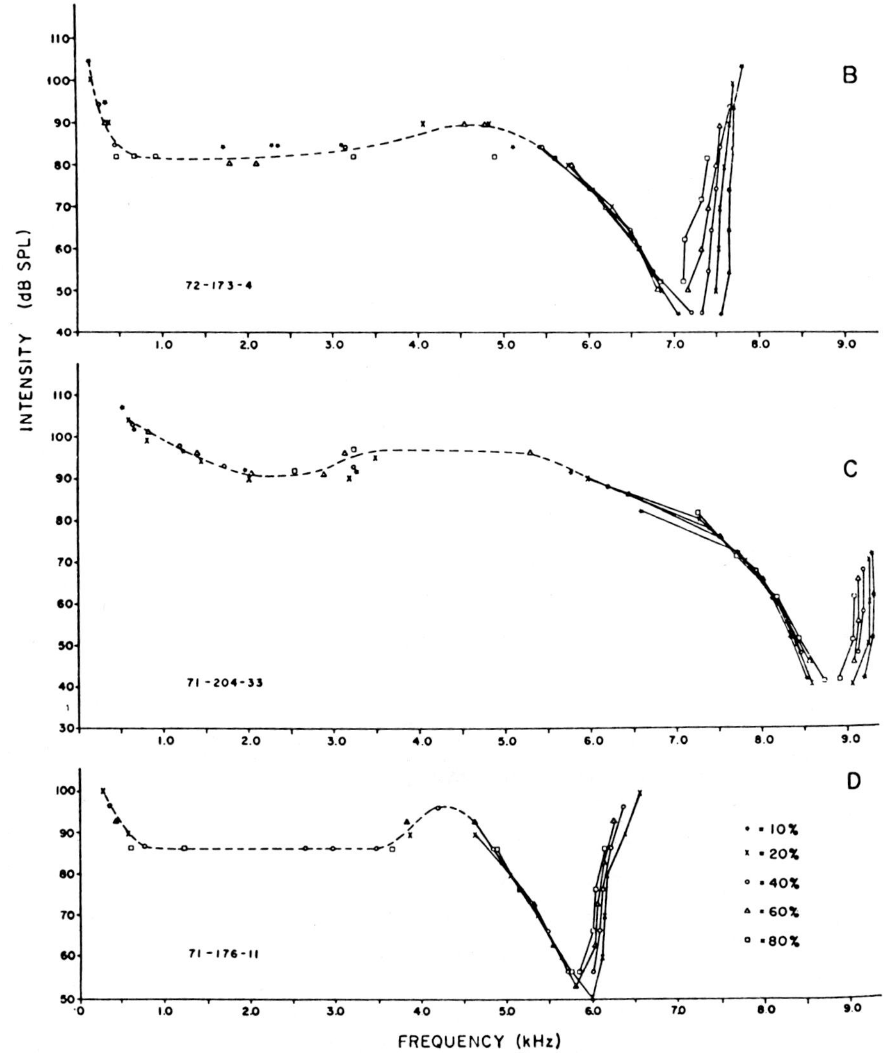

Fig. 8. Isorate contours for three nerve fibers with best frequencies between 6 and 9 kHz from the squirrel monkey. Curves are shifted vertically toward the 20% curve for best fit just below best frequency. For clarity, point at low frequences are not jointed by straight lines; rather a single representative curve is drawn. For each fibre, indicated rates are the increases, above its spontaneous rate, given in percentages of its dynamic range (defined here as maximum rate minus mean spontaneous rate). Note the lack of fit between curves for frequencies above CF. From Geisler et al (1973) *J. Neurophys. 37,* 1156-1172, by permission of the authors.

Such a resistance change has been observed in the scala media by Kurakawa (1965) Johnstone et al. (1966), Strelioff et al. (1971), Geisler et al. (1977). We have measured resistance changes intracellularly by injecting sinusoidal current and measuring the potential change with a lock-in amplifier during exposure to a swept pure tone stimulus. The results are illustrated in Figure 10. Note that the receptor

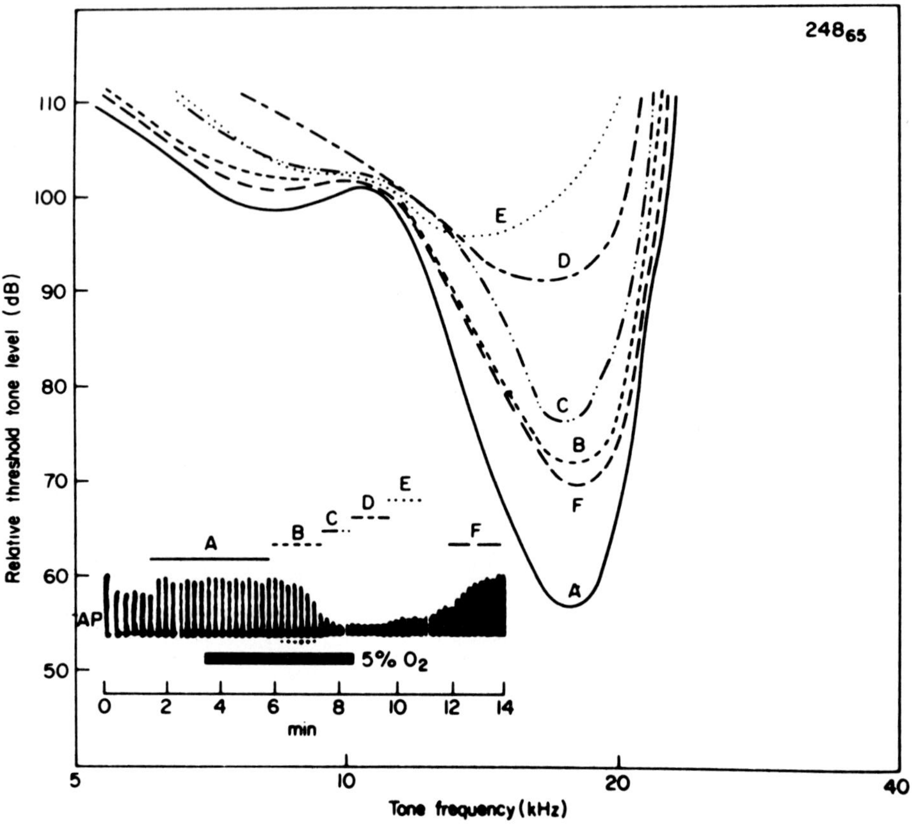

Fig. 9. Effect of hypoxia on the tuning of a single auditory nerve fibre in the cat. Inset shows time course of gross cochlear AP response amplitude to click stimuli of constant intensity presented at a rate of 1/10s. Black bar indicates duration of administration of 5% O_2 in N_2O. Bars over the AP record indicate the time during which determinations of the FTC for the fibre, illustrated in the main figure, were taken. The curves were determined from counts of the spike activity evoked during 60ms tone bursts (shaped to avoid artefacts) of frequency and intensity by an on-line computer to cover the frequency-intensity space of the figure in randomised order. The solid curve is the control FTC. The upper dotted curve is the FTC of the fibres at the height of the hypoxia, as judged from the AP record. The middle dashed curve was obtained during partial recovery of the cochlea from the hypoxia. (These curves have not been corrected for the characteristics of the sound system and therefore represent relative thresholds.) From Evans (1975) *Symp. Zool. Soc. Lond. 3,* 133-165, by permission of the author.

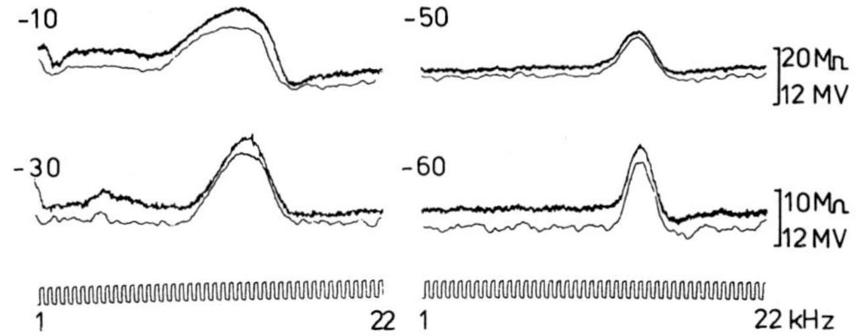

Fig. 10. DC potential change (upper trace) and resistance change (lower trace) recorded simultaneously from a presumed inner hair cell in response to a linearly swept pure tone. The numbers by the side of each pair of traces indicate the attenuation of the sound system, the frequency scale indicates 500 Hz intervals.

potential has a peak around CF and that the resistance change follows the potential change exactly. This is further demonstrated by the plot of resistance vs voltage in Figure 11. Similar plots were made for 8 other hair cells and their slopes were found to have a mean of 0.62 ± 0.18mV/MΩ (Russell and Sellick, 1978). At high SPLs (c. 100 dB) the resistance of the hair cell decreases by about 50% in those cells in which the total membrane resistance was measured.

THE BASIS OF FREQUENCY ANALYSIS IN THE COCHLEA

On the basis of our observations, two types of models can be excluded from forming the basis of the "sharpening" process of fibers in the auditory nerve. The tuning properties of auditory nerve fibers can be fully accounted for by those of the individual inner hair cells and, therefore, the possibility can be excluded that the FTCs of nerve fibers are due to interaction between each other (Zwislocki, 1974). Simultaneous measurements of resistance change and the DC component of the receptor potential recorded from inner hair cells demonstrate that they exactly mimic each other. Hence all of the potential change can be accounted for by the resistance change in the hair cell membrane. This excludes the possibility that the potential change is modified by an external source via electrotonic spread (Manley, 1977), unless such a potential source has exactly the same frequency response as the hair cell, and the resulting addition amounts to a change in gain of an existing finely tuned mechanism. Thus we are left with the conclusion that inner hair cells are mechanically tuned.

A comparison between hair cell FTCs and measurement of basilar membrane vibration in the same region of the guinea pig cochlea from which our recordings were made (Johnstone and Boyle, 1967; Wilson and Johnstone, 1975) reveal several important differences. The low frequency slopes of the mechanical FTCs are close to zero compared with the 45-253 dB/octave slopes of the hair cell FTCs. The high frequency slopes of the hair cell FTCs are steeper than those of the mechanical FTCs, being 340-500 dB/octave and 60-245 dB/octave respectively. The basilar membrane vibrations are linear between 40-120 dB SPL (the largest range over which the linearity was tested), while the intensity functions for the hair cell potentials at CF over this range are almost fully saturated. However the mechanical and hair cell FTCs show common CF or cut-off frequencies (Russell and Sellick, 1977b, 1978).

How might these differences in the tuning properties of the basilar membrane and those of hair cells be reconciled since we believe cochlear hair cells to be mechanically tuned? It is conceivable that the lack of similarity between guinea pig cochlea mechanical measurements and hair cell measurements are due to damage sustained by the basilar membrane when the mechanical measurements were made. For example, we have found that damage to the cochlea causing raised AP thresholds for tones above 10 kHz produced a reduction of the saturation effect around CF and a marked reduction in the low frequency slope (cell 211, Table 1, Fig. 12b). However, Evans and Wilson (1975) measured the basilar membrane response and FTCs from single fibers in the auditory nerve concurrently in the cat and found normal neural FTCs coexisting with basilar membrane responses that are essentially the same as those measured in the guinea pig.

A likely basis for reconcilliation is Davis' (1957) model of transduction in the organ of Corti. According to this, and from measurements in other acoustico-lateralis receptors (Harris et al., 1970; Flock, 1965, 1971), the excitatory stimulus is a shearing displacement of the sensory hairs on the apical surface of the hair cells. Thus the excitatory displacement in the organ of Corti occurs between the tectorial membrane and the reticular laminar, ie. at right angles to the measured vibration of the basilar membrane.

We have a direct measure of the tuning properties of this shear displacement in the tuning properties of the AC component of the receptor potential, which is generally accepted to reflect the mechanical stimulus to the hair cells as it does in hair cells in other sense organs (Flock, 1971; Weiss et al., 1974; Hudspeth and Corey, 1977; Sand et al., 1975). Thus the effective shear displacement in the first turn of the guinea pig (and cat) cochlea does not reflect the vibration of the basilar membrane.

A different picture has emerged from measurements of basilar membrane motion at the 6-8 kHz region of the squirrel monkey with the Mössbauer technique by Rhode (1971). He found two important effects which contrast with the guinea pig data. Firstly, the low-frequency amplitude slope was not smooth but had a region of slope about 30 dB/octave near CF. Secondly, he found a substantial nonlinearity at the CF and down the high frequency slope. The lower frequencies were linear (Fig. 5a). These are qualitatively similar to the nonlinearities observed in the

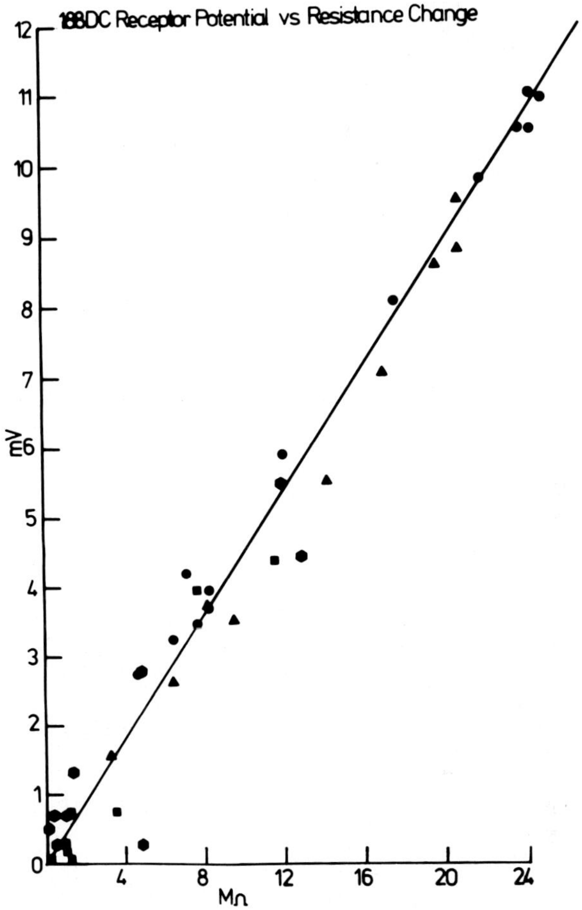

Fig. 11. Relationship between receptor potential and resistance change from a presumed inner hair cell in response to a swept pure tone.

hair cell receptor potential. However, the measurements do not account for the neural and hair cell FTCs quantitatively. The difference is most noticeable in the frequency region just below CF where the basilar membrane measurements lack a sharp valley of about 40 dB that always occurs in the neural data. The difference is not due to the data being collated at different SPLs as shown by Geisler et al. (1974), who compared 80% isorate neural contours with isoamplitude mechanical measurements made at similar SPLs.

The similarities between Rhode's data and the receptor potential measurements is most striking when the predictions of a model devised by Kim et al. (1973)

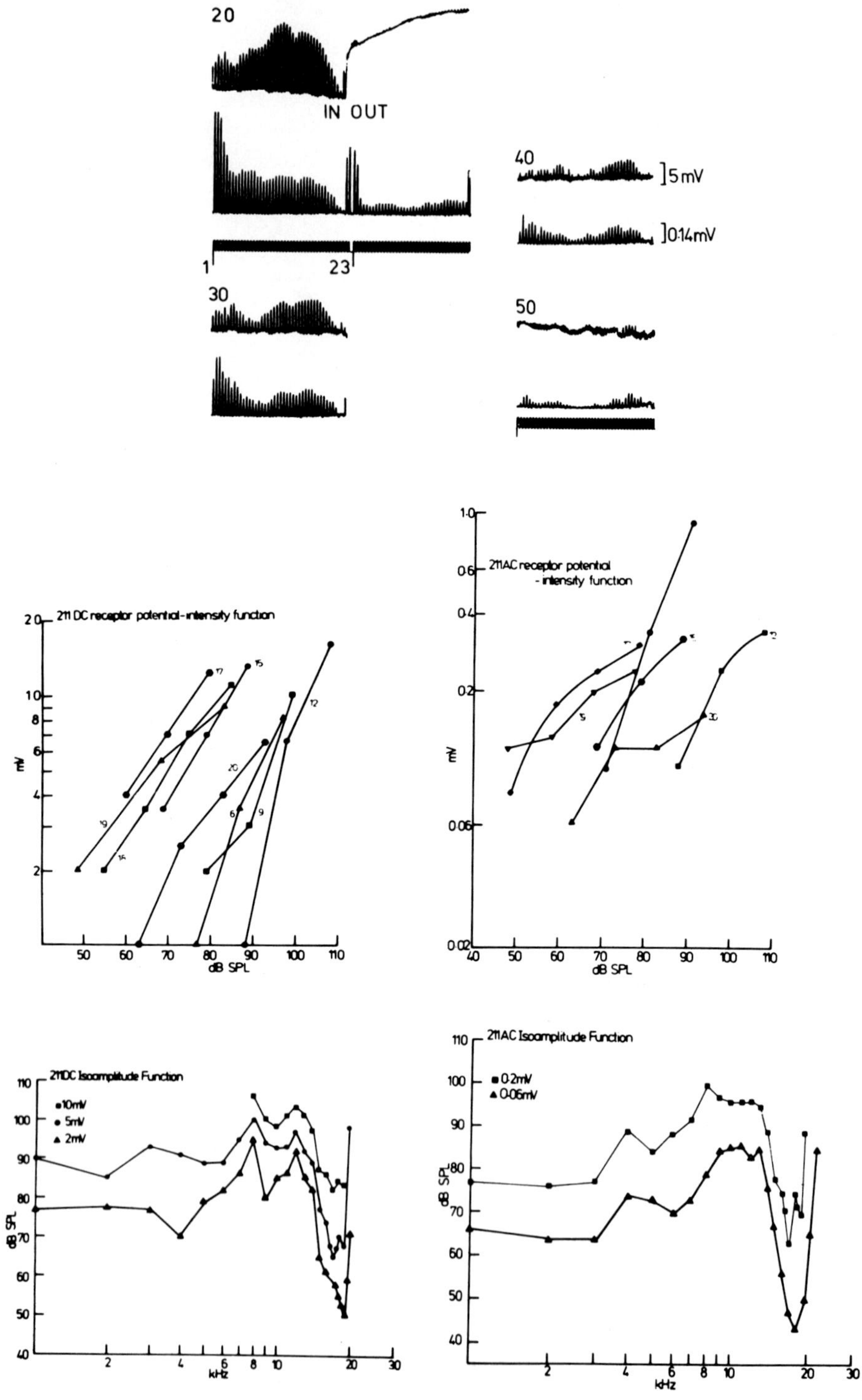
20
IN OUT
1
23
30
40
]5 mV
]0·14mV
50
211 DC receptor potential-intensity function
mV
dB SPL
211AC receptor potential - intensity function
mV
dB SPL
211DC Isoamplitude Function
10mV
5mV
2mV
dB SPL
kHz
211AC Isoamplitude Function
0·2mV
0·06mV
dB SPL
kHz

based on Rhode's data are considered (Fig. 5). Intensity functions predicted by the model for frequencies around CF are remarkably similar to those for the intracellular receptor potential and predict a decrease in most effective frequency (CF) with increasing SPL due to a cross over of the intensity functions at high SPL. Hence, to a limited extent in the squirrel monkey, vibration of the basilar membrane in the 6-8 Hz region may reflect the shear displacement to the hair cells.

LABILITY OF TUNING

Evans (1972) reported that when recordings were made from the auditory nerve in the guinea pig under conditions where the cochlear blood supply was impaired through low systemic blood pressure the FTCs had high thresholds, were broadly tuned and resembled basilar membrane tuning curves. Robertson and Manley (1974), Evans and Klinke (1974) and Evans (1975b) showed that the neural FTC could be "detuned" reversibly by making the animal hypoxic. As can be seen from Figure 9 "detuning" consisted of a reduction of the threshold at CF by about 35 dB whereas the threshold of the low frequency tail was altered to smaller degree. This results in a broadening of the FTC since the CF threshold moves close to the level of the low frequency tail. In the extreme, a shift in CF towards low frequencies was observed. Robertson and Manley found a linear relationship between Q_{10dB} and threshold at CF, reflecting the broadening of the FTC with increased CF threshold (Fig. 7). Similar effects could be produced by instilling cyanide or furosamide into the scala tympani (Evans and Klinke, 1974). The fact that neural FTCs could be detuned by metabolic manipulation of the cochlea so that they resembled the more broadly tuned basilar membrane mechanical response lead to the hypothesis of a labile second filter situated in series with the mechanical filter of the basilar membrane (Evans, 1975b).

Many of the recordings that we have made from hair cells in the cochlea display the "detuned" characteristics described above and this is usually the result of surgical damage inflicted during exposure of the basilar membrane. The AP threshold to frequencies above 10 kHz are raised by as much as 40 dB and it is noted that the extracellular summating potential recorded during the approach through the organ of Corti is markedly reduced. The response to high SPL is similar to that recorded for sensitive cells as shown in Figure 1a; however, as the SPL is reduced

Fig. 12a. DC (upper trace) and AC (lower trace) receptor potentials of 80ms tone bursts from an insensitive cell. Legend as for Figure 1.

b. Intensity functions for the DC and AC component of the receptor potential. The numbers by the side of each curve indicate frequency in kHz.

c. Isoamplitude curves for the DC and AC component of the receptor potential.

the tuned response at CF disappears. The isoamplitude curves for these cells (Fig. 12c) are similar in shape to those of the insensitive cells found by Robertson and Manley (Fig. 7). We suggest that these cells are analogous to the fibers recorded under pathological conditions.

Since we have not yet carried out the procedure of making the animal anoxic during recording, it is difficult to tell what happens to the potentials during hypoxic detuning. However it is interesting to speculate from the receptor potential intensity functions how the neural FTCs could change their shape during hypoxia. We have previously speculated (Russell and Sellick, 1977a, 1977b) that detuning could be explained by simple reduction of the receptor potential or a rise in the threshold of the afferent synapse. From the data we had at the time which consisted of relatively detuned cells, an increase in the amplitude criterion of the FTC above 2mV resulted in movement into the saturated region of the CF intensity function so that the tip of the FTC moved up more rapidly than the low frequency tail resulting in a broadening of the FTC. This contrasted to the finding of Evans (1975c) that for higher rate criterion the neural FTC became narrower, ie. the Q_{10dB} increased. Now that we have data from more sensitive cells we see that this is indeed the case and that the increase in Q_{10dB} with increasing amplitude criterion occurs in a region where the intensity functions with frequencies below CF are still linear but where those above CF have reached saturation as explained above. Hence an increase in amplitude criterion produces first an increase in Q_{10dB} while the CF intensity function is linear and then a rapid decrease as the amplitudes reach the saturated region of the CF intensity function. It therefore follows that the relationship between Q_{10dB} and threshold that Robertson and Manley observed could not be produced by a reduction of receptor potential amplitude or increase in afferent threshold alone.

However, it is likely that a reduction in receptor potential amplitude occurs during hypoxic detuning. Manley and Robertson (1976) used an electrode in scala media to measure the endocochlear potential and SP while simultaneously monitoring single unit threshold. They found that during hypoxia the unit threshold at CF increased by 50 dB and this was accompanied by a decrease in endocochlear potential and summating potential of 30mV and 75% respectively. If neural threshold corresponds to a receptor potential of 2mV then, from the intensity functions, a 75% decrease in amplitude of receptor potential would result in a loss of threshold of 20-30 dB at CF. It should be emphasized that this figure is critically dependent upon the magnitude of the receptor potential at neural threshold and it is conceivable that this may increase radically during hypoxia thus increasing the threshold loss.

The other mechanism that we have to invoke to explain the lability of tuning must have the effect of moving the intensity curves around CF towards higher SPLs as is seen to happen for the detuned cell in Figure 12 in comparison with these sensitive cells illustrated in Figure 3a and b and in the neural rate functions during hypoxia (Evans, 1975a). This would have the effect of increasing the threshold at CF and reducing the Q_{10dB} simultaneously. Such an effect could be produced by detuning the mechanical stimulus to the top of the hair cells. Thus we suggest that detuning of the neural FTCs is the result of at least two mechanisms, a reduction in the magnitude of the receptor potentials across the frequency spectrum and a detuning of the mechanics that produce the stimulus to the hair cells.

Abnormal or detuned FTCs have been recorded from animals after treatment with Kanamycin, an antibiotic which has been shown to selectively destroy the outer hair cells (Kiang et al., 1970; Dallos et al., 1977; Evans and Harrison, 1976). It has been suggested (Dallos et al., 1977) that the outer hair cells interact in some way with the inner hair cells in order to produce normal FTCs. The present study has little to say about the role of outer hair cells except to exclude either neural or electrotonic interactions.

Acknowledgements

We thank Professor Brian Johnstone and Dr. Thomas Collett for their valued criticism of the manuscript, and Miss Wendy Randall for excellent technical assistance. This research was supported by a research grant from the M.R.C. and an equipment grant from the charities panel of the Reader's Digest.

REFERENCES

Adrian, E.D. The microphonic action of the cochlea in relation to theories of hearing. In: *Report of a Discussion on Audition, Phys. Soc. London,* 1931, p. 5-9.

Békésy, G.von, *Experiments in Hearing,* New York: McGraw Hill, 1960.

Brown, K.T. and Flaming, D.G. Instrumentation and technique for bevelling fine micropipette electrodes. *Brain Res. 86:* 172-180, 1975.

Dallos, P. *The Auditory Periphery.* New York: Academic Press, 1973.

Dallos, P., Ryan, A., Harris, D., McGee, T. and Ozdamar, O. Cochlear frequency selectivity in the presence of hair cell damage. In: *Psychophysics and Physiology of Hearing,* edited by E.F. Evans and J.P. Wilson. London: Academic Press, 1977, p. 249-261.

Davis, H. *Biophysics and Physiology of the inner ear. Physiol. Rev. 37:* 1-49, 1957.

Duifhuis, H. Cochlear nonlinearity and second filter; possible mechanism and implications. *J. Acoust. Soc. Am. 59:* 408-423, 1976.

Evans, E.F. The frequency response and other properties of single fibers in the guinea pig cochlear nerve. *J. Physiol. Lond. 226:* 263-287, 1972.

Evans, E.F. The sharpening of cochlear frequency selectivity in the normal and abnormal cochlea. *Audiology 14:* 419-442, 1975a.

Evans, E.F. Normal and abnormal functioning of the cochlear nerve. *Symp. Zool. Soc. Lond. 3:* 133-165, 1975b.

Evans, E.F. Cochlear Nerve and Cochlear Nucleus. In: *Handbook of Sensory Physiology. V/2,* edited by W.D. Keidel and W.D. Neff. Berlin, Heidelburg, New York: Springer-Verlag, 1975c, p. 1-108.

Evans, E.F. Frequency selectivity at high signal levels of single units in cochlear nerve and nucleus. In: *Psychophysics and Physiology of Hearing,* edited by E.F. Evans and J.P. Wilson. London: Academic Press, 1977, p. 185-192.

Evans, E.F. and Klinke, R. Reversible effects of cyanide and furosamide on the tuning of single cochlear fibers. *J. Physiol. Lond. 242:* 129-131P, 1974.

Evans, E.F. and Wilson, J.P. Cochlear tuning properties: concurrent basilar membrane and single nerve fiber measurements. *Science 190,* 1218-1221, 1975.

Evans, E.F. and Harrison, R.V. Correlation between cochlear outer hair cell damage and deterioration of cochlear nerve tuning properties in the guinea pig. *J. Physiol. Lond. 256:* 43-44P, 1976.

Flock, Å. Electron microscopic and electrophysiological studies on the lateral line canal organ. *Acta Otolaryngol.* Suppl. *199:* 1-90, 1965.

Flock, Å. Sensory transduction in hair cells. In: *Handbook of Sensory Physiology, 1,* edited by W. Lowenstein. Berlin, Heidelberg, New York: Springer-Verlag, 1971, p. 396-441.

Flock, Å., Jorgensen, M. and Russell, I.J. The physiology of individual hair cells and their synapses. In: *Basic Mechanisms in Hearing,* edited by A.R. Møller. New York: Academic Press, 1973, p. 273-306.

Geisler, C.D., Rhode, W.S. and Kennedy, D.T. Responses to tonal stimuli of single auditory nerve fibers and their relationship to basilar membrane motion in the squirrel monkey. *J. Neurophysiol. 37:* 1156-1172, 1974.

Geisler, C.D., Mountain, D.C., Hubbard, A.E., Adrian, H.O. and Ravindran, A. Alternating electrical-resistance changes in the guinea pig cochlea caused by acoustic stimuli. *J. Acoust. Soc. Am. 61:* 1557-1566, 1977.

Harris, G.G., Frischkopf, L.S. and Flock, Å. Receptor potentials from hair cells in the lateral line. *Science 167:* 76-79, 1970.

Honrubia, V. and Ward, P.H. The longitudal distribution of cochlea microphonic potentials inside the cochlea duct. *J. Acoust. Soc. Am. 44:* 951-958, 1968.

Hudspeth, A.J. and Corey, D.P. Sensitivity, polarity and conductance change in the response of vertebrate hair cells to controlled mechanical stimuli. *Proc. Natl. Acad. Sci. 74:* 2407-2411, 1977.

Johnstone, B.M., and Boyle, A.J.F. Basilar membrane vibration examined with the mossbauer technique. *Science 158:* 389-390, 1967.

Johnstone, B.M., Johnstone, J.R. and Pugsley, I.D. Membrane resistance in endolymphatic walls of the first turn of the guinea pig cochlea. *J. Acoust. Soc. Am. 40:* 1398-1404, 1966.

Johnstone, J.R. Properties of ganglion cells from the extreme basal region of guinea pig cochlea. In: *Psychophysics and Physiology of Hearing,* edited by E.F. Evans and J.P. Wilson. London: Academic Press, 1977, p. 89-99.

Kiang, N.Y., Moxon, E.C. and Levine, R.A. Auditory-nerve activity in cats with normal and abnormal cochleas. In: *Sensorineural hearing loss,* edited by G.E.W. Wolstenholme and J. Knight, London: Churchill, 1970, p. 241-268.

Kim, D.O., Molnar, C.E. and Pfeiffer, R.R. A system of non-linear differential equations modeling basilar-membrane motion, *J. Acoust. Soc. Am. 54:* 1517-1529, 1973.

Kurakawa, S. Experimental study of electrical resistance of basilar membrane in guinea pig. *J. Oto-Rhino-Laryngol. Soc. Jap. 68:* 1177-1195, 1965.

Manley, G.A. Frequency dependent extracellular interaction between hair cells as a possible mechanism for cochlear frequency sharpening. In: *Psychophysics and Physiology of Hearing,* edited by E.F. Evans and J.P. Wilson. London: Academic Press, 1977, p. 139-146.

Manley, G.A. and Robertson, D. Analysis of spontaneous activity of auditory neurones in the spiral ganglion of the guinea pig cochlea. *J. Physiol. Lond. 258:* 323-336, 1976.

Nieder, P. Addressed delay line theory of cochlear organization. *Nature 230:* 255-257, 1971.

Pinto, L.H. and Pak, W.L. Light-induced changes in photoreceptor membrane resistance and potential in Gecko retinas. *J. Gen. Physiol. 64:* 26-48, 1974.

Rhode, W.S. Observations of the vibration of the basilar membrane in squirrel monkeys using the Mossbauer technique. *J. Acoust. Soc. Am. 49:* 1218-1231, 1971.

Robertson, D. Cochlear neurons; frequency selectivity altered by perilymph removal. *Science 186:* 135-155, 1974.

Robertson, D. and Manley, G.A. Manipulation of Frequency analysis in the cochlear ganglion of the guinea pig. *J. Comp. Physiol. 91:* 363-375, 1974.

Rose, J.E., Brugge, J.F., Anderson, D.J. and Hind, J.E. Phase locked response to low-frequency tones in single auditory nerve fibers of the squirrel monkey. *J. Neurophysiol. 30:* 769-793, 1967.

Russell, I.J. and Sellick, P.M. The tuning properties of cochlear hair cells. In: *Psychophysics and Physiology of Hearing,* edited by E.F. Evans and J.P. Wilson. London: Academic Press, 1977a, p. 71-87.

Russell, I.J. and Sellick, P.M. Tuning properties of cochlear hair cells. *Nature 267:* 858-860, 1977b.

Russell, I.J. and Sellick, P.M. Intracellular studies of hair cells in the guinea pig cochlear. (Submitted for publication, 1978).

Sachs, M.B. and Abbas, P.J. Rate versus level functions for auditory nerve fibers in cats; tone burst stimuli. *J. Acoust. Soc. Am. 56:* 1835-1847, 1974.

Sand, O., Ozawa, S. and Hagiwara, S. Electrical and mechanical stimulation of hair cells in the mudpuppy. *J. Comp. Physiol. A 102:* 13-26, 1975.

Schroeder, M.R. and Hall, J.L. Model for mechanical to neural transduction in the auditory receptor. *J. Acoust. Soc. Am. 55:* 1055-1060, 1974.

Spoendlin, H. Innervation patterns in the organ of Corti of the cat. *Acta Otolaryngol. 67:* 239-254, 1969.

Steele, C.R. A possibility for sub-tectorial membrane fluid motion. In: *Basic Mechanisms in Hearing,* edited by A.R. Mφller. New York: Academic Press, 1973, p. 69-90.

Strelioff, D., Haas, G. and Honrubia, V. Sound induced electrical impedance changes in the guinea pig cochlea. *J. Acoust. Soc. Am. 51:* 617-620, 1971.

Tonndorf, J. Shearing motion in scala media of cochlear models. *J. Acoust. Soc. Am. 32:* 238-244, 1960.

Weiss, T.F., Mulroy, M.J. and Altman, D.W. Intracellular responses to acoustic clicks in the inner ear of the alligator lizard. *J. Acoust. Soc. Am. 55:* 606-621, 1974.

Wilson, J.P. and Johnstone, J.R. Basilar membrane and middle-ear vibration in guinea pig measured by capacitive probe. *J. Acoust. Soc. Am. 57:* 705-723, 1975.

Zwislocki, J.H. A possible neuro-mechanical frequency analysis in the cochlea. *Acustica 31:* 354-359, 1974.

DISCUSSION

Brownell: Did you record from outer hair cells? If so, did they display large resting membrane potentials? Bobbin (*Arch. Otolaryngol. 102:* 45-48, 1976) and others (for review, see Fex in *Handbook of Sensory Physiology, Vol. V/1,* Springer-Verlag, 1974) have been unable to associate outer hair cells with negative DC shifts, leaving open the possibility that outer hair cells may be electrically transparent. A small resting membrane potential would be consistent with Dr. Catherine Smith's comment earlier in this symposium, that the outer hair cell plasma membrane appears "leaky".

Russell: We have never managed to dye-mark outer hair cells and have, therefore, so far failed to obtain morphological correlates of our recordings from the outer hair cell region.

Spoendlin: How do your results fit with Evans' findings of the highly tuned segment of the tuning curve?

Russell: It really comes down to the role of the outer hair cells. We think one of the roles of outer hair cells is to mechanically tune inner hair cells but we don't know how. It may follow from Flock's (1977) finding that stereocilia are stiff and are probably composed of actin-like filaments, and that their stiffness may be controlled by intracellular calcium levels. If this is so, then their mechanical properties would be metabolically labile. So perhaps what we are dealing with here is with a metabolically labile mechanical filter. I don't find any basis for discrepancy between our results and Evans (1973) and I can imagine a metabolically labile mechanical filter.

Nuttall: Some of the data you have would indicate that you had to get measurements over a long period of time from a single cell. Would you care to comment on how difficult it is to hold a cell, and how you overcame these difficulties?

Russell: Peter Sellick was a young man when he started this project. Our success rate is low and in the last four months of recording we have had perhaps a dozen really good cells, even though we experiment almost every day. We have recorded from many cells for only a few seconds; however, we have recorded from the ones we have reported here for at least five minutes and up to half an hour, with constant resting potentials. The properties of the recording electrode are the major limiting factors.

Bennett: Do you see any electrical response of these cells when you stimulate them? How many are there, or what is the IV relationship?

Russell: We have never measured IV relationships on the cochlear hair cells. There is a paper by Hudspeth and Corey (1977) who recorded calcium spikes from hair cells in the hearing organ of the frog, when they exposed the hair cells to a very unusual environment resembling perilymph, with a high calcium concentration. It may be that the electrical properties of the hair cells in Hudspeth and Corey's preparation were changed by their unusual environment.

Galambos: Would you reiterate that tangential motion theory you ended up with.

Russell: I simply wanted to say that if one believes that the AC component of the receptor potential was an electrical analogue of the mechanical displacement of the tops of the hair cells, then our results would indicate that the mechanical displacement at the top of the hair cells, the shear displacement, was different from that of the basilar membrane motion. It was far sharper.

Galambos: Is this idea of yours the same as Békésy's, or different?

Russell: We have not ruled out any of his theories, as far as I can see.

Galambos: Didn't Békésy also postulate tangential motion somewhere near the peak?

Russell: Yes, as far as I can remember, but he thought that the up-and-down motion of the basilar membrane closely resembled the shear displacement.

Bennett: These are beautiful records, and they lay to rest some of the speculations that I was making this morning, but not all of them. There would still be hope for regenerative responsiveness in tuning out in the low-frequency cells, and I gather you are only looking at the high-frequency ones. Have you looked at the low-frequency cells in the apical portion?

Russell: No, we haven't.

Bennett: One thing is very intriguing, and you may have some information on it. The carbon microphone theory in its simplest form suggests you should get an AC signal in the cell unless the hairs, the mechanosensory portion, are all the way pushed over so it is completely shut. If that were true, which your records are suggesting, because you are not seeing any AC signal – or are you?

Russell: Very slight.

Bennett: All right. So it is major AC, and it can be AC associated with DC pulses rather than a hyperpolarization that you would expect to see with the onset of a singleness of opposite phase with the carbon microphone theory. If the carbon microphone were already shut you would expect to see some nonlinearity as you get over to the point where it really opened. Maybe you have an answer to that.

Russell: We would need to record the responses of cells at low frequencies, below their electrical cut-off frequencies, in order to investigate this point; this is something we have not done.

Trahiotis: Could you say something about the phase relationship between the outer potential and the stimulus?

Russell: No. The problem there is that we don't know the phase rolloff of our microelectrodes, so we are able to make only relative phase changes for different amplitudes at fixed frequencies.

COCHLEAR ELECTROPHYSIOLOGY

Peter Dallos

Northwestern University

Most contemporary workers in the field of hearing accept, at least as a departure point, the basic notions of the resistance modulation scheme of the cochlear function as formulated by Davis (1965). This familiar model can be reviewed with the aid of Figure 1 where a sketch of the cross section of the cochlea is overlaid with its electrical equivalent circuit. It is assumed that "biological batteries" maintain a resting potential difference between scala media and the interior of hair cells (only an outer hair cell is shown in the figure) and that the inherent electrical properties of the various cochlear boundaries may be represented as constant resistances. It is further assumed that a mechanical deformation of the hair cell causes its electrical resistance to be altered, thus the hair cell is represented as a variable resistor. When this latter resistance is changed, the current flowing in the circuit is necessarily altered. This variable, stimulus-dependent, current component through the hair cell is the receptor current. When measuring anywhere in the circuit one could detect voltage drops due to the receptor current, these may be called receptor potentials. One usually distinguishes two receptor potential components, the ac cochlear microphonic (CM) and the dc summating potential (SP). The final assumption of the resistance modulation scheme is that the receptor current initiates and regulates synaptic transmission between hair cell and afferent neurons by controlling the release of synaptic transmitter substances from the infranuclear zone of the hair cells.

Virtually all components of this scheme have been studied in detail. Some of these are now well understood, others are still under intense scrutiny. There are several recent publications that summarize facets of cochlear physiology (Eldredge, 1974; Fex, 1974; Johnstone and Sellick, 1972; Dallos, 1973a, 1973b, 1975, 1978). These works are recommended for detailed study of the physiological properties of the cochlear transducer. The present communication is confined to a brief cataloguing of the salient features of the resistance modulation scheme and of some unresolved issues related to these, as well as a somewhat more detailed treatment of the gross receptor potentials. Many of the former topics are considered by others during this Symposium, and the latter has great importance to those who seek to relate the evoked electrical activity of the cochlea to auditory function.

In Davis' scheme the biological batteries are identified with the stria vascularis

ISBN 0-12-514960-3

and with the ordinary inside-negative polarization of the hair cells. The marginal cell layer of the stria is presumably specialized to move potassium into the sodium out of the endolymph filling the cochlear duct. This process is thought to be accomplished by an active electrogenic membrane pump that generates a high positive potential at its scala media pole. This potential, together with one of opposite

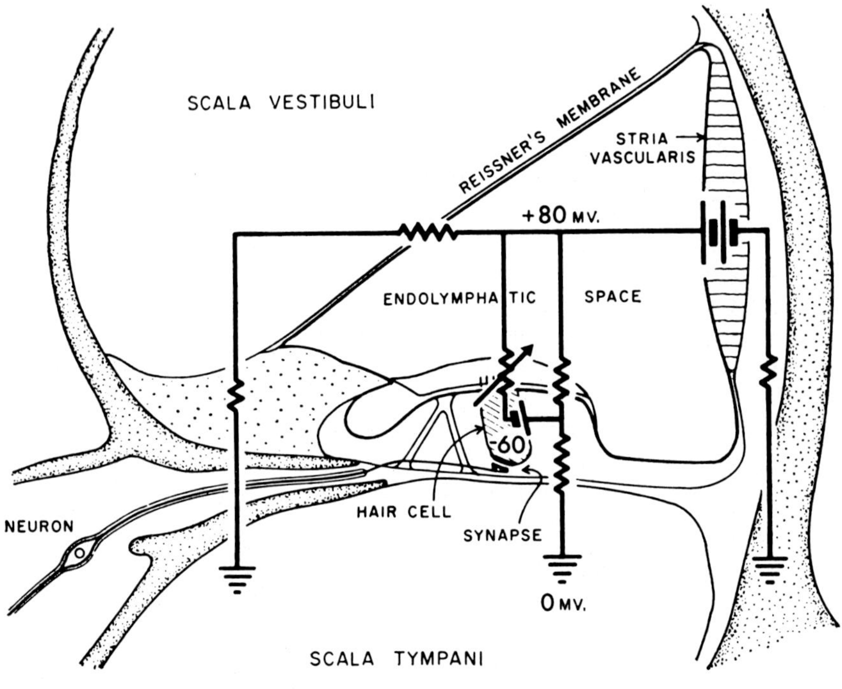

Fig. 1. Cross section of the cochlear canal with a simplified electrical network analog superimposed upon it (from Davis, 1965).

polarity sum to produce the familiar endocochlear potential (EP) measured within the endolymphatic space. The EP is between +70 and +100 mV with respect to neural tissue. It is usually assumed that the negative dc potential that affects the EP is the K^+ diffusion potential (see Johnstone and Sellick, 1972) across the membranes that bound the scala media. Other suggestions, however, have also been made (Sitko et al., 1976).

The intracellular negativity of the hair cells (60 to 80 mV) is maintained by the active sodium-potassium pump of their membranes. The older notion that there is an intercellular negative resting potential within the organ of Corti is now thought unlikely (see Fex, 1974). As a result of the various resting potentials within the cochlear space, a voltage gradient of up to 180 mV is established across the apical poles of the hair cells. In the Davis-scheme this potential difference provides the immediate electro-motive force that maintains a resting current through the receptor cells. The existence of an actual ionic resting current is not essential for the operation of the model but it is more parsimonious. It is most commonly thought that the resting current is carried by K^+ ions that are in abundance in the endolymph, however, at least in lateral line hair cells calcium is shown to be necessary for transduction (Sand, 1975). The identity, and in fact the existence, of a steady-state ion flux into the receptor cells is under active scrutiny.

The means of modulation of the resting current, in other words the detailed mechanism of hair cell transduction, is one of the least understood aspects of cochlear physiology. Several contributions to this Symposium relate to the subject of hair cell physiology, thus a further treatment here is unwarranted. The control of synaptic transmitter release by the receptor current is another poorly understood topic on which only limited indirect information is available (Flock, 1971; Fex, 1974).

The gross manifestation of the resistance modulation process is the receptor potential that can be measured from within or from the vicinity of the cochlea. This response reflects the sum of contributions from all active receptor cells and thus its quantitative relationship to the transmembrane potential of any individual hair cell is tenuous. The difficulties in estimating individual hair cell responses from the gross receptor potential stem from numerous causes. Among these are the graded (in amplitude and phase) excitation pattern of the receptors, possible differences in the excitation of inner and outer hair cells, the complex electrical network properties of the three-dimensional cochlear space, and the inherently nonlinear nature of the hair cell transduction process (Whitfield and Ross, 1965; Kohllöffel, 1971; Weiss et al., 1971; Dallos, 1973a). The more localized the pick-up area of the recording electrode(s), the more closely does the recorded gross response approximate the output of a limited number of hair cells. The most successful method of recording gross responses, the so called differential electrode technique, was introduced by Tasaki et al. (1952). The further removed the recording electrode is from the organ of Corti, the less quantitative information may be gleaned from the recording thus obtained. Assuming now that optimal techniques are used, one may inquire how the recorded gross receptor potentials relate to mechanical intracochlear events that precede them and to neural events that follow them.

In Figure 2 the ac and dc components of the potential gradient across the cochlear partition approximately 4 mm from the stapes are shown when the sound pressure at the eardrum is kept at a constant and moderate level throughout the frequency range. The CM (ac) response component, when measured at low sound levels, reflects the displacement magnitude (and also phase) of the cochlear partition in the vicinity of the recording electrodes. A comparison of the pattern shown here with the mechanical measurements of partition displacement in the same species (guinea pig) yields a remarkably good correspondence (Dallos, 1973b; Wilson, 1974). One measure of this agreement is the similarity of the high frequency cut-off frequencies in the CM and mechanical response curves. In Figure 3 median CM cut-off frequencies are shown for three cochlear locations along with

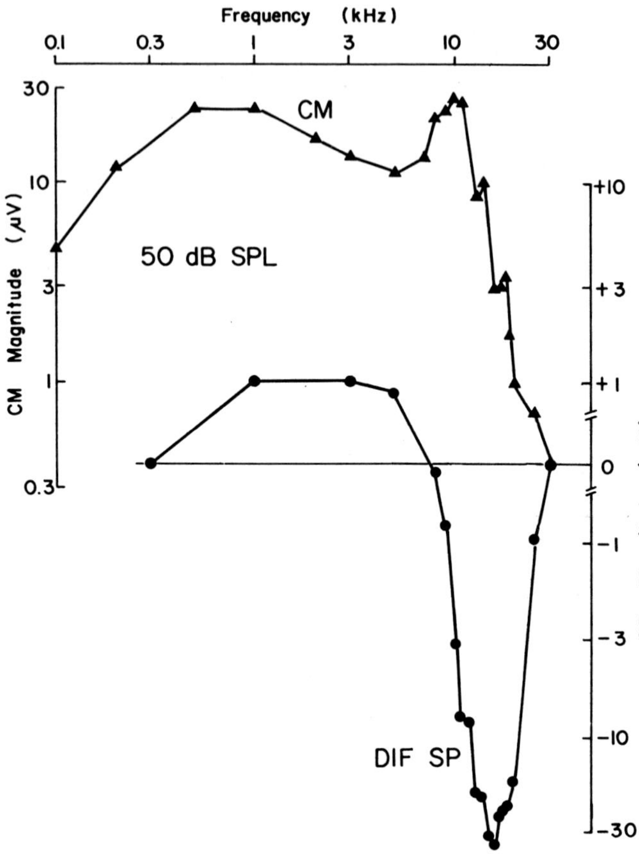

Fig. 2. Cochlear microphonic (CM) and summating potential (DIF SP) recorded from a first turn electrode pair in the guinea pig's cochlea at a constant 50 dB sound pressure level. (From Dallos 1973b).

individual mechanical cut-off frequencies from the work of Wilson and Johnstone (1972). The latter data points clearly fit the extrapolation of the straight line described by the CM data. Thus one may conclude that the gross CM reflects the salient properties of the basilar membrane displacement pattern. The same discrepancies that have been noted between the tuning characteristics of single auditory nerve fibers and basilar membrane displacement (Evans and Wilson, 1973) also exist between CM and neural responses. It is then possible that the CM represents the output characteristics of the "first filter" of the cochlea. Aside from the CM frequency response pattern, other characteristics of the ac receptor potential also indicate that this response arises in an earlier stage of transduction than what is reflected in the neural discharge patterns. Experiments with two-component signals are particularly useful to dramatize these differences. Numerous properties of the distortion component $2f_1$-f_2 are such that they are not compatible with those seen in the neural response (Dallos, 1969). The suppression of the CM response to a given input in the presence of a second signal (interference phenomenon) also possesses characteristics unlike the parallel phenomenon in the neural response (two-tone suppression) (Dallos et al., 1974).

The frequency response of the dc potential gradient across the cochlear partition is very different from that of the CM. At frequencies below the best frequency of the recording location (where the travelling wave peaks) the SP is positive. In the conventional terminology this means that scala vestibuli is positive with respect to scala tympani. As frequency increases an abrupt transition from SP^+ to SP^- is seen. Figure 2 clearly shows that the SP^- component is narrowly tuned. Various experiments with two-tone interactions indicate that the SP^+ response behaves very similar to the CM (Dallos and Cheatham, 1977, unpublished data). In contrast, the SP^- component appears to be a more specialized response and its tuning properties suggest that it may be more closely related to neural excitation than the CM. The particular discrepancy between CM and SP^-, in which the latter appears to have higher cut-off frequencies than the former, might be a consequence of the complex network properties of the mammalian cochlea. It is worth noting that in the rela-

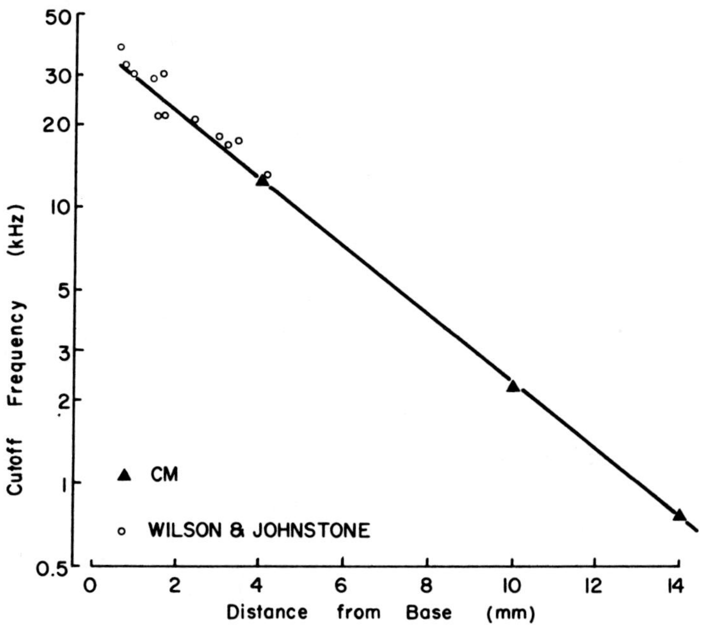

Fig. 3. Median cut-off frequencies in turns one, two, and three for CM (▲). For comparison the mechanical cut-off frequencies obtained in individual animals by Wilson and Johnstone (1972) are also shown (o). (From Dallos, 1973b).

tively straight cochlea of the pigeon the CM and SP are tuned to the same frequency (Pierson and Dallos, 1976). The narrow tuning of the SP⁻ is seen only at low sound pressure levels. While at its peak-frequency and SP⁻ grows linearly with signal intensity, the low frequency transition between SP^+ and SP^- moves to ever lower frequencies. Thus the bandwidth of SP^- increases radically with sound level. The patterns of families of SP^- versus frequency plots at various intensities are highly reminiscent to groups of auditory nerve discharge rate curves under similar conditions (for example Rose et al., 1971 compared with Dallos et al., 1970).

Acknowledgement

This work is supported by grants from the NINCDS and a John Simon Guggenheim Fellowship.

REFERENCES

Dallos, P. Combination tone $2f_1$-f_h in microphonic potentials. *J. Acoust. Soc. Am. 46:* 1437-1444, 1969.

Dallos, P. *The Auditory Periphery. Biophysics and Physiology.* New York: Academic Press, 1973a.

Dallos, P. Cochlear potentials and cochlear mechanics. In: *Basic Mechanisms in Hearing,* edited by A. Møller. New York: Academic Press, 1973b, p. 335-372.

Dallos, P. Cochlear potentials. In: *The Nervous System, 3. Human Communication and its Disorders,* edited by E. Eagles. New York: Raven Press, 1975, p. 69-80.

Dallos, P. Peripheral mechanisms of hearing. In: *Handbook of Physiology. Sensory Processes,* edited by I. Darian-Smith. Bethesda: American Physiological Society, 1978 (To be published).

Dallos, P., Cheatham, M.A. and Ferraro, J. Cochlear mechanics, nonlinearities, and cochlear potentials. *J. Acoust. Soc. Am. 55:* 597-605, 1974.

Dallos, P., Schoeny, Z.G. and Cheatham, M.A. Cochlear summating potentials: composition. *Science 170:* 641-644, 1970.

Davis, H. A model for transducer action in the cochlea. *Cold Spr. Harb. Symp. Quant. Biol. 30:* 181-190, 1965.

Eldredge, D.H. Inner ear-cochlear mechanics and cochlear potentials. In: *Handbook of Sensory Physiology. V/1. Auditory System: Clinical and Special Topics,* edited by W.D. Keidel and W.D. Neff. Berlin, Heidelberg, New York: Springer-Verlag, 1974, p. 549-584.

Evans, E.F. and Wilson, J.P. The frequency selectivity of the cochlea. In: *Basic Mechanisms in Hearing,* edited by A. Møller. New York: Academic Press, 1973, p. 519-551.

Fex, J. Neural excitatory processes of the inner ear. In: *Handbook of Sensory Physiology. V/1, Auditory System: Clinical and Special Topics,* edited by W.D. Keidel and W.D. Neff. Berlin, Heidelberg, New York: Springer-Verlag, 1974, p. 585-646.

Flock, Å. Sensory transduction in hair cells. In: *Handbook of Sensory Physiology. I. Principles of Receptor Physiology,* edited by W.R. Loewenstein. Berlin, Heidelberg, New York: Springer-Verlag, 1971, p. 396-441.

Johnstone, B.M. and Sellick, P.M. The peripheral auditory apparatus. *Quart. Rev. Biophys. 5:* 1-57, 1972.

Kohllöffel, L.U.E. Studies of the distribution of cochlear potentials along the basilar membrane. *Acta Otolaryngol.* Suppl. *288:* 1-66, 1971.

Pierson, M. and Dallos, P. Re-examination of avian cochlear potentials. *Nature 262:* 599-601, 1976.

Rose, J.E., Hind, J.E., Anderson, D.J. and Brugge, J.F. Some effects of stimulus intensity on response of auditory nerve fibers in the squirrel monkey. *J. Neurophysiol. 34:* 685-699, 1971.

Sand, O. Effects of different ionic environments on the mechano-sensitivity of lateral line organs in the mudpuppy. *J. Comp. Physiol. 102:* 27-42, 1975.

Sitko, S.T., Strelioff, D. and Honrubia, V. Source and maintenance of the endocochlear potential. *Trans. Am. Acad. Ophthalmol. Otolaryngol. 82:* 328-335, 1976.

Tasaki, I., Davis, H. and Legouix, J.-P. The space-time pattern of the cochlear microphonics (guinea pig), as recorded by differential electrodes. *J. Acoust. Soc. Am. 24:* 502-518, 1952.

Weiss, T.F., Peake, W.T. and Sohmer, H.S. Intracochlear potential recorded with micropipets. II. Responses in the cochlear scalae to tones. *J. Acoust. Soc. Am. 50:* 587-601, 1971.

Whitfield, I.C. and Ross, H.F. Cochlear microphonic and summating potentials and the outputs of individual hair cell generators. *J. Acoust. Soc. Am. 38:* 126-131, 1965.

Wilson, J.P. Basilar membrane vibration data and their relation to theories of frequency analysis. In: *Facts and Models in Hearing,* edited by E. Zwicker and E. Terhardt. Berlin, Heidelberg, New York: Springer-Verlag, 1974, p. 56-63.

Wilson, J.P. and Johnstone, J.R. Capacitive probe measure of basilar membrane vibration. In: *Symposium on Hearing Theory.* Eindhoven: IPO, 1972, p. 172-181.

DISCUSSION

Trahiotis: Peter, how do these observations square with some of Zwislocki's ideas about inhibitory . . . .

Dallos: Not at all. I think that this is an important point. These experiments that deal with selective destruction of one population of hair cells and the maintenance of another population are difficult experiments, not to do, but to interpret. All we can hope for is that the cell population that remains in the cochlea actually functions the way it is supposed to, and there is no way of directly proving that.

The particular slide (Fig. 1) where I had the comparison between cochlear microphonic and summating potential obtained from outer hair cells alone versus inner hair cells alone, is probably the best piece of evidence that in fact the remaining cells do function. Why do I say that? Both of those preparations were obtained with the same method, namely, Kanamycin intoxication of the animal. In relatively modest doses of Kanamycin outer hair cells were eliminated in the basal part of the cochlea, while inner hair cells remained intact throughout, as determined with light microscopy. This situation yielded severe reduction of the receptor potentials. With extremely heavy doses of Kanamycin, the inner hair cells disappeared first from the apex before the outer hair cells, even though about 60% of the outer hair cells were gone as well. This is an incredibly damaged cochlea, yet the cochlear microphonic and summating potential in this situation recorded from the remaining hair cells (from the fourth turn) were near normal. That implies to me that in the converse situation when recording from inner hair cells alone, what you do see is probably real, and thus that there are significant sensitivity differences between the two hair cell populations.

There is no way of proving this, but if you make the assumption that the data reflect the actual operation of the cells (normal cells) then what seems to be needed

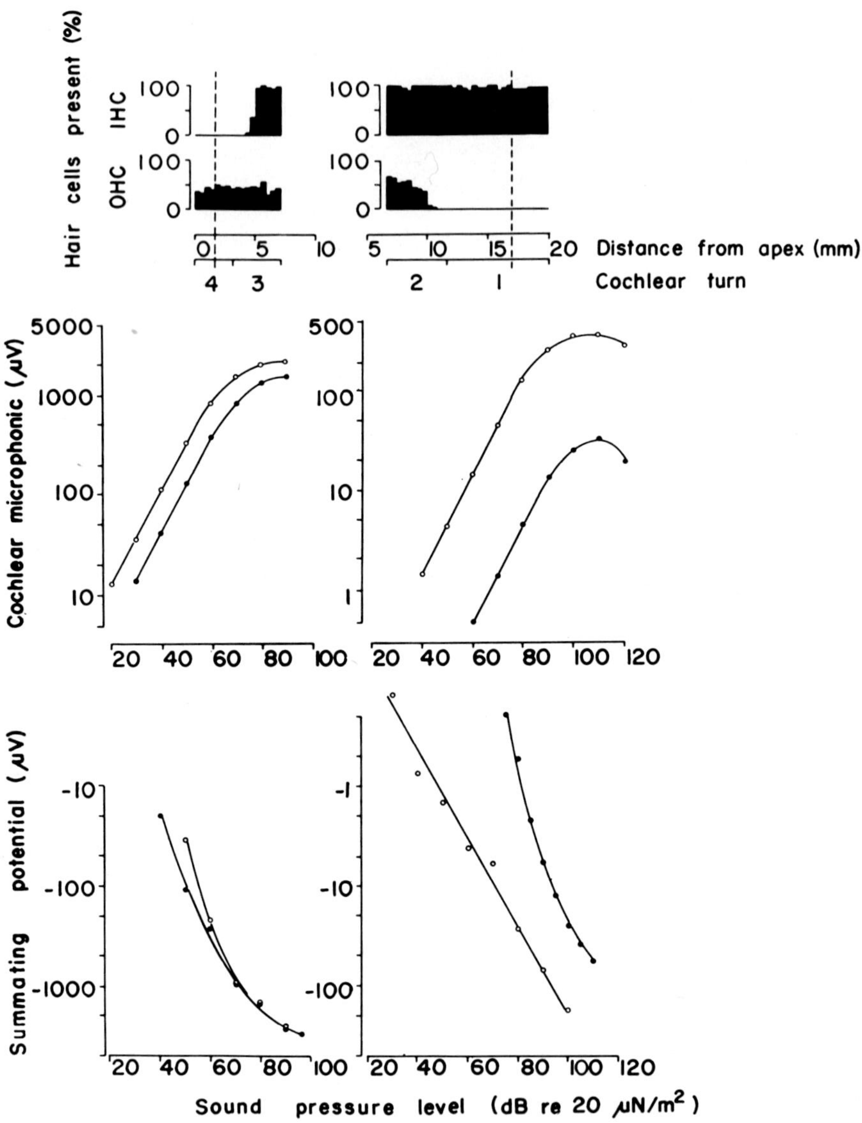

Dallos Discussion Figure 1

Cochleograms and physiological results from two representative Kanamycin damaged cochleas. Top row: Cochleograms showing the percentage of hair cells present as a function of distance from the apex. On the left side only the relevant fourth and third turns are shown (guinea pig) while on the right side only the second and first. Vertical interrupted line shows the location of the recording electrodes (in basal turn differential electrode method, in fourth turn micropipette in scala media). Middle row: Cochlear microphonic magnitude functions compared between normal median (o) and the two experimental animals (•). Bottom row:

is not some sort of subtractive mechanism–in other words, you don't want to take something away from what the afferent dendrites produce, on the contrary, what you want is to boost their sensitivity so that they should be able to operate at low levels. Apparently the frequency selectivity is already there at the inner hair cell level (Russell and Sellick, this volume) or at the afferent fiber level in the absence of outer hair cells (Dallos and Harris, *J. Neurophysiol.*, 1978, in press). What we need is a great deal of sensitivity to make the operation at low levels possible.

Galambos: As I understand it you see the internal hair cells as being responsible for the center frequency in the tuning curve, and the outer hair cells as providing the gain. We have heard that perhaps only 5% of the afferents come from the outer hair cells. How does this 5% provide gain to the 95%, and where does this happen? Do you conceive of this interaction occurring at the cochlear level or the central level?

Dallos: Clearly it is at the cochlear level. I don't have any better ideas about that than any of my colleagues who spoke before. The inner hair cell receptor potential is apparently sharply tuned in the normal cochlea, so that has to occur at or prior to the hair cell level.

Now, it can happen several different ways. One would be that the outer hair cells that generate the majority of receptor potentials, but whose neural output (if in fact there is one) is a minor component of the neural outflow from the cochlea–outer hair cells might have developed to provide an environment to the inner hair cells in which they could generate both frequency selectivity and sensitivity. This environment might be provided by direct electrical interaction. The inner hair cells might function as some sorts of quasi-electro receptors. Or it could be that outer hair cells in fact produce a local mechanical change in the organ of Corti, and clearly such a change would directly influence the inner hair cells. But it certainly has to happen at the hair cell level and not at the neural level, I think.

Bodian: Is it clear what is the effect of kanamycin destruction of outer hair cells upon the tectorial membrane? It is clear that the outer hair cells are very intimately associated with the tectorial membrane. In fact, when there is retraction, pieces of the tectorial membrane are pulled off. With the outer hair cells destroyed, what happens to the tectorial membrane?

Dallos: As well as anybody can tell, the tectorial membrane is there and is unaffected. After outer hair cells are destroyed the indentations at the bottom of the tectorial membrane from where the cilia are removed stay clearly visible for many months (D. Lim, private communication, 1977) thus the membrane itself had not changed. However, in the normal state the outer hair cell cilia provide strong coupling, and that coupling is gone. That could be an extreme manifestation of this mechanical influence that outer hair cells might have.

Summating potential magnitude functions compared between normal median (o) and the two representative animals (•). SP^- and DIF SP^- functions are shown for the fourth and first turns respectively. Stimulus frequencies are as follows: First turn, for both CM and SP: 8000 Hz; fourth turn, for CM 200 Hz, for SP 400 Hz (from Dallos, P., and Cheatham, M.A., *J. Acoust. Soc. Amer., 60:* 510-512, 1976).

Thornton: If you got this fine tuning maintained by the inner hair cells so you still have this reasonably sharp and defined tip would you like to comment on the interpretation of recruitment with outer hair cell damage with reference to the explanations Ted Evans has used, where you have only a broad pattern explaining recruitment phenomena? If you still have fine tuning, how is this going to work?

Dallos: I don't think that there is a serious conflict there. We have a threshold change at the best frequency and recruitment would then imply that immediately above threshold you bring in a large number of basal fibers. The sharply tuned tip segments of these fibers are very short, 15 dB maybe, thus there is no conflict.

Goldberg: Peter, maybe we can pull some of the papers together. Russell started his paper by suggesting various models for sharp tuning; I believe they were electrical interactions, neural interactions or straight mechanical interactions on the inner hair cells.

Since you favor that the outer hair cells are not there just to balance the organ of Corti, can you or Ian talk about what kind of interaction would be consistent? Off the top of my head I would guess that a mechanical sharpening would be, but that an electrical interaction--well, nothing is ever ruled out, but the fact is he has conductive changes in his inner hair cells which do parallel the receptor potential and don't seem to need an external source of current to explain the receptor potentials, which we saw were sharp.

Dallos: I am somewhat at a loss to see why the electrical interaction would be ruled out on the basis of the work of Ian and Peter. What I am suggesting here is a gain change. If the outer hair cells would generate a great deal of dc current flowing in that particular region and that creates some effect--I am talking very loosely, as every one of you is painfully aware--some effect upon the inner hair cell. That effect is already incorporated in the recording and cannot be separated by merely looking at the resistance change.

INTERPRETATION OF EVOKED NEURAL RESPONSES: FACTS AND ILLUSIONS RELATED TO THE METHODS FOR RECORDING WHOLE-NERVE ACTION POTENTIALS

Donald H. Eldredge

Central Institute for the Deaf

The title of this symposium is "Evoked Electrical Activity in the Auditory Nervous System." The whole-nerve action potential (AP) recorded from the cochlea of an experimental animal is an example of such evoked electrical activity. However, if we compare these potentials in some detail to our knowledge of the cochlear microphonic (CM) responses and to the characteristics of the responses of single auditory neurons, several problems concerning the interpretations of the events underlying AP responses appear. These are related to the physical configurations of the recording electrodes, to the space-time relations of the Békésy traveling wave, and to the spectral properties of the signals used to evoke responses.

GENERAL METHODS

Electrocochleography in the guinea pig or the chinchilla has several advantages over electrocochleography in man. First, the tympanic membrane is left undisturbed because it is possible to open the auditory bulla for the placement of electrodes. Secondly, two active electrodes may be used instead of one. These are placed, as shown in Figure 1, one in scala vestibuli and one in scala tympani on either side of the cochlear partition. The reference electrode is usually placed on the soft tissues of the wound in the neck that had been used to expose the auditory bulla. The bony cochlea and the air around it are good insulators compared to the body fluids. Accordingly the current path between the active electrodes and the reference electrode will be the cochlear fluids and the neural and vascular channels between the cochlea and the rest of the body fluids by way of the internal auditory meatus. As indicated to the right in Figure 1, the CM voltages at the active electrodes are out of phase because the principal source of CM is located between the electrodes. In contrast the AP are in phase at the active electrodes. To the extent that the AP common to the two electrodes is equal and in phase, when we record the potential difference between the active electrodes, that is subtract the voltage

ISBN 0-12-514960-3

recorded in scala tympani from that recorded in scala vestibuli, the AP will be reduced or eliminated. The CM traces reported in an earlier chapter (Eldredge, 1978) were recorded in this manner.

When we add or average the potentials at the two active electrodes the opposite result is obtained. To the extent that the CM components are equal in magnitude and opposite in phase, they are reduced or eliminated and the AP appears in a relatively pure form. The results of both of these electrical operations are shown in Figure 2. The acoustic signal was a wide-band click at 60 dB SPL, peak equivalent. The three CM responses were recorded differentially from pairs of electrodes in each of the three cochlear turns in chinchilla. The AP trace was the average recorded from the active electrodes in the first or basal turn. Each trace is an average of eight responses to improve the ratio of signal to noise. A small remnant of CM_1 can be detected in the AP trace and in the CM_2 trace. Also there is a hint of some CM_2 in the CM_3 trace. These slightly less than perfect electrode placements are common and, if anything, tend to support the above statements about the nature of these methods of measurement.

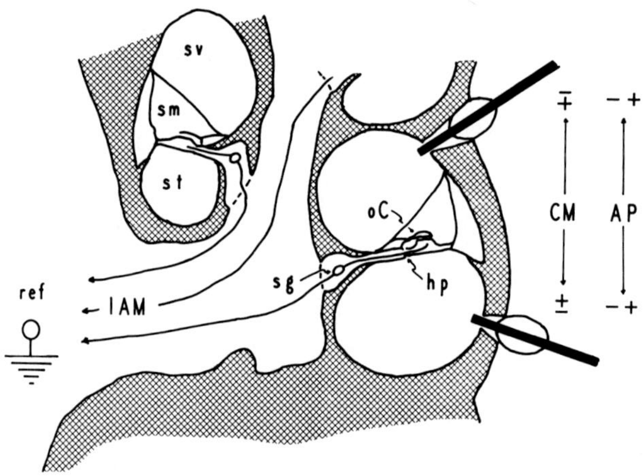

Fig. 1. Diagram showing locations of intracochlear electrodes in relation to bony cochlea and the cochlear partition. Symbols to the right indicate that CM appears in opposite phases and AP in the same phase at these electrodes. hp, habenula perforata; IAM, internal auditory meatus; oC, organ of Corti; ref, effective location of reference electrode; sg, spiral ganglion; sm, scala media; st, scala tympani; sv, scala vestibuli.

AP RESPONSES FROM NORMAL EARS

The AP trace shown in Figure 2 is typical. There are two prominent negative waves, N_1 and N_2, separated by a small positive deflection. The peak of the N_1 shows a latency of about 1 msec with respect to the CM_1 and the peak of N_2 is about 1 msec later. What is the nature of N_1 and N_2? What are the sources of N_1

and N_2? Why do we not see more evidence of later neural activity? Note that CM_2 is delayed nearly as much as N_1 and that CM_3 is concurrent with and in part follows N_2. Kiang's (1965) report of the responses of single auditory neurons in the cat to wide-band clicks serves to emphasize this problem. The neurons most sensitive to high frequencies do respond with latencies appropriate to N_1 and sometimes also respond at a time appropriate to N_2. But as the most sensitive or characteristic frequency of the neuron under study becomes lower, latency is systematically lengthened in a manner consistent with the Békésy traveling wave. Kiang recorded post-stimulus time histograms of the probabilities of neural responses as functions of time after presentation of the click. For units with characteristic frequencies below about 5 kHz there were epochs of high probability of responses alternating with epochs of low probability of response in a manner that corresponds roughly to the oscillations in the CM responses shown in Figure 2. The period of these fluctuations in probability of responses corresponds to the period of the characteristic frequency of the neuron. Neurons with low characteristic frequencies have latencies as long as 4-6 msec. There is no convincing evidence of such activity in Figure 2.

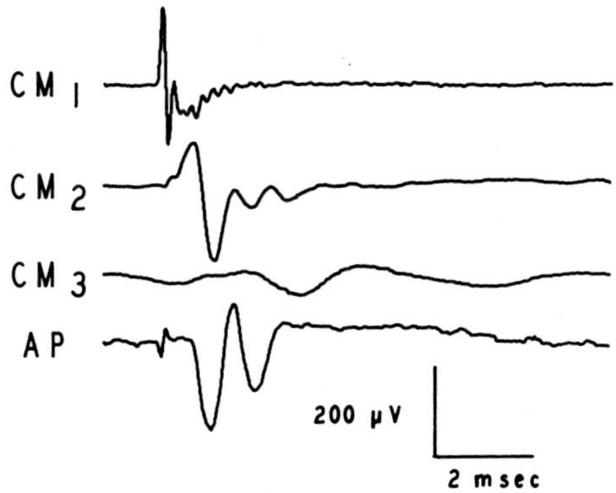

Fig. 2. CM and AP responses to a wide-band click at 60 dB SPL, peak equivalent. Responses recorded from the first, second and third cochlear turns are identified by corresponding numbers. Note small portions of CM, in traces for CM_2 and for AP, and of CM_2 in the trace for CM_3. Otherwise the waveforms are quite distinctive and the AP response is completed before the CM_3 response ends. Eight of each response was summed to enhance the ratio of signal to noise.

Selective Masking of AP

For some years we have used a method of selective masking of the AP that appears to shed some light on the above problem (Teas, et al., 1962). Essentially the same approach has been and is being applied to human electrocochleography, for example by Elberling (1974) and by Eggermont, et al., (1976), so it appears appropriate to review this approach in this symposium. The basic method is illustrated in Figure 3. On the right appear a set of measured AP traces and on the left are AP traces derived from pairs of the measured traces. First the level of a wide-band noise is adjusted so that it will fully mask the AP response to a wide-band click or, as in Figure 3, so that it will mask the AP as much as possible without interfering with the CM response. Then, with the click alone alternating with the click with noise, a number of samples of each response are summed into separate sections of computer memory. It is useful and physiologically appropriate to define whole-nerve AP as that portion of the waveform that can be masked by noise. This can be found by subtracting in the computer point-by-point the top waveform on the right, with wide-band noise, from the second waveform measured without noise. The resulting waveform is shown on the left in Figure 3 just under the waveform for CM_1. It appears as a characteristic whole-nerve AP with residual, uncancelled CM removed.

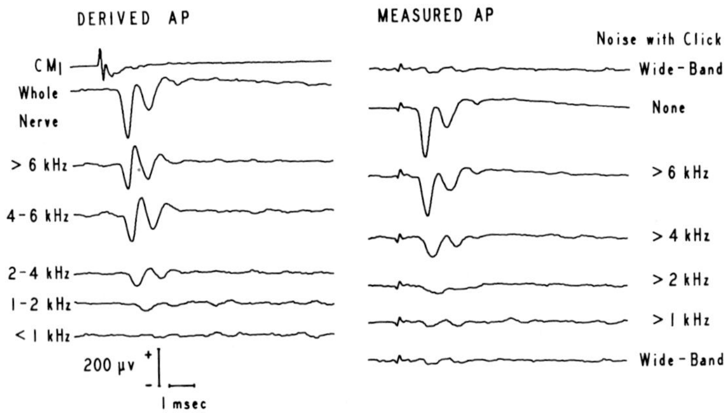

Fig. 3. Set of AP responses that illustrates the method of analysis by selective masking. Each waveform on the right is a response to a wide-band click at 60 dB SPL, peak equivalent, in the kind of high-pass or wide-band noise indicated with each trace. On the left the whole-nerve waveform is the point-by-point difference between the AP with no noise and that with wide-band noise. The waveform labeled ">6 KHz" is the difference between the response with no noise and the response with 6-kHz high-pass noise. The other traces on the left were similarly derived as differences between adjacent traces on the right. See text for details.

In the next step the spectrum level of the wide-band noise is maintained, but the noise is high-pass filtered at 6 kHz. Sets of responses to the click are collected while alternating no noise with the 6 kHz high-pass noise. The average response in the presence of the 6 kHz high-pass noise is shown by the third waveform on the right in Figure 3. The response that is not present and has been masked by this noise can be calculated by subtracting the response in the presence of this noise from the response to the click alone and is shown as the third trace on the left. By changing the filter settings to provide successively 4 kHz, 2 kHz and 1 kHz high-pass noises it is possible to infer from successive differences between traces each additional part of AP that disappears or is masked by the progressive addition of lower frequencies to the masking noise. These waveforms are shown on the left in Figure 3 as the 4-6 kHz, 2-4 kHz, 1-2 kHz and <1 kHz traces.

Each of the derived waveforms appears as a usual sort of AP. Four features are of special interest. First, the waveform corresponding to those neurons masked by frequencies above 6 kHz appears as the bulk of the earliest portion of the whole-nerve AP. Second, the latencies of the increments masked by successively lower frequencies are systematically longer. This is consistent with our understanding that noise at lower frequencies should mask responses more apically in the cochlea and that these more apical responses should include some delays introduced by the traveling wave. Third, even the waveform masked by the extension of the high-pass frequency from 2 kHz down to 1 kHz does not have a latency so long as those reported by Kiang (1965) for neurons with the lowest characteristic frequencies and there is little or no synchronized neural activity masked by frequencies below 1 kHz.

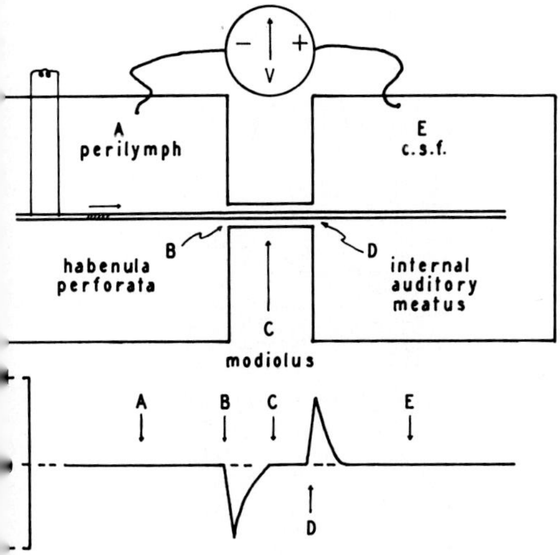

Fig. 4. Above, model for the electrical configuration of a monopolar electrode in cochlear perilymph as in Fig. 1 and below, corresponding properties of a unit neural response as seen by the active electrode in the perilymph. The voltage waveform and the places of propagated neural depolarization are matched by the sets of letters.

The fourth observation is perhaps the most important. We expect the neural responses masked by frequencies above 6 kHz to be best synchronized because the velocity of the traveling wave along the basilar membrane is greatest in the basal turn. The waveform for the AP component masked by frequencies above 6 kHz is strongly diphasic. If this waveform is a summation of many synchronous responses from individual primary auditory neurons, then the waveform for these individual responses as seen by this configuration of electrodes should also be diphasic.

Model for Diphasic AP

A model for the electrode configuration of Figure 1 is shown in the diagram of Figure 4. This model suggests that no potential is observed by electrodes in the volume conductors of the cochlear fluids, including the perilymph, or in the general tissue fluids, including the cerebrospinal fluid, when the depolarization of an action potential is in either of these areas. However, the bridge of salt solutions between these areas is constricted at the habenula perforata, the modiolus, and the internal auditory meatus. When a depolarization is present at either end of this series of constrictions, an electrode in the pool of fluids most closely associated with that end will show a negative potential consistent with the electrical currents of the depolarization and the impedances to the electrodes. Thus, as indicated in Figure 4, the electrode in the perilymph will first show no voltage, then be negative with respect to an electrode in the tissue fluids, perhaps be neutral, then be positive with respect to the electrode in the tissue fluids, and finally again be neutral. For this model the specific temporal patterns will depend on the rate of propagation of the

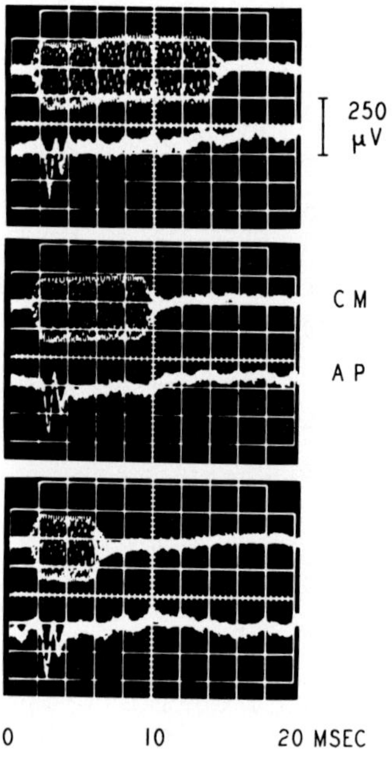

Fig. 5. CM and AP (guinea pig) in response to a 7-kHz tone with rise and fall times of 1 msec and plateau durations of about 4, 8, and 12 msec. Note absence of dc during tone and slow positive potential with termination of tone. (Teas, Eldredge and Davis, 1962)

depolarization, the rate of repolarization, and the effective impedances seen by the electrodes. The total movement of charge should be the same at either end of the constriction. Thus, to the extent that the effective impedances seen by the electrodes are similar, the integrals of voltage in time should also be the same for both the negative and the positive phases. The positive phase may follow the negative phase with a delay as shown in Figure 4 or it may follow more closely superimposed on the tail of the negative phase as implied by the waveform of the AP component masked by 6 kHz high-pass noise shown in Figure 3.

Note that in Figure 3 the components masked by successively lower frequencies become progressively less diphasic. This reflects the loss of synchrony as the traveling wave slows in the midcochlear regions. Here the positive phases of the earlier responses are more and more being offset by the negative phases of later responses. As noted earlier, the components masked by frequencies below 1 kHz show little or no synchrony in these traces.

This model implies two relations for the AP response to a burst of high-frequency tone. In the steady-state period following the onset response, the continuing asynchronous neural activity should show no direct current offset because the same amount of negative charge will appear at the internal auditory meatus as at the habenula perforata. However, when the tone is gated off, the last events should be the depolarizations at the internal auditory meatus. These will appear as a positive voltage at the active electrodes. In Figure 5 the CM and AP responses to a 7 kHz tone burst clearly show both of these predicted features. While the tone is on, the AP trace is not distinguishable from zero voltage and there is a clearly defined positive potential associated with termination of the tone.

Kiang, et al., (1976) have used an ingenious method to record the average responses of a single neuron as recorded by an electrode on the round window of cat. The appearance of a spontaneous unit discharge at a microelectrode on the fiber of a single primary auditory neuron was used to index the averaging of the voltage at the round window. By averaging some 10,000 to 80,000 indexed segments of these waveforms, they were able to see clear responses. The published waveforms are not all quite so strongly diphasic as implied by the waveforms shown here, but are enough so to support the interpretation suggested here.

Legouix and Pierson (1974) reported other measures on guinea pig that tend to support this model for the interpretation of whole-nerve AP. They recorded AP from electrodes in the first and also from the third turns of the cochlea while the auditory nerve was rendered more or less inactive at the internal auditory meatus by the application of a solution of isotonic potassium chloride. They observed that the positive phase of the AP decreased and the waveform assumed a more triangular shape with the initial peak followed by a voltage that decayed over a period of about 1 msec. They also found that the values of the later portion of this waveform were relatively higher for the electrodes in the third turn compared to those in the first turn and concluded that the electrodes in the third turn were significantly better oriented anatomically with respect to the late neural activity arising more apically than were the electrodes in the basal turn.

From the observations described so far we can conclude that there must be some reasonably well synchronized onset of neural activity in order to elicit one of these evoked responses. Otherwise even high rates of random activity yield zero net voltage. However, the appearance of the nicely synchronized N_1 is also largely an artifact of the diphasic nature of the basic unit response. So, although such synchrony is necessary, its appearance is enhanced by the following positive potential which cuts short a slower negative wave. This model also casts some doubt on the nature of the N_2 response. Earlier Tasaki (1954) and Teas et al. (1962) interpreted N_2 responses as the second response in the same neurons. Both Tasaki's measurements and some of those reported by Kiang (1965) show that some units with high characteristic frequencies do indeed respond in this manner. However, the report by Legouix and Pierson (1974) suggests that the delineation of an N_2 may also be largely an artifact of the positive phase of the earliest units to respond. Pugh et al. (1973) reported that the magnitude of N_2 is to some extent positively correlated with neural activity arising from more apical regions of the cochlea and that its magnitude can vary independently from the magnitude of N_1.

Even though the responses of primary auditory neurons are well locked to the phases of tones at low frequencies, it remains very difficult to demonstrate AP responses arising from apical neurons. The longitudinal CM gradients for a tone at 500 Hz in Figure 8 of Eldredge (1978) suggest three reasons why the appropriate synchrony is difficult to achieve. To begin, the excitatory half-cycle of 1 msec already invites some temporal dispersion. Then, between the second and third turns the phase is changing so rapidly that there is little chance for real synchrony. Finally, there are good voltages in the basal turn which are relatively more in phase. At higher signal levels neurons in the basal turn will respond with short-latency synchronized responses (Deatherage et al., 1959) that obscure any less well-synchronized responses from apical regions that may actually be present. Weak, poorly synchronized responses with long latencies appropriate to the apical turn have been reported in man by Davis and Hirsh (1976). At suprathreshold levels they found these to be obscured by a frequency following response with short latencies appropriate to the basal turn.

AP RESPONSES FROM ABNORMAL EARS

For some time we have used the technique of selective masking of AP elicited by wide-band click on chinchillas with temporary or with permanent loss of hearing following exposures to noise. We see interesting, even enticing, changes in the responses, but so far have not been able to tie up the relations among behavioral threshold shifts, cochlear potentials, and anatomical injuries in the nice neat packages we had been seeking. Even so a few examples can serve to indicate some of the possibilities. The responses shown in Figure 6 were recorded from a chinchilla that had been exposed to an octave band of noise with a center frequency of 4 kHz at a level of 108 dB SPL for 3.5 hours. This exposure produced permanent shifts of behavioral auditory thresholds of 5-10 dB from 0.125 to 1.0 kHz, 30 dB at 1.4 kHz, 45 dB at 2 kHz, 50 dB at 2.8 kHz, 35 dB at 4 kHz, 25 dB at 5.7 kHz and then about 20 dB from 8 kHz to 16 kHz. There was scattered loss of outer hair cells beginning at the round window for a distance of 4.9 mm, complete loss of the organ of Corti for the next 2 mm, and then a gradual return to near-normal in the next 3 mm. The wide-band click was presented at 75 dB SPL, peak equivalent, to collect the responses shown in Figure 6. No part of this AP was masked by frequencies above 4 kHz. The CM_1 waveform was clear but not entirely normal. The latency from CM_1 to the onset of AP was 1.0 msec instead of the normal 0.6 msec and the latency to the peak of N_1 was 1.6 msec instead of a normal 0.9 msec. The AP responses at 75 dB SPL were maximal for this ear. When the signal levels were increased to 85, 95, and 105 dB SPL the same basic patterns were observed but noise in the form of uncancelled CM continued to grow with level. This example was chosen for illustration because the AP responses were still quite clear. Other ears with similar exposures to noise have shown even greater behavioral threshold shifts, more anatomical injuries, and much smaller and noisier AP responses.

Several features of normal AP responses and of the patterns of abnormal responses are indicated in Figure 7. Average peak AP voltages plus and minus one standard deviation as functions of peak equivalent sound pressure level for the wide-band click are shown for the whole-nerve, the greater than 6 kHz component, the 4-6 kHz component, and the 2-4 kHz component. These functions grow monotonically to a maximum and then decrease. Note that the whole-nerve response appears to be dominated by the 4-6 kHz component at 40 and 50 dB SPL and by the greater than 6 kHz component at higher levels.

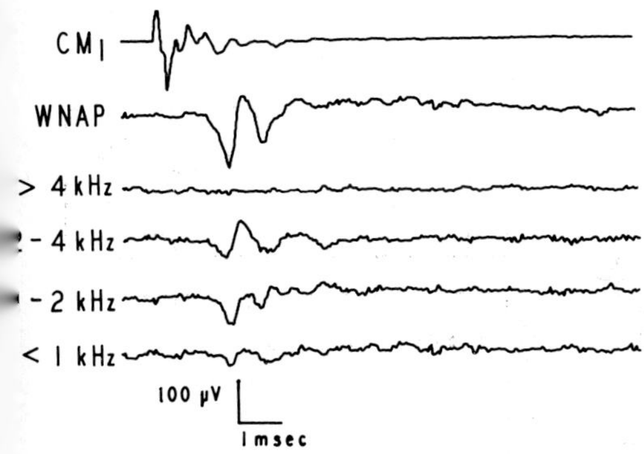

Fig. 6. CM_1 and selectively-masked AP responses to a wide-band click at 75 dB SPL, peak equivalent, from a chinchilla with permanent threshold shifts and cochlear injury following exposure to noise. No part of these AP responses was masked by frequencies above 4 kHz. See text for details.

In spite of the large standard deviations, so far few noise-exposed chinchillas have given responses that lie entirely within one standard deviation of normal. Several examples are shown here in Figure 7. The function labeled H-3 was normally sensitive at 30-50 dB SPL but then clearly low in voltage at higher levels. The function labeled H-5 begins with normal sensitivity but never grows at a normal rate. The functions labeled L-1 and B-15 combine small shifts in threshold sensitivity with slower than normal rate of growth at first, then followed by rapid growth of voltage with level in a manner suggestive of recruitment. In spite of the considerable sensitivity of these AP responses to minor cochlear changes as reported by Eldredge et al. (1973) and in spite of the potentially revealing changes in the input-output functions for components of AP, so far it has not been possible to relate these in a satisfactory way to specific acoustic injuries to the organ of Corti.

COMPLEX SIGNALS

Because the essentially diphasic nature of the unit response conceals the existence of continuous neural activity, the *sine qua non* of whole-nerve AP is synchronized, coherent responses by the individual neurons. The wide-band click, a complex signal, is one way to accomplish this in part. Even here there are problems because resonances of earphones and in the ear canal can lead to signals that are

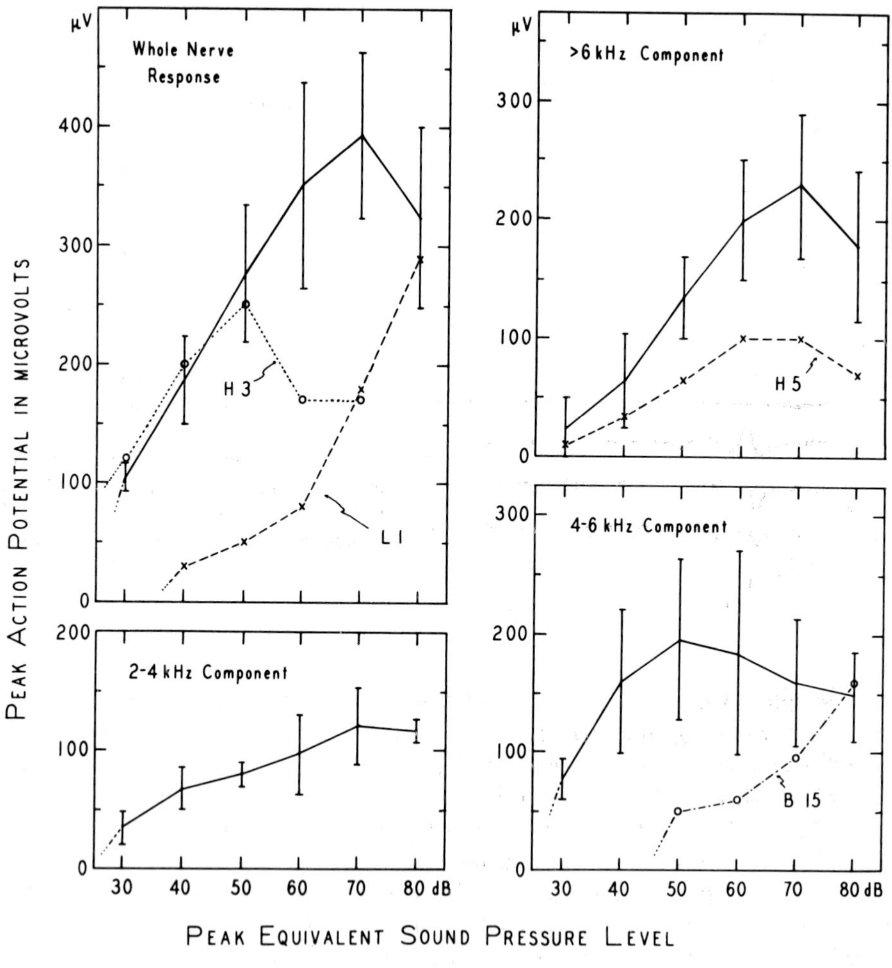

Fig. 7. Mean normal values plus and minus one standard deviation for peak AP in microvolts as a function of peak equivalent SPL. Separate panels are used for whole-nerve AP and the >6 kHz, 4-6 kHz, and 2-4 kHz components. Four examples of abnormal functions are also shown. See text for details.

equivalent to a tone-pip riding on a wide-band click. The smooth input-output function for normal AP shown in Figure 7 depends on adequate damping within the speculum connecting the earphone to the ear canal. In the absence of this damping the functions show inflections.

In his monograph Davis (1976) spelled out the nature of these acoustic problems and also discusses the compromises that are necessary when tonal signals are used to elicit AP responses. When tones are gated on or off there is always some spread of acoustic energy to other frequencies. With care these ratios can easily be 40 dB and useful frequency selectivity of responses can be demonstrated. However, as signal level is increased so that these other components exceed threshold, something new is added to the effective signal and also to the response.

A worst-case example of this problem is shown in Figure 8. Differential records of CM from the first, second and third turns of a guinea pig are shown in response to a 6 kHz tone gated on to and off from full amplitude at zero crossings in

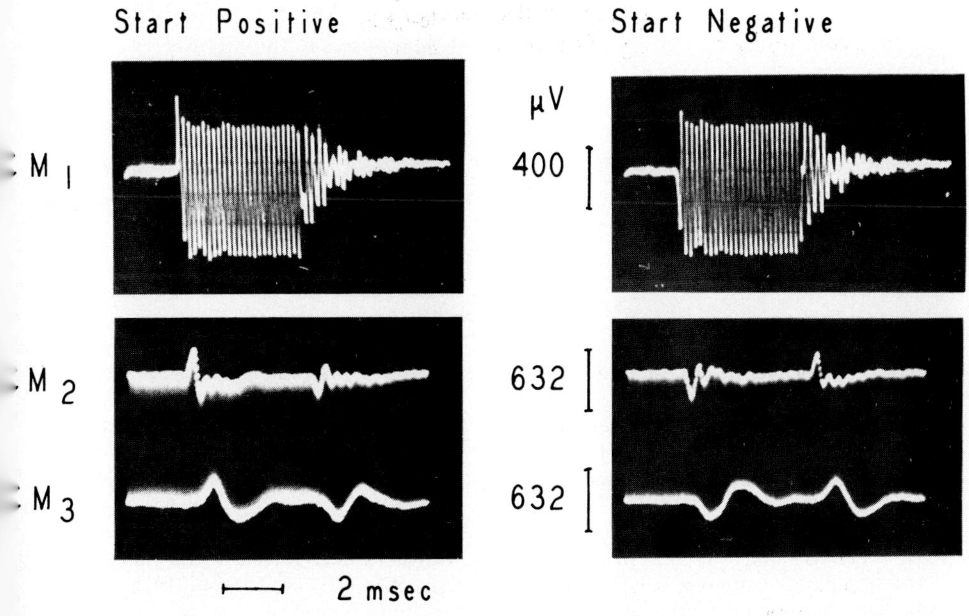

Fig. 8. CM recorded from three cochlear turns in guinea pig in response to a 6-kHz tone at 85 dB SPL gated on and off at zero crossings. Note the well-developed click responses in the second and third turns.

the electrical waveform to the earphone. Both onset and offset transients travel with usual delays and without any 6 kHz component to the second and third turns. The voltages in the second and third turns are only about 6 dB below those in the first. More common relations are shown in Figure 9 of Eldredge (1978). Here the small slow wave in the third turn is not likely to be significant at 41 dB SPL. At higher levels not only may the slow wave in the third turn become significant, but significant wide-band energy may be introduced in the basal turn by the transition from zero to the first peak of the onset waveform. Accordingly even the most well-behaved AP responses will usually show discontinuities of amplitude and latency as signal levels are increased and new components are introduced.

SUMMARY

The unit response basic to whole-nerve AP appears to be diphasic. Thus to see AP there must be synchronous responses and often the appearance of synchrony will be enhanced as the positive phase cuts short the appearance of later neural activity. Only neurons from regions of the cochlea most sensitive to frequencies above about 1 kHz show enough synchrony to contribute significantly to AP and these neurons can also be better synchronized by low frequencies than can neurons arising more apically.

An AP response can be absent either because there is no neural activity or because it is asynchronous. Thus the presence of a response should carry more weight than the absence.

Acoustic signals designed to enhance neural synchrony are spectrally complex and entail some compromises between synchrony and frequency selectivity. The effective use and interpretation of the whole-nerve AP is at best difficult and requires continuing awareness of the different weaknesses in the method.

Acknowledgement

The preparation of this manuscript was supported by Grant No. NS 03856 from the National Institute of Neurological and Communicative Disorders and Stroke to the Central Institute for the Deaf.

REFERENCES

Davis, H. Principles of electric response audiometry. *Ann. Otol. Rhinol. Laryngol.* Suppl. *28:* 1-96, 1976.

Davis, H. and Hirsh, S.K. The audiometric utility of brain stem responses to low-frequency sounds. *Audiology 15:* 181-195, 1976.

Deatherage, B.H., Eldredge, D.H. and Davis, H. Latency of action potentials in the cochlea of the guinea pig. *J. Acoust. Soc. Am. 31:* 479-486, 1959.

Eggermont, J.J., Spoor, A. and Odenthal, D.W. Frequency specificity of tone-burst electrocochleography. In: *Electrocochleography,* edited by R.J. Ruben, C. Elberling and G. Salomon. Baltimore, London, Tokyo: University Park Press, p. 215-246, 1976.

Elberling, C. Action potentials along the cochlear partition recorded from the ear canal in man. *Scand. Audiol. 3:* 13-19, 1974.

Eldredge, D.H. Electrical equivalents of the Békésy traveling wave in the mammalian cochlea. (ibid.) 1978.

Eldredge, D.H., Mills, J.H. and Bohne, B.A. Anatomical, behavioral, and electrophysiological observations on chinchillas after long exposures to noise. *Oto-Rhino-Laryngol. 20:* 64-81, 1973.

Kiang, N.Y.S. *Discharge Patterns of Single Fibers in the Cat's Auditory Nerve.* Cambridge: MIT Press, 1965.

Kiang, N.Y.S., Moxon, E.C. and Kahn, A.R. The relationship of gross potentials recorded from the cochlea to single unit activity in the auditory nerve. In: *Electrocochleography,* edited by R.J. Ruben, C. Elberling and G. Salomon. Baltimore, London, Tokyo: University Park Press, 1976, p. 95-115.

Legouix, J.P. and Pierson, A. Investigations on the sources of the whole-nerve action potentials recorded from various places in the guinea-pig cochlea. *J. Acoust. Soc. Am. 56:* 1222-1230, 1974.

Pugh, J.E.Jr., Anderson, D.J., Burgio, P.A. and Horowitz, M.R. The origin of N_2 of the cochlear nerve action potential. *J. Acoust. Soc. Am. 53:* 325, 1973.

Tasaki, I. Nerve impulses in individual auditory nerve fibers of guinea pig. *J. Neurophysiol. 17:* 97-122, 1954.

Tasaki, I., Davis, H. and Legouix, J.-P. The space-time pattern of the cochlear microphonics (guinea pig) as recorded by differential electrodes. *J. Acoust. Soc. Am. 24:* 502-519, 1952.

Teas, D.C., Eldredge, D.H. and Davis, H. Cochlear responses to acoustic transients: an interpretation of whole-nerve action potentials. *J. Acoust. Soc. Am. 34:* 1438-1459, 1962.

DISCUSSION

Durrant: With regard to the positive after-potential, which exists at the turn-off of the stimulus, I think it may contribute more to electrocochleography than we yet know. I wonder if you feel that it is purely the result or the aftermath of the AP, as such; and if that is true, would you expect the influence of changing rise-fall time on the positive after-potential and the N_1 of the whole-nerve action potential to be the same?

Eldredge: There are several different possibilities that must be considered in relation to this topic. First, if you gated the tone on and off more slowly, you will also lose the N_1 response. If you can make an asymmetrical gating with a normal rise time and a longer fall time, then you will lose synchrony at the off and so reduce the positive phase without losing N_1. But there is another problem because in a closed acoustic system there is a certain amount of acoustic decay time which is in addition to the electrical fall time. I have never been able to distinguish clearly the quantitative relations between the two decays. If you use an open acoustic system there will be later echoes unless the acoustic absorption of the room and its contents is enough to make it anechoic.

Another possibility I have considered, but neither demonstrated nor ruled out, is that some of the positive potential represents activity in those units of the cochlear nucleus which are tucked close to the internal auditory meatus. For this interpretation the reference electrode has become the "active" electrode and negative voltages here again appear as positive potentials at the normally active electrodes. The several possibilities are not mutually exlusive. With this electrode configuration, when you stop the signal the positive phases of previously active units must run their course in time. Echoes may introduce complexity and activity in the cochlear nucleus could add positive potentials.

Durrant: Over the past year or so I have started looking at the after-potential in detail to get a little better description of how it depends on various factors. Some of the preliminary observations would suggest that there might be a certain independence between at least a part of what we are thinking of as this positive after-potentiation. It is somewhat subtle. One of the subtleties is that you do have a difference in the influence of rise-decay. You can have some very long rise-decay times and still get a substantial after-potential at times when you do not have much N_1. Secondly, regardless of fall time, the after-potential is always peaking out right when the stimulus to the cochlear partition is going totally to zero. So, it is really fascinating in that it is a completely off after-response. Another thing is that with very sharp rise-decay you also have an "off-N_1", but you can eliminate it with any significant rise-decay while you still have substantial after-potentials.

The other observation is that in some animals you see also a rather long-lasting negative potentiation following the positive after-potentiation. I don't know whether any part of this is recording artifact, but there is quite a bit of activity going on, I think, surrounding the initial stages of the excitation of the nerve, following the stimulus turn-off. I am looking forward to some more interesting facts as we get our teeth further into the study of the after-potential.

UNIT ACTIVITY UNDERLYING THE N_1 POTENTIAL

Francisco Antoli-Candela, Jr.

Centro Especial "Ramon y Cajal," Madrid

Nelson Y. S. Kiang

Harvard Medical School

INTRODUCTION

One objective of electrocochleography is to assess the functional state of the auditory nerve by examining certain components of electric responses recordable in human subjects. With clicks or other acoustic transients as stimuli, characteristic waveforms are observable from many locations such as scalp, ear canal, or otic capsule. One common component of all these waveforms is the compound action potential of the auditory nerve, the first peak of which is called N_1. A theoretical expression relating the compound action potential to single-unit activity in the auditory nerve was formulated in 1958 (Goldstein and Kiang, 1958). In this formulation, the two physiological measurements needed to synthesize a theoretical compound action potential are poststimulus time (PST) histograms of single-unit activity and the waveforms of unit discharges as seen by the gross electrode (N_0). Since then, it has become routine in animal experiments to collect PST histograms that describe the time patterns of discharges in single auditory-nerve fibers responding to controlled sounds (Kiang et al., 1965). More recently, N_0's have been measured for the cat (Kiang et al., 1976). Unfortunately, these measurements require long samples of unit activity, leaving limited time to obtain other data, such as PST histograms, from the same units. A full-scale test of the theory awaits comparison of measured compound action potentials with ones synthesized from single-unit data from the same animal. Meanwhile, it is still instructive to see how PST histograms of unit activity change under conditions that alter the gross responses. This is a report of such a study using clicks as stimuli and anesthetized cats as experimental animals. Because this meeting is intended to serve partially as an introductory review of auditory evoked potentials, sufficient background material has been included so that the non-specialist can follow the main arguments without being forced to consult a long list of papers either on N_1, or auditory-nerve responses.

ISBN 0-12-514960-3

METHODS

The general techniques are as described in Kiang et al. (1965), except that the experiments were conducted in a different chamber (Vér et al., 1975). Adult cats were anesthetized with dial-urethane (75 mg/kg) and a closed acoustic system inserted into the left external auditory meatus. The sound source was a 1″ Brüel & Kjaer condenser microphone used as an earphone. A ¼″ condenser microphone in a probe tube system was used for acoustic calibrations. Tuning curves for single units were obtained by an automated procedure described in Kiang et al. (1970). Clicks were produced by delivering 100μsec pulses at a rate of 10/sec to the earphone. Stimulus levels are expressed in dB re a 100V pulse to the earphone, which generates a click that is approximately 108 dB peak SPL.

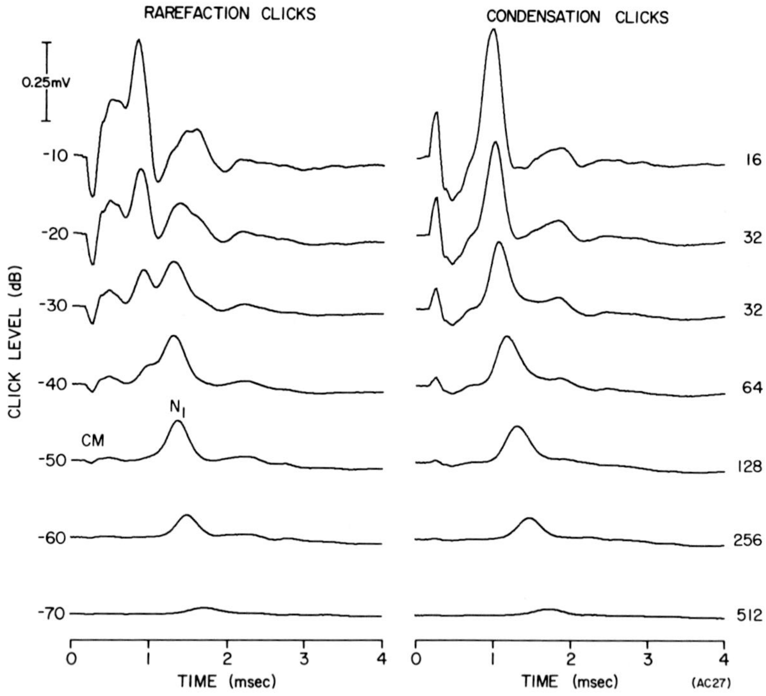

Fig. 1. Gross responses recorded near the round window of the cochlea for rarefaction and condensation clicks at seven click levels. Each trace is an average of the responses to the number of clicks indicated in the right-hand column. Upward deflections in this and subsequent figures indicate negativity of the round window electrode relative to the headholder. The recordings were made in the following order: first, rarefaction clicks at the lowest level (-70 dB), then condensation clicks at -70 dB, then rarefaction clicks at -60 dB, etc. For the -50 dB rarefaction trace, the cochlear microphonic potential is labeled CM, and the first negative neural potential is labeled N_1. Zero time for each trace is the onset time of the electric pulse delivered to the earphone. The sound conduction time from the earphone to the tympanic membrane is approximately 0.1 msec.

After tracheotomy, the bulla was opened and the middle-ear septum removed. A wire electrode placed on the bone near the round window was used to record the round window (RW) potentials. In some experiments a second wire electrode was placed on the nerve in the internal auditory meatus near the microelectrode penetrations. The microelectrodes used for single-unit recordings were 2M KCl-filled pipets. The reference lead for all recordings was the headholder.

The gross potentials shown in this paper are 30-second averages of responses recorded concurrently with the unit recordings used in constructing poststimulus time (PST) histograms. The passband of the recording system for gross electrodes

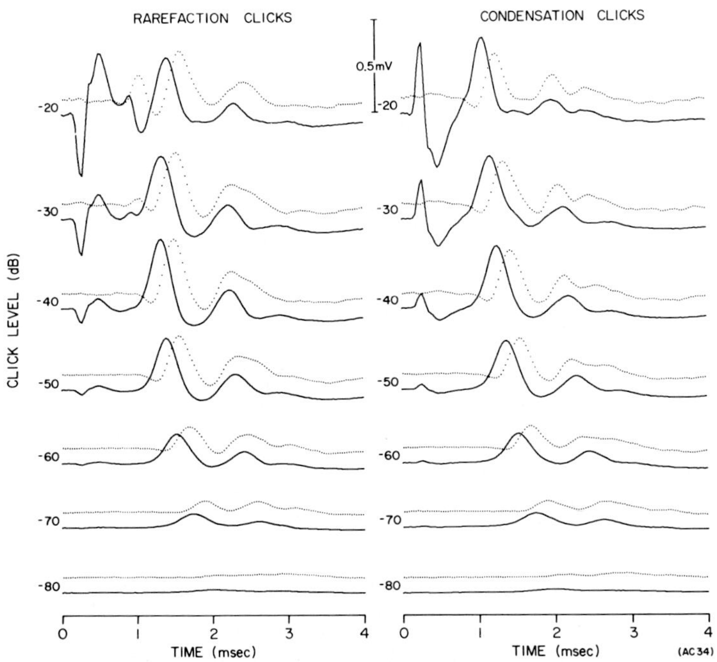

Fig. 2. Gross potentials recorded simultaneously from the bone near the round window (solid traces) and in the internal auditory meatus (dotted traces). Each trace is an average of between 16 and 512 responses to clicks. In most of the RW recordings, the early deflections represent the cochlear microphonic (CM) components which are negligible in the meatus recordings. In all traces, the N_1 in RW recordings occurs approximately 0.2 msec earlier than N_1 in meatus recordings. This difference probably represents the time needed for conduction of spikes from the site of spike origin in the cochlea to the recording electrode site in the internal auditory meatus. Although the spike conduction time may be slightly different for units of different CF, the differences are small enough that in all subsequent figures relating gross and unit responses, the former are plotted with a delay of 0.2 msec, with respect to the PST histograms.

was 7.5-20,000 Hz, and averages were made with a time resolution of 20-30μsec. Whenever many sequentially recorded units are to be related to gross potentials, there is a problem in displaying the results compactly because there can be small changes in the size and shape of the gross potential over the course of a long experiment. For this reason, the gross responses for Figures 11 through 15 and 17 were selected because they were approximately equal in amplitude to the average of the largest and smallest gross potentials obtained during the recording of the unit activity. The total range of amplitudes for the gross potentials was almost always within 10% of the average for each cat. The only exception was Cat AC36, where a 50% range in amplitudes was noted.

The unit-discharge patterns are displayed as PST histograms calculated from 30-second samples of data. The horizontal scale (time after the electric pulses are delivered to the earphone) has a bin width of 50μsec. Vertical scales are normalized to instantaneous discharge rate expressed in spikes/sec.

RESULTS

Characteristics of Gross Neural Responses

Electrical recordings from the bone near the round window in an anesthetized cat show a series of complex waves in response to clicks (Fig. 1). At low-click levels, a single peak of approximately 1¾ msec latency is seen. As the click level increases, the waveform of responses becomes more complicated with both earlier and later components appearing. Some of the earlier components reverse in polarity as click polarity is reversed. Others do not, although they may change in appearance. The reversible components, the cochlear microphonic (CM) potentials, do not involve auditory-nerve fiber activity, since they are not substantially different even after most of the nerve degenerates. Some of the other components disappear after the nerve degenerates and are therefore thought to be neural in origin (Rawdon-Smith and Hawkins, 1939; Kiang and Peake, 1960).

In order to compare gross neural potentials with unit discharge patterns, it is necessary to decide in all cases which components of the gross responses are neural. Recordings from the internal auditory meatus with gross electrodes (Fig. 2) show mainly the "neural" components so that changes in waveform and latency with click level can be measured without contamination by CM components that may overlap with the neural components. This recording location also has the advantage of being closer to the site of the single-unit recordings. Unfortunately, the potentials recorded in the nerve tend to differ in waveform as a function of electrode position. Also, the gross electrode sometimes damages the nerve sufficiently to change the potentials recorded during the experiment.

Thus, for stable recordings of gross potentials, a better choice for electrode location is the bone near the round window where the responses are large and the chances of injuring the nerve or cochlea are small. For such recordings, it is possible to cancel CM potentials by averaging responses to condensation and rare-

peak (arrows), to domination by this new, early peak, which occurs even before the first part of the split N_1. This progression takes place at different click levels for the three units. The threshold values for the broad, low-frequency tails are related to the CF; that is, the higher the CF, the higher the threshold for the tail of the tuning curve and the higher the click level at which a particular pattern is seen in the PST histogram.

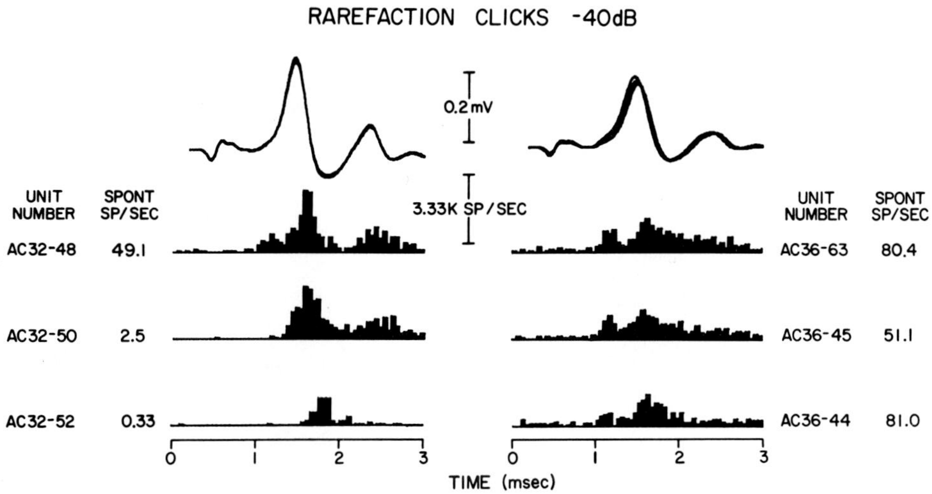

Fig. 7. Response patterns to clicks for 6 units in the auditory nerve and concomitant gross responses. The 3 poststimulus time (PST) histograms on the left are for the three units whose tuning curves are shown in Figure 5B. Their CF are approximately 5.5 kHz, and their spontaneous discharge rates are shown on the left. The PST histograms on the right are for three units with high spontaneous discharge rates from a different cat. From top to bottom, these 3 units have CF of 5.7, 6.2, and 5.7 kHz, respectively. The simultaneously recorded gross RW responses for the two groups of units are shown above the histograms as superimposed averages. The three gross responses on the left are virtually identical. The three averaged gross responses on the right have nearly identical CM and a smaller N_1 for the three units in descending order.

A more detailed click-level series for a unit with a high (>18 spikes/sec) spontaneous discharge rate is shown in Figure 9. There is a rough correspondence between the PST histogram shapes and the gross potential waveforms. At low-click levels, the histograms have a broad peak with approximately the same duration and timing as N_1. There is some activity around the time of later deflections in the gross response. At a click level of -40 dB, an earlier peak can be seen in the histogram around the time that an inflection point appears on the rising edge of N_1. At -30 dB, there is a definite peak in the gross response near the time of the early peak in the histogram. At this click level, the early peak in the histogram has become the tallest peak. At still higher-click levels, the earliest peak in the gross neural poten-

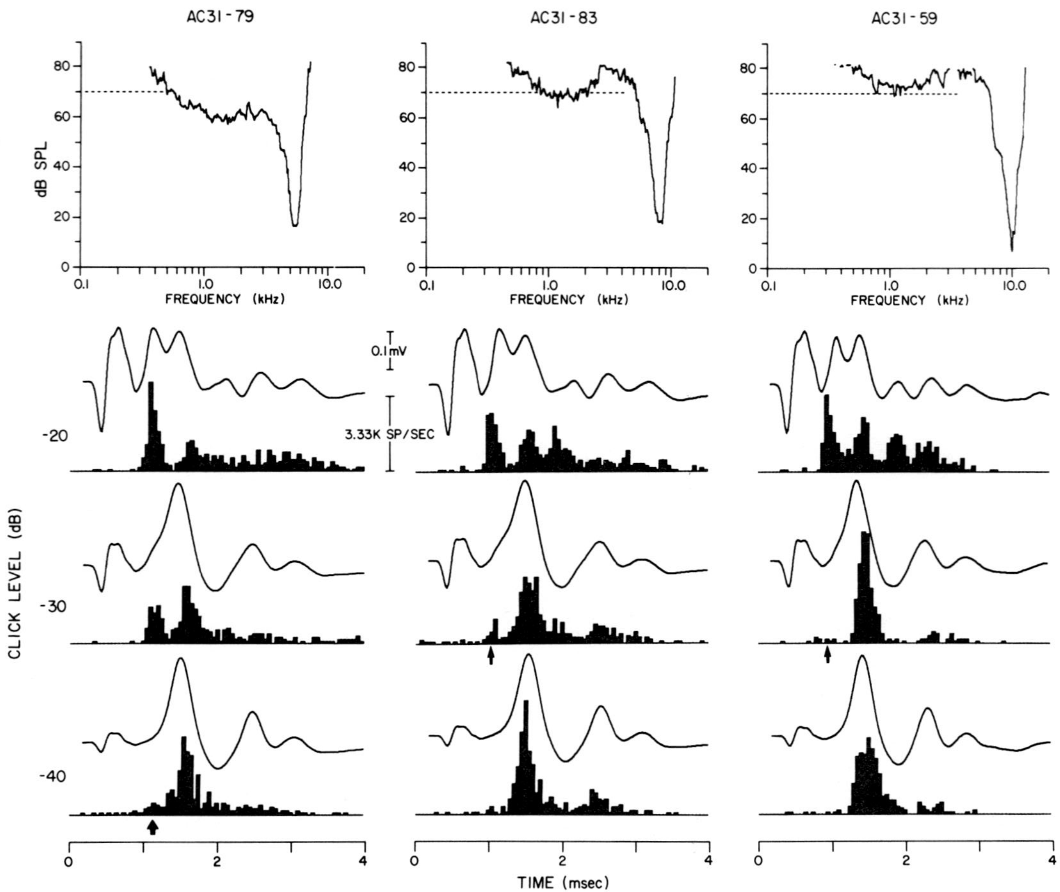

AC31-79
AC31-83
AC31-59
dB SPL
FREQUENCY (kHz)
0.1mV
3.33K SP/SEC
CLICK LEVEL (dB)
-20
-30
-40
TIME (msec)

Fig. 8. Response patterns at three click levels for 3 units with high (> 18 spikes/sec) spontaneous discharge rates whose tuning curves are different. At the top of the figure are shown tuning curves for the 3 units whose CF are 5.5, 8.1, and 10.0 kHz, respectively. The dotted horizontal line provides a convenient reference level to compare the tails of the tuning curves. Below each tuning curve are the PST histograms for the responses of that unit to three levels of rarefaction clicks. The click levels are given with the lowest level at the bottom and the highest at the top. Just above each histogram is the simultaneously-obtained averaged gross response for each stimulus condition. The arrows below the histograms point to an early, small peak which, at higher click levels, will become the earliest and largest peak.

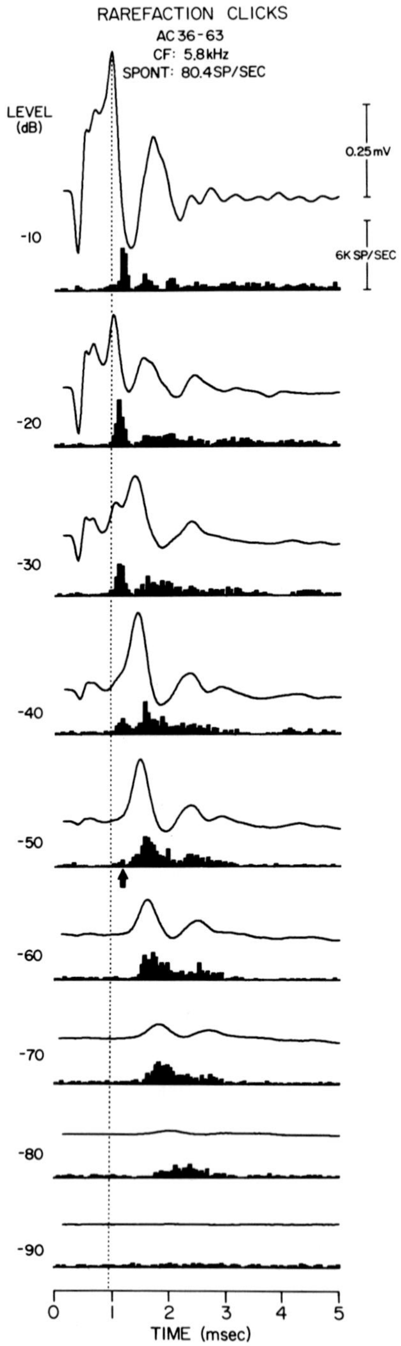

Fig. 9. Response patterns of a unit with high spontaneous discharge rate to clicks at nine different levels. The gross responses were obtained simultaneously with each PST histogram. The arrow points to the first appearance of an early peak as the click level is increased in 10 dB steps. The time at which N_1 is maximal for the highest click level is indicated by a dotted vertical line.

tials becomes the dominant peak, and there is a hint of an even earlier peak in the histogram at -10 dB click level.

Figure 9 showed that the PST histograms of a unit whose CF is 5.8 kHz can parallel the shape of the gross neural potentials to a considerable degree. Figure 10 shows PST histograms for 5 units with different CF. For Unit 36-40, with a CF of 1.7 kHz, there are detectable responses at -90 dB. At -80 dB, the earliest peak has a latency slightly longer than 3 msec, and the later peaks appear at approximately 0.6 msec (1/CF) intervals. As click level increases, new peaks, both earlier and later, appear but the old peaks remain with approximately the same latencies as for lower-level clicks. At the highest click level (-10 dB), the earliest peak occurs later than does the earliest peak at -20 dB. The sequence of changes in the PST histograms as click level increases is that a small, early peak appears, grows rapidly within a 20 dB range to be the largest peak, only to be displaced as the largest peak by yet another earlier peak. For Unit 36-1, with a CF of 2.3 kHz, a similar sequence occurs. The interpeak time is, of course, 0.44 msec (1/CF) instead of 0.6 msec. At levels above -50 dB, the first peak is the largest, with the later peaks appearing more subdued than at lower-click levels. For Unit 36-63, the responses have already been described (Fig. 9). It is interesting that at -10 DB, there appear to be multiple peaks at intervals of approximately 0.4 msec, so that on the basis of this histogram alone, one might have erroneously concluded that this unit had a CF of 2.5 kHz. For Unit 36-33, with a CF of 9.5 kHz, the emergence of an earlier peak at -30 dB correlates with the splitting of N_1 into two distinct peaks. The growth of the first peak of N_1, relative to the second with further increases in click level, matches well the growth of the new, early peak in the histograms. For Unit 36-57, with a CF of 23 kHz, there are few, if any, responses below -20 dB, when a single short latency peak is seen in the histogram. At -10 dB, there are two peaks with an interpeak time of approximately 1 msec. The response pattern of this unit is of special interest because what little energy there is in the 100μsec click at 23 kHz is further attenuated by the acoustic system and the middle ear, so the responses to high-level clicks may well be due to the low-frequency components of the click, rather than components near 23 kHz. In examining the histograms for all these units, one notes that for units with CF below 10 kHz the earliest peak begins to emerge at click levels that are approximately 30 dB above the levels at which each unit begins to show responses to the clicks.

Although data such as are contained in Figure 9 suggest that response patterns in certain units may resemble the waveforms of the gross neural potentials, one would require data for many units in order to see how the gross potentials relate to the overall distribution of activity in the auditory nerve. Figure 11 shows such data for units with high (>18 spikes/sec) spontaneous discharge rates, and Figure 12 shows similar data for fibers with medium (0.5-18 spikes/sec) spontaneous discharge rates in the same cat. As is well known, all the high-CF units tend to have an early peak at nearly the same time, while the low-CF units show a systematically increasing latency with decreasing CF. Moreover, as the N_1 splits into two peaks at click levels between -40 and -20 dB, the PST histograms of the

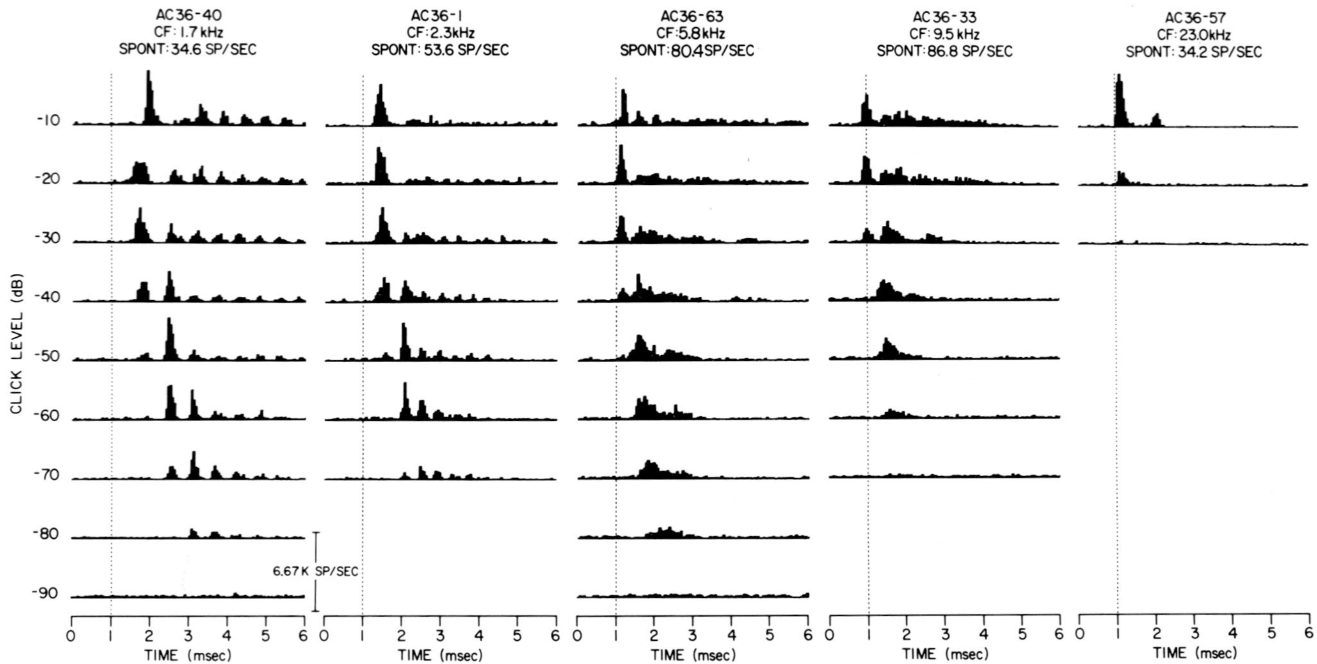

Fig. 10. Response patterns for 5 units in one animal to a click level series. Each column contains PST histograms for 1 unit at different click levels (highest level at the top). A set of gross responses for this animal is available in Figure 9. The dotted vertical line is at 1 msec.

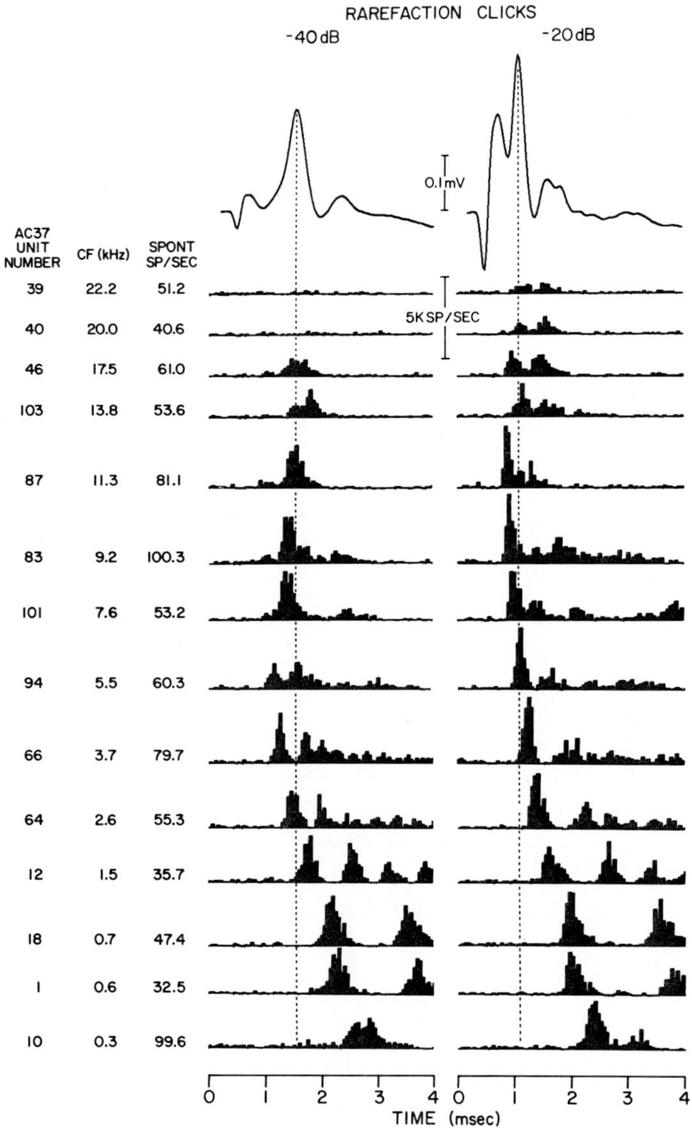

Fig. 11. PST histograms for 14 units in one animal to rarefaction clicks at two levels. All of these units had high spontaneous discharge rates and were selected to have a wide range of CF. The histograms are arranged in order of descending CF. Gross responses for the two click levels are shown at the top. Dotted vertical lines are drawn from the N_1 peaks in the gross response.

highest-CF units also show split peaks. Both in terms of synchrony and in the amount of discharge, the major contributions to the earliest gross neural potential seem to be from units with CF between 4 and 14 kHz, with this range being extended as the stimulus level increases.

Displays exemplified by Figures 11 and 12 are useful in showing not only which units are discharging, but also the strength of the discharge. If one were willing to sacrifice the latter information, a more panoramic picture of activity in the nerve could be obtained by plotting isorate neurograms. An isorate neurogram is a plot showing unit activity above a particular discharge rate taking place within the neural population as a function of poststimulus time. In the present case, the neural population can be ordered according to CF which presumably indicates the locus of innervation by each fiber along the length of the cochlea.

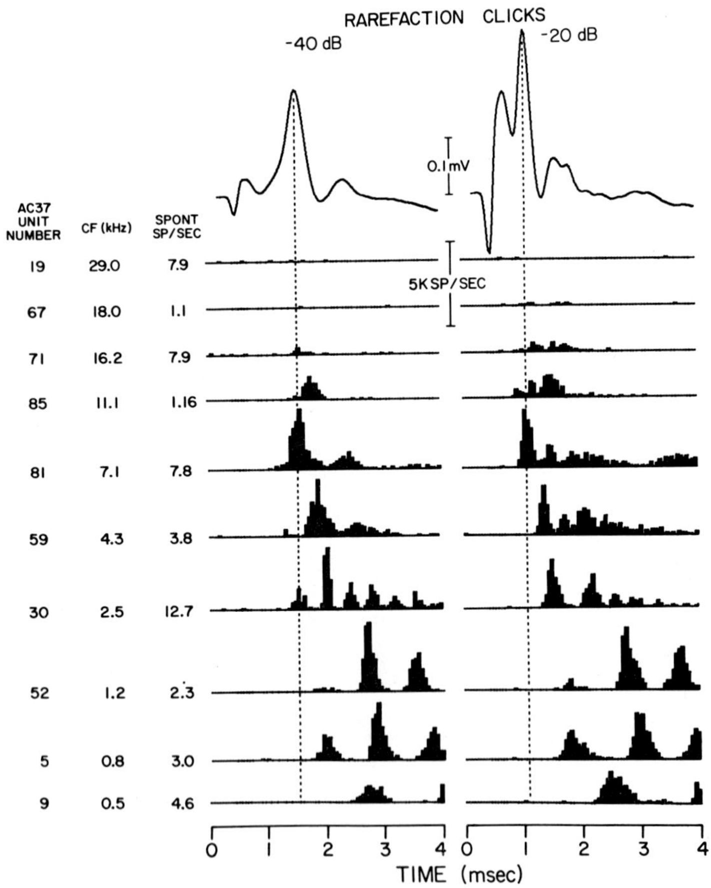

Fig. 12. Response patterns to rarefaction clicks at two levels for 10 medium (0.5 - 18 spikes/sec) spontaneous discharge rate units. This figure is arranged in much the same way as Figure 11 which is for units with high spontaneous discharge rates (> 18 spikes/sec).

Figure 13 shows how isorate neurograms are constructed from PST histograms of single-unit activity. Neurograms for three different rate criteria are shown for each of two rarefaction click levels. The click levels were chosen so that at the lower level (-40 dB), the N_1 is still a single peak; whereas at the higher level (-20 dB), the N_1 is split into two peaks. For the highest rate criterion (A), the neurograms show that the peaks of activity for units with CF above 3-4 kHz are well synchronized with one another, while for units with lower CF, the peaks occur systematically later for units of decreasing CF. The timing of the tallest peak in the histograms of the high-CF units seems to match that of N_1. (As explained in the caption for Figure 2, the time scales of the histograms are shifted forward by 0.2 msec.)

Another interesting aspect of Figure 13 is that if the rate criterion is set at a relatively low value, as in C, responses occur for many milliseconds after the click is delivered, even for high-CF units. These late responses have repeatable time structure and could result from long-lasting mechanical "ringing" of the acoustic system, the middle ear, and the inner ear.

Figure 14 shows how isorate neurograms can change as a function of click level. The main contribution to N_1 appears to come from units with CF above 3-4 kHz. After N_1 splits into two peaks, these high-CF units also show two peaks in the PST histograms. This point is seen more clearly in Figure 15, which shows data for a cat in which more units with CF above 10 kHz were studied. The peaks in N_1 appear to correspond with vertical columns of activity in the neurogram indicating synchronized discharges.

One can occasionally find vertical columns of activity that line up with later peaks in the gross response (Fig. 13). However, this is not as clear as the match of unit activity with the peaks of N_1. Apparently, auditory-nerve units can contribute to N_2 (as suggested by Tasaki, 1954), but it may not be the only, or even the major, component.

It is instructive to compare responses to condensation and rarefaction clicks because click polarity affects N_1 without changing the stimulus level. Figure 16 shows some PST histograms and gross responses for both rarefaction and condensation clicks for three units. For the units with CF of 5.4 and 8.1 kHz, the PST histograms show peaks that correlate roughly with the shape of N_1. For rarefaction clicks, the splitting of the N_1 peak corresponds to the appearance and growth of an earlier peak in the PST histograms. For condensation clicks, the N_1 does not split, and only a single dominant peak is evident in the PST histograms. The unit with a CF of 0.3 kHz obviously cannot contribute to N_1 at all.

DISCUSSION

Single-Unit Behavior Underlying N_1

Although most of the points made here are known from earlier work (Kiang et al., 1965), they are presented here in a more systematic and complete way. In

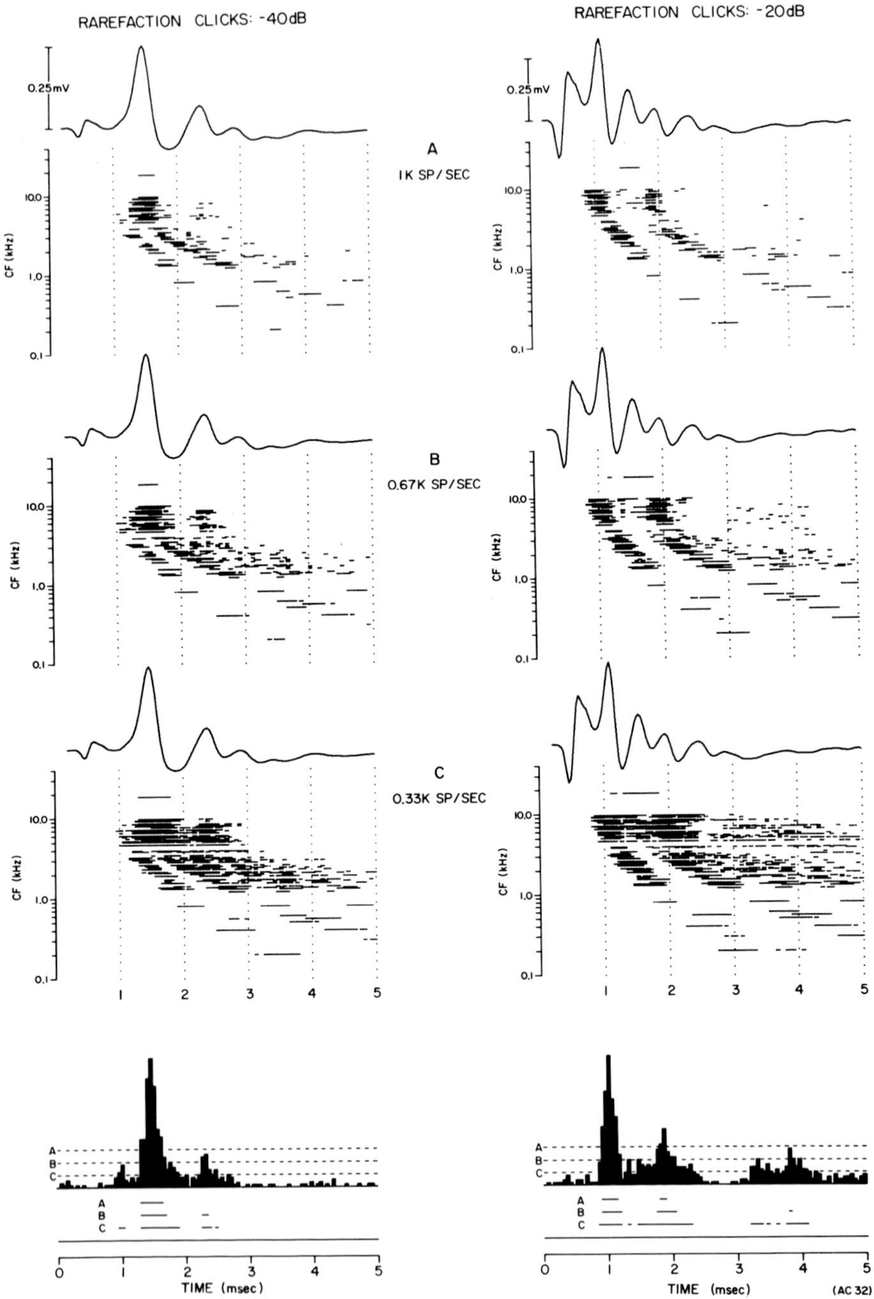

Fig. 13. Construction of isorate neurograms. At the bottom of the figure are shown histograms of the responses of 1 unit to clicks at two levels. A height discriminator is set at discharge rates corresponding to a specific number of spikes/sec. Three rates (A, B, and C) are shown as examples. Below each histogram are three sets of horizontal bars that correspond to

the neurogram display, vertical columns of activity indicate synchronized discharges in groups of auditory-nerve fibers and appear to be correlated with peaks in the gross neural responses. At low-click levels, the fibers that contribute most to N_1 are those with CF between 4-10 kHz. As the click level increases, more and more units with higher CF begin to contribute. Some units with lower CF show earlier peaks of activity that can also contribute to N_1. It is clear, however, that units with CF lower than 1 kHz never contribute significantly to N_1 at any click level.

It is the interaction of stimulus variables with unit properties that determines how much each unit contributes to N_1. Thus, the relatively small contribution of units with CF above 10 kHz results from an interplay of factors such as the spectrum of the 100μsec click, the characteristics of the sound generating system, the transfer function of the middle ear, and the properties of the sensorineural apparatus. Units with CF below 1-2 kHz have response latencies that are progressively longer with lower CF. Thus, their peak activities do not align in vertical columns in a neurogram and do not sum to give a sizeable gross response.

As rarefaction click level increases to certain levels, two peaks approximately 0.2 msec apart appear in place of a single N_1 peak. A similar phenomenon is seen for the PST histogram peaks that occur near the time of N_1. At still higher rarefaction click levels, the earlier of these two peaks dominates and there is a return to a single N_1 peak with, of course, a shorter latency than at lower-click levels. There is a similar change in the PST histograms of single units with CF between 4 and 10 kHz. Thus, the changes in N_1 appear to parallel changes in the activity of units with CF between 4 and 10 kHz under the present experimental conditions. This is not to deny that there are changes in the relative contribution of units with changes in click level. It is clear that at high-click levels, for instance, units with CF above 10 kHz will contribute significantly to N_1.

The changes in unit discharge patterns as click level changes are not yet understood on theoretical grounds. At a qualitative level, it is easy to see how the broadening of tuning curves at high-stimulus levels should be an important factor in determining the responses to complex stimuli such as clicks. The change from operating in a sharply tuned range to a broadly tuned one most certainly will affect the impulse response of the unit. The theory of how auditory-nerve units respond to transient stimuli leads to complications that have only begun to be explored (Gray, 1967; Smith, 1973; Harris, 1977). Clicks are not only transient signals, they are also broadband. Many complicated non-linear effects have been demonstrated

the times for which the discharge rate exceeds the three discriminator rates respectively. The neurogram is constructed by plotting these horizontal bars for units of different CF in order to display the distribution of activity over the whole nerve. For each of the two click levels, -40 dB and -20 dB, three separate neurograms are shown. The neurograms A, B, and C were obtained with rate thresholds set at 1000, 666, and 333 spikes/sec, respectively. The same 54 units are represented in each neurogram. A representative averaged gross response from the same cat is shown above each neurogram.

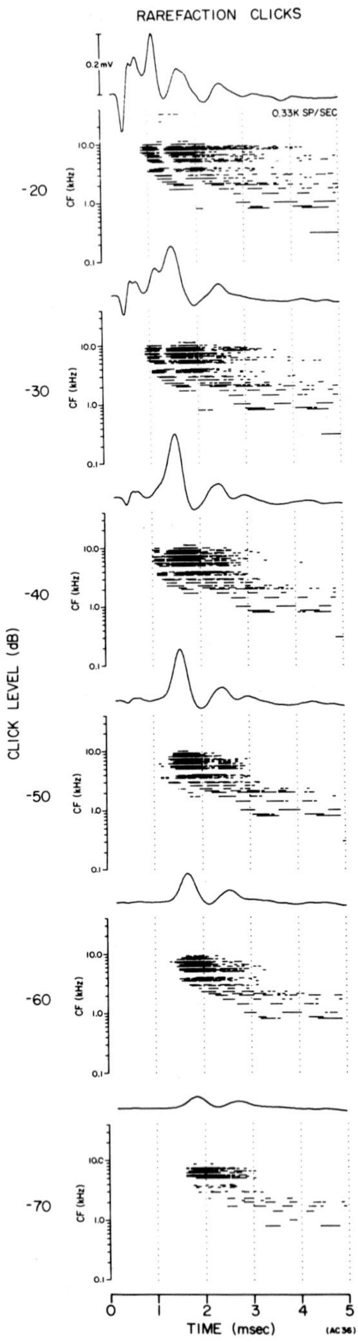

Fig. 14. Isorate neurograms based on 39 units in 1 animal. Responses to six levels of clicks are shown along with a set of gross RW responses taken at the beginning of the experiment. Few data were obtained for units with CF above 10 kHz in this experiment.

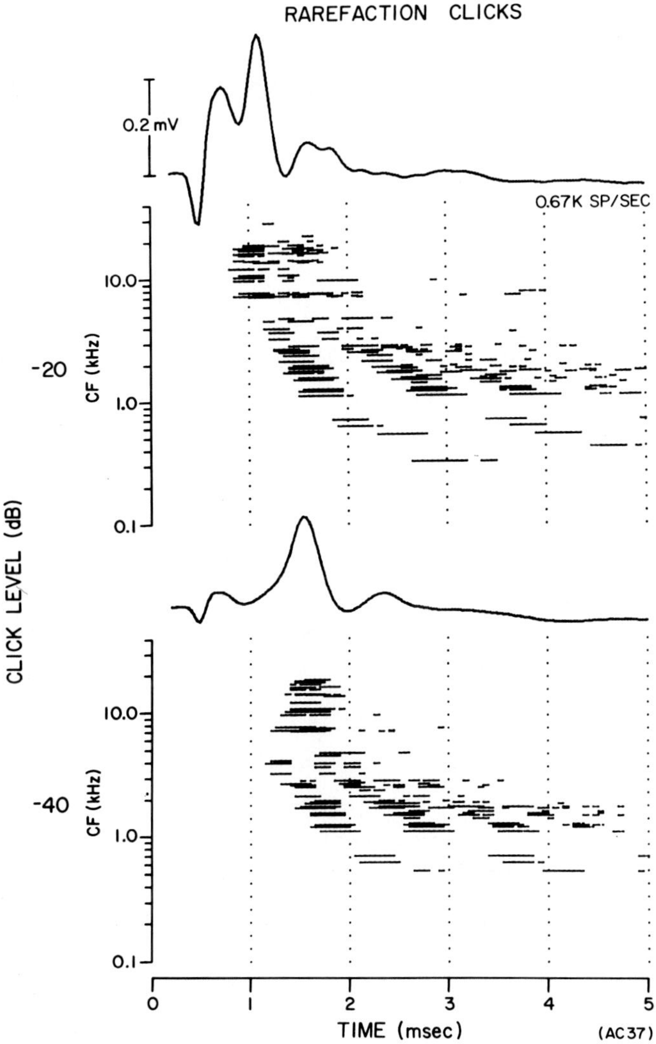

Fig. 15. Isorate neurograms for 2 click levels. Seventy-one units are represented in each neurogram. More units with CF above 10 kHz were studied in this animal than in Cat AC36 (Fig. 14).

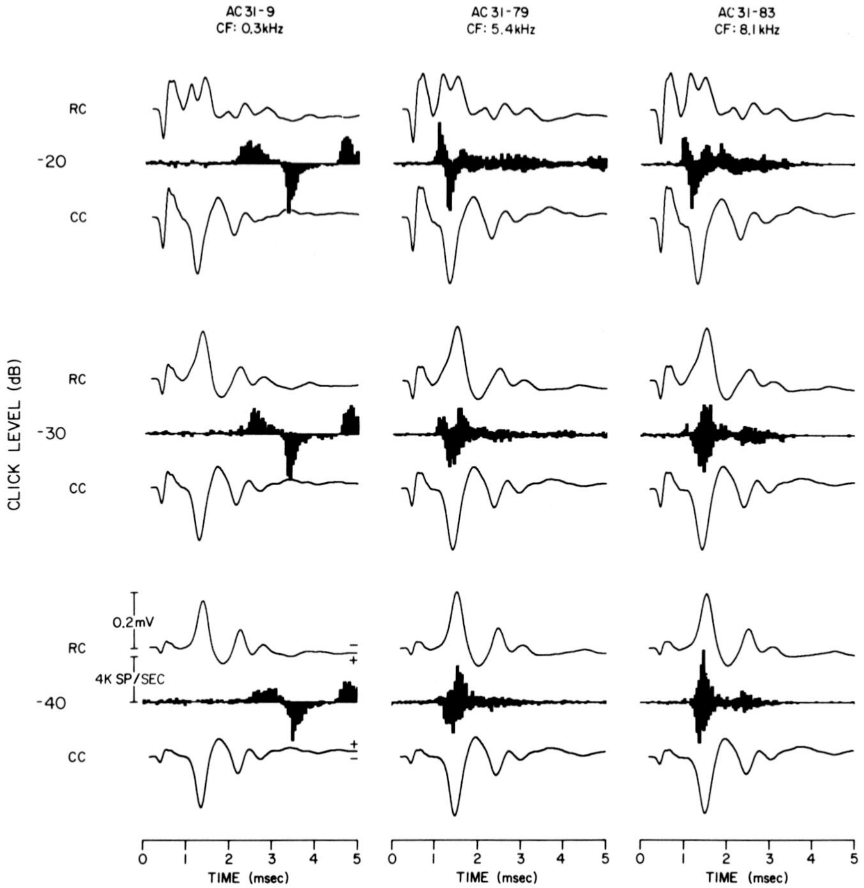

Fig. 16. Simultaneously recorded gross RW potentials and responses of 3 units to rarefaction and condensation clicks. The CFs of these units are shown on the top of each column. The PST histograms for condensation clicks (CC) are inverted and placed under the PST histograms for rarefaction clicks (RC). Similarly, the gross responses to condensation clicks were inverted and placed below the corresponding histograms. Responses for three click levels are shown.

for single-unit responses to two tones (Sachs and Kiang, 1968; Goldstein and Kiang, 1968; Kiang et al., 1969; Kiang and Moxon, 1972). The importance of such effects in responses to broadband stimuli has not been adequately evaluated.

Modelling Gross Neural Potentials

There have been many attempts to account for the complex changes in N_1 as click level changes. Early efforts predated single-unit data for the auditory nerve so that proposed explanations were necessarily based on hypothetical behavior of auditory-nerve units (Frishkopf and Rosenblith, 1958; Davis, 1961; Peake and

Kiang, 1962). Curiously enough, long after single-unit data became available (Kiang et al., 1965), the thinking of most electrocochleographers continued to be based on hypothetical conjectures about auditory units (Elberling, 1973; Yoshie, 1973; Eggermont and Odenthal, 1974). More recently, some workers have begun to incorporate some of the single-unit data into their schemes (deBoer, 1975; Özdamar and Dallos, 1975; Elberling, 1976), but these theoretical formulations are still far from satisfactory in the light of present data.

While it is obvious that existing information will not suffice to model gross responses quantitatively from unit responses, it must also be clear that modern experimental methods are capable of generating such data. Simplistic theories based on fancied differences in neuronal populations must be replaced by quantitative assessments of how the single units are influenced by all the stimulus and physiological variables that need to be specified in order to account for gross neural potentials.

It might be thought that a more insightful model could be generated in terms of the component stages preceding auditory-nerve activity. Although some of the earlier stages are becoming fairly well understood, the stages in the cochlea are still only loosely described. The primary difficulty in thinking about how cochlear mechanisms generate auditory-nerve responses is that there are too many free-floating possibilities. To explore all the arguments assigning various phenomena to specific stages in the mechanical, sensory, and neural sequence would require a monograph in itself. Even such fundamental questions as to whether there are two or more populations of sensory cells that have very different response properties; whether the different sensory cells interact; how the hair cells relate to the nerve cells; and whether different nerve cells can influence one another; remain equivocal. While it may be fascinating to speculate on the various theoretical possibilities, the confusion between conjectures and facts in the current literature plagues the beginning student.

Fortunately, at the auditory-nerve level, one can continue to build a quantitative theory of the gross neural responses in terms of single-unit activity without completely understanding the mechanisms that generate such activity.

Implications for Electrocochleography

The dangers in interpreting potentials recorded from abnormal human ears must certainly be apparent when the understanding of even normal neural potentials is not yet firm. Even assuming that the recordings are of purely neural origin (by no means a safe assumption in many clinical situations), the problem of adequate stimulus control must be considered. The tuning curves of auditory-nerve fibers is not only determined by cochlear processes but also by all the preceding stages in the external and middle ears, to say nothing of the acoustic system (Kiang et al., 1967). In the case of patients with hearing disorders, one cannot assume that all these previous stages are functioning normally, even if sensorineural defects are clearly indicated. Furthermore, even within the cochlea, abnormalities at mechanical, sensory, or neural stages can all eventually result in altered activity of single units in the nerve. There is abundant evidence that a variety of complex changes can occur in the tuning curves of auditory-nerve fibers after insults to the cochlea (Kiang et al., 1970; Kiang, Liberman and Levine, 1976). Although it is theoretically possible that tests may be developed for the differential diagnosis of various levels of disorders, it may also be that similar electrocochleographic recordings can result from different underlying abnormalities.

Notwithstanding all these intricate warnings, the clinician does have immediate problems and needs to know what can be decided from electrocochleographic data. As a general principle, it is probably safest to avoid involved interpretations unless it directly affects treatment or money matters. If surgical intervention is to be considered, if rehabilitation training is to be planned, or if other kinds of tests need to be ordered, then one must proceed on a "best guess" basis. Gross distinctions in assigning defects to brain or ear can frequently be made with some confidence. Conductive vs sensorineural losses can sometimes be assessed, when other tests are inapplicable. Perhaps the diagnosis of specific conditions such as Menière's disease or acoustic tumors can also be aided.

The point is that few of these practical applications require interpretation at a detailed cellular level. The clinician can correlate electrocochleographic recordings and disease entities in a straightforward empirical manner, insisting only that the correlations be validated on their own merits. To couch interpretations and make recommendations in terms of presumed underlying mechanisms is probably premature and certainly unnecessary. With further advances in knowledge, it may become possible to use clinical electrocochleography in a more satisfactory way.

Acknowledgements

Supported by NIH Grants 1 PO1 NS13126, 1 RO1 NS01344, and 1 RO1 NS11000.

REFERENCES

Davis, H. Peripheral coding of auditory information. In: *Sensory Communication,* edited by W.A. Rosenblith. Cambridge: MIT Press, 1961, p. 119-141.

de Boer, E. Synthetic whole-nerve action potentials for the cat. *J. Acoust. Soc. Amer. 58:* 1030-1045, 1975.

Derbyshire, A. and Davis, H. The probable mechanism for stimulation of the auditory nerve by the organ of Corti. *Amer. J. Physiol. 113:* 476-504, 1935.

Eggermont, J.J. and Odenthal, D.W. Action potentials and summating potentials in the normal human cochlea. *Acta Otolaryng.* Suppl. *316:* 39-61, 1974.

Elberling, C. Transitions in cochlear action potentials recorded from the ear canal in man. *Scand. Audiol. 2:* 151-159, 1973.

Elberling, C. Simulation of cochlear action potentials recorded from the ear canal in man. In: *Electrocochleography,* edited by R.J. Ruben, C. Elberling and G. Salomon. Baltimore: University Park Press, 1976, p. 151-168.

Frishkopf, L.S. and Rosenblith, W.A. Fluctuations in neural thresholds. In: *Symposium on Information Theory in Biology,* edited by H.P. Yockey, R.L. Platzman and H. Quastler. New York: Pergamon Press, 1958, p. 153-168.

Goldstein, J.L. and Kiang, N.Y.S. Neural correlates of the aural combination tone $2f_1 - f_2$. *Proc. IEEE, 56:* 981-992, 1968.

Goldstein, M.H., Jr. and Kiang, N.Y.S. Synchrony of neural activity in electric response evoked by transient acoustic stimuli. *J. Acoust. Soc. Amer. 30:* 107-114, 1958.

Gray, P.R. Conditional probability analyses of the spike activity of single neurons. *Biophys. J. 7:* 759-777, 1967.

Harris, D.M. *Forward Masking and Recovery from Short-Term Adaptation in Single Auditory-Nerve Fibers.* Research Report, Auditory Research Laboratory (Audiology), Northwestern University, Evanston, Illinois, 1977.

Kiang, N.Y.S. The use of computers in studies of auditory neurophysiology. *Trans. Amer. Acad. Ophthalmol. Otolaryngol. 65:* 735-747, 1961.

Kiang, N.Y.S., Baer, T., Marr, E.M. and Demont, D. Discharge rates of single auditory-nerve fibers as functions of tone level. *J. Acoust. Soc. Amer. 46:* 106, 1969.

Kiang, N.Y.S., Liberman, M.C. and Levine, R.A. Auditory-nerve activity in cats exposed to ototoxic drugs and high-intensity sounds. *Ann. Otol. Rhinol. Laryngol. 75:* 752-768, 1976. Also in *Trans. Amer. Otol. Soc., Inc. 64:* 79-95, 1976.

Kiang, N.Y.S. and Moxon, E.C. Physiological considerations in artificial stimulation of the inner ear. *Ann. Ctol. Rhinol. Laryngol. 81:* 714-731, 1972.

Kiang, N.Y.S., Moxon, E.C. and Kahn, A.R. The relationship of gross potentials recorded from the cochlea to single unit activity in the auditory nerve. In: *Electrocochleography,* edited by R.J. Ruben, C. Elberling and G. Salomon. Baltimore: University Park Press, 1976, p. 95-115.

Kiang, N.Y.S., Moxon, E.C. and Levine, R.A. Auditory-nerve activity in cats with normal and abnormal cochleas. In: *Sensorineural Hearing Loss,* edited by G.E.W. Wolstenholme and J. Knight. London: J. And A. Churchill, 1970, p. 241-268.

Kiang, N.Y.S. and Peake, W.T. Components of electrical responses recorded from the cochlea. *Ann. Otol. Rhinol. Laryngol. 69:* 448-459, 1960.

Kiang, N.Y.S., Sachs, M.B. and Peake, W.T. Shapes of tuning curves for single auditory-nerve fibers. *J. Acoust. Soc. Amer. 42:* 1341-1342, 1967.

Kiang, N.Y.S., Watanabe, T., Thomas, E.C. and Clark, L.F. *Discharge Patterns of Single Fibers in the Cat's Auditory Nerve.* Research Monograph No. 35. Cambridge: MIT Press, 1965.

Özdamar, Ö. and Dallos, P. Input-output functions of cochlear whole-nerve action potentials: interpretation in terms of one population of neurons. *J. Acoust. Soc. Amer. 59:* 143-147, 1975.

Peake, W.T. and Kiang, N.Y.S. Cochlear responses to condensation and rarefaction clicks. *Biophys. J. 2:* 23-34, 1962.

Rawdon-Smith, A.F. and Hawkins, J.E. The electrical activity of a denervated ear. *Proc. Royal Soc. Med. 32:* 496-507, 1939.

Rosenblith, W. Auditory masking and fatigue. *J. Acoust. Soc. Amer. 22:* 792-800, 1950.

Rosenblith, W.A. and Rosenzweig, M.R. Electrical responses to acoustic clicks: influence of electrode location in cats. *J. Acoust. Soc. Amer. 23:* 583-588, 1951.

Sachs, M.B. and Kiang, N.Y.S. Two-tone inhibition in auditory-nerve fibers. *J. Acoust. Soc. Amer. 43:* 1120-1128, 1968.

Smith, R.L. *Short-Term Adaptation and Incremental Responses of Single Auditory-Nerve Fibers.* Special Report, Laboratory of Sensory Communication, Syracuse University, Syracuse, New York, 1973.

Tasaki, I. Nerve impulses in individual auditory nerve fibers of guinea pig. *J. Neurophysiol. 17:* 97-122, 1954.

Vér, I.L., Brown, R.M. and Kiang, N.Y.S. Low-noise chambers for auditory research. *J. Acoust. Soc. Amer. 58:* 392-398, 1975.

Yoshie, N. Diagnostic significance of the electrocochleogram in clinical audiometry. *Audiology 12:* 504-539, 1973.

DISCUSSION

Davis: You have given us some wonderful information, and some very good advice particularly along toward the end. My question is, what would you recommend for the best acoustic spectrum, the best clicks to use, in order to get not only reasonably simple physiological action but also standardization across laboratories and across clinics in order to compare one thing with another? This may be something that can be brought under control, but I think it is often disregarded far too much.

Kiang: Our clicks are generated by delivering a 100 msec pulse to a 1 in. condenser earphone. The calibration is given in some of our previous papers. Ideally what you would like to deliver is an acoustic stimulus which would appear at the transducer level to be a simple stimulus. But that is hard to achieve without a way to measure the stimulus at that level. My guess is that the simplest thing to do in order to produce some consistent activity is to use a stimulus that can easily be duplicated anywhere. Of course, if you wish to study the system more carefully, other signals would have to be used also. The big problem at the moment is that people want to say something more than whether the system is entirely out of commission or not. At the same time they use a wide variety of different acoustic systems in different kinds of rooms. Under these conditions, talking about one particular stimulus that will give the most information for all purposes is not reasonable. In terms of standardization the best practical bet is to adopt a stimulus that can be generated easily, reproducibly and cheaply. At least then results in different laboratories can be compared.

Dallos: This is a comment on what Dr. Davis is asking. I think that the best click to use is no click at all! At least in animal models one can show quite clearly that properly shaped tone bursts are much simpler than clicks, and they provide audiometric information. One does not need to introduce great complexity in explanations to correlate single unit responses to them with the waveform of the action potential; in fact they correlate very well (Ö. Özdamar, Doctoral Thesis, Northwestern University, Evanston, 1976).

Nielsen: Most of your data were of rarefaction clicks. I noticed in one slide you combined the rarefaction and condensation clicks. In that slide the low levels it looked as if the condensation click led the rarefaction click in time, ie. it had a shorter latency. Does that happen very often?

Kiang: At low levels the latency of responses where high CF units is the same for both rarefaction and condensation clicks. This will not be true, of course, for low CF units.

Nielsen: At high levels?

Kiang: At high levels the situation is more complicated. The high CF units will respond to low frequency components in the stimuli. The tail of the tuning curves becomes more important.

Nielsen: And those are the situations in which you may get condensation leading rarefaction?

Kiang: At certain levels the response to condensation clicks can lead their responses to rarefaction clicks. Certainly.

Trahiotis: I have a question for Dr. Dallos. Are you saying that you have data that unequivocally show that if you do use tone pips the source of the action potential is not in the basal fibers, even though the base would be ringing at that low frequency?

Dallos: No question about that (see Özdamar, Ö. and Dallos, P., *J. Acoust. Soc. Am., 59:* 143-147, 1976, and Dallos, P. and Cheatham. M.A., *J. Acoust. Soc. Am., 59:* 591-597, 1976).

Kiang: I agree with that so long as the sound levels are low. One important point is that in the normal animal, the contribution of each single unit action potential has a roughly biphasic shape. Given the CF vs. latency curve for click responses, the contributions of the low CF units will cancel each other and not contribute significantly to the compound action potential.

But now in an abnormal ear, that is missing the high CF units, you will actually see a contribution from some of the low CF units near the edge of the lesion because their activity will not be canceled by the responses of the high CF units.

Moore: You showed mainly recordings from the round window. I wonder if you have used the electrode to monitor potentials from the external auditory meatus?

Kiang: In cats if the electrode is on the promontory the neural potential is smaller than but otherwise similar to the neural potential from the round window. In working with Montandon we stuck some electrodes in the ear canal, and they looked very much like the round window action potentials except that they were very much more attenuated.

Moore: Does the gross response line up with the PST histograms?

Kiang: Yes. The latencies are similar to the round window neural potential. If you look in our paper with Montandon you will find those recordings and will see how they line up. The N_1 everywhere outside of the skull lines up. Some of the later potentials can differ in appearance with electrode location.

ELECTROCOCHLEOGRAPHY (I)

Moderator: *Gerhard Salomon*

RECORDING AND ANALYSIS TECHNIQUES

Stanley Zerlin and Ralph F. Naunton

University of Chicago

INTRODUCTION

Electrocochleography refers to the recording of sound-evoked activity from the auditory periphery and has, in our experience, been of inestimable value in the assessment of patients unresponsive to conventional techniques.

In this paper we consider the two electrical indices most commonly associated with the periphery - the whole-nerve potential (AP) and the cochlear microphonic (CM).

Our primary aim is to suggest some methods of analysis that permit finer discriminations of the ECoG data, and thus provide better assessments of hearing in particularly difficult cases.

Our discussion limits itself to data derived from transtympanic recordings, and we begin by considering the effect of electrode placement.

RECORDING

Effect of Electrode Location

While the position of the transtympanic needle is necessarily limited to a small region of the promontory, the reference and ground electrodes can assume a variety of locations.

It is thus of interest to see how placement of reference and ground electrodes will influence the recorded potential; consequently, a small study was done to evaluate this variable.

Disc electrodes were positioned on the earlobe, forehead and vertex of a normal hearing, young adult subject. A transtympanic electrode was then positioned on the promontory under local anesthesia.

By means of wired connectors that were inserted quickly between the electrode leads and the amplifier input, the various disc electrodes were made to serve as either reference or ground points. One ear of the listener was then stimulated with wideband clicks at sensation levels of 70 and 10 dB at a 10 per second rate.

Results are summarized in Figure 1. The center column illustrates the various electrode configurations. The promontory electrode (arrow) serves as the "active" lead throughout; in the topmost head, earlobe is reference and forehead ground; in the middle head, vertex is reference and earlobe ground; and in the lowest head,

ISBN 0-12-514960-3

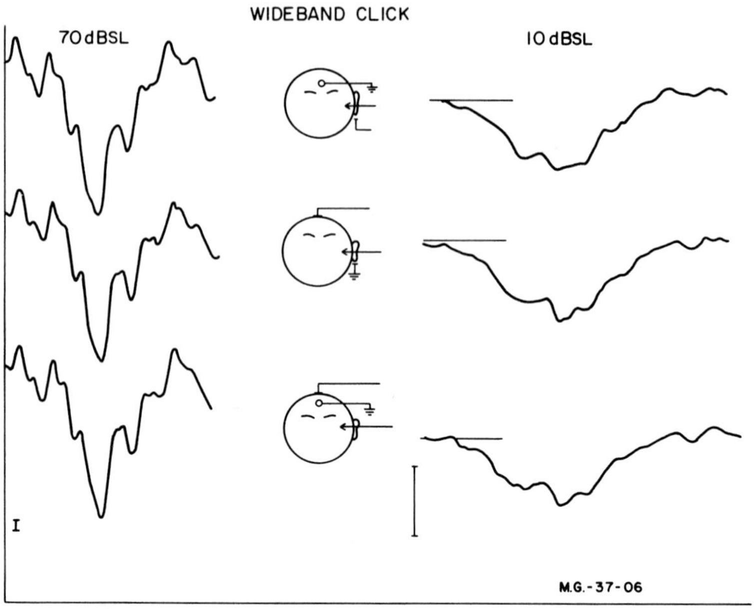

Fig. 1. Effects of different electrode locations on the amplitude of the whole nerve response. Promontory electrode (arrow) remains stationary; positions of reference and ground electrodes vary, as indicated. Vertical calibrations at the bottom of the columns represent one microvolt. Note that the various positionings of reference and ground electrodes do not influence amplitude of the AP.

vertex is again reference with forehead acting as ground. In the adjoining columns, labeled 70 dB and 10 dB, AP waveforms resulting from the different electrode configurations are shown. The vertical calibrations at the bottom of the two columns each represent one microvolt.

The results of Figure 1 show, first, that the amplitude and configuration of the whole-nerve response at 70 dB remain unchanged as the positions of reference and ground electrodes are varied. Careful measurement of the three amplitudes show small differences on the order of what would be expected from repeated measurements of the same condition.

The N_1 responses at the 10 dB level also remain essentially unchanged across the different combinations; this suggests that the ECoG threshold derived from a transtympanic recording is virtually independent of the location of the ground and reference electrodes, when they are in the region of the upper head.

ANALYSIS

CM Extraction

In electrocochleography, cancellation of the cochlear microphonic is ordinarily achieved by alternately reversing the polarity of the stimulus. If the CM

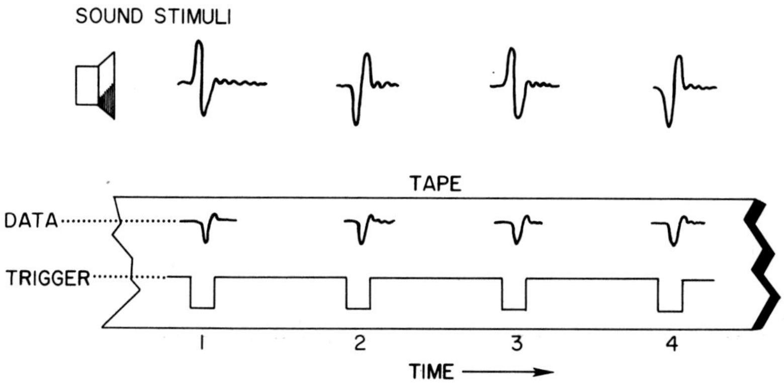

Fig. 2. Basic format of the recording technique, indicating (top) the reversing of stimulus polarity on alternate presentations and (below) the recording, on magnetic tape, of evoked response data (data channel) and of timing pulses coincident with stimulus presentations (trigger channel).

is to be preserved, some modern averagers are able to sum separately, on line, the responses to the two opposite polarities (The AP response is then visualized by simply adding the two traces).

We achieve a similar result by storing all evoked responses on magnetic tape and, on playback, instructing the computer to sum independently all the responses to the two polarities. The basic format for sound generation and recording is illustrated in Figure 2. Figure 3 (top) shows an AP to third-octave click (Zerlin and

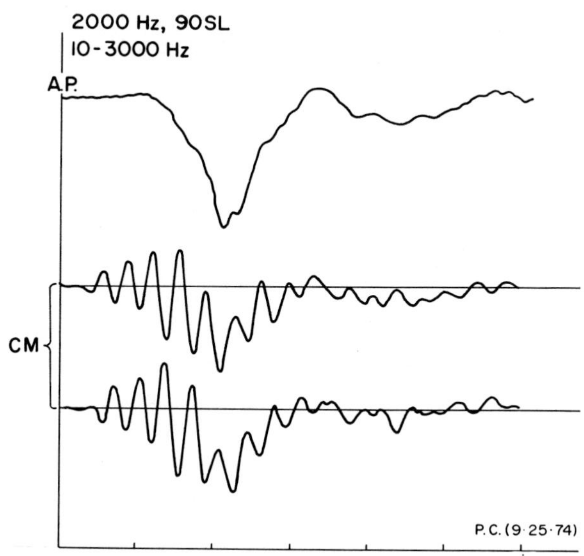

Fig. 3. Top: A 2000 Hz AP to third-octave click resulting from the summation of all recorded responses.

Below: The extraction of 2000 Hz CM from the same recording by having the computer sum separately the responses to stimuli of the same polarity. Note the presence of AP in CM.

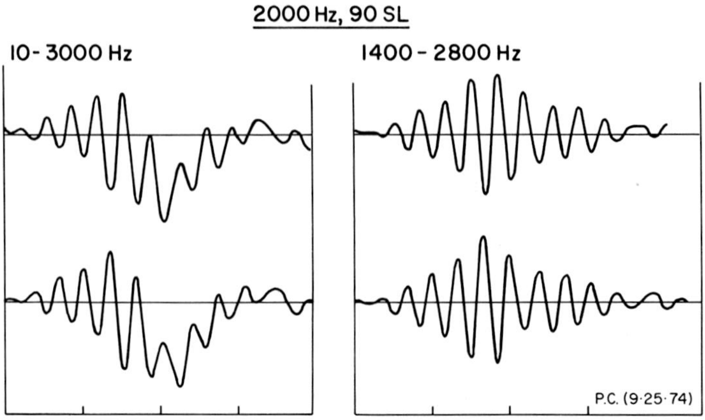

Fig. 4. Left panel: The mixture of 2000 Hz AP and CM, seen in Figure 3. Right panel: Elimination of AP by filtering the recorded responses through an octave-band filter centered at 2000 Hz.

Naunton, 1975) that results from summing responses to both polarities, and below, the effects of extracting the two opposite polarities of CM from that recording. Figure 4, left panel, repeats the CM seen in Figure 3; note the AP contained in the waveform, and that the recording passband is wide, extending from 10 - 3000 Hz.

Elimination of the AP can usually be accomplished by passing the recorded material through a passband filter. Experience has shown that a one octave filter centered around the microphonic frequency is satisfactory. The right panel of Figure 4 shows that octave filtering eliminates the frequencies comprising the AP.

Of greater importance is the use of octave filtering in visualizing the CM at lower levels of stimulation. Figure 5 shows, in the left panel, the decreasing visibility of a 500 Hz CM as the sensation level is reduced. Note that the recording passband is from 10 - 3000 Hz. While still apparent at 70 dB, the CM is lost at 50 dB. The right panel shows the same recorded material passed through an octave filter with passband 350-700 Hz. CM is still evident at 50 dB although questionable at 30 dB.

(It should be borne in mind that filtering will also introduce time delays, and that measurements of absolute response latency would be influenced by these delays).

Another possible technique is that of subtraction, illustrated in Figure 6. Shown in the upper traces are the alternate-polarity responses to a 1000 Hz click. In the lowest trace, one of the polarities has been inverted and added to the other. While the technique will not eliminate AP that follows the individual cycles (as in this case at 1000 Hz), the AP is generally cancelled at higher frequencies, where the nerve does not synchronize to individual cycles.

Techniques for Validating the AP

The superior signal-to-noise-ratio offered by the transtympanic recording does not always guarantee an unambiguous result. On occasion, doubt may arise con-

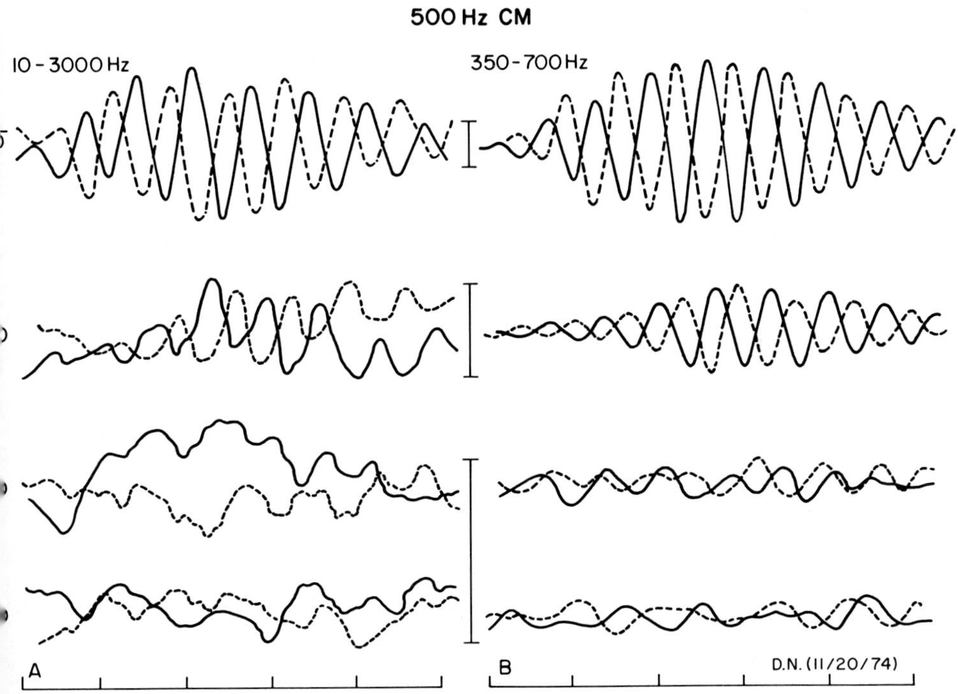

Fig. 5. Use of octave filtering to improve the visibility of the CM. Left panel: Unfiltered CM at 500 Hz (both polarities). Right panel: Same recorded material processed through an octave filter centered at 500 Hz.

cerning whether a response is real or the result of artifact.

To this end, we have developed techniques or criteria designed to increase or decrease confidence in questionable waveforms.

Latency Norms

The primary criterion involves the use of latency norms for evaluating the N_1 response. We have, retrospectively, collected a series of cases of children whose hearing had been evaluated in our laboratory and whose ECoG thresholds to third-octave clicks showed normal sensitivity at all frequencies.

Between 25 and 30 such ears were collected and the mean N_1 latencies calculated; those means are shown as a function of frequency and sensation level in Figure 7 and indicate the systematic changes in latency that are to be expected: for each frequency, latency decreases as sensation level increases, and latency decreases as frequency changes from 1000 to 8000 Hz. Note also that the latency separations

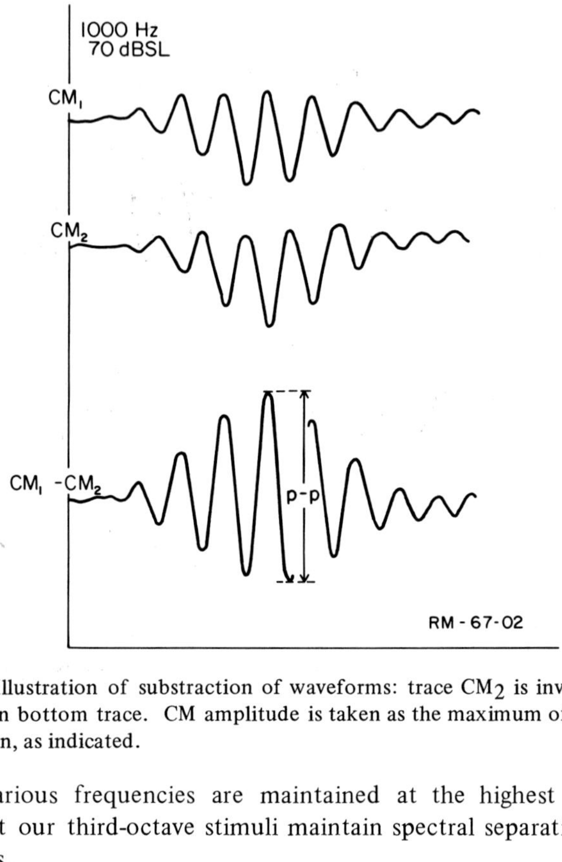

Fig. 6. Illustration of substraction of waveforms: trace CM_2 is inverted and added to CM_1, resulting in bottom trace. CM amplitude is taken as the maximum of the resulting peak-to-peak excursion, as indicated.

among the various frequencies are maintained at the highest sensation levels, suggesting that our third-octave stimuli maintain spectral separation even at quite high intensities.

These data form a useful basis for evaluating poor or ambiguous responses obtained in the clinic. However, they do not necessarily reflect true neural latencies at the lower sensation levels: it may be seen for example, that N_1 latencies at 1 and 2 kHz exceed 4-5 msec at levels below about 50 dB.

These latency estimates are long with respect to estimates of human whole-nerve latency found in the literature. (See, for example, Elberling (1974), who measured the derived AP latency using a technique based on masking procedures that allows neural activity from specific segments of the membrane to be evaluated.)

The unmasked AP latencies that we report have a more complicated origin, but we can begin to explain our excessively long latencies in the following way: at high click intensity, neural excitation will occur early on the sharply-rising segment of the stimulus waveform. As click intensity decreases, however, the leading edge

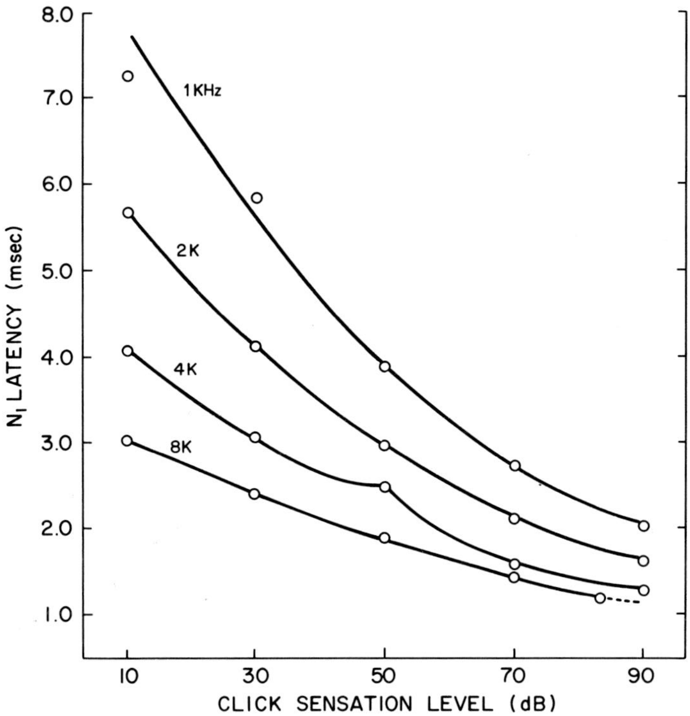

Fig. 7. Mean N_1 latency as function of click frequency and sensation level as determined from 25-30 young ears. The ears were considered normal in that all showed ECoG thresholds of normal sensitivity in the range 1000-8000 Hz.

of the stimulus waveform becomes gradually more shallow, and neural excitation will be delayed until the waveform reaches an appropriate amplitude. Since our stimulus waveforms are third-octave clicks that rise to maximum amplitude in three cycles, it is clear that low-intensity clicks may not produce neural excitation until the envelope maximum is reached, that is at the peak of the third cycle. In the case of the 1 kHz click, this means that the stimulus will have completed three cycles (3 msec) before neural excitation begins. Since we characteristically measure N_1 latency from the first rarefaction wave, it can be seen that this method of measurement will, at lower frequencies at low intensity, engender long N_1 latencies.

In Figure 8, the data are replotted on a logarithmic ordinate and are seen to describe essentially straight lines. (Note that the sensation levels presented are with reference to auditory thresholds for the third-octave clicks as determined on a group of normal young listeners in our laboratory.)

Not shown in these figures are the ranges of latency, taken as plus and minus one standard deviation around the mean. Generally speaking, we would accept responses falling inside the calculated ranges and reject those falling outside. The picture is not necessarily that simple, however, as Figure 9 illustrates: these are the

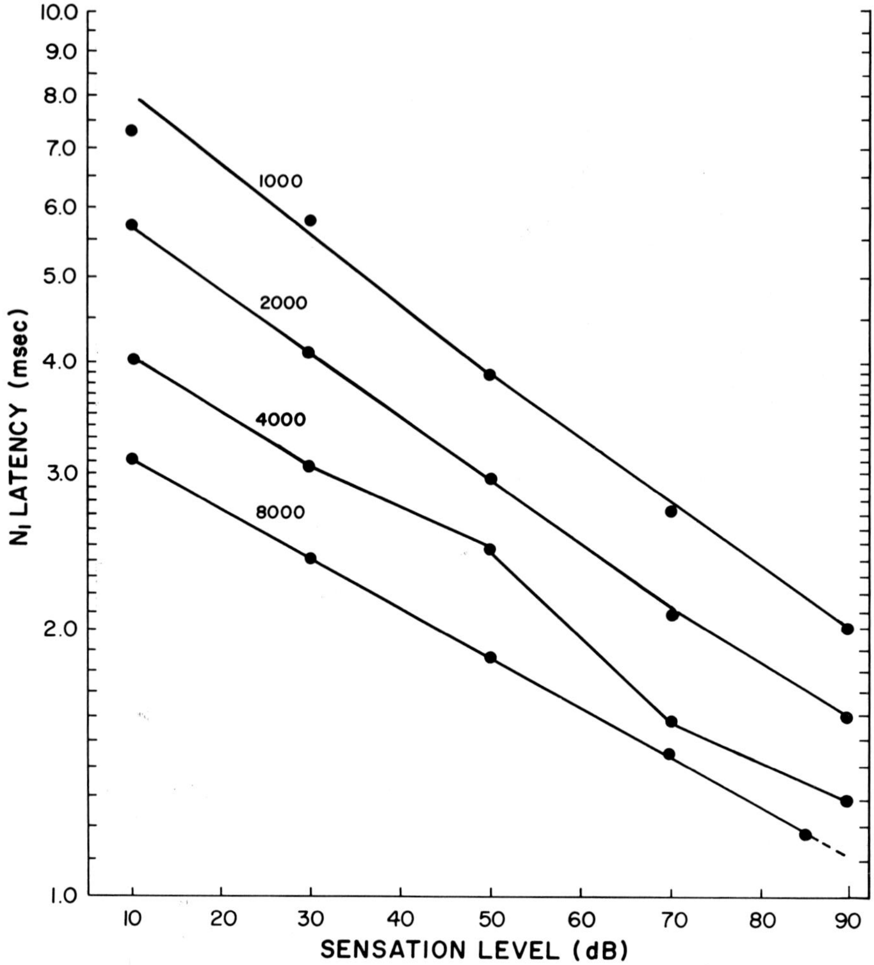

Fig. 8. Same data as Figure 7 plotted on a log ordinate.

ECoG results of a recently evaluated young patient. The ranges of N_1 latency are seen as the dashed lines accompanying each trace; the filled circles represent mean values. Note that the presumed responses increase in latency as level decreases; note also that none fall within the latency limits just described. However, the systematic increases in latency with decreasing level provide a form of face validity and the results would be considered legitimate, at least at the higher levels.

(The latency norms are based on ears with normal sensitivity; a conductive loss, for example, might account for the longer latencies seen here.)

Response Subdivision

We continue with the same example to introduce another technique used for validation of the AP. In Figure 9, the 1000 Hz responses at 45 dB and below were

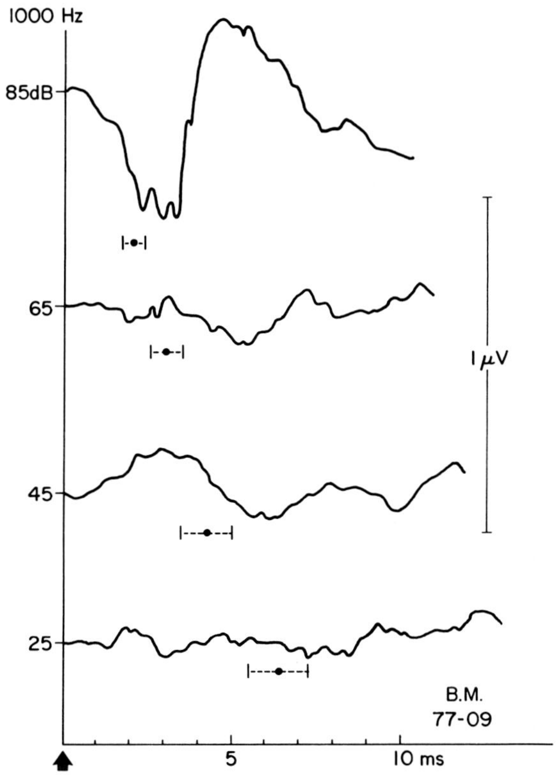

Fig. 9. ECoG responses of a young patient at 1000 Hz. The filled circles and horizontal dashed lines accompanying the waveforms indicate, respectively, the means and standard deviations of normal N_1 latencies for those conditions of stimulation: See text for additional details.

suspect because of excessive movement of the subject during this portion of the test. Some suspicion existed that movement artifact may have generated the response at 45 dB, and that the threshold lay above 45 dB, rather than below it.

As a check, the recorded responses were played back and, rather than summing the total of 500 individual responses, the computer was instructed to sum sequentially in 4 blocks of 125 responses each. That is, because four independent segments of memory are available, we had the computer sum the first 125 responses on the first trace, the second 125 on the second trace, and so on. If the results then showed all 4 traces to contain AP waveforms with similar latencies and amplitudes, we would consider the response valid, since it would indicate the overall waveform to be the result of an ongoing neural process.

The analysis can be furthered by instructing the computer to add, successively, the first block of 125 to the second, that new block of 250 to the third, and so on. That form of cumulative addition is illustrated in Figure 10. The example concerns the questionable 45 dB response, seen in Figure 9. The response shows a cumulative growth over time, increasing number, indicating without question that

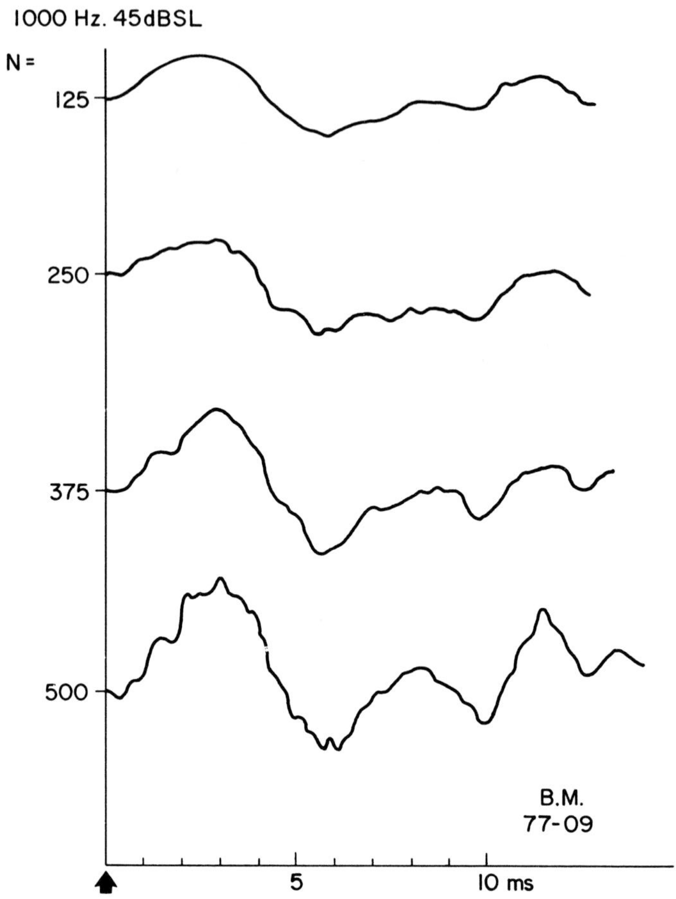

Fig. 10. Checking the validity of a questionable response by means of cumulative summation. The response here is the 45dB response seen in Figure 9. Note that as number of samples increase, the AP features (seen near 5 msec) increases systematically in amplitude. See text for further explanation.

the final waveform is the result of steady neural activity and not of a transient artifact.

Two further figures serve to amplify this technique. Figure 11 shows the ECoG results at 2000 Hz for a young child. Responses below 50 dB were in question because of the exaggerated latency and amplitude of the waveform at 30 dB and because of the bizarre shape seen at 10 dB.

In Figure 12, left panel, the 30 dB response of Figure 11 has been subdivided into blocks and cumulated. The steady growth of the response over time (increasing N) indicates its reputability. The 10 dB analysis is shown in the right panel: here the total N of 500 has been subdivided into 4 blocks of 125 each. No response

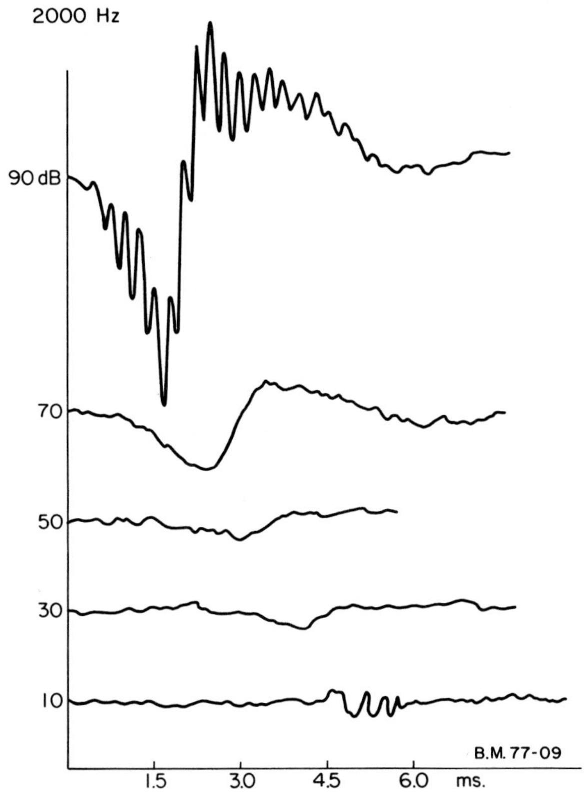

Fig. 11. ECoG waveforms of a young child. Responses below 50 dB were suspect because of the unusual configurations of both traces.

is seen common to all segments; rather, an artifact occurring somewhere in the third block is responsible for the questionable feature at the lowest level.

Evidence of Cochlear Microphonic

A final criterion for response evaluation lies in the use of the cochlear microphonic and may be of occasional use when evaluating the severely or profoundly deaf.

In processing the ECoG data of a number of profoundly deaf children, we have invariably found some CM present at the very high intensities of 100-110 dB SL (re normal). However, at very high levels of stimulation it is possible to mistake stimulus artifact for the cochlear microphonic, and precautions must be taken to assure the CM's validity. These precautions are treated in the paper "CM in the Clinical Diagnosis" (ibid).

A few examples will serve to illustrate the method. Figure 13, left panel displays the AP responses of a severely hard-of-hearing child; the right panel displays

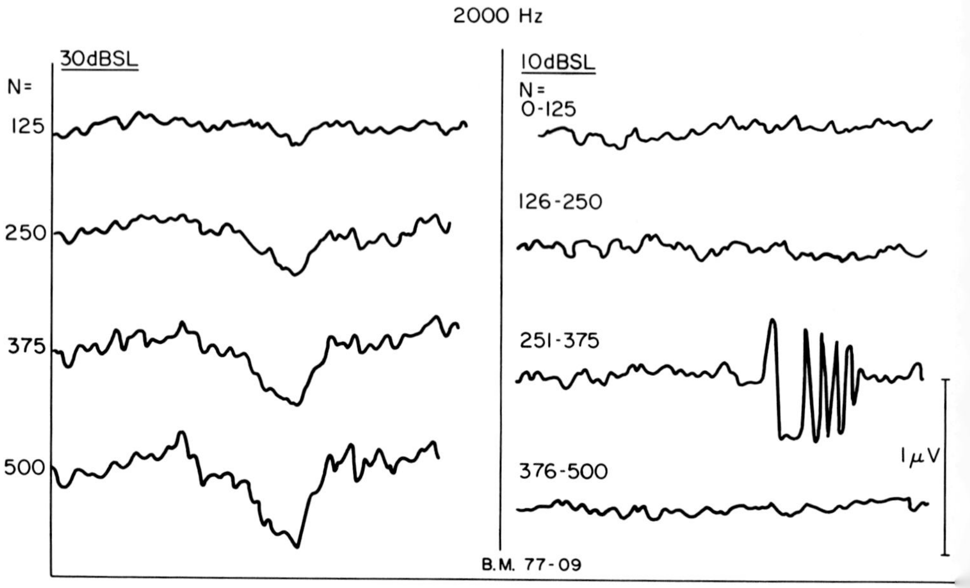

Fig. 12. Analysis of the questionable 30 dB and 10dB responses of Figure 11. Left panel: Cumulative summation of the 30dB response indicates its validity. Right panel: Breakdown of 10 dB recording into blocks of 125 each indicate no consistent response present; merely an artifact that occurred during the third block.

the corresponding CM's (CM's have been filtered, and one polarity inverted and added to other, as previously described). Both AP and CM amplitudes at 100 dB are far smaller than those from normals; the CM is on the order of 1μV, while normal young adults yield microphonic amplitudes of some 25-50μV at levels of 90 dB.

It is clear that CM amplitude decreases with decreasing levels of stimulation, but is is doubtful whether AP threshold can be predicted from the CM. In this instance, for example, the CM is still visualized at 50 dB while AP threshold, we know from other means, is in the vicinity of 80 dB.

Another example, shown in Figure 14 again compares AP and CM from another severely hard-of-hearing child, this time at 1000 Hz. Here, 100 dB yields a valid AP; lower levels do not yield definite responses, and threshold would be estimated at about 95 dB. Here, however, the CM becomes indistinguishable between 80 and 90 dB.

In the severely deaf, examples such as these permit the potentially useful observation that, while the CM can be seen at levels below those corresponding to AP threshold, AP is not seen when CM is absent.

In testing the residual hearing of some severely or profoundly impaired

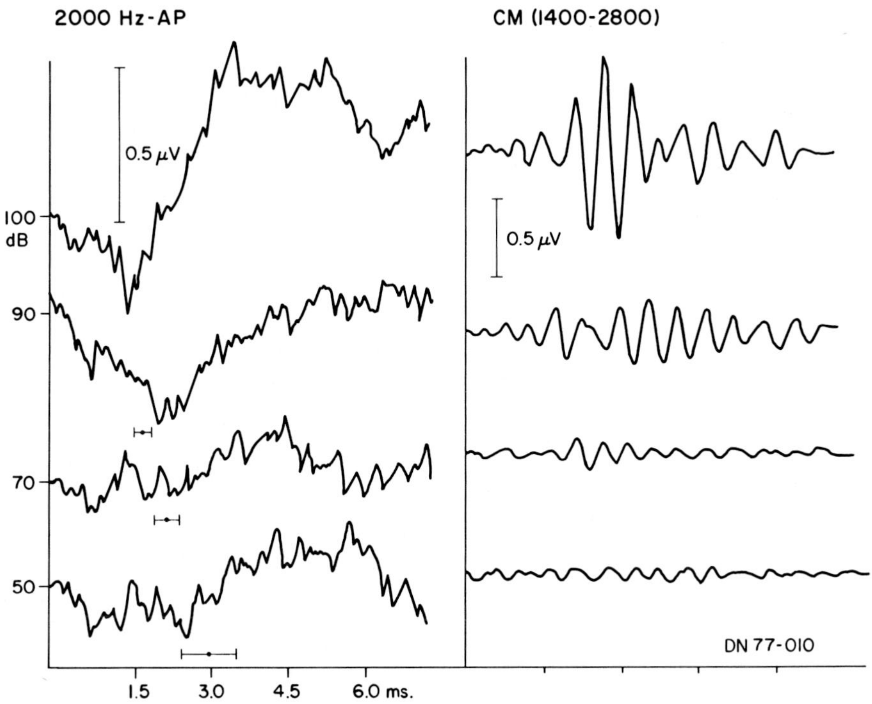

Fig. 13. Examples of AP and CM from a severely hard-of-hearing child. Both AP and CM amplitudes are much smaller than those from a normal ear. In this instance, the CM can be seen at levels considerably below the AP threshold.

children the presence or absence of the CM may make the difference between certainty and uncertainty in the evaluation.

Acknowledgements

This work supported by PHS/NIH grant No. 5-P50-NS03358-15.

REFERENCES

Elberling, C. Action potentials along the cochlear partition recorded from the ear canal in man. *Scand. Audiol. 3:* 13-19, 1974.

Zerlin, S. and Naunton, R.F. Physical and auditory specifications of third octave clicks. *Audiology 14:* 135-143, 1975.

DISCUSSION

Trahiotis: How do you handle the problem that as you go lower in frequency with the third octave filter, when you get down around 1000 cycles it is

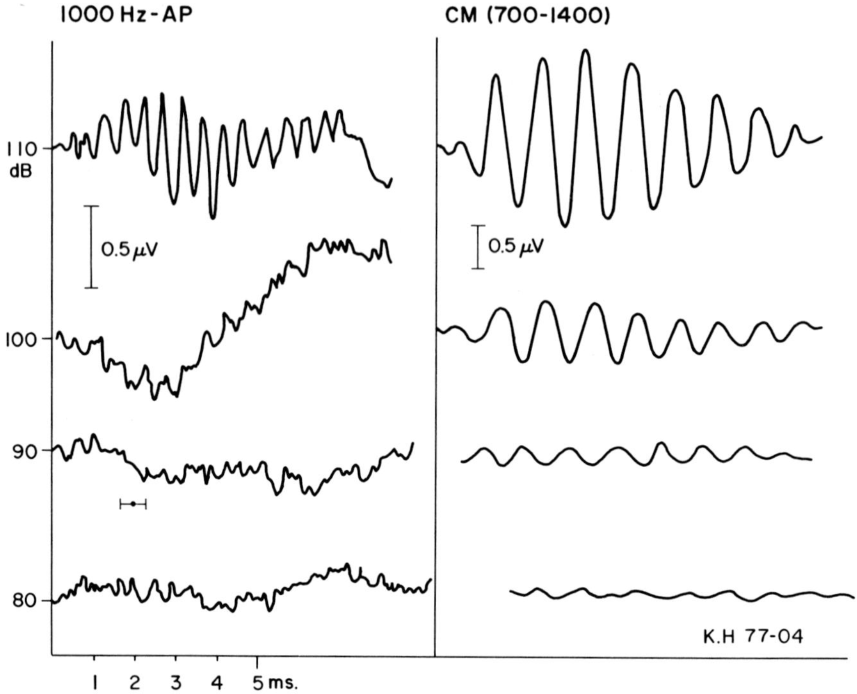

Fig. 14. Examples of AP and CM from a second child, diagnosed as severely hard of hearing. Here, CM is absent at 80 dB, and AP threshold is at about 95 dB. See text for further discussion.

230 cycles wide and you might have a 4 msec rise time, and when you go down to 500 you have a very long rise time? Aren't you just looking at the physical filter?

Zerlin: Perhaps to some extent. I used the first observable negative-going excursion as the starting point. I agree the slopes will change with respect to the high frequencies. At low frequencies it may take the stimulus a little longer to get to an excitatory level. The data show latencies which, at least at moderate levels, are right in the line with other data; they follow nicely psychoacoustic and single nerve data.

Greeley: What is the duration of the pulse that you are hitting the filter with?

Zerlin: 100 μsec. It doesn't matter all that much. Sometimes we use 50μsec. If you make it too wide you get two pulses, but within limits broadening the pulse width simply increases the amplitude of the filtered waveform.

STIMULUS-RESPONSE RELATIONS FOR PROMONTORY-RECORDED COMPOUND ACTION POTENTIALS IN NORMAL AND RECRUITING EARS

Josef J. Eggermont

University Hospital, Leiden

INTRODUCTION

Compound action potential (AP) parameters depend in various ways on the characteristics of the sound stimulus. The relationships used most often in electrocochleography (ECoG) are the AP-amplitude and AP-latency dependency on stimulus intensity (Yoshie, 1968; Aran et al., 1971; Elberling and Salomon, 1971; Eggermont et al., 1974). These stimulus-response relations have been described for normal ears and various types of ear pathology (for a recent review see Eggermont, 1976a), and in due course applied to the diagnosis of hearing disorders (Yoshie, 1973; Hermans et al., 1975). The reliability of the diagnosis depends to a great extent on the composition of the reference groups of pathological conditions of the ear and on the way in which these groups are studied. Although a high-intensity click stimulates almost the whole cochlea, the click threshold invariably corresponds with the lowest threshold in the audiogram, so that additional information provided by more frequency-specific stimuli is needed (Yoshie, 1973; Eggermont et al., 1974; Naunton and Zerlin, 1976).

The use of tonebursts permits reliable objective audiograms (Spoor and Eggermont, 1976) and more or less frequency-specific estimates of the presence of recruitment (Eggermont, 1977a). The intensity of the stimulus, whether click or toneburst, determines to a high degree which part of the cochlea contributes dominantly to the compound AP (Elberling, 1974; Eggermont, 1976b).

All these considerations already played a role in animal experimentation in the late 50's and early 60's, when the compound AP was almost the only available approach for the study of neural responses to sound. A method of deriving narrow-band APs (NAP), assignable to specific parts of the cochlea, was then devised on the basis of a high-pass noise masking technique (Teas et al., 1962); this introduced a new dimension, since the dependency of AP-amplitude and latency on the site of

ISBN 0-12-514960-3

generation could now be studied. More recently, this method has been adopted in human electrocochleography (Elberling, 1974) and extended to the analysis of toneburst-evoked APs (Eggermont, 1976b). In time it will probably provide us with a method of relating AP-recordings in man to single-fiber data from normal and pathological animal ears.

One of the last masking methods to be introduced into electrocochleography is tone-on-tone masking. This technique makes it possible to derive compound AP tuning curves (Dallos and Cheatham, 1976; Eggermont, 1977b). These curves resemble those obtained from single fibers and are thought to give information about the peripheral frequency selectivity of the human cochlea, both normal and pathological. The above mentioned stimulus-response relations for APs and NAPs will be described briefly in this paper and discussed with respect to their value in the diagnosis and description of hearing disorders.

METHODS

Recording is carried out with a needle electrode placed transtympanically on the promontory with reference to the ipsilateral earlobe or mastoid; the ground electrode is placed on the forehead. The responses are amplified (20,000 - 100,000 times) by a preamplifier (PAR 113, 10,000 times) with a pass band of 10 Hz-10 kHz and a wide-band main amplifier (2 - 10 times; 0.1 Hz - 30 kHz). The preamplifier is connected to the electrodes via a safety input stage. The responses are averaged (DL micro 4 system, Data Laboratories) and recorded with an XY recorder (Brians). For stimulation with clicks and tonebursts an exponential horn loud speaker is used. The masking noise or the continuous tone masker are presented via the same speaker. The sound pressure level is monitored at the entrance of the ear canal, by means of a 1/8 inch condensor microphone (Bruel and Kjäer, type 4138) for calibration purposes and to control the combined stimulus-masker output to avoid non-linear distortion (for details concerning the methods, see Spoor, 1974 and Eggermont, 1976b).

RESULTS

Simple Stimulus Conditions

For 2 kHz toneburts as stimuli, AP amplitudes plotted as a function of intensity for 27 normal ears and 25 recruiting ears are shown in Figure 1. The group of recruiting ears was selected from a series of patients suffering from Menière's disease and having audiometric thresholds of between 45 and 65 dB at 2 kHz. This Figure illustrates a few characteristic points; first, the relatively large spread in amplitude values found for a given toneburst intensity in normal as well as recruiting ears. This range of amplitude values typically amounts to a factor of 10, and is thought to be caused by the large differences in electrode-promontory resistances and the shunt resistances from the middle ear mucosa in the various ears. Secondly,

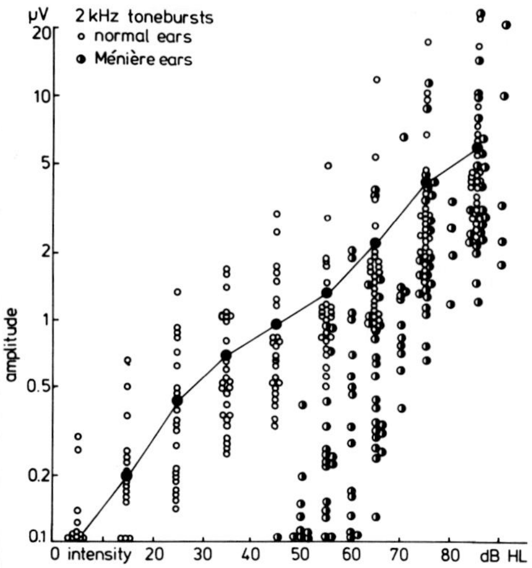

Fig. 1. Input-output properties for normal and recruiting ears. The mean values for each intensity used in the normal ears are interconnected. It is observed that for Menière ears the amplitude at high stimulus intensities is generally in the normal range.

despite the threshold elevation of about 55 dB HL, the high intensity output for the recruiting ears lies in the same range as for the normal ears. This phenomenon mimics loudness recruitment and is therefore considered to be of value in diagnosing recruitment (Portmann et al., 1973; Eggermont, 1977a). It must be kept in mind, however, that a steep input-output curve alone is not sufficient; a high output value (in the normal amplitude range) at high stimulus levels is also required. If this latter criterion is not taken into account, and especially if the amplitude-intensity curve is plotted as a percentage of, for example, the output at 90 dB, errors in interpretation may occur (Montandon et al., 1975).

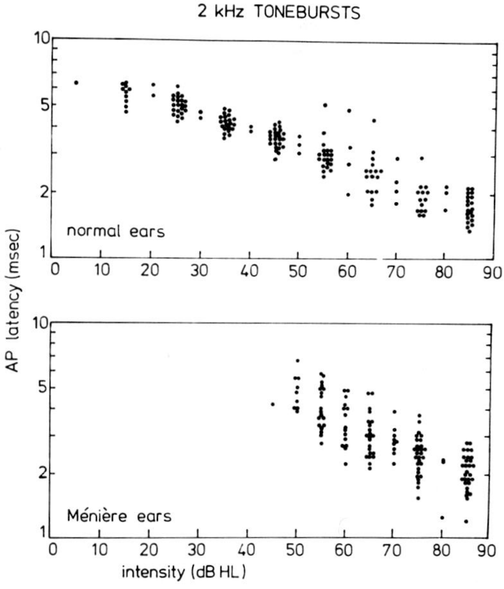

Fig. 2. Latency-intensity relationships for normal and recruiting ears. For the same ears as in Figure 1 the latency values have been plotted. The Menière ears tend to have higher latencies than the normal ears at corresponding intensities.

Another stimulus-response curve frequently used is the latency-intensity curve. Figure 2 shows a collection of data for 2 kHz tonebursts for the group of normal ears and the group of recruiting ears. It is evident that the AP-latency increases with decreasing intensity, and for 2 kHz tonebursts as stimuli, covers a range of approximately 1.5 to 7 msec. At high stimulus intensities the latency values for the normal ears spread over a range of about 1 msec, and at near threshold values this range may be even larger. For the Menière's ears the latencies tend to be larger at each intensity value than for the normal ears. The considerable spread in latency value raises doubts about the reliability of using the latency-intensity function as the sole criterion for estimating the amount of conductive hearing loss, especially when the loss is less than 30 dB. Reports indicating a slightly smaller spread in latency values, obtained with click stimuli, have also been published (eg. Cullen et al., 1972).

Complex Stimulus Conditions

1. High-pass Noise Masking of Click-evoked APs

By combining wide-band clicks with masking noise high-passed at various cut-off frequencies about ½-octave apart, and then subtracting responses obtained in the presence of high-pass noise with a given cut-off frequency from those obtained at a ½ octave higher cut-off frequency, it is possible to derive narrow-band APs. These NAPs are thought to originate from ½-octave-wide regions (-3 dB) along the cochlear partition. These regions are about 3 mm wide for the human cochlea and are innervated by 2000-2500 radial nerve fibers.

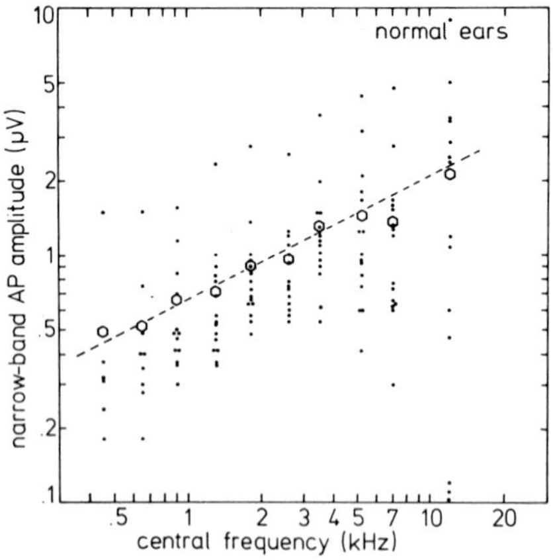

Fig. 3. Narrow-band action potential amplitudes as a function of central frequency for normal ears. For each central frequency the mean amplitudes have been drawn in. The dotted line has a slope of -3 dB/octave and is visually fitted to the mean values.

A plot of NAP amplitudes obtained in 15 normal human ears in response to clicks of 90 dB p.e. SPL (Fig. 3) gives an impression of the synchronized activity evoked by these clicks in various parts of the cochlea. As for the compound AP amplitude, the individual NAP values differ by a factor of up to 10 at a given central frequency (CF). For the basalmost region of the cochlea, represented by these parts of the APs that are masked by a 12 kHz high-pass noise, even much larger differences in amplitudes are found. Since this region is not normally covered by audiometry, its status does not influence the diagnosis of "normal" ear.

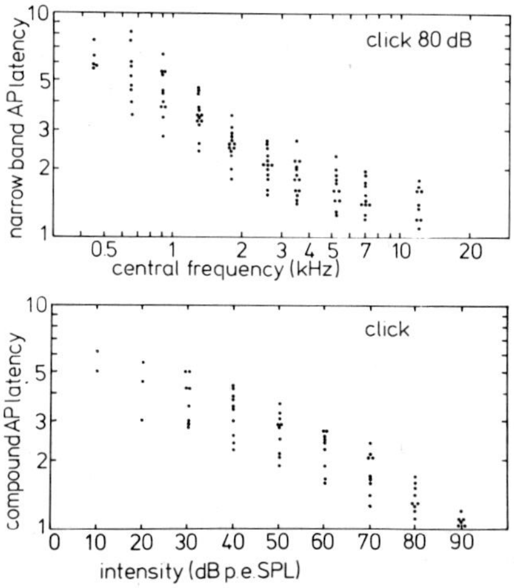

Fig. 4. Latency-intensity and latency-place relationships in normal ears. The upper part of the Figure show the dependency of narrow-band AP latency on central frequency for a click level of 80 dB pe SPL. The lower part shows for the same group of ears the latency-intensity function. A comparison of both parts of the Figure suggests that latency changes as a function of intensity can be explained in terms of changing excitation pattern along the cochlear partition.

However, as the data show, three ears barely show a detectable NAP and only eight lie in the normal range. The mean values calculated for each CF show a tendency to increase by 3 dB/octave with ascending CFs. The dashed line which is a visual fit to the mean values, shows the corresponding slope. This behavior is typical for a high-intensity click; at lower click levels (below 70-80 dB p.e. SPL) the NAP amplitudes drop rapidly for low and high CFs but remain relatively constant in the 2-3 kHz region (Eggermont, 1977a). The 3 dB/octave increase for the NAP amplitude suggests a dependency on the energy of the click in these particular ½-octave bands, since the click spectrum is flat over almost the entire frequency range of the various narrow bands.

When the NAP latencies for normal ears are plotted as a function of the central frequency (in this case for a click intensity of 80 dB p.e. SPL in roughly the same group of ears as that of Figure 3), which is shown in the upper half of Figure 4, the latency increases monotonically at descending CFs. For comparison, the compound AP latency for 9 of these 13 normal ears is plotted as a function of click intensity and shown in the lower half of Figure 4. Here it can be seen that the latency range at 80 dB p.e. SPL (lower half) corresponds with that at CF = 12 kHz in the NAP plot (upper half), from which it can be concluded that the click AP at 80 dB p.e. SPL represents mainly activity from the basalmost part of the cochlea. At 30 dB p.e. SPL (lower half of Figure 4), however, the range of latencies corresponds with that for a central frequency of 1.3 kHz (where an 80 dB click was used). This indicates that going from high intensity (80 dB) to a relatively low intensity (30 dB), the region dominantly contributing to the AP shifts from the basalmost part of the cochlea to more apical regions, presumably the 2 kHz range. Therefore stimulus-response relations for wide-band clicks are not likely to give a clear picture of the functioning of the cochlea.

2. High-pass Noise Masking of Toneburst-evoked APs: Input-Output Properties

For tonebursts, the NAP-amplitude and latency distributions as a function of CF can be obtained using the same masking paradigm as for click stimulation. The most characteristic difference shown by the amplitude distribution, even at the higher toneburst levels, is the limitation of excitation toward lower CFs. For a 2 kHz toneburst the region of excitation does not pass below about 600 Hz, whereas a click produces excitation beyond that point. With this single restriction all the results obtained for click stimulation are also valid for toneburst stimulation. The input-output behavior for the various narrow-band regions in response to a 2 kHz toneburst shows some interesting points, as can be seen in Figure 5 (right). The whole-nerve AP input-output curve and three NAP input-output curves are shown. It is evident that the NAP curves become steeper for higher CFs. The group of fibers in the narrow-band region with a CF of about 3.5 kHz obviously have a threshold value of about 45 dB for 2 kHz toneburst stimulation, but slight increases in toneburst intensity recruit more fibers than for narrow-band regions having a lower threshold value. This phenomenon resembles the pattern observed for ears showing loudness recruitment for part of the frequency range. The example shown on the left in Figure 5 represents a low-frequency hearing loss (500 Hz, 45 dB;

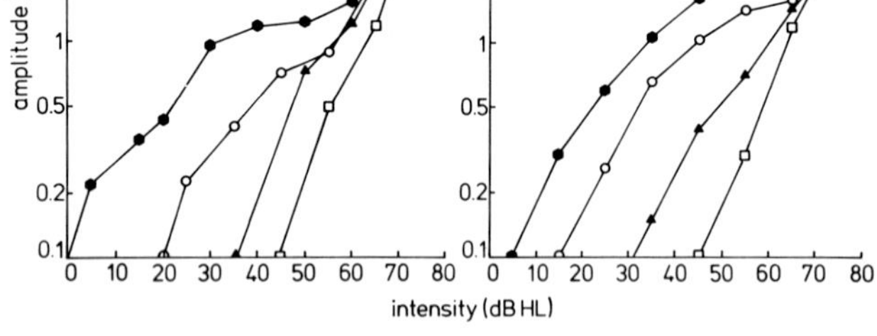

Fig. 5. Input-output curves for compound action potentials and narrow band action potentials. The AP amplitude-intensity functions for various tone-burst stimuli in a recruiting ear with low frequency hearing loss indicate that independent of threshold value the output at 70-80 db HL reaches the same level. This leads to an increase in steepness of the input-output curves. The NAPs in a normal ear for 2 kHz tone-bursts (right-hand side of the Figure) as a function of central frequency show the same tendency. An increase in threshold is associated with a steeper input-output curve, leading to the same high-intensity amplitude.

1000 Hz, 35 dB, 2000 Hz and above 0 dB) with normal hearing at the middle and high frequencies. The 2 kHz input-output curve for the whole-nerve AP indicates this normal behavior. At descending frequency there is an increase in threshold value corresponding with a steepening of the input-output curves, ie., more fibers are recruited per 10 dB intensity increment than for frequencies where the threshold lies at a more normal level. However, this holds only for reference to the threshold value (dB SL), since in the absolute sense the amplitude increment as a function of intensity seems to be a function of the intensity value itself and does not differ for normal or recruiting ears (Eggermont, 1977a).

Comparison of the two sides of Figure 5 indicates that in a normal cochlea the group of fibers having a CF about 1 octave higher than the toneburst frequency behave in the same way as fibers at the toneburst frequency in a pathological

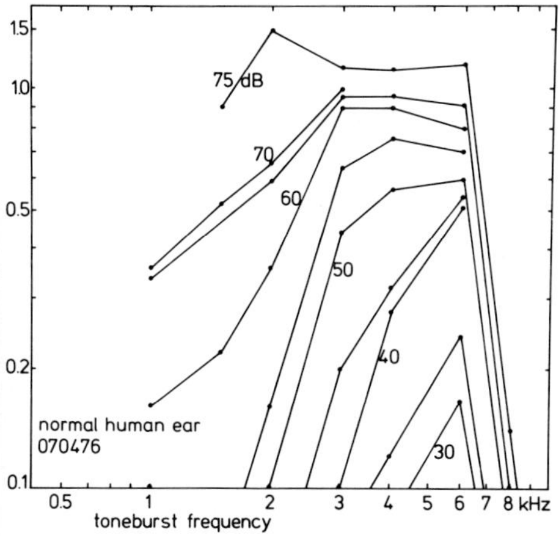

Fig. 6. Iso-intensity contours for narrow-band action potentials in a normal ear. For the narrow band responses evoked in the narrow-band masked by 4 kHz high-pass noise but not by 6 kHz high-pass noise, amplitudes obtained at the same intensity level for tonebursts of various frequency are connected. This shows contours which are qualitatively comparable to those obtained for the firing rate in single auditory nerve fibers (cf Rose et al., 1971).

cochlea that have the same threshold elevation. This suggests that the recruitment phenomenon is due either to activation of more basally located nerve fibers or to a change in the properties of the fibers having a CF roughly equal to the toneburst frequency.

3. *High-pass Noise Masking of Toneburst-evoked APs: Iso-intensity Contours*

Another way of showing stimulus-response properties for a particular narrow-band is analogous to the iso-intensity contours for single auditory nerve fibers (Rose et al., 1971). In these plots the number of firings per second is plotted as a function of the tone frequency and intensity. Spike counts at the same SPL for various tone frequencies give iso-intensity contours for that particular nerve fiber. An equivalent in electrocochleography would be a plot of the NAP amplitude for a given narrow-band, evoked by tonebursts of various frequencies and intensities. In Figure 6 the NAP amplitude is plotted as a function of toneburst frequency for the masking situation 6 kHz high-pass and 4 kHz high-pass in a normal ear. Here it should be noted that at low toneburst levels only a 6 kHz toneburst is capable of

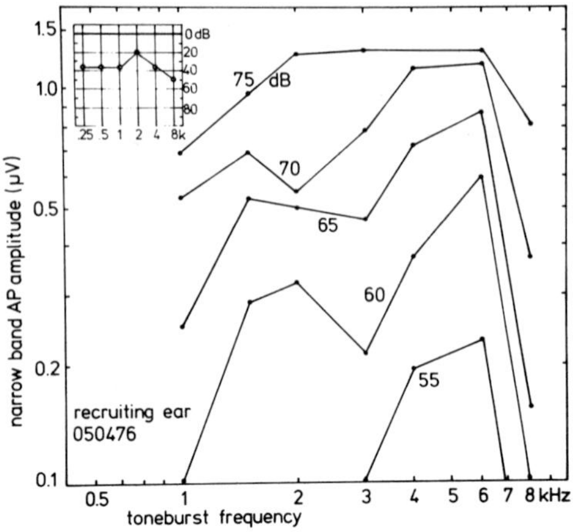

Fig. 7. Iso-intensity contours for narrow-band action potentials in a recruiting ear. For the narrow band 6-4 kHz the audiogram shows a hearing loss of about 40 dB. At 50 dB HL it was impossible to detect any NAP in that particular narrow-band; however, at 60 dB the iso-intensity contour is already of the same extension as in the normal ear. This demonstrates that the physiological correlate of loudness recruitment is already detectable in the ½-octave-wide narrow-band region.

evoking an NAP (the high-passed noise is 6 dB down at 6 kHz). As the intensity level is raised, NAPs are also evoked by toneburst frequencies below that value, but an 8 kHz toneburst only evokes some activity at relatively high levels (75 dB HL). Figure 6 shows a qualitative correspondence with the data from single fibers. However, it would be going too far to relate (onset) NAP amplitude to the number of firings per second in the single nerve fiber. The same recordings were carried out in a recruiting ear (Fig. 7). At 50 dB no NAP was detectable, but a 5 dB increase in intensity is sufficient to produce an excitation comparable to that given by 35 dB in a normal ear (cf Fig. 6). At 65 dB the output across the entire frequency range is already normal and reaches amplitudes equal to those in a normal ear. This suggests that recruitment is a phenomenon occurring within small regions of the cochlea, at least if there is some relation between steepening of input-output curves and loudness recruitment.

Fig. 8. Tuning curves in man and animal. The well known single fiber tuning curves (e.g. Kiang et al., 1967) recorded in normal hearing cats can be mimicked in man using a tone-on-tone masking paradigm. By plotting those frequency-intensity combinations of a continuous masking tone which just abolish the audibility of the test tone presented at 10 dB above threshold one obtains a psychoacoustic tuning curve. Taking as criterion the detectability of the AP evoked by the test tone burst one obtains an AP-tuning curve. All three curves bear great resemblence.

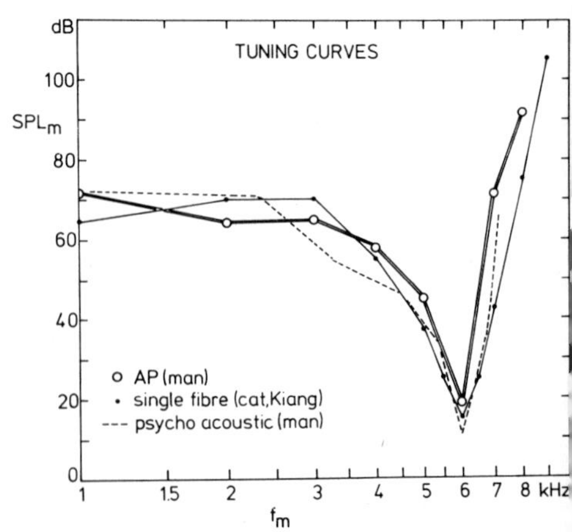

4. Tone-on-tone Masking Curves

By masking APs evoked by a 5 or 10 dB SL toneburst in normal ears, with continuous tones varying in frequency and intensity one obtains a tone-on-tone masking curve showing great similarity to single-fiber tuning curves. Hence they have been called AP-tuning curves (Dallos and Cheatham, 1976; Eggermont, 1977b).

Instead of taking the detectability of an AP as the masking criterion one can judge the audibility of the toneburst and thus obtain psychoacoustic tuning curves (Small, 1959; Zwicker, 1974). In Figure 8 a tuning curve obtained by Kiang et al. (1967) for a single nerve fiber in the cat is shown together with a psychoacoustic tuning curve and an AP-tuning curve, both obtained in normal human ears with the same short tonebursts used as test stimuli. Comparison shows the close agreement

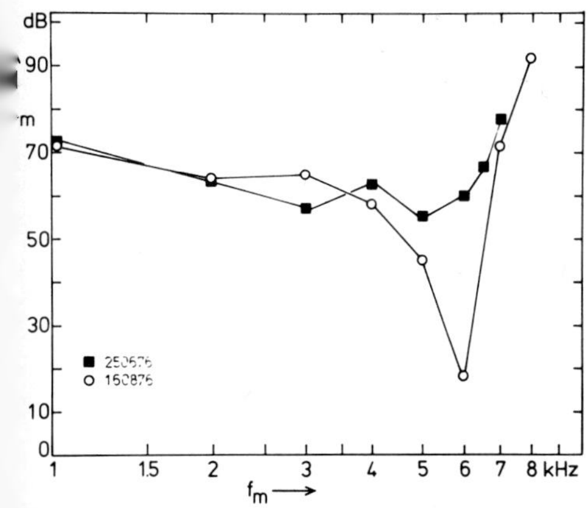

Fig. 9. AP-tuning curves in normal and recruiting ears. The characteristic two-segment tuning curve found in normal ears is changed into a broadly tuned one for a recruiting ear. This parallels the change observed in single fiber tuning curves in animals exposed to noise or to ototoxic drugs.

between the psychoacoustic and AP-tuning curves in man on the one hand and their similarity to the single fiber tuning curve in the cat on the other. It may therefore be assumed that at least in normal ears either the psychoacoustic tuning curves or the AP-tuning curves, offer an adequate substitute for single fiber tuning curves. When these tone-on-tone masking effects are measured in recruiting ears one invariably obtains broad tuning curves, ie., the two-segment tuning curves loose their sharp tip. This is also found psychoacoustically for APs and, as is well known, in single-fiber tuning curves (Kiang et al., 1970). Figure 9 shows an AP-tuning curve obtained in a recruiting ear (having a flat, 50 dB, hearing loss) and one for a normal ear. When the tone-on-tone masking procedure is performed at the same toneburst intensity in a normal ear, sharp masking curves are always obtained. The finding of broad tuning curves therefore indicates cochlear dysfunction. AP-tuning curves obtained with a tone-on-tone masking procedure may be compared with those derived from the iso-intensity contours (cf Figs. 6 and 7) for a constant output criterion. AP-tuning curves are always sharper than those derived from the NAP-iso-intensity contours, the general trend, however, is the same.

DISCUSSION

The survey of stimulus-response relations given in the preceding pages serves to indicate how these relations can be used in electrocochleography, the basic objective being to relate compound AP input-output properties to findings in more restricted regions of the cochlea, ie., the narrowband APs. This requires the interpretation of intensity-dependent phenomena found for click- or toneburst-evoked AP in terms of changing activity along the cochlear partition. The second group of stimulus-response relations discussed here points to the interpretation of narrowband APs on the basis of a similarity with single fiber stimulus-response relationships. Because electrophysiological measurements in man rely upon the whole-nerve AP and the anatomical basis of the hearing disorder is generally far from clear, any interpretation of such findings should be based on reasonable approximations of single-fiber data obtained in animals in which controlled pathological changes have been induced. Narrow-band action potentials may be considered to provide these approximations, since the NAP waveform resembles (for high CFs) that of the contribution of the single auditory nerve fiber recorded from the round window (Kiang et al., 1976; Eggermont, 1976b), and the NAP latency as a function of CF shows the same trend as the model latency of the first peak from the PST-histograms of single fibers (Kiang et al., 1965; Eggermont, 1976a). In addition, the other NAP stimulus-response relations parallel those found for single fibers: they show saturation (cf Figs. 5-7) and the input-output curves become steeper if the toneburst frequency lies below the central frequency, a phenomenon which has also been observed for single fibers (see Sachs and Abbas, 1974). On the whole the narrow-bands behave like "large" fibers, whose properties resemble those of a single fiber in many respects. Low-intensity tonebursts produce only a limited spread of activity along the cochlear partition, which can be observed under high-pass noise masking (Eggermont, 1976b): the AP thus evoked does not differ from the corresponding NAP at the same intensity level. Tone-on-tone masking procedures show the striking similarity between AP-masking curves and single-fiber tuning curves.

It is hoped that the revival of the use of whole-nerve APs, combined with the improved understanding of the phenomena occurring at the single fiber level, will result in greater reliability of clinical diagnosis and a better understanding of human auditory pathology.

REFERENCES

Aran, J.M., Perlerin, J., Lenoir, J., Portmann, C. and Darrouzet, J. Aspects theoretiques et pratiques des enregistrements électrocochleographiques selon la methode établie à Bordeaux. *Rev. Laryngol. Otol. Rhinol.*, Bord. Suppl. *92:* 601-644, 1971.

Cullen, J.K., Ellis, M.S., Berlin, C.I. and Lousteau, R.J. Human acoustic nerve action potential recording from the tympanic membrane without anesthesia. *Acta Otolaryngol. 74:* 15-22, 1972.

Dallos, P. and Cheatham, M.A. Compound action potential (AP) tuning curves. *J. Acoust. Soc. Am. 59:* 591-597, 1976.

Eggermont, J.J. Electrocochleography. In: *Handbook of Sensory Physiology. V/III,* edited by W.D. Keidel and W.D. Neff. New York: Springer-Verlag, 1976a, p. 625-705.

Eggermont, J.J. Analysis of compound action potential responses to tone bursts in the human and guinea pig cochlea. *J. Acoust. Soc. Am. 60:* 1132-1139, 1976b.

Eggermont, J.J. Electrocochleography and recruitment. *Ann. Otol. Rhinol. Laryngol. 86:* 138-149, 1977a.

Eggermont, J.J. Compound action potential tuning curves in normal and pathological human ears. *J. Acoust. Soc. Am.* (In press), 1977b.

Eggermont, J.J., Odenthal, D.W., Schmidt, P.H. and Spoor, A. Electrocochleography. Basic principles and clinical application. *Acta Otolaryngol.* Suppl. *316:* 1-84, 1974.

Elberling, C. Action potentials along the cochlear partition recorded from the ear canal in man. *Scand. Audiol. 3:* 13-19, 1974.

Elberling, C. and Salomon, G. Electrical potentials from the inner ear in man in response to sounds generated in a closed acoustic system. *Rev. Laryngol. Otol. Rhinol.* Bord. Suppl. *92:* 691-708, 1971.

Hermans, J., Eggermont, J.J., Hagedooren, J. and Odenthal, D.W. Probabilistic differential diagnosis of auditory dysfunction on the basis of electrocochleography. *Meth. Inf. Med. 14:* 87-95, 1975.

Kiang, N.Y.S., Moxon, E.C. and Levine, R.A. Auditory-nerve activity in cats with normal and abnormal cochleas. In: *Sensorineural hearing loss,* edited by G.E.W. Wolstenholme and J. Knight. London: Churchill, 1970, p. 241-268.

Kiang, N.Y.S., Moxon, E.C. and Kahn, A.R. The relationship of gross potentials recorded from the cochlea to single unit activity in the auditory nerve. In: *Electrocochleography,* edited by R.J. Ruben, C. Elberling, and G. Salomon. Baltimore: University Park Press, 1976, p. 95-115.

Kiang, N.Y.S., Sachs, M.B. and Peake, W.T. Shapes of tuning curves for single auditory-nerve fibers. *J. Acoust. Soc. Am. 42:* 1341-1342, 1967.

Kiang, N.Y.S., Watanabe, T. Thomas, E.C. and Clark, L.F. *Discharge patterns of single fibers in the cat's auditory nerve.* Cambridge: MIT Press, 1965.

Montandon, B, Shepard, N.T., Marr, E.M., Peake, W.T. and Kiang, N.Y.S. Auditory nerve potentials from ear canals of patients with otological problems. *Ann. Otol. Rhinol. Laryngol. 84:* 164-173, 1975.

Naunton, R.F. and Zerlin, S. Human whole-nerve responses to clicks of various frequencies. *Audiology 15:* 1-9, 1976.

Portmann, M., Aran, J.M. and Lagourge, P. Testing for recruitment by electrocochleography. *Ann. Otol. Rhinol. Laryngol. 82:* 36-43, 1973.

Rose, J.E., Hind, J.E., Anderson, D.J. and Brugge, J.F. Some effects of stimulus intensity on response of auditory nerve fibers in the squirrel monkey. *J. Neurophysiol. 34:* 685-699, 1971.

Sachs, M.B. and Abbas, P.J. Rate versus level functions for auditory-nerve fibers in cats: toneburst stimuli. *J. Acoust. Soc. Am. 56:* 1835-1847, 1974.

Small, A. Pure tone masking. *J. Acoust. Soc. Am. 31:* 1619-1625, 1959.

Spoor, A. Apparatus for electrocochleography. *Acta Otolaryngol.* Suppl. *316:* 25-36, 1974.

Spoor, A. and Eggermont, J.J. Electrocochleography as a method for objective audiogram determination. In: *Hearing and Davis: Essays honoring Hallowel Davis,* edited by S.K. Hirsh, D.H. Eldredge, I.J. Hirsh and S.R. Silverman. St. Louis: Washington University Press, 1976, p. 411-418.

Teas, D.C., Eldredge, D.H. and Davis, H. Cochlear responses to acoustic transients: an interpretation of whole-nerve action potentials. *J. Acoust. Soc. Am. 34:* 1438-1459, 1962.

Yoshie, N. Auditory nerve action potential responses to clicks in man. *Laryngoscope 78:* 198-215, 1968.

Yoshie, N. Diagnostic significance of the electrocochleogram in clinical audiometry. *Audiology 12:* 504-539, 1973.

Zwicker, E. On a psychoacoustical equivalent of tuning curves. In: *Facts and Models in Hearing,* edited by E. Zwicker and E. Terhardt. New York: Springer-Verlag, 1974, p. 132-141.

ELECTROCOCHLEOGRAPHY: BEHAVIORAL THRESHOLD COMPARISONS

Ralph F. Naunton and Stanley S. Zerlin

University of Chicago

INTRODUCTION

In the past twenty-five years many attempts have been made to develop accurate objective methods of measuring auditory function, - procedures that could be used in the evaluation of subjects unable or unwilling to cooperate in more conventional tests of hearing. There was a flurry of interest in psychogalvanic skin resistance testing (PGSR), then in EEG audiometry, in cortical audiometry and finally in electrocochleography (ECoG). ECoG is, in our experience, very close to being an ideal objective hearing test method; but the precise role of brainstem evoked response audiometry (BSERA), as a threshold-seeking device for the difficult-to-test child, remains uncertain (Eggermont et al., 1974).

In this presentation we will briefly describe some of our experiences using ECoG techniques to derive near-conventional threshold audiograms in both adults and children. We shall do no more than touch upon the use of ECoG as a differential diagnostic tool, although it certainly provides information on the electrical activity of the inner ear and first order neuron hitherto available only in animals (Naunton and Zerlin, 1976).

TECHNIQUE

We use a transtympanic electrode, with two ear-lobe surface electrodes; a third surface electrode (vertex) is added in older children so that BSER testing can be carried out as a diagnostic measure should the cochleogram appear to be normal or near-normal. Iontophoretic topical anesthesia is used in adults; intramuscular and/or intravenous Ketamine is used in infants and children. Tests are carried out first using unfiltered clicks, then with 1/3rd octave filtered clicks of center frequencies 0.5, 1.0, 2.0, 4.0 and 8.0 kHz (Zerlin and Naunton, 1975). Five-hundred clicks are presented at a rate of ten per second for each frequency-intensity setting, working down in intensity from 90 dB to 10 dB SL in 20 dB steps. If no electrical activity is seen in response to the 90 dB stimulus, the sensation level is increased in the next run by 20 dB. If in older children as the first ear is tested it becomes

ISBN 0-12-514960-3

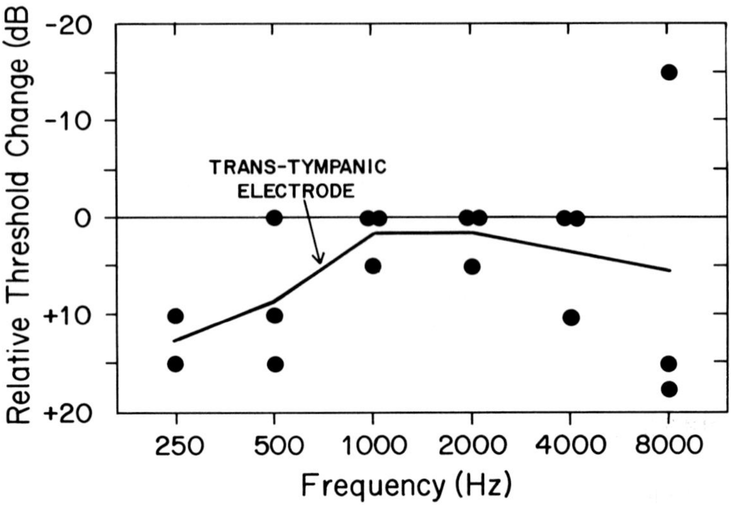

Fig. 1. Comparison between behavioral thresholds with and without transtympanic electrode in place (three normal subjects, third-octave click stimuli).

abundantly clear that hearing is near-normal, the second ear is not tested but a BSER examination is carried out using broadband clicks.

This modus operandi has emerged as a result of a number of considerations; thus on-line evaluation of the results is never regarded as final, the electrical responses always being tape-recorded and evaluated later in detail; and complete response-latency studies on ears that prove to be normal have provided important data at the various test frequencies, - data of value in the identification of the responses of the abnormal inner ear.

The only adverse reactions probably attributable to Ketamine that we have encountered in testing approximately one-hundred and fifty children have been in one child who developed a marked cutaneous erythema that faded rapidly at the conclusion of the test, and in another child who developed intermittent glottic spasm. In no case has the test had to be discontinued because of adverse reactions. Clearly one would prefer not to use general anesthesia of any type but many children and infants cannot be examined without general anesthesia and, as in so many and varied types of examination in this age group, the diagnostic information provided by the test amply justifies the means. Moreover, in this same group of subjects such simple examinations and procedures as otoscopy and removal of wax are commonly difficult or impossible without anesthesia; we are able, as we prepare the anesthetized child for ECoG, to clean the ears, examine the drums and carry out myringotomy and middle ear aspiration whenever it is indicated. Routinely, we bring each tested child back for otoscopy two weeks after the examination; no child has failed to heal at the site of transtympanic electrode passage through the drum.

THE MECHANICAL EFFECT OF THE ELECTRODE

Concern has been expressed that the transtympanic electrode, held in place through the otherwise intact drum, might limit drum mobility and thus produce an apparent hearing impairment. Conventional threshold tests were therefore carried out on three young adult volunteers, using the loudspeaker-generated click stimuli we normally use in electrocochleography; the threshold tests were carried out first without and then with the transtympanic electrode in place. The resulting threshold comparisons suggest that the electrode has little affect on the center and higher frequencies while at 500 Hz there may be a threshold elevation of the order of 10 dB; the results at 8 kHz were equivocal (Fig. 1).

SUBJECTS TESTED

Our experience in the past several years has been limited largely to three types of subject;

1. Infants "at risk" for hearing impairment;
2. Older difficult-to-test children;
3. Adults.

The infants at risk for hearing impairment have included such examples as infants recently recovered from meningitis, infant children of parents with a strong family history of deafness and infants with multiple congenital anomalies involving

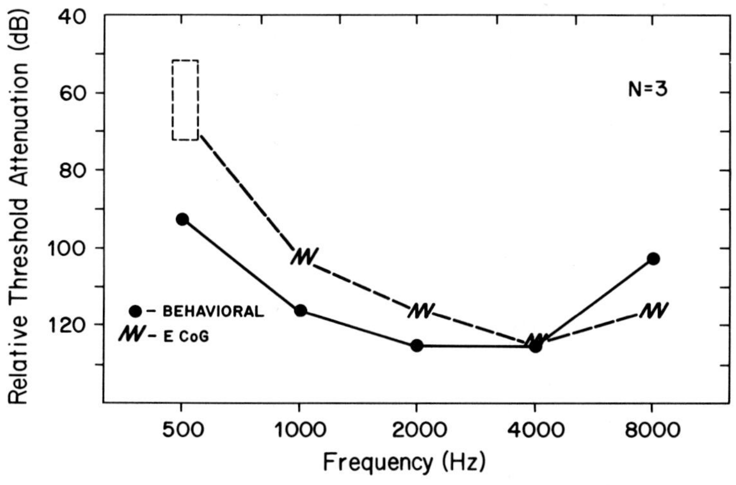

Fig. 2. Comparison between behavioral and ECoG thresholds (three normal subjects, third-octave click stimuli). Rectangle indicates expected range of ECoG thresholds at 500 Hz.

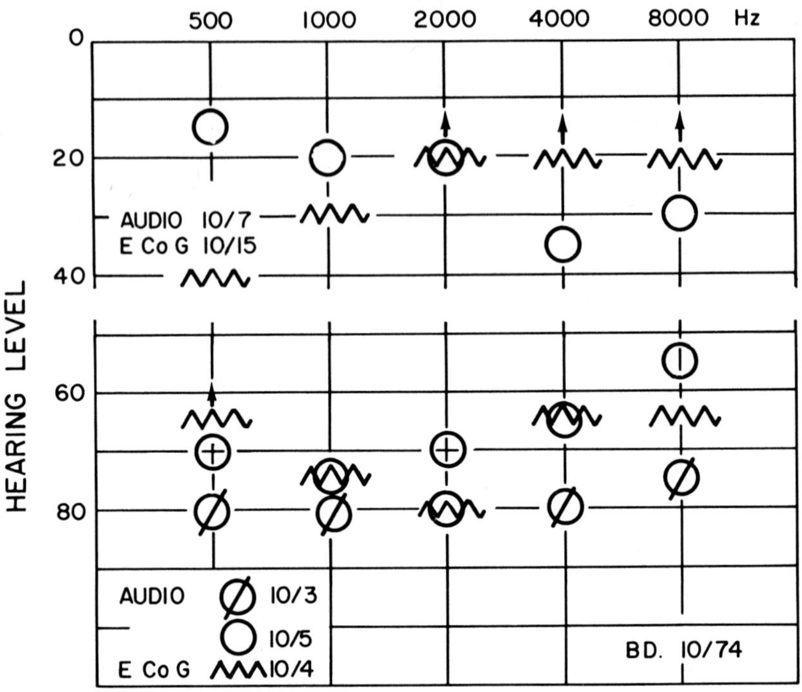

Fig. 3. Sudden deafness in a young adult male; comparison between conventional audiometry and ECoG carried out when hearing was impaired (lower section of audiograph) and as it recovered (upper section).

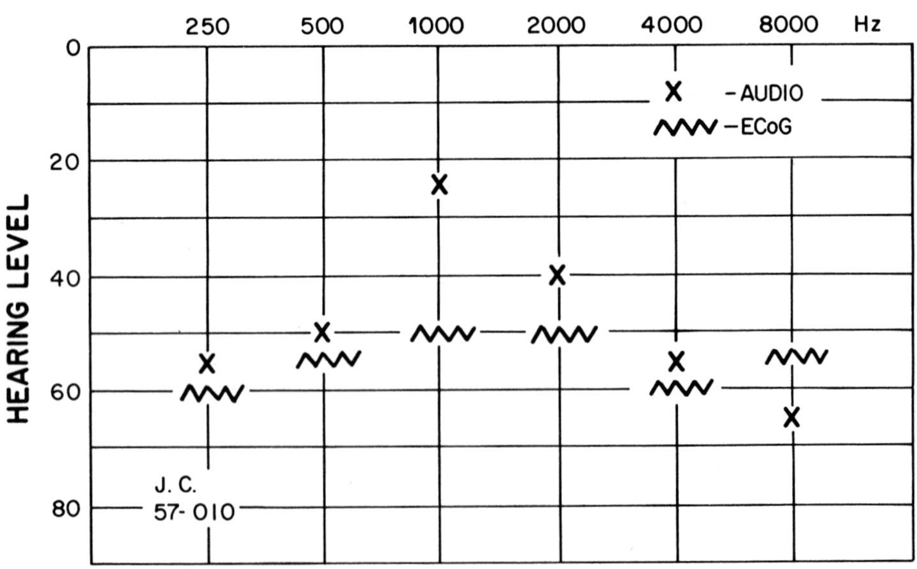

Fig. 4. Menière's Disease; comparison between conventional audiometry and ECoG.

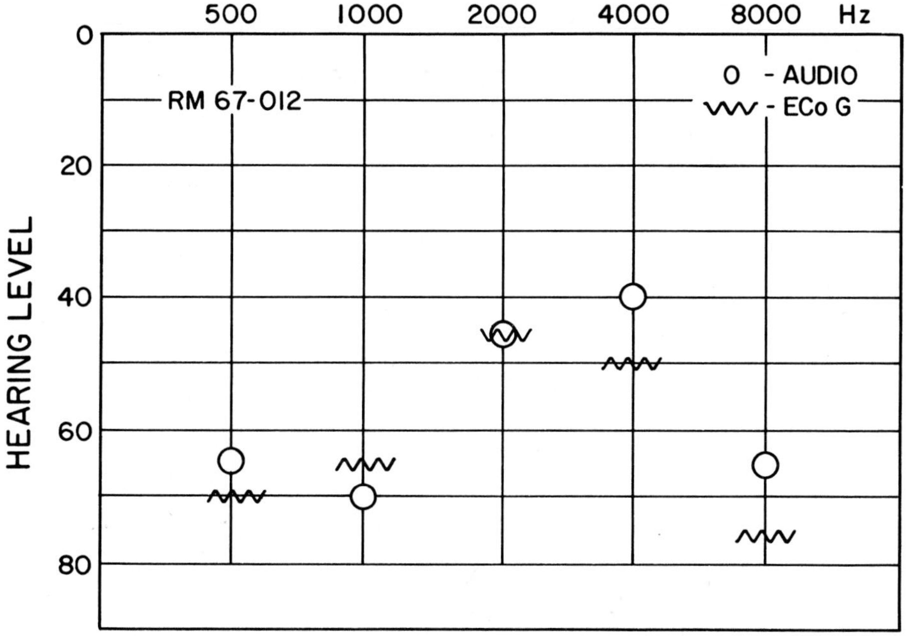

Fig. 5. Menière's Disease; comparison between conventional audiometry and ECoG.

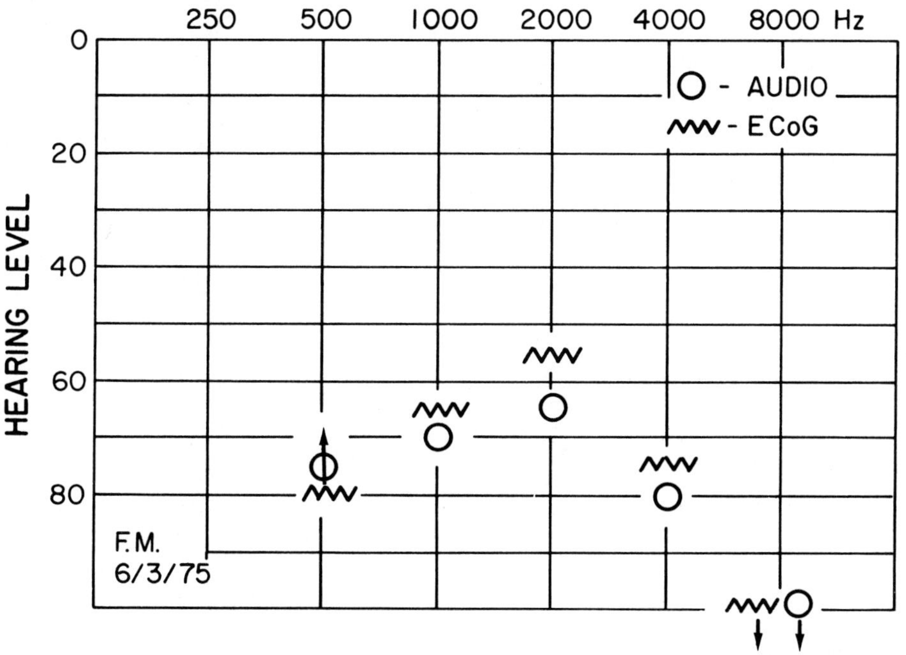

Fig. 6. Sensorineual deafness of unknown etiology in an adult; comparison between conventional audiometry and ECoG.

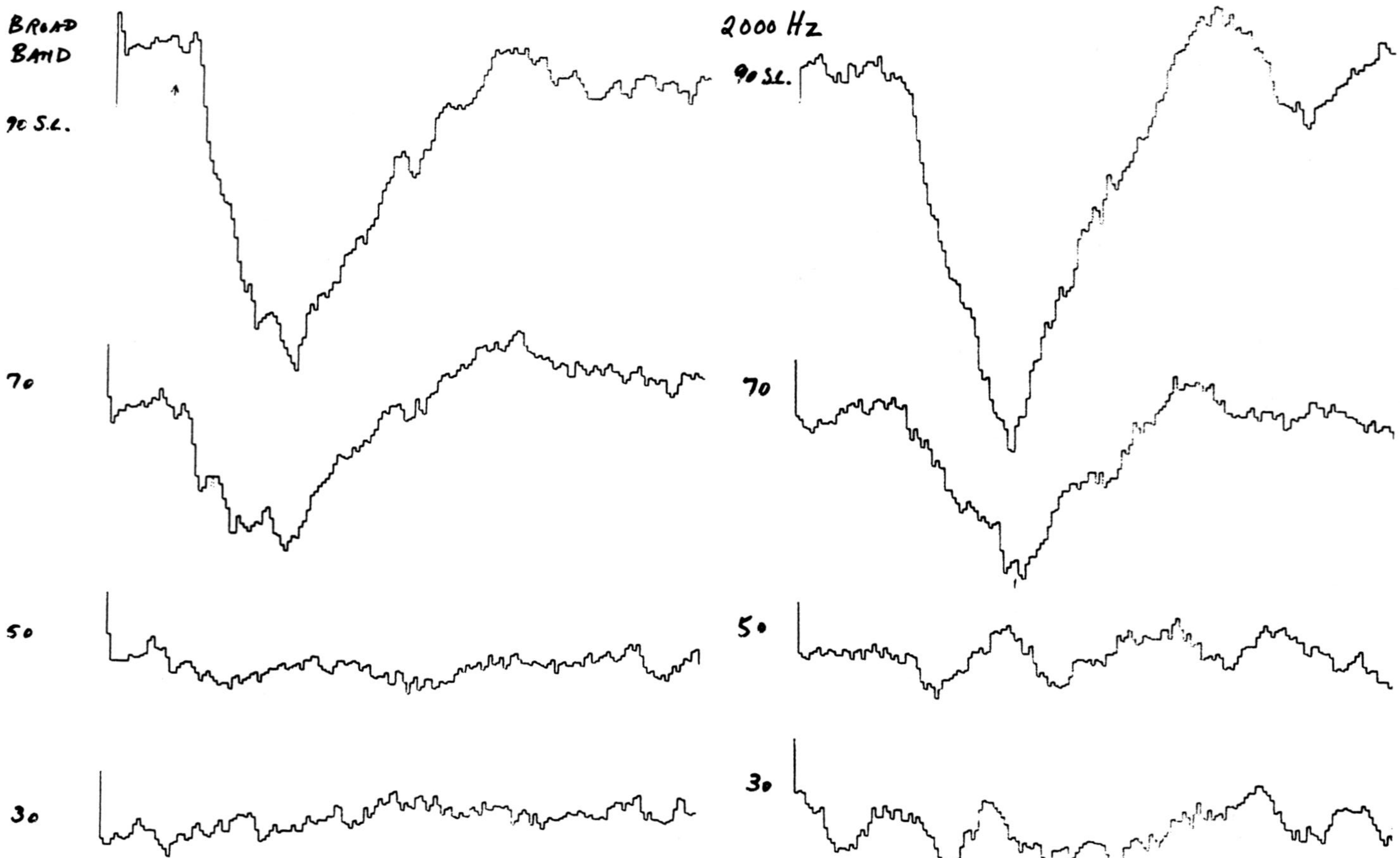

BROAD BAND
90 S.L.
70
50
30
2000 Hz
90 S.L.
70
50
30

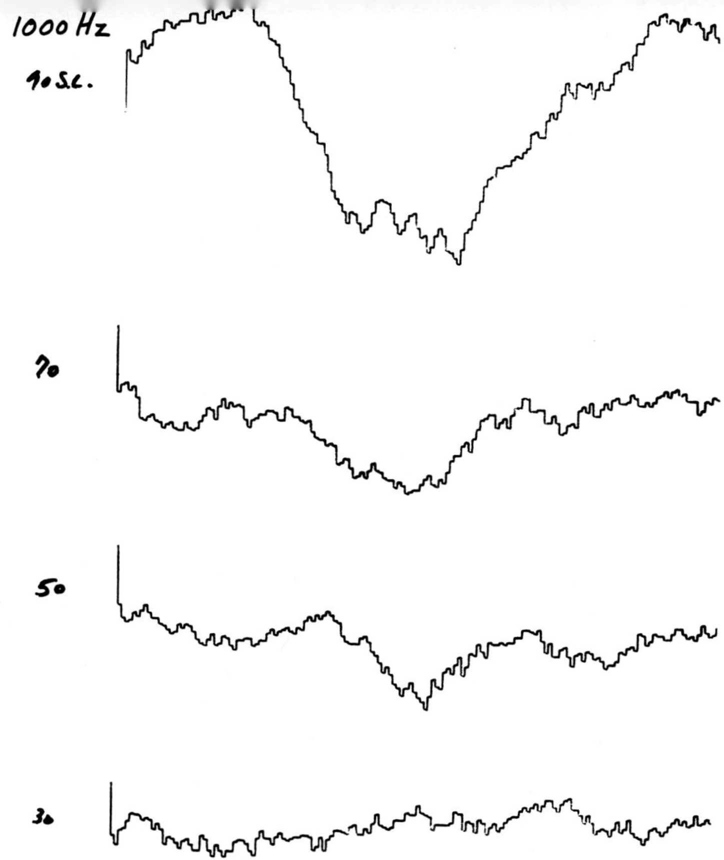

Fig. 7, 8, & 9. Retrocochlear lesion in adult female; summated AP at various sensation levels (re normal) of broadband click (7), 2000 Hz (8) and 1000 Hz clicks (9).

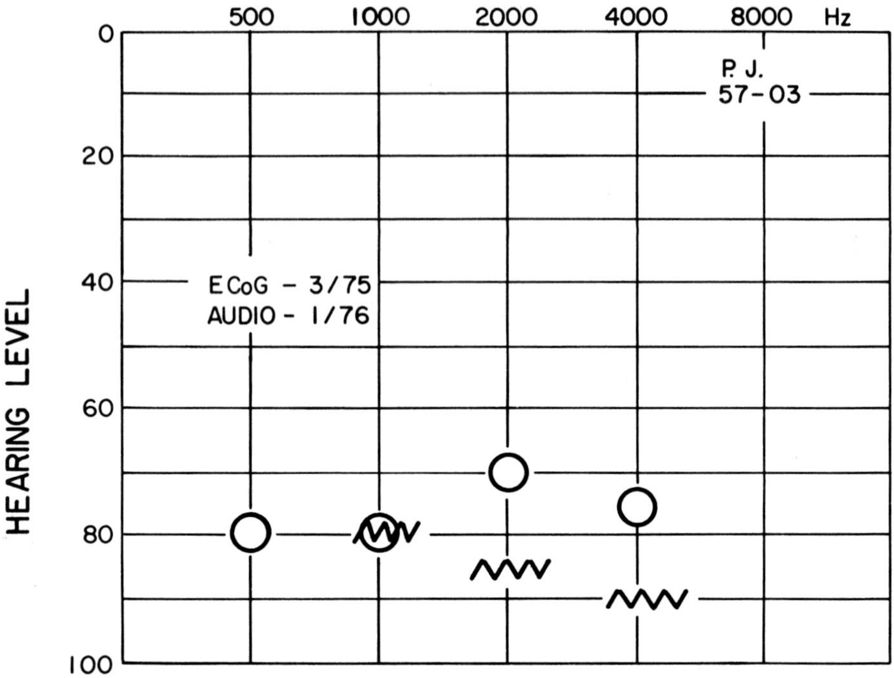

Fig. 10. Comparison between ECoG at age 30 months and conventional audiogram taken ten months later.

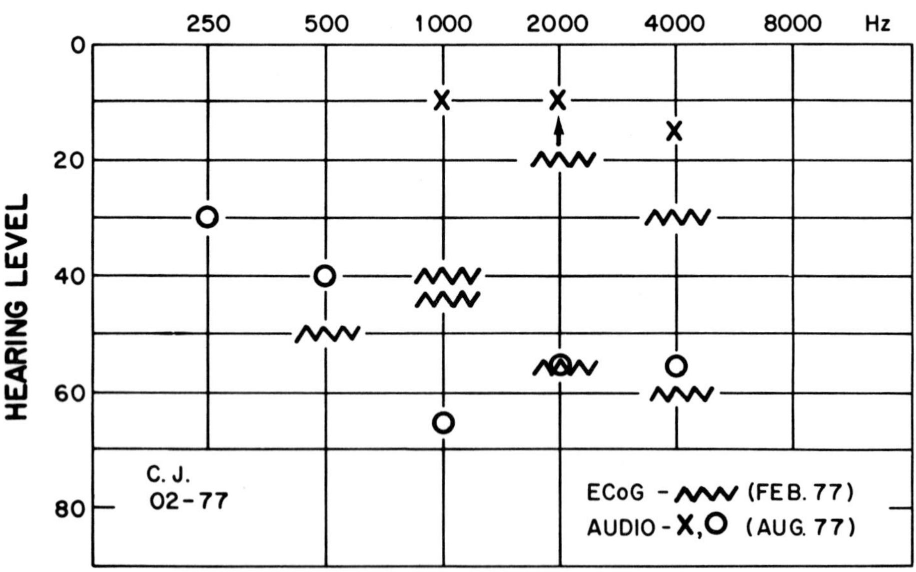

Fig. 11. Comparison between ECoG at age 18 months and conventional audiogram taken six months later.

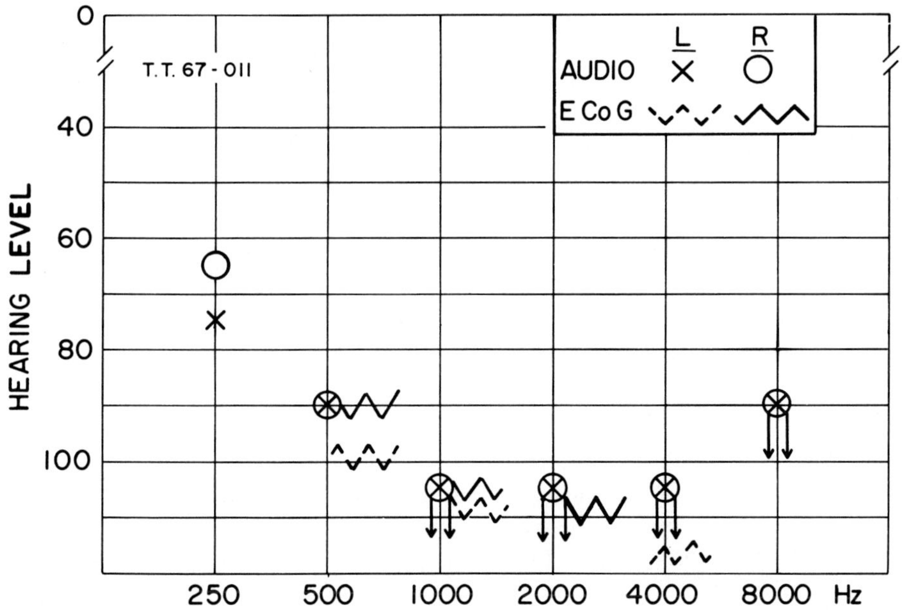

Fig. 12. Comparison between conventional audiometry and ECoG in a ten-year-old, the validity of whose conventional test result was doubted by several audiologists.

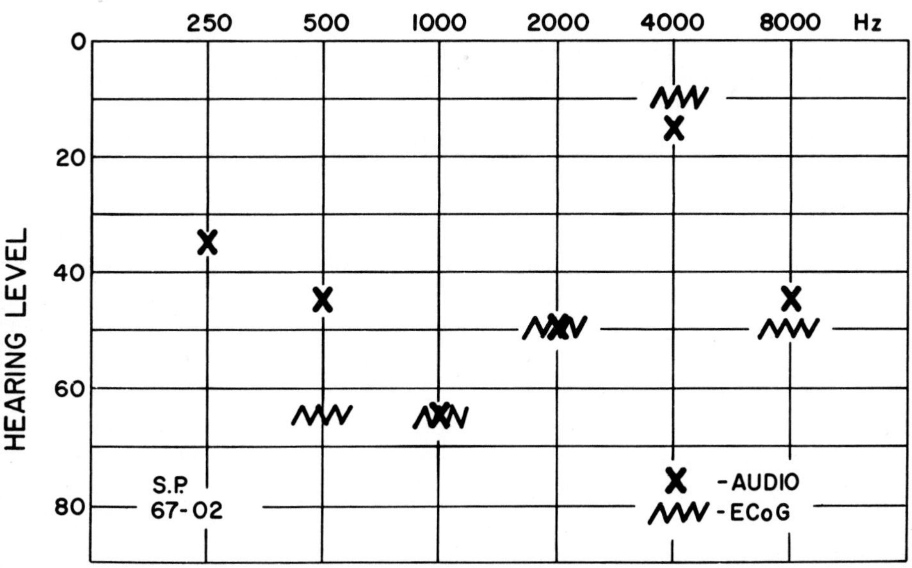

Fig. 13. Comparison between conventional audiometry and ECoG in a nine-year-old, the validity of whose conventional test result was doubted by several clinicians.

the head and neck areas. In all instances conventional hearing test methods had been attempted first and ECoG recommended and carried out only when observation and conventional test methods supported the possibility of deafness.

The older children we have tested have included those where retardation was probable or certain, and hyperactive children. The common factor has been inability to permit conventional audiometry. We have also tested a number of children where audiologists or clinicians have differed markedly in their estimates of residual hearing.

Normal and hearing impaired adult volunteers were tested extensively as our experience with this test modality began and as we sought to validate our test technique. We continue to use ECoG in adults in perplexing clinical situations as a diagnostic measure.

ECoG-BEHAVIORAL COMPARISONS IN NORMAL ADULTS

Three normal adult volunteers were tested behaviorally and by ECoG (one ear only), each of three within single sessions, using only the ECoG test stimuli. The results (Fig. 2) permitted comparison of the two types of test results and indicate that our ECoG technique tends to *underestimate* hearing acuity at 500, 1000 and 2000 Hz. At 4000 Hz the two methods agree while at 8000 Hz electrocochleography *overestimates* hearing acuity. These observations are taken into account as we interpret clinical ECoG's, and express the test results as threshold evaluations.

ECoG-BEHAVIORAL COMPARISONS IN HEARING-IMPAIRED ADULTS

Electrochochleography in adult clinical cases has been of value in malingerers, has served as a differential diagnostic tool (particularly with retrocochlear lesions) but has also provided additional opportunities of comparing ECoG and behavioral testing techniques. These comparisons have usually conformed well with the general relationships shown in Figure 2 and will be illustrated by several representative examples.

Figure 3 shows the results of several conventional hearing tests and ECoGs carried out on an adult male who initially complained of sudden unilateral deafness but whose hearing gradually recovered during treatment. Behavioral audiograms and ECoGs were taken while the hearing was impaired and following recovery, and are drawn for comparison on the same audiograph. The two test methods clearly compare favorably. In this instance, we were also able to demonstrate that both the CM and the N_1 responses increased in amplitude as the ear recovered, suggesting that whatever the nature of the disease process, hair cells were involved either alone or in addition to the first-order neuron.

Figures 4 and 5 compare the ECoG and conventional audiograms of two clinical subjects with Menière's disease, while Figure 6 shows the same comparison in a case of severe sensorineural deafness of uncertain origin. In each instance the comparison is favorable and supports the contention that our technique commonly allows compilation of a conventional threshold audiogram.

The next case illustrates the situation where disparity between conventional threshold audiometry and ECoG testing serves to identify a retrocochlear lesion. This patient had suffered sudden loss of hearing, total in one ear (the one subsequently tested by ECoG) and severe in the other. Careful and extensive clinical work-up, including brain scan and chest x-ray, revealed no clue to the diagnosis, but ECoG testing demonstrated clear CM and AP over a considerable range of stimulation levels and frequencies in the ear that was totally deaf, - clear indication of retrocochlear damage (Figs. 7, 8 and 9). Further evaluation revealed a Pancoast's tumor not demonstrable by standard chest x-rays and, as the presumed metastatic disease in the posterior fossa extended, the brain scan became positive (Morrison et al., 1976).

ECoG-BEHAVIORAL COMPARISONS IN INFANTS AND CHILDREN

Follow-up of the infants and children we have tested has been incomplete because many of the children are still too young to give us reliable conventional audiograms for comparison, others are grossly retarded and may never be evaluated by conventional means. We have anecdotal information on many; for example, the child whose ECoG in the first year was normal and who later began to develop speech; or the grossly retarded child whose ECoG was also normal and who subsequently began to obey simple spoken commands but who remains speechless. In other instances we are able to be more precise; for example, Figures 10 and 11 show the results of two such children where conventional testing was initially impossible, ECoG tests were carried out and sometime later as the children matured, conventional tests became feasible. Figures 12 and 13 compare ECoG and conventional test results carried out on two other children; in these, ECoG tests were ordered because the audiologists or clinicians who had previously examined the child remained very uncertain of the validity of their conventional behavioral test findings.

Follow-up of the children we have tested has revealed a few disagreements but none serious enough to invalidate treatment or habilitation plans.

FUTURE TECHNICAL CONSIDERATIONS

The emergence of BSER and claims concerning its value as a threshold-seeking technique, raise the possibility that, whenever it is feasible, BSER testing should be attempted before carrying out ECoG under general anesthesia. Many of the children we have tested could not have been examined by BSER even under sedation because of hyperactivity or mental retardation. In other children, this approach may be of value.

CONCLUSIONS

Our experience leads us to conclude that electrocochleography has proved its worth as a threshold-seeking and diagnostic method of high validity and reliability.

Electrocochleography is now in routine use and is providing valuable diagnostic information not otherwise accessible.

Acknowledgement

This work supported by PHS/NIH grant #5-P50-NS 03358-15.

REFERENCES

Eggermont, J.J., Odenthal, D.W., Schmidt, P.H. and Spoor, A. Electrocochleography: basic principles and clinical application. *Acta Otolaryng.* Supp. *316:* 1-84, 1974.

Morrison, A.W., Gibson, W.P.R. and Beagley, H.A. Transtympanic electrocochleography in the diagnosis of retrocochlear tumors. *Clin. Otolaryng. 1:* 153-167, 1976.

Naunton, R.F. and Zerlin, S. Basis and some diagnostic implications of electrocochleography. *Laryngoscope 86:* 475-482, 1976.

Zerlin, S. and Naunton, R.F. Physical and auditory specification of third-octave clicks. *Audiology 14:* 135-143, 1975.

DISCUSSION

Rapin: I would like to state that Ketamine is a pretty safe anesthetic except in children with severe seizures. One child given this drug for electroretinography developed very severe myoclonus lasting for many hours. One needs to be aware of this possibility.

You said that in severely retarded children one could not test with brain stem potentials. We don't find recording of either brain stem or late potentials to be a problem in these patients. We sedate them with other drugs (chloral hydrate, chlorpromazine, and/or promethazine), not Ketamine, and test them without difficulty.

Naunton: Your point about Ketamine is an important one. When, as on several occasions, we have tested children with histories of seizures we have prescribed Valium ahead of time; as a result we have had no difficulties. Regarding your comment about brain stem testing in the retarded child, we are beginning to test all types of children under Ketamine by both ECoG and BSER.

Galambos: It is interesting to encounter an individual who is both a cochleogrammer and a brain stemmer. Theoretically the brain stem response can reveal a selective responsivity to frequency like that you report from the ECoG, and so in principle what you see with a transtympanic electrode should as readily be seen with a surface electrode on the mastoid. Have you, in a normal subject compared the results obtained by the cochleogram with those obtained using the brain stem response? My guess is that each would give a similar correlation with the audiogram.

Naunton: We are now testing adults by both methods but have not yet compared threshold-seeking accuracy in the two.

We have the conviction that ECoG is giving us a good deal of information that brain stem testing does not provide, in directions other than threshold evaluation.

Galambos: Could you say what that good deal of information is?

Naunton: Notice that I carefully did not say it was giving us a good deal of information of clinical importance. I think enough has been said already about the type of information. It may be that this will prove to be clinically significant; certainly it seems very attractive to have some additional information about the inner ear, –information which, in the case of CM, increases our threshold-finding accuracy.

Berlin: I would like to respond to Dr. Galambos's question and then share some related experiences as both a cochleogrammer and brain stemmer.

First, ear-by-ear specific information, if you don't know what thresholds are, is hard to extract. When you are on the ear, as in cochleography, you know you are getting a response from that ear alone. In a very young child cochleography provides information bearing on hearing aid prescription.

Second, we use cochleography to measure cochlear reserve either by bone conduction or air-conducted clicks, looking for masking dilemmas, and we find cochleography extremely powerful in that respect.

Third, we have seen a few cases where, had we used brain stem recording alone we would have diagnosed the child as deaf, but where cochleography showed the child was not. One happened to be an autistic child.

We found one unusual case that was refractory to all our techniques, a patient who showed no cochleogram to a broad band click, but we ultimately found he had nearly normal hearing outside the traditional range of audiometry, and somehow or other we are going to have to modify our spectral content in the tone bursts to assess responsivity above that.

To summarize in response to your point, we do get ear-specific information, cochlear reserve information, and hearing aid selection information from cochleography that we don't easily get from brain stem. In support of brain stem audiometry our experience has been in extremely young infants, 2, 3 or 4 weeks old, who are at risk or adopted children. Brain stem has turned out to be safer for us, a lot easier to do, and just as informative with respect to the screening process. We are not wedded to just one. The combination of all techniques has been productive for us.

Galambos: Just one point. It is easy to visualize wave I, which is the auditory nerve response, by brain stem audiometry.

Berlin: Not at low levels.

Galambos: Not at low levels; that is correct. But here wave V takes it place.

Moore: I have a little problem with your 500 and 1000 Hz data. I wonder if you have computed over the approximately 150 subjects that you have tested, any correlational coefficients between thresholds for 500 and 1000 Hz. The fact that you are using very high intensity levels at 500 and 1000 Hz, leads me to believe that your data are not really frequency-specific at those frequencies.

Also, have you conducted masking experiments for the AP responses at 500 and 1000 Hz, in an attempt to explicate your data at those frequencies. It appears that data at those frequencies do not correlate well with the behavioral thresholds.

Naunton: Without doubt it is more difficult to estimate the threshold at 500 than it is, for example, at 2000 Hz; we have made comparative tests and simply made visual comparisons on a considerable number of adults where we have dependable behavioral thresholds, some with high tone sensorineural losses, some with flat audiograms and some with low tone losses; and the correlation between ECoG audiograms and conventional audiograms has been good.

Moore: If you look at the spectra of your one-third octave clicks, which I admit are somewhat more frequency-specific than using a short tone burst with a rapid rise time, you will find a rather wide band width. We collected data at 1000 to 4000 Hz. A narrow band masking noise, centered at 4000 Hz, was routed to the same ear as the 1000 Hz signal. We succeeded in masking the AP response, which indicates to me that there is considerable spread from the 1000 Hz signal into the 4000 Hz region of the basilar membrane. On the other hand, when we placed a 1000 Hz narrow band noise in the ipsilateral ear in an attempt to mask out the AP generated by the 4000 Hz signal, we were not successful The stimulus we used was a 3 msec tone burst with a 100μsec rise/fall time. The cutoff of the filters were 48 dB per octave for the narrow band noise.

Naunton: I don't have a slide to illustrate the spectrum, and we have not used masking on clinical subjects, but the stimulus is a third-octave wide at 3 dB with a 50 dB per octave rejection rate (70 dB in two octaves), this was confirmed by sound-spectrum analysis.

Durrant: What did you do with your normative data that showed the ECoG discrepancy with the behavioral data? Do you correct your threshold measurements to take that gap into account?

Naunton: Yes, we do.

Durrant: One technical point. I wonder if it would be better, for the sake of directness, to call your intensity levels "HL" (hearing level; or "HTL", hearing threshold level) and then specify what your standard is, just as we would say ISO. We all know what that means. The use of HL, instead of using the "SL" terminology would be less ambiguous. The definition of SL is very clear, and a lot of people are still using "SL" to mean individual sensation levels.

Naunton:. That is a good point.

Wiederhold: How often and how frequently can you use transtympanic recording? Is there a problem with scarring of the tympanic membrane?

Naunton: When we take our transtympanic electrode out we often cannot see the hole it made. Moreover, when we check the ears a few days after the test, as is our routine, the drum always looks completely normal, so I doubt if there is any scarring at all. When we began to do this work we used paid student volunteers to a considerable extent. One impecunious student had his right ear tested three times, and then pointed out that he also had a left ear. His right ear shows no sign of scars.

Wiederhold: One other point that may be of value. We have been using Ketamine in cats, recording from them once a week, and we found that some cats became tolerant to Ketamine. I have heard that other people around the country have found this also. After three or four sessions, we have to nearly double the dose to keep them down.

Payne: I would like to know what information you need that you collect at low levels, that you can get at higher levels, that you would use in fitting a hearing aid or when you are having a masking dilemma. What kinds of masking dilemmas do you have with low level losses?

Berlin: If we had a patient with approximately 60 to 70 dB hearing level, our air conducted clicks are barely intense enough to elicit a response from him by air conduction, and sometimes we need to know his responses by bone conduction. When you put a bone conduction oscillator on a patient with brain stem electrodes in place, aside from the artifact problem, which is horrendous--you never know which ear is contributing to the cochlear response. This is the kind of patient where you need a high intensity stimulus by either air or bone, and our air conduction stimulus is not powerful enough to guarantee we get a large response. At that point we don't know which ear is doing the hearing. If we simply use the earphones at the 90 to 100 dB level we still don't know where it is coming from by brain stem response.

As far as the hearing aid is concerned, working with young children 6 to 9 or 14 months of age, there was no other way we could get ear-specific information at our level of expertise at the time, when we were into cochleography, to separate one ear or the other.

You must understand where we were coming from, the cochleography was always done first and brain stem audiometry second. First, in our experience we were doing cochleography when the first few papers on brain stem audiometry were out, so we didn't know it at the start. We found it useful to go on with that. We may not in the future.

To answer your question, this is one case. As for our practice with separating ears by hearing aids, it has been our practice to do that, and we have found it useful and productive that way. We may want to stop if we can get valid data by brain stem. We have limited experience. I didn't mean to convince you to do it our way, because I am not sure our way is absolutely correct, nor do I have an emotional investment in it. It is simply a longstanding history of doing it that way.

Salomon: There is one instance more: Where you have a cochleogram with a better threshold than the BSER, it is an indication that there is a tumor on the eighth nerve. In that case a cochleogram gives specific clinical information.

Thornton: What we would like to know about our patients is the measure of their perception. What we end up with are measures of detection. We are talking about electrophysiological measures of detection that can reflect the audiogram. This leads to the argument that the nearest you can get to reflecting the audiogram would involve trying to measure responses from the highest neurological level.

What worries me more than arguments about which technique is best concerns the general premise that different places with different facilities will be better suited to different techniques. What we are really after is a choice of techniques to suit the facility and, more importantly, a choice of an electrophysiological method or combinations of method to suit the patient.

In no other branch of medicine does one select one test to the exclusion of others. We routinely record transtympanic results. We use early neurogenic, late cortical responses, etc., depending on whether we suspect a central lesion or not. I think it is disturbing in this field, to hear arguments leading to a technique-oriented methodology as opposed to what we should be thinking of, which is a patient-oriented methodology.

ELECTROCOCHLEOGRAPHY (II)

Moderator: *F. Blair Simmons*

We have recently gathered such data in guinea pigs (GP) using particular techniques described elsewhere (Aran and Erre, 1977). We also happened to obtain cochleas with discrete and localized lesions different from those usually resulting from the classical oto-destructive agents (noise and drugs) and very useful in studies of the relations between patterns of VIIIth nerve APs and patterns of destruction along the basilar membrane. A few examples of such data are now presented and discussed.

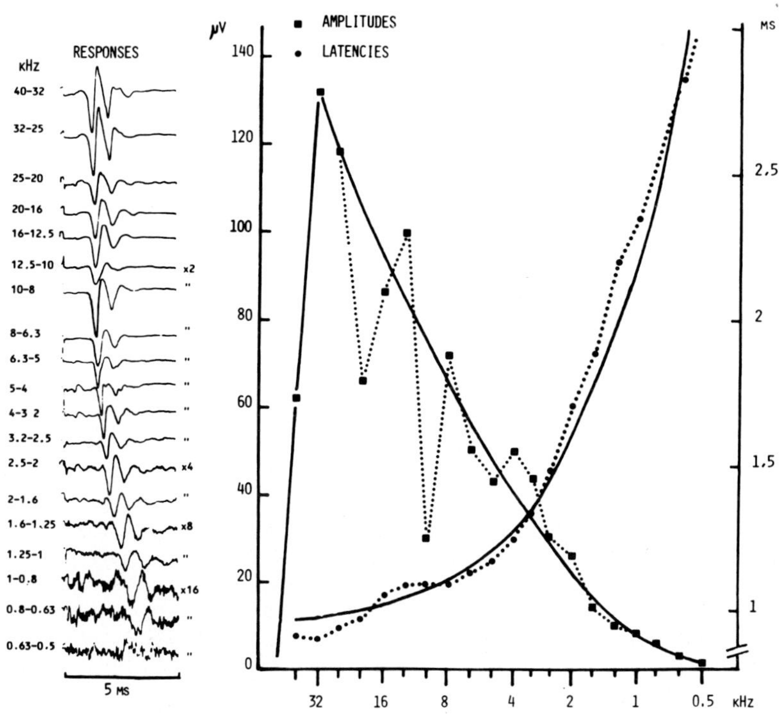

Fig. 3. Third octave derived APs obtained by using high-pass noise masking, from 40 kHz to 500 Hz. Rarefaction click, 65 dB peSPL (50 dB HL). Noise level adjusted so that unfiltered noise (white) completely masks the AP response to the click.

Left: Waveforms. Note the presence of a second peak constantly around 0.75 ms after the first in all the responses which, as indicated by Eggermont (1976b), could be due to repetitive firing or contribution of the cochlear nucleus. However, if it were repetitive firing, as shown in PST histograms (Kiang 1965), the second peak should not appear for high frequencies and the time interval between the two peaks should increase with decreasing frequency. Thus it seems as if it was a contribution from the cochlear nucleus since then the synaptic delay could be constant.

Right: Corresponding amplitudes and latencies. Note the importance of the high frequency derived APs. Note also the two amplitude points at 10 and 20 kHz corresponding to the troughs in the spectrum of the 0.1 ms rectangular click. Latencies are more precisely measured than amplitudes. The latency function, presumed to represent the traveling wave along the basilar membrane can be expressed as: L (latency in msec) = 0.946 + 1.295/F (frequency in kHz) with a determination coefficient $r^2 = 0.974$.

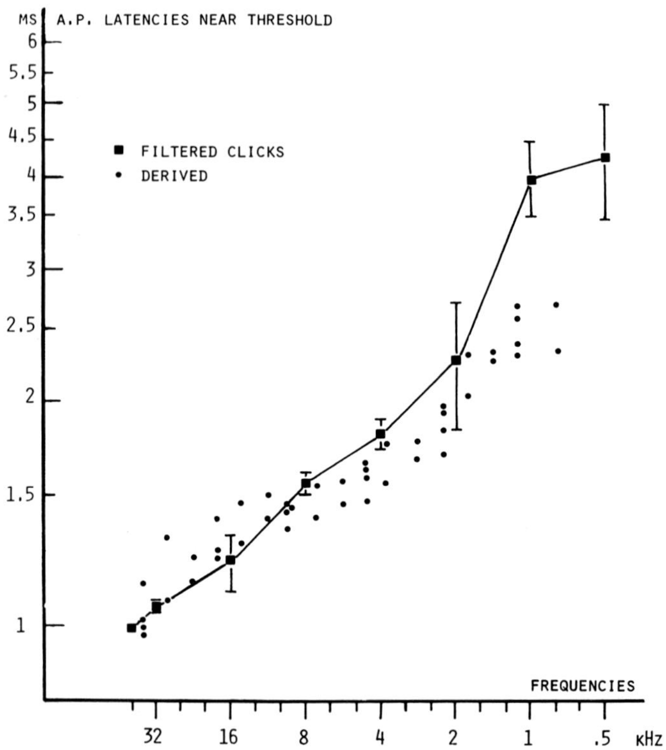

Fig. 4. Comparison of the response latencies to filtered clicks (FC) with that of the derived APs to rarefaction click near threshold in normal GPs. For FCs the mean values are determined at levels less than 5dB above threshold; they are plotted with their standard deviations. The latencies are measured between the maximal peak of the third octave FC (third wave) and the most negative peak on the response. For derived APs, since thresholds were not systematically determined, latencies of responses in various normal GPs obtained to low intensity click levels are displayed directly. Log time scale.

Experiments were performed in awake GPs with a stainless steel wire electrode chronically implanted on the round window membrane according to a technique currently used in our laboratory (Portmann et al., 1966; Aran and Darrouzet, 1975; Aran and Charlet De Sauvage, 1976). Screws fixed in the skull at the vertex served as reference and ground. The three electrodes are soldered to a socket fixed on the animal skull with dental cement. At the beginning of each recording session in the freely moving GP, a polarized Bruel and Kjaer condenser microphone (½ inch) is used as an earphone; it is coupled to the GP's ear through a 10 cm silastic tube sealed into the external meatus with histoacryl. Thresholds of averaged APs to 1/3rd octave filtered clicks ranging from 0.5 to 40 kHz are determined (AP audiograms). Responses to broad-band click (0.1 msec) as well as to the 20 filtered clicks (FC) are recorded and stored on digital magnetic tape. Moreover 20 derived APs, corresponding to the frequencies from 500 Hz to above 40 kHz are now systemat-

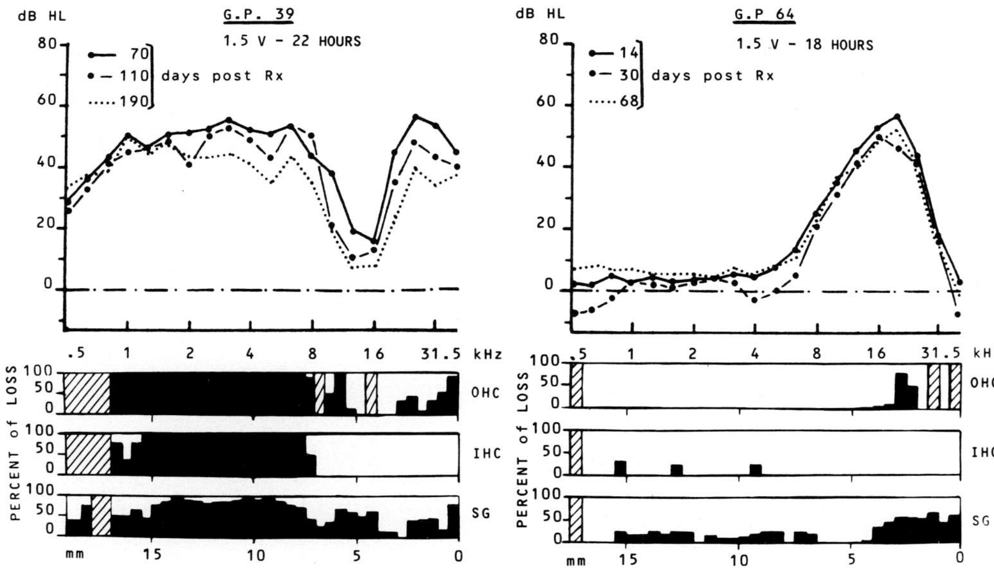

Fig. 5. Thresholds of the APs to the 20 FCs as a function of frequency (AP audiograms) and percent of losses (solid black areas) of outer hair cells (OHC), inner hair cells (IHC) and spiral ganglion neurons (SG) as a function of distance from the base on the basilar membrane (histocochleograms) in two GPs exposed to dc current (constant 1.5 V applied between round window and cortex–round window negative–giving 20 to 40 μA for the durations indicated). The last AP audiograms were performed the day before sacrifice. Note the opposite situations for the two GPs corresponding to similarly localized preserved or damaged areas.

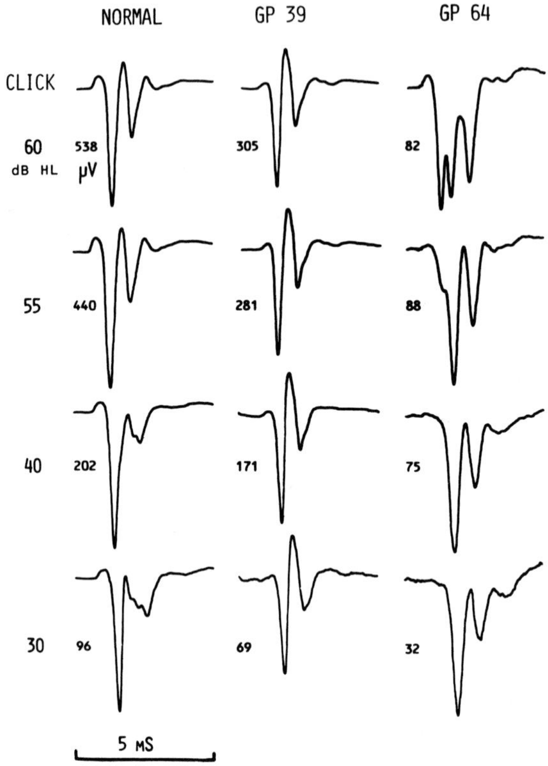

Fig. 6. Comparison of averaged AP waveforms in the normal and the two GPs of Figure 5 for various click levels (clicks of alternated polarity). Note the constantly diphasic response for GP 39 and the double-peaked N_1 at 60 dB for GP 64, originating probably from the sides of the impaired 20 kHz area. The peak-to-peak amplitude of each response is indicated in μV.

ically obtained in the normal as well as in the pathological GPs, using the technique of high-pass masking noise (Teas et al., 1962). For this purpose a Schlumberger FAB 48 active filter with a 96 dB/octave slope and a 58 dB suppression level was used.

In order to be able to relate the electrophysiological observations to the histopathology along the basilar membrane, a long period after any ototoxic treatment is needed for the sensorineural elements to degenerate so as to give a clear picture when observed microscopically. Optical and electron microscopic observations are required. The cochleas were fixed and prepared as for electron microscopy but were decalcified in order to permit serial sections and reconstruction as in Guild's method (Guild, 1921). The decalcified cochleas, embedded in low viscosity Spurr resin (Spoendlin and Brun, 1974), were cut on an LKB pyramitome with a glass knife large enough to section the entire cochlea. 10μm sections, taken every 100μm, were placed on glass plates in liquid Spurr which was again polymerized in an oven. Such slides are quickly obtained and can be observed by light microscopy for reconstruction of the entire cochlea. Every 100μm, a thicker section (20-30μm) was made, dissected and mounted on a pyramide for thin sections and electron microscopy.

With these techniques we were able to confirm, in the normal guinea pig, some basic mechanisms of cochlear function. For instance in Figure 3 derived action potential responses for a 65 dB peSPL rarefaction click are presented together with amplitude and latency functions. Latencies of the derived APs and that of the AP responses to the various filtered clicks near threshold are compared in Figure 4, the agreement appearing very good except at low frequencies. These and other data indicate that the click is progressively exciting the entire basilar membrane; however, the contribution of the basal part of the cochlea in response to the click above 40 dB HL (55 dB peSPL) is enormous with respect to that of the

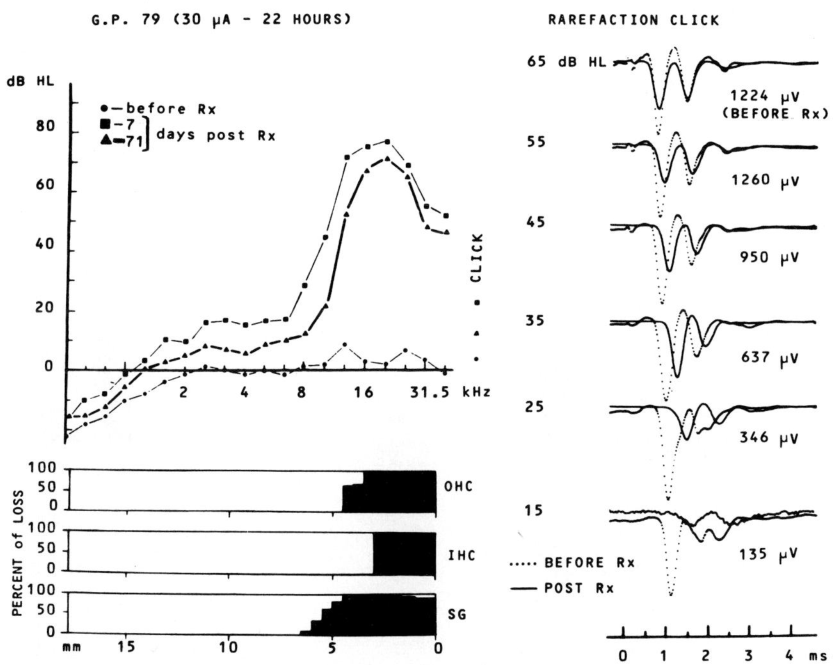

Fig. 7.

Left: CAP audiogram and histocochleogram of GP 79 exposed to constant dc current (30 μA) between round window and cortex (round window negative) during 22 hours.

Right: Responses before (. . . . . . .) and 71 days after (———) the treatment at various levels of the rarefaction click. The amplitudes of the responses before are indicated in μV, amplification for the corresponding traces post-℞ is 2x greater except for 15 dB HL where it is 6x greater.

Note the modified diminution rate of N1 amplitude, together with the increase in latency with decreasing click intensity post-℞, which indicate that the basal part of the cochlea is not responding to the low intensity clicks. Note also the different ratios between N1 and N2 amplitudes before and after treatment. See also data for this GP in Figures 9 and 10.

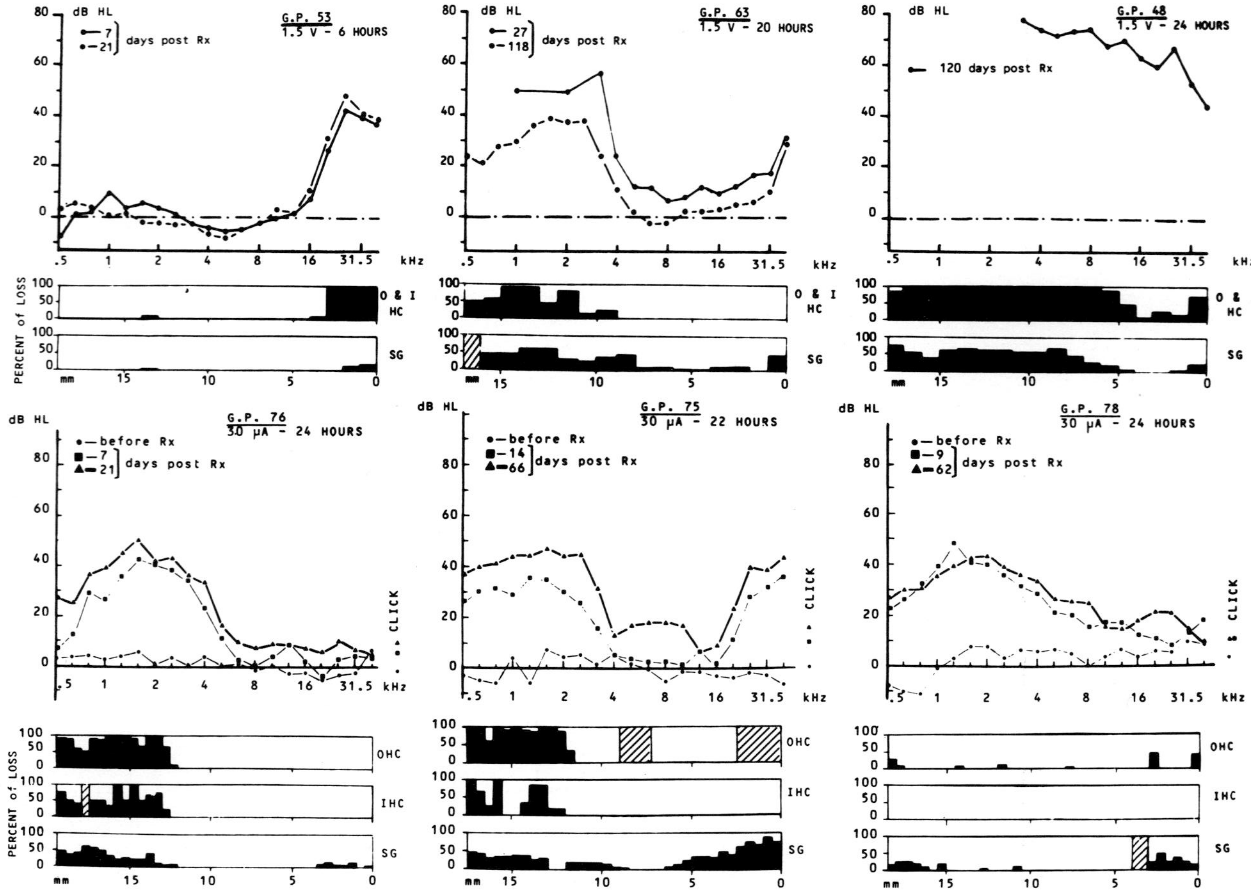

G.P. 53
1.5 V - 6 HOURS
dB HL
7
21
days post Rx
kHz
PERCENT of LOSS
O & I HC
SG
mm
G.P. 63
1.5 V - 20 HOURS
27
118
days post Rx
G.P. 48
1.5 V - 24 HOURS
120 days post Rx
G.P. 76
30 μA - 24 HOURS
before Rx
7
21
days post Rx
CLICK
OHC
IHC
G.P. 75
30 μA - 22 HOURS
before Rx
14
66
days post Rx
G.P. 78
30 μA - 24 HOURS
before Rx
9
62
days post Rx

Fig. 8. AP audiograms and corresponding histocochleograms for 6 additional GPs treated with dc current between round window and cortex (round window negative) for the various indicated durations, and using constant voltage (upper row) or constant current (lower row). In the first row percent of hair cell loss (outer + inner) is globally represented. Destruction–solid black area. Preparation artifact–cross-hatched areas.

other turns (Fig. 3 and also Fig. 10); filtered clicks near threshold in the normal excite the area of the basilar membrane corresponding to the center frequency of each filtered click (Fig. 4), in agreement with the observations of Naunton and Zerlin in the human (1976).

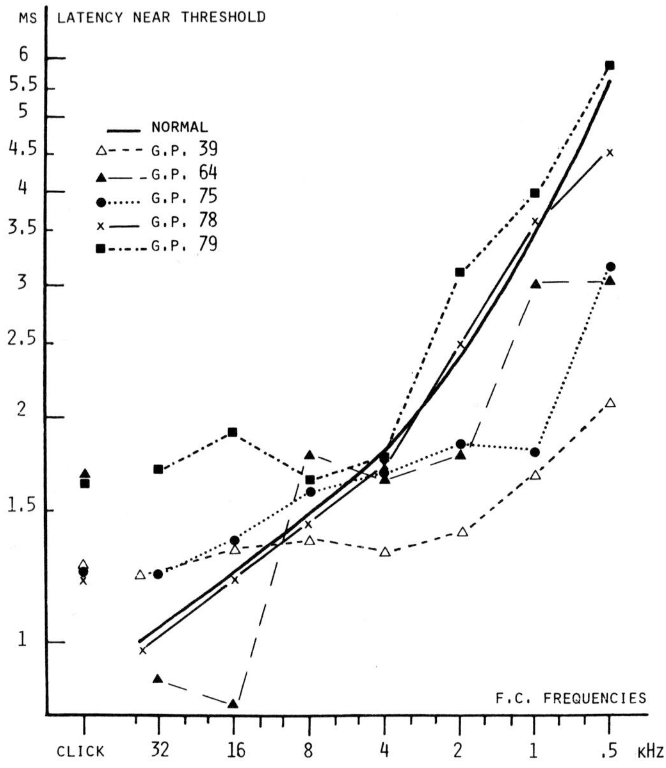

Fig. 9. Comparison of latencies (log scale) of responses to FCs of different frequencies between the normal (smoothed curve) and various pathological GPs (see AP audiograms and histocochleograms on Fig. 5 for GPs 39 and 64, Fig. 7 for GP 79, and Fig. 8 for GPs 75 and 78).

GP 39: The constant latency, except for the lowest frequencies, confirms that only one area is responding to any frequency; this latency of about 1.25 msec is that corresponding to around 16 kHz in the normal.

GP 64: Latencies of the responses are shifting toward that of the nearest preserved area: for the 16 kHz FC, the latency is that of 32 kHz; for the 8 kHz FC, it is that of 4 kHz.

GP 75: Latencies are more constant since the most sensitive area is between 16 and 4 kHz.

GP 78: Exhibits normal latencies. Since the thresholds are more or less elevated and the cochlea appears almost normal, there could be a transmission loss which was not obvious during dissection.

GP 79: Latencies for high frequencies are that of 8–4 kHz; from there on to the low frequencies, the latencies are normal.

Examples of pathological conditions are presented in Figures 5 to 10. These conditions resulted from a process originally used to evaluate damage caused by electric currents applied to the cochlea as might occur with inner ear prostheses. In two series of experiments dc current was applied between round window (RW) and cortex (RW negative), in the same waking guinea pigs, for durations ranging from 6 to 24 hours; voltage was constant (1.5 V, current varying between 20 and 40μA) in the first series, or constant current of 30μA in the second series in which electrode resistance and AP responses were continuously monitored during the entire exposure (Aran et al., 1977).

The results are very different from one guinea pig to another, either with constant current or constant voltage, with respect to patterns of AP responses and of destructions along the basilar membrane. The great variations in the effects cannot yet be explained. However such differences are of interest in our present concern with AP waveform analysis.

GPs 39 and 64 present with opposite conditions (Fig. 5). GP 39 should be convenient for the study of the response of a small area of the basilar membrane alone, which is the area preserved around 3mm (16 kHz), while GP 64 should allow the study of the effect of a localized destruction on the basilar membrane at about the same location. Responses to the click in these two GPs as compared to the normal are very explicit (Fig. 6). For GP 39 the response is well synchronized and has a constant waveform, while for GP 64 the pattern changes considerably with click intensity, particularly around 60 dB where N_1 is divided in two peaks, one earlier and one later than the normal N_1 which could correspond to responses originating on either side of the impaired 20 kHz area.

Another example is presented in Figure 7. For this guinea pig (# 79) there is an important elevation of threshold for high frequencies, with a slope of about 60 dB/octave from 8 to 16 kHz, corresponding to total destruction of outer and inner hair cells and of the spiral ganglion from 0 to about 5 mm from the base. In this GP comparison of AP waveforms in response to the rarefaction click before (normal) and after treatment shows how the pattern is modified by the lesion.

Additional examples of pathological cochleas after such electrical treatment are represented in Figure 8. They display various conditions such as very high frequency loss (GP 53), loss only of low frequencies (GP 76), preserved middle frequencies (GPs 63 and 75), extensive loss but remaining high frequencies (GP 48) and finally small-to-moderate losses from high to low frequencies (GP 78). A particular set of AP and histopathological data corresponds to each guinea pig.

It is important to note that in all the cochleas, thresholds, although sometimes elevated, can be determined for any frequency while some areas of the basilar membrane are totally destroyed. However, latencies of the responses to the filtered clicks near threshold for elevated thresholds are different from normal (Fig. 9). They correspond to those of the nearest intact area on the basilar membrane, stimulated by these filtered clicks at high intensity as a result of the envelope of the frequency spectrum of the third octave clicks and the mechanical properties of the basilar membrane. Thus, after taking into consideration the latencies of the responses to filtered clicks near threshold, the results can be better evaluated and then agree well with the histopathological data (see correspondances between Fig. 8 and 9).

The responses above threshold are more intricate. For the FCs we know that excitation spreads towards the base and the latencies are mixed. For the derived APs in principle no such prolbem should appear. However, as shown by Eggermont

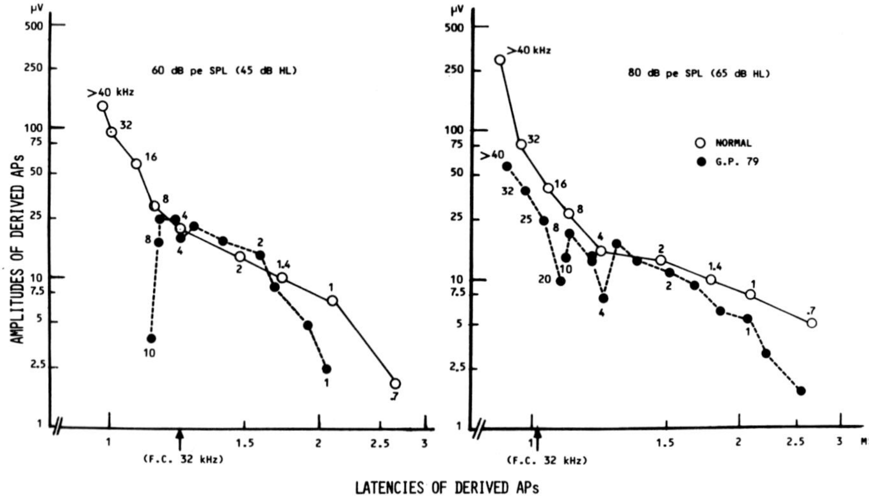

Fig. 10. Amplitudes of derived APs as a function of their latency for 2 levels of the rarefaction click in GP 79 (see Fig. 7 and 9). At low intensity level, the absence of derived APs of very short latency confirms the impairment of the first millimeter on the basilar membrane. Although in this area the organ of Corti appears completely destroyed, leaving the basilar membrane empty, short latency derived APs, with the greatest amplitudes, can be recorded, while there is still no response between 20 and 10 kHz. They contribute to the unmasked AP response at high click intensity (see traces in Fig. 7). Frequencies of FCs corresponding to each point are indicated.

(1976b) the latencies of the derived APs are intensity-dependent above mid-range frequencies. There we enter the problem of coding of intensity. Moreover in GP 79, where the basal part of the cochlea appears completely destroyed in the first millimeters, although data at threshold for FCs and derived APs are in perfect agreement with this situation, at higher intensities both show responses with short latencies which seem to correspond to the highest frequency area of the normal, on the hook of the basilar membrane. While no derived APs can be recorded from the 20-10 kHz area, clear derived APs above 20 kHz are obtained for high intensity click (Fig. 10). In agreement with this finding, the latency of the 32 kHz FC at high intensity is short. However it is possible that some remaining sensorineural structures are present at the beginning of the basilar membrane which is always very difficult to evaluate, although in such a case it was impossible to demonstrate any remaining cells, the basilar membrane appearing completely empty, even without pillars.

It is impossible to go further into this matter since data for each GP should be discussed. However the main conclusion would be that relations of AP waveforms with cochlear histopathology, although sometimes obvious, are not always simple, and that methods of analysis as well as modeling experiments may help in understanding phenomena but must first be tried extensively on animals before being proposed for analysis of human electrocochleographic data.

Acknowledgements

This work was supported in part by I.N.S.E.R.M. Grants No. 17.75.40.05 and 75.1.193.6.

The authors are greatly indebted to R. Charlet de Sauvage, J.-P. Erre and A. Guilhaume for their valuable help.

REFERENCES

Aran, J.-M. The electrocochleogram: recent results in children and in some pathological cases. *Arch. Klin. Exp. Ohren Nasen Kehlkopthellkd. 198:* 128-141, 1971.

Aran, J.-M. Clinical measures of eighth nerve function. *Adv. Oto-Rhino-Laryngol. 20:* 374-394, 1973.

Aran, J.-M. Patterns of electrochleographic responses observed in the guinea pig during ethacrynic acid intoxication. *Neurosci. Let. 2:* 335-338, 1976.

Aran, J.-M., Cazals, Y. and Charlet de Sauvage, R. Short and long term effects of dc currents applied to the cochlea: electrophysiological and histological observations. *V. Symposium über Cochleaforschung,* edited by D.D.R. Halle and H. Jakobi. (In Press).

Aran, J.-M. and Charlet de Sauvage, R. Evolution of CM, SP and AP during ethacrynic acid intoxication in the guinea pig. *Acta Otolaryngol. 83:* 153-159, 1977.

Aran J.-M. and Darrouzet, J. Observation of click-evoked compound VIII nerve responses before, during and over seven months after kanamycin treatment in the guinea pig. *Acta Otolaryngol. 79:* 24-32, 1975.

Aran, J.-M. and Erre, J.-P. Long-term recordings of endocochlear potentials. In: *Technological Basis of Auditory Investigations,* edited by H. A. Beagley. In preparation.

Aran, J.-M., Pelerin, J., Lenoir, J., Portmann, C. and Darrouzet, J. Aspects théoriques et pratiques des enregistrements électrocochléographiques selon la méthode établie à Bordeaux. *Rev. Laryngol. Otol. Rhinol.,* Bord. *92:* 601-644, 1971.

Biondi, E., Dacquino, G. and Grandori, F. Acoustic nerve action potential and single fibers activity generation: an equivalent neuron approach. *Labaratorio di Controlli Automatici, Relazione Interna* 74-3, 1974.

Biondi, E., Dacquino, G. and Grandori, F. Mathematical modeling of cochlear electrical activity and its possible application to a diagnostic methodology. Paper presented at the 89th A.S.A. Meeting, Austin, Texas, 1975.

Charlet de Sauvage, R. and Aran, J.-M. Clinical value of adaptation measurements in electrocochleography. In: *Electrocochleography,* edited by R.J. Ruben, C. Elberling and G. Salomon. Baltimore: University Park Press, 1976, p. 169-181.

Chinn, J. and Miller J. Animal model of acoustic neuroma. *Arch. Otolaryngol. 101:* 222-226, 1975.

Daigneault, E.A., Brown, R.D. and Blanton, J.F. Alterations of round window recorded N_1 by selective sections of the cochlear and vestibular nerves. *Acta Otolaryngol. 70:* 254-259, 1970.

Davis, H. Biophysics and physiology of the inner ear. *Physiol. Rev. 37:* 1-49, 1957.

de Boer, E. Synthetic whole-nerve action potentials for the cat. *J. Acoust. Soc. Am. 58:* 1030-1045, 1975.

Eggermont, J.J. Electrocochleography. In: *Handbook of Sensory Physiology. V/3. Auditory System: Clinical and Special Topics,* edited by W.D. Keidel and W.D. Neff. Berlin, Heidelberg, New York: Springer-Verlag, 1976a, p. 625-705.

Eggermont, J.J. Analysis of compound action potential responses to tone bursts in the human and guinea pig cochlea. *J. Acoust. Soc. Am. 60:* 1132-1139, 1976b.

Eggermont, J.J., Odenthal, D.W., Schmidt, P.H. and Spoor, A. Electrocochleography: basic principles and clinical application. *Acta Otolaryngol.* Suppl. *316:* 1-84, 1974.

Elberling, C. Stimulation of cochlear action potentials recorded from the ear canal in man. In: *Electrocochleography,* edited by R.J. Ruben, C. Elberling and G. Salomon. Baltimore: University Park Press, 1976, p. 151-168.

Elberling, C. Deconvolution of action potentials recorded from the ear canal in man. In: *Disorders of the Auditory Function II,* edited by S.D.G. Stephens. London: Academic Press, 1977, p. 109-117.

Elberling, C. and Salomon, G. Action potentials from pathological ears compared to potentials generated by a computer model. In: *Electrocochleography,* edited by R.J. Ruben, C. Elberling and G. Salomon. Baltimore: University Park Press, 1976, p. 439-455.

Evans, E.F. and Klinke, R. Reversible effect of cyanide and furosemide on the tuning of single cochlear fibers. *J. Physiol.,* London *242*: 129-131P, 1974.

Goldstein, R., McRandle, C.C. and Rodman, L.B. Site of lesion in cases of hearing loss associated with Rh incompatibility: an argument for peripheral impairment *J. Speech Hear. Disord. 37:* 447-450, 1972.

Goodhill, V. Auditory pathways lesions resulting from Rh incompatibility. In: *Deafness in Childhood,* edited by F. McConnell and P.H. Ward. Nashville: Vanderbilt University Press, 1967, p. 215-228.

Guild, S.R. A graphic reconstruction method for the study of the organ of Corti. *Anat. Rec., 22:* 141-157, 1921.

Gunn, C.K. Hereditary acholuric jaundice in a new mutant strain of rats. *J. Hered. 29:* 137, 1938.

Hallpike, C.S. and Hood, J.D. Observations upon the neurological mechanism of the loudness recruitment phenomenon. *Acta Otolaryngol. 50:* 472-486, 1959.

Hieke, D. and Hoke, M. Modeling of the formation of the compound action potential of the auditory nerve. In: *Sondersforchungsbereich 88, Teratologische Forshung und Rehabilitation Mehrfachbehinderter,* Vol. I, edited by M. Hoke and G. von Bally. University of Münster, 1976, p. 141-150.

Johnson, L., Sarmiento, F., Blanc, W.A. and Day, R. Kernicterus in rats with an inherited deficiency of glucuronyl transferase. *A.M.A. J. Dis. Child. 97:* 591-608, 1959.

Kiang, N.Y.S. *Discharge Patterns of Single Fibers in the Cat's Auditory Nerve.* Cambridge: M.I.T. Press, 1965.

Kiang, N.Y.S., Moxon, E.C. and Levine, R.A. Auditory-nerve activity in cats with normal and abnormal cochleas. In: *Sensorineural Hearing Loss,* edited by G.E.W. Wolstenholme and J. Knight. London: Churchill, 1970, p. 241-268.

Kimura, R.S. Experimental pathogenesis of hydrops. *Arch. Oto-Rhino-Laryngol. 212:* 263-275, 1976.

Kimura, R.S. and Schuknecht, H.F. Membranous hydrops in the inner ear of the guinea pig after obliteration of the endolymphatic sac. *Pract. Otol. Rhinol. Laryngol. 27:* 343-354, 1965.

Konishi, T. and Kelsey, E. Cochlear potentials and electrolytes in endolymph in experimentally induced endolymphatic hydrops of guinea pigs. In: *Electrocochleography,* edited by R.J. Ruben, C. Elberling and G. Salomon. Baltimore: University Park Press, 1976, p. 295-313.

Kupperman, R. Cochlear adaptation, central influences. *Acta Otolaryngol. 73:* 130-140, 1972.

Naunton, R.F. and Zerlin, S. Human whole-nerve response to clicks of various frequency. *Audiology 15:* 1-9, 1976.

Oshima, W., Suzuki, M., Shida, S. and Machino, M. Some findings on the inner ear after experimental obliteration of the endolymphatic duct and sac of guinea pigs. In: *Inner Ear Biology,* edited by M. Portmann and J.-M. Aran. Colloque INSERM, Vol 68. In Press.

Peake, W.T. and Kiang, N.Y.S. Cochlear responses to condensation and rarefaction clicks. *Biophys. J. 2:* 23-34, 1962.

Portmann, M. and Aran, J.-M. Relations entre "pattern" électrocochléographique et pathologie rétro-labyrinthique. *Acta Otolaryngol. 73:* 190-196, 1972.

Portmann, M., Aran, J.-M. and Coste, C. Vérification expérimentale sur l'animal de quelques aspects électrocochléographiques de la pathologie humaine. *Acta Otolaryngol. 75:* 132-142, 1973a.

Portmann, M., Aran, J.-M. and Lagourgue, P. Testing for recruitment by electrocochleography. Preliminary results. *Ann. Otol. Rhinol. Laryngol. 82:* 36-43, 1973b.

Portmann, M., Aran, J.-M. and Le Bert, G. Mise en place définitive d'une électrode sur la fenetre ronde du cobaye. *C.R. Soc. Biol. 160:* 551-556, 1966.

Schuknecht, H.F. and Woellner, R.C. An experimental and clinical study of deafness from lesions of the cochlear nerve. *J. Laryng. Otol. 69:* 75-97, 1955.

Spoendlin, H. and Baumgartner, H. Electrocochleography and cochlear pathology. *Acta Otolaryngol. 83:* 130-135, 1977.

Spoendlin, H. and Brun, J.-P. The block-surface technique for evaluation of cochlear pathology. *Arch. Oto-Rhino-Laryngol. 208:* 137-145, 1974.

Spoendlin, H. and Suter, R. Regeneration in the VIII Nerve. *Acta Otolaryngol. 81:* 228-236, 1976.

Teas, D.C., Eldredge, D.H. and Davis, H. Cochlear responses to acoustic transients: and interpretation of whole-nerve action potentials. *J. Acoust. Soc. Am. 34:* 1438-1459, 1962.

ELECTROCOCHLEOGRAPHY IN ADULTS

H.A. Beagley and W.P.R. Gibson
Royal National Throat, Nose and Ear Hospital

Transtympanic electrocochleography (ECoG) is now established as a safe and reliable procedure and has found a definite place in the clinical investigation of adult patients. It is used occasionally for threshold estimations, but more commonly for the diagnosis and differential diagnosis of cochlear and retrocochlear lesions, as well as for some lesser applications, as follows:

1. Threshold estimations in some cases of non-organic hearing loss (NOHL).
2. Investigation of sudden hearing loss.
3. Monitoring the effects of potentially ototoxic drugs.
4. Diagnosis of acoustic neuroma.
5. Diagnosis of Menière's disease.

THRESHOLD DETERMINATION

Transtympanic ECoG is rarely used for this purpose as there are other techniques available such as ERA (audiometry based on the vertex or V-potential) which is reliable in most adults and is frequency-specific. However, in a few cases of NOHL where ERA was unsatisfactory because of poor cooperation, with the patient interfering with the headphones or electrodes or wriggling and moving incessantly, ECoG was carried out with excellent results. Figure 1 shows the traces from such a case.

SUDDEN HEARING LOSS

Cases of profound deafness of sudden onset present serious problems of management and a wide diagnostic net is generally cast. In this hospital, ECoG is usually carried out after the more conventional tests have been done. Sometimes ECoG has provided useful information; for example, many of the bilateral cases tested have had absent action potential (AP) but a well marked cochlear microphonic (CM) to reasonably low stimulus intensity levels (70 - 80 dB HL) suggesting that the problem is predominantly a neural one. Cases of round window rupture have been discovered in the course of these tests, usually by a process of exclusion,

ISBN 0-12-514960-3

and have been duly repaired. Acoustic neuroma sometimes presents as a sudden hearing loss and ECoG can give information of crucial importance in many of these cases. M.D. Graham (personal communication) in a series of 70 cases of sudden hearing loss reports that 6 (9%) were due to acoustic neuroma.

MONITORING OF POTENTIALLY OTOTOXIC DRUGS

ECoG has been found useful in monitoring the effects of certain potentially ototoxic drugs. Wilson and Ramsden (1977) have demonstrated marked AP and CM changes in a case treated by Tobramycin. ECoG carried out on patients receiving treatment with new and potentially ototoxic drugs may be useful in assessing the dangers of using such medications.

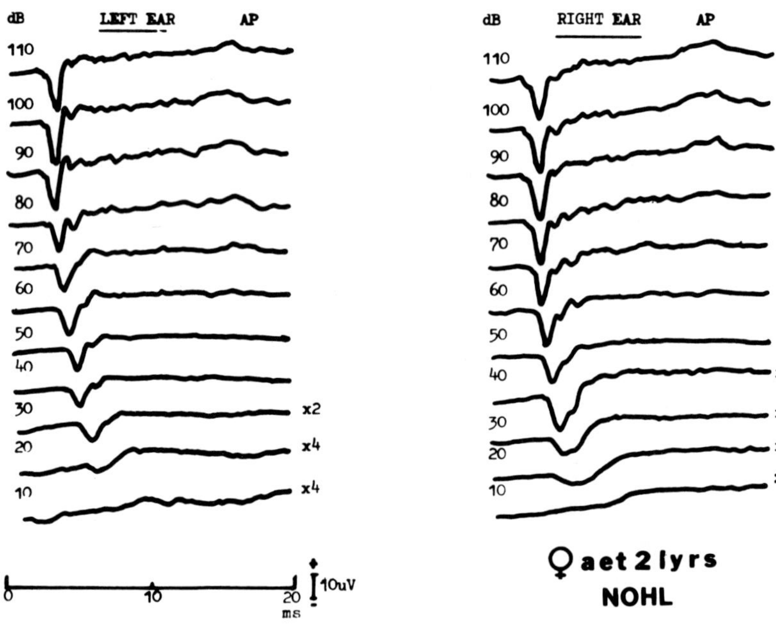

Fig. 1. This 21 year old female was suspected of having non-organic hearing loss (NOHL). Because of restlessness and poor cooperation the ERA traces were of very poor quality. ECoG was carried out with sedation (I.V. diazepam) and the traces shown above were obtained.

DIAGNOSIS OF ACOUSTIC NEUROMA AND SIMILAR TUMORS

It is in this field that ECoG finds its main application in adults. The tumor develops from the neurilemma of the auditory nerve, usually the superior vestibular division, but occasionally another division or even the cochlear nerve itself. Pressure of the tumor, especially when laterally placed in the internal auditory meatus (IAM), causes a neural type of hearing loss, and other cochlear effects due to vascular changes; ECoG in such cases will yield much pertinent information. Acoustic neuromas fall into two main categories; those laterally placed in the IAM cause early unilateral audiometric changes and should be detected early; those placed medially, in the cerebellopontine angle, tend to be more silent in the early stages and present later, often with symptoms suggestive of a cerebellopontine angle tumor with brainstem compression as well as audiometric changes.

It is now generally accepted that any sensorineural hearing loss which is unilateral, especially if it is progressive and associated with tinnitus, should be regarded as the result of an acoustic neuroma until proved otherwise. In this way the condition is more likely to be diagnosed and treated early. The classical audiometric findings such as tone decay, speech discrimination loss, stapedial reflex decay and even radiology can be misleading; this explains the advantages of ECoG which is the most useful test available apart from contrast radiography (pantopaque meatography). Computerized tomography (CT or CAT scan) is usually unsuccessful in confirming the presence of acoustic neuromas less than 2 cm in diameter, and those situated in the IAM. CT however, is very useful in the larger medially placed neuromas and is also very useful in showing the presence of such conditions as hydrocephalus which it is important to recognize prior to surgery.

Four distinct ECoG findings are characteristic of acoustic neuroma, but it must be stressed that these findings give no assurance as to the histological identity of the tumor. Usually it is an acoustic neuroma (Schwannoma or neurilemmoma) but other space-occupying lesions in the same region such as facial nerve neuroma, meningioma, angioma or basilar artery ectasia, can cause similar changes. This does not invalidate the general findings as each of these represents a pathologic state and is a tumor in the general sense.

The first of the four characteristic ECoG pictures consists of absent AP or diminished AP with a large CM. The AP in the normal subject can be traced down to the region of the subjective threshold, whereas the CM in most normal subjects usually cannot be traced lower than about 60 dB HL. In a neuroma case there may be no AP to be seen at maximal intensities (about 110 dB) or it may have a high threshold (about 90 dB); but the CM may be clearly visible at, for example, 60-70 dB. Moreover, in acoustic neuromas the CM tends to be large in amplitude and is easily recognized visually. Such a CM which can be detected easily at intensity levels where the AP has disappeared suggests the presence of a neural lesion which has suppressed AP generation in the nerve fibers, but that many cochlear hair cells have been spared to produce a microphonic potential. This state of affairs is compatible with the presence of an acoustic neuroma, especially a large medially-placed one in which cerebellopontine signs may also be present (Figure 2).

In most modern ECoG equipment the AP and CM can be obtained separately. This is done by means of a two-memory averager into which are multiplexed alternate responses from the patient's cochlea elicited by stimuli which alternate in polarity. By taking sums and differences of the two memory contents it is possible to inspect the AP and the CM separately.

The second of the characteristic ECoG pictures is absence of subjective hearing but an evident AP. This is very strong evidence in favor of acoustic neuroma. The hypothesis here is that the tumor causes a complete neural block at some point along the cochlear nerve which prevents the AP from being transmitted centrally. Thus it cannot pass along the auditory tracts and is not detected by the patient as an audible stimulus. But peripheral to the neural block the cochlear nerve continues to function as shown by the presence of a typical AP. Although this is very strong evidence in favor of the presence of acoustic neuroma, it is essential to eliminate the possibility of non-organic hearing loss, which can be confirmed by ERA, or of the presence of another discrete and total lesion of the appropriate segment of the auditory pathways, such as tumor pressing on the homolateral cochlear nucleus or the lateral lemniscus just cephalic to the cochlear nucleus.

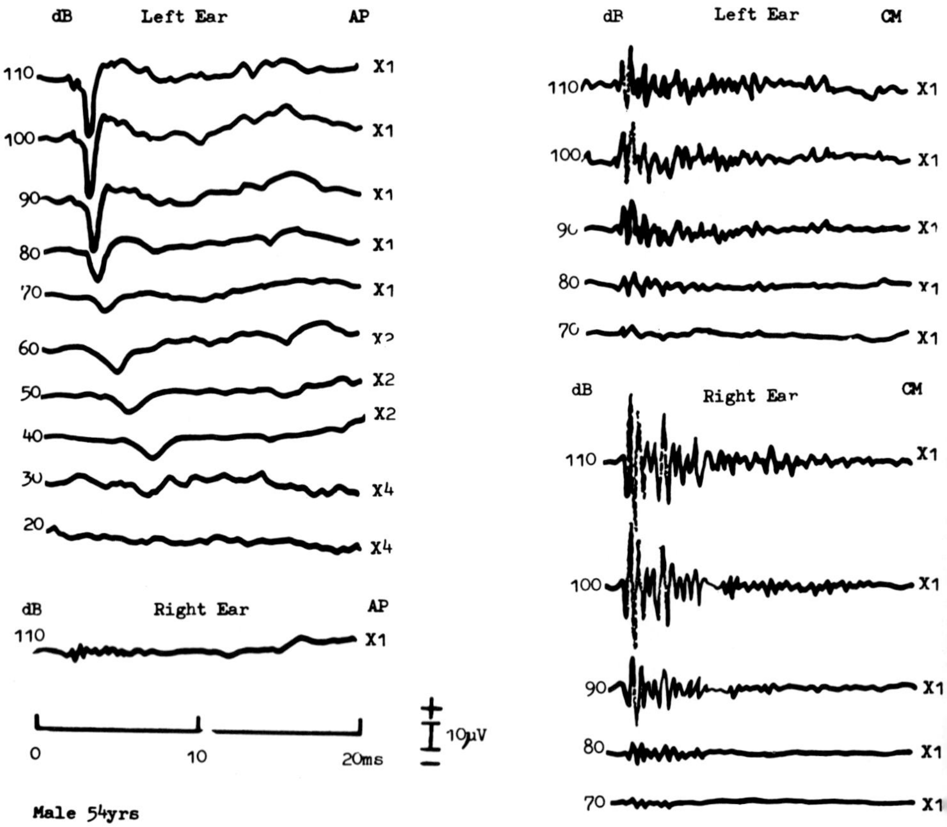

Fig. 2. This patient who was deaf in the right ear showed no AP on the right when ECoG was carried out but there was a large CM present showing that there is some remaining cochlear (hair cell) activity. A large right acoustic neuroma was removed subsequently.

A third characteristic ECoG picture is where the ECoG threshold is lower than the subjective, ECoG showing greater auditory acuity than the conventional pure tone audiogram (PTA). Figure 3 shows the PTA and the ECoG thresholds for a patient who had symptoms vaguely suggestive of acoustic neuroma. This finding was crucial in the decision to carry out contrast radiological studies which showed non-filling of the IAM; a small acoustic neuroma was removed subsequently. The patient had noticed vague symptoms for several years and ECoG lead the way to complete diagnosis and treatment. Gibson and Beagley (1976) reported that 19 (27%) of 71 acoustic neuromas showed ECoG thresholds at least 15 dB more sensitive than subjective audiometry (Figure 3).

The fourth and final characteristic ECoG picture is that of a widened and distorted AP; it is frequently seen in early laterally placed neuromas. In these cases there is appreciable remaining hearing and the tumor is usually a small one situated within the IAM where it causes pressure on, and dysfunction of the cochlear nerve. The experiments of Teas et al., (1962) have shown that the compound AP is generated by the combined activity of the cochlear nerve fibers both within the modiolus and within the IAM. Legouix and Pierson (1974) have shown that deactivation of the nerve fibers centrally (at the IAM) by instilling KCl converts the normally diphasic AP of the guinea pig to a widened monophasic waveform. Beagley et al., (1977) have indicated experimentally that a similar deactivation of cochlear fibers at the IAM is the probable explanation of the widened AP observed when an acoustic neuroma is present in this situation, (Figures 4 to 6).

The presence, therefore, of a widened AP which may be as wide as 5 to 20 milliseconds is consistent with the presence of an acoustic neuroma. Other conditions in which a similar widened AP can be recorded include deafness resulting from kernicterus where, it is postulated, a similar neural block exists, and in the case of other tumors such as neuroma of the facial nerve which similarly causes pressure and dysfunction of the cochlear nerve. A different form of widening of the AP is seen in some cases of Menière's disease; the characteristic of this waveform and its differential diagnosis are discussed below.

ECoG IN MENIÈRE'S DISEASE

Much is known of the causes and the symptoms of this condition yet much remains unknown. The characteristic symptom-complex of vertigo, balance disturbance without loss of consciousness, tinnitus and fluctuating hearing loss is well known to all clinicians yet such is the vagueness of the condition that most clinicians develop their own criteria as to what constitutes Menière's disease. It is generally accepted that disturbance of the endolymph circulation is involved, usually with hydrops of the endolymphatic system, yet this adds little of real value to our basic understanding of the condition. Electrocochleography has something to offer in this field, and in the differential diagnosis between unilateral Menière's disease and acoustic neuroma.

The most typical ECoG sign in Menière's disease is a widened multipeaked AP

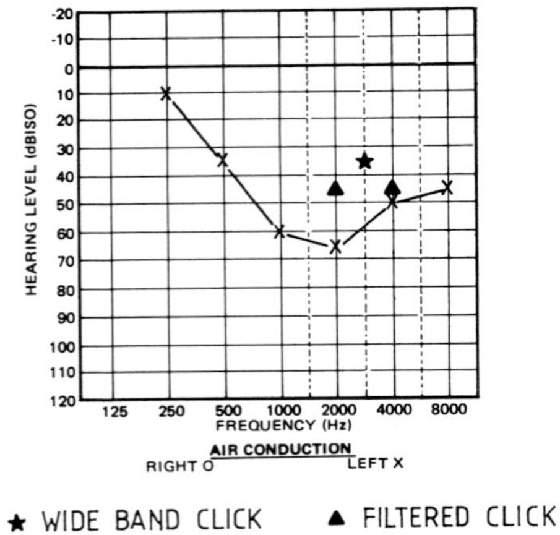
HEARING LEVEL (dBISO)
-20
-10
0
10
20
30
40
50
60
70
80
90
100
110
120
125
250
500
1000
2000
4000
8000
FREQUENCY (Hz)
AIR CONDUCTION
RIGHT O
LEFT X
★ WIDE BAND CLICK
▲ FILTERED CLICK

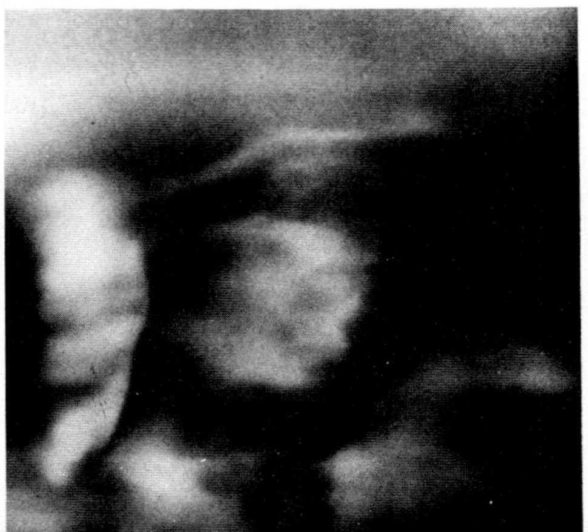

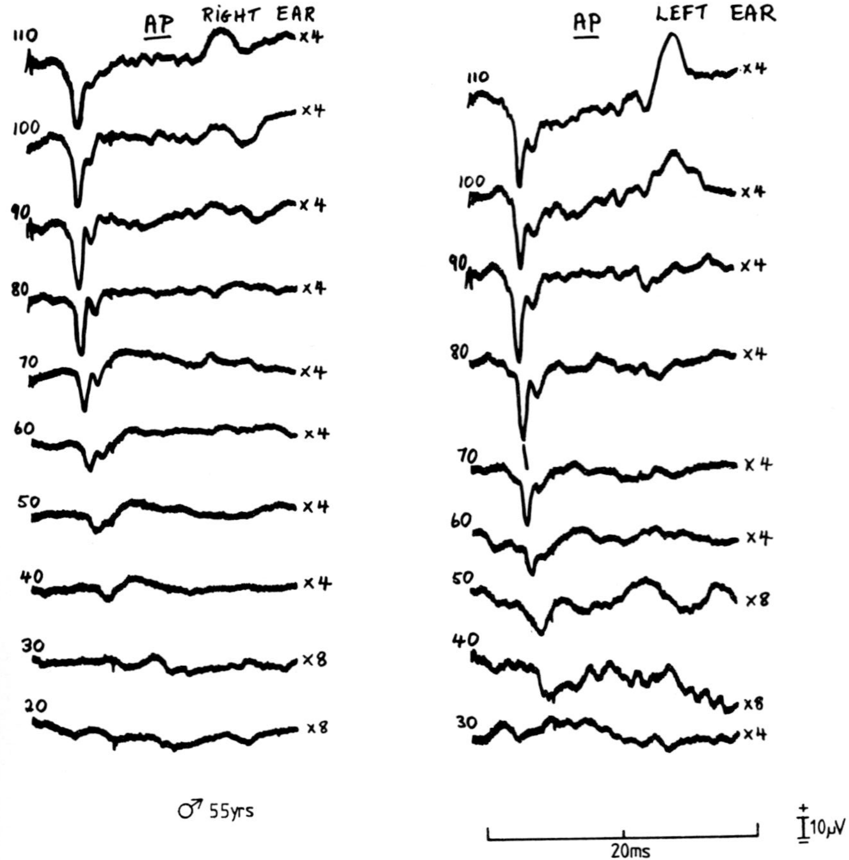
AP RIGHT EAR
110
100
90
80
70
60
50
40
30
20
x4
x8
AP LEFT EAR
♂ 55yrs
20ms
10μV

Fig. 3. This 55 year old male had vague symptoms of vertigo and hearing loss for many years. The ECoG (right) showed a slightly abnormal left AP trace suggestive of acoustic neuroma. In addition, the ECoG threshold for wide band clicks and tone-bursts was lower than the subjective threshold (top left). This was very suggestive of acoustic neuroma; contrast radiography (bottom left) was carried out and showed a meatal filling defect. An acoustic neuroma was removed subsequently.

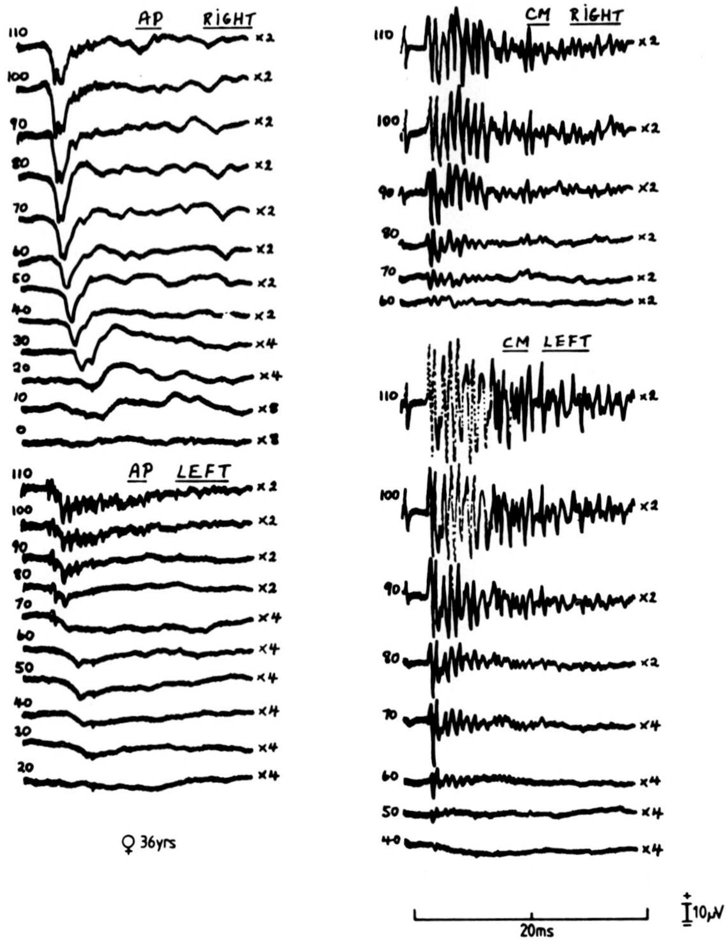

Fig. 4. Traces from a 36 year old female. Acoustic neuroma on the left was considered to be a possibility and the ECoG shows the typical widened AP which can be traced down to at least 30dB in spite of her subjective threshold being 90dB. Note the very large CM which is not completely cancelled in the high intensity AP traces. An acoustic neuroma, or similar space occupying lesion, was reported on the basis of these traces; an acoustic neuroma was later removed.

(Brackmann and Selters, 1976). The CM tends to be rather small in amplitude and distorted and there is usually a well marked negative summating potential (-SP) as Eggermont showed (1976a). Occasionally there is a positive spike immediately before the negative AP peak (Aran and Portmann, 1976) which has been attributed to a +SP; this may indeed be so especially when there is a loss of basal hair cells. However, it may be also due simply to uncancelled microphonic deflections.

While it is possible to confuse the multipeaked and widened AP of Menière's

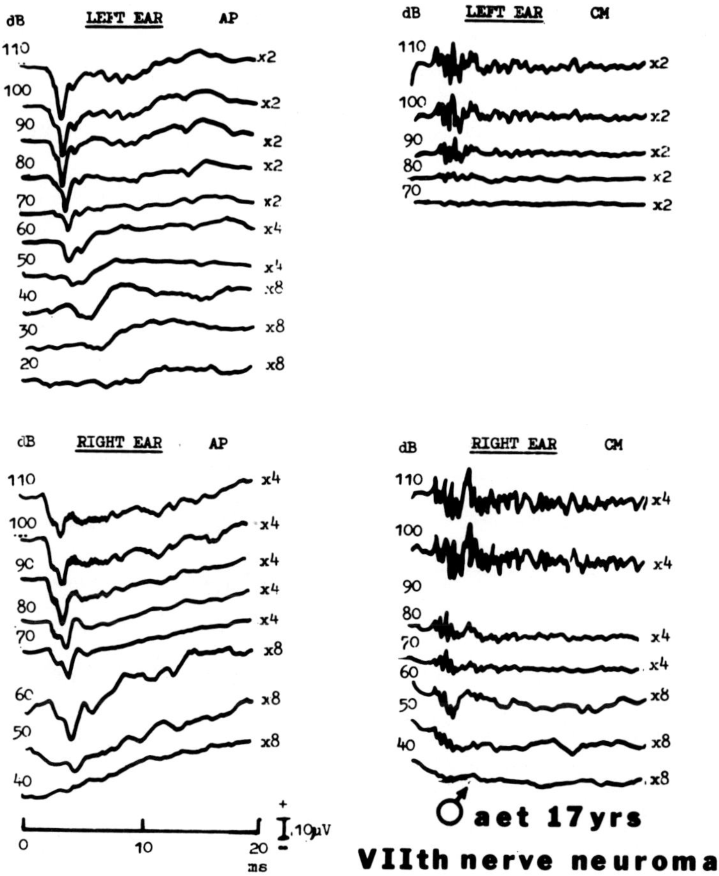

Fig. 5. This 17 year old male was suspected of having an acoustic neuroma because of history of progressive right sided hearing loss and tinnitus. There was in fact no subjective hearing in the right ear when the ECoG was done. The right AP shows a widened, distorted AP visible to about 50dB. Contrast radiography showed a meatal filling defect and at operation a facial nerve neuroma was removed.

disease with the widened AP seen in acoustic neuroma, attention to the details of the waveform will usually allow the two to be distinguished. The multipeaked AP is brought about mainly by a large -SP which displaces the whole AP in a negative direction so that it does not regain the baseline level for a few milliseconds and the N_2 and N_3 peaks, if present, are observed as part of the ascending limb of the widened AP. To clarify this matter it is usual to eliminate the AP leaving the -SP which can then be subtracted from the unadapted waveform, revealing the true AP waveform. Eggermont (1976a) used a technique of adaptation to achieve this effect, whereby the AP is eliminated by increasing the repetition rate, thereby inducing fatigue-like diminution of the AP. However, if wideband clicks are used, a repetition rate of 2 - 4,000 clicks per second is required for complete AP suppression and this is not practicable with averaging systems. It is therefore better to use tone bursts eg. 2 kHz tone with 8 complete cycles delivered 50 or 100 times per second. This is generally effective in causing maximal, but not necessarily total, AP adaptation. The remaining waveform, mainly -SP, is then subtracted from the unadapted waveform produced by tone bursts delivered at the rate of 5 or 10 per second in which the AP will be very conspicious. In averagers with a divided memory and appropriate switching this can be done instantly leaving the AP as

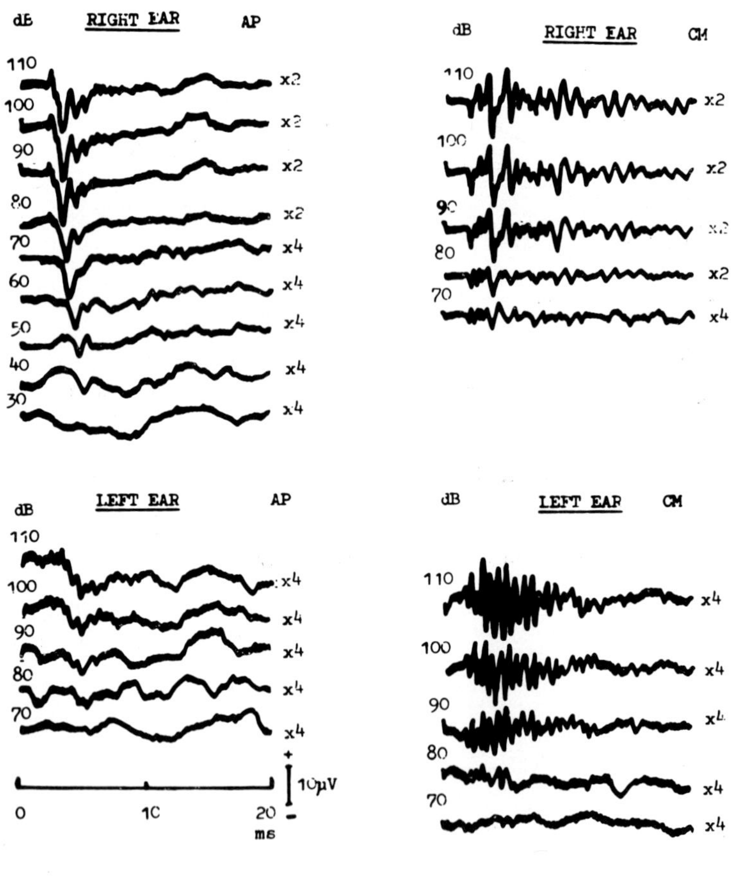

♂ 49yrs Lt Acoustic Neuroma

Fig. 6. An example of left acoustic neuroma. The right ear was normal apart from a 4 kHz notch due to industrial noise exposure.

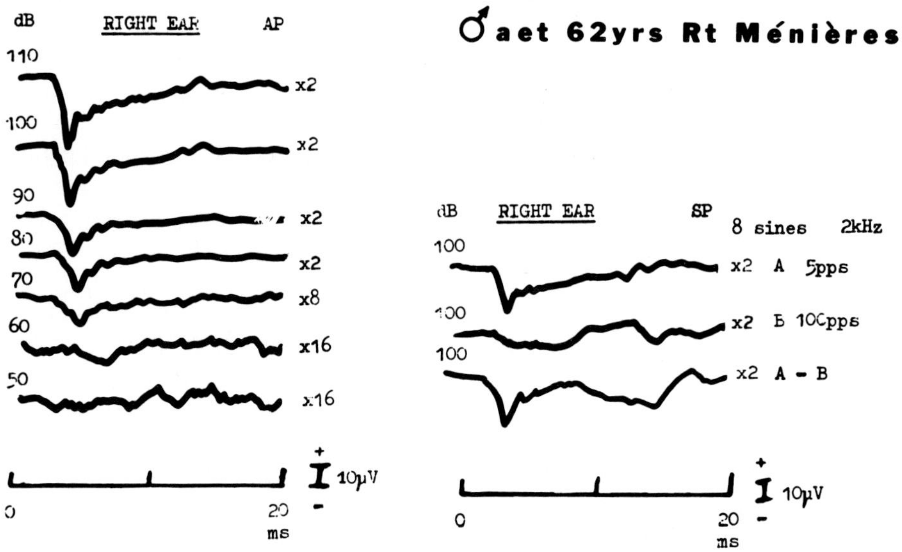

Fig. 7. This 62 year old male suffered from right sided Menière's disease. Note the large –SP and the widened, multipeaked AP. When the –SP is subtracted a fairly normal AP is seen in A – B.

Figure 7 shows. However, there is one constant problem with this technique as Eggermont (personal communication) has shown, namely, that sometimes the AP is not fully adapted to the point of extinction and when this happens the reduced AP deflection (N_1) is increased in latency relative to the unadapted situation and subtraction of the partly adapted waveform leads to a spurious or enhanced diphasic AP waveform as shown in Figure 8, which can be misleading in some neuroma cases where a monophasic AP is expected.

DIFFERENTIAL DIAGNOSIS OF MENIÈRE'S DISEASE AND ACOUSTIC NEUROMA

The problems of differential diagnosis are maximal when one is faced with a widened monophasic AP in one ear only, which could be the result of an early acoustic neuroma or unilateral Menière's disease. It is usually found that careful inspection of the waveforms gives most of the information required to differentiate between them and Figure 9 shows a Menière's AP waveform with multiple peaks as well as the characteristic widened monophasic AP waveform of early acoustic neuroma. Such classical examples present no serious diagnostic problems.

To assist in differentiating between the two conditions two separate techniques, adaptation and high-pass masking proposed by Eggermont, as well as certain other observations which will now be mentioned, can be useful. The technique of narrow-band analysis by successive high-pass masking offers the best theoretical possibility of clinching the diagnosis where there is a widened AP in acoustic neuroma. In this condition there is almost certainly a monophasic instead of the diphasic unit response as a result of the absence of the central contribution from the cochlear nerve fibers. When the monophasic unit responses are convoluted the widened AP typical of acoustic neuroma is seen. Successive high-pass masking by Eggermont's method should give a good idea of the underlying unit response and this should be monophasic in early neuroma cases. In practice however, the method may be difficult and uncertain and it may be better to rely on direct observations.

The use of adaptation of the AP to separate the -SP mentioned earlier is valuable particularly in Menière's with multipeaked waveforms. The essentially normal AP which remains is very clear when total adaptation is achieved. However, incomplete adaptation may occur which on subtraction causes an objectionable artifact, namely a falsely diphasic AP, and no reliance should be placed in this finding. The essential problem remains to differentiate a conspicious -SP from the widened AP of acoustic neuroma. One important observation relates to the time of onset of the negative deflection. If it is a true -SP it should start with the onset of the cochlear microphonic and be practically coterminous with it when tone-burst stimulation is used. A rather low frequency tone-burst eg. 8 cycles of a 2 kHz sinusoid, seems the best stimulus to elicit a -SP in Menière's disease, probably because it will cause its maximal deflection at a wider and more lax part of the basilar membrane than would a high frequency tone-burst such as 8 kHz. The -SP

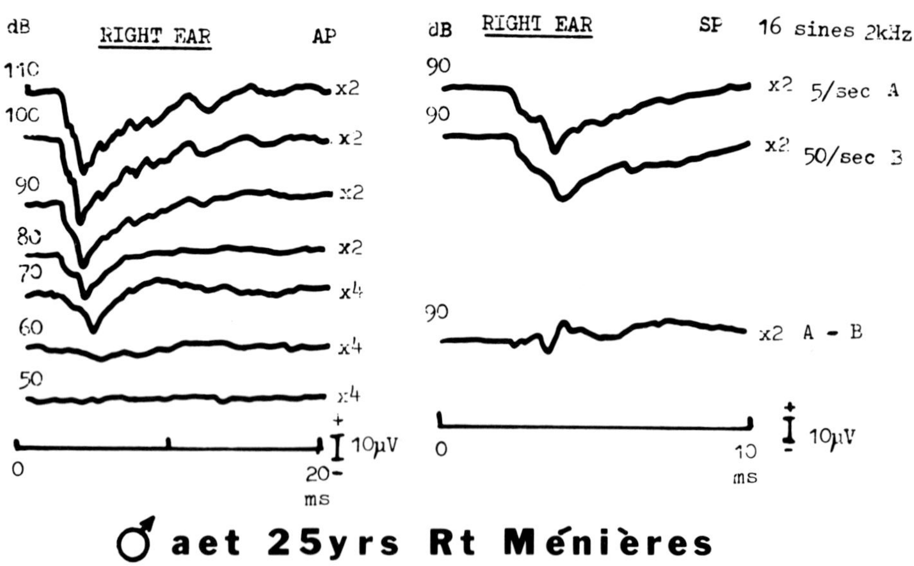

Fig. 8. This shows the notched, multipeaked AP with a large –SP that is seen in Menière's disease. Adaptation was incomplete (trace B) and subtraction leads to the spurious diphasic AP waveform seen in A – B.

can then be removed by the adaptation technique and a normal AP should be seen. It is postulated that the widened notched waveform is due to -SP and the clearly separated N_2 and N_3 peaks are the result of the hydrops impeding the traveling wave so that the successive peaks tend to be seen individually rather than being incorporated more closely with the N_1 peak.

The widened waveform of acoustic neuroma on the other hand commences a finite time, 0.5 to 1.0 msec, after the commencement of the CM and it is certainly not co-terminous with it but persists well after the termination of the CM and is quite independent of the duration of the stimulus, whether a click or a tone-burst as Figure 9 shows. An 8 kHz tone-burst is very useful for eliciting this response. The onset delay of the widened negative waveform of acoustic neuroma and its prolongation long beyond the duration of the stimulus suggests that it is of neural origin, probably the result of convolution of monophasic unit potentials. There is little difficulty in distinguishing this from the multipeaked Menière's waveform, except when the presumed neuroma waveform commences at the same time as the CM. This is attributed to the presence of -SP as well as widened AP of the neuroma type. The obvious way to separate these two potentials would be to cause the widened AP to adapt, and to substract the remaining -SP. But unfortunately the widened AP of neuroma is sometimes very resistant to adaptation. This, it is

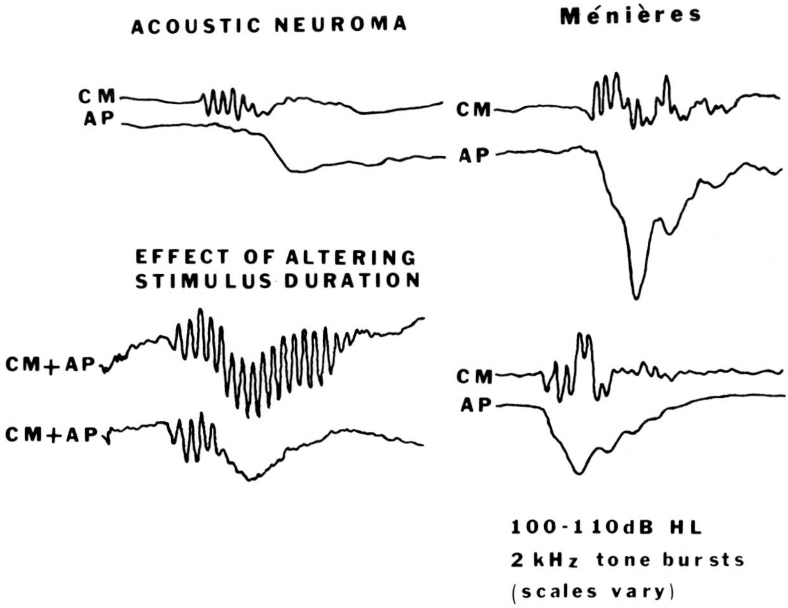

Fig. 9. The widened, notched, multipeaked AP waveforms of Menière's (right upper and lower) can usually be distinguished from the widened AP of acoustic neuroma. Note the distorted CM often seen in Menière's and the fact that the AP/–SP trace starts at the time of the onset of the CM and ends more or less at the same time. However, the widened AP waveform of acoustic neuroma starts after the onset of the CM, and its width (duration) is independent of the duration of the stimulus as shown by the CM duration (left upper and lower).

proposed, is due to the widened monophasic unit responses, presumably with their conduction velocity reduced and probably poorly synchronized, failing to produce the well-timed volleys that would be more susceptible to adaptation. Charlet de Sauvage and Aran (1976) and Yoshie and Ohashi (1971) have discussed abnormal adaptation in retrocochlear conditions.

There are two minor stratagems that can be tried to eliminate -SP when adaptation cannot be achieved:

a. by using high frequency (8 kHz) rather than lower frequency (2 kHz) tone-bursts, as the latter are more likely to produce a -SP.
b. by reducing the intensity of the tone-bursts progressively; at 80 or 70 dB HL the -SP is much less conspicuous or may be absent altogether.

In this clinic some 130 acoustic neuromas have been identified and removed surgically and the success rate for positive identification by ECoG is about 90%. The only diagnostic procedure to exceed this success rate is contrast radiography with pantopaque but this is a highly invasive and unpleasant investigation for the patient. It is proposed that ECoG should first be carried out and contrast studies done only if the likelihood of a tumor being present is considerable and if surgical removal is likely to be undertaken subsequently.

REFERENCES

Aran, J.-M. and Portmann, M. Applied cochlear electrophysiology. In: *Scientific Foundations of Otolaryngology,* edited by R. Hinchcliffe and D. Harrison. London: Heinemann, 1976, p. 303-312.

Beagley, H.A., Legouix, J.-P., Teas, D.C. and Remond, M.-C. Electrocochleographic changes in acoustic neuroma. *Clin Otolaryng.* (In Press, 1977).

Brackmann, D.E. and Selters, W.A. Electrocochleography in Ménière's disease and acoustic neuromas. In: *Electrocochleography,* edited by R.J. Ruben, C. Elberling and G. Salomon. Baltimore: University Park Press, 1976, p. 315-329.

Charlet de Sauvage, R. and Aran, J.-M. Clinical value of adaptation measurements in electrocochleography. In: *Electrocochleography,* edited by R.J. Ruben, C. Elberling and G. Salomon. Baltimore: University Park Press, 1976, p. 169-181.

Eggermont, J.J. Summating potentials in electrocochleography: relation to hearing disorders. In: *Electrocochleography,* edited by R.J. Ruben, C. Elberling and G. Salomon. Baltimore: University Park Press, 1976, p. 67-93.

Eggermont, J.J. Electrocochleography. In: *Handbook of Sensory Physiology. V/3. Auditory System: Clinical and Special Topics,* edited by W.D. Keidel and W.D. Neff. Berlin, Heidelberg, New York: Springer-Verlag, 1976, p. 625-705.

Eggermont, J.J. (Personal communication).

Gibson, W.P.R. and Beagley, H.A. Transtympanic electrocochleography in the investigation of retrocochlear disorders. *Rev. Laryngol. Otol. Rhinol.,* Bord. Suppl. *97:* 507-516, 1976.

Graham, J.M. (Personal communication).

Legouix, J.-P. and Pierson, A. Investigations on the sources of whole-nerve action potentials recorded from various places in the guinea-pig cochlea. *J. Acoust. Soc. Am. 56:* 1222-1225, 1974.

Teas, D.C., Eldredge, D.H. and Davis, H. Cochlear reponses to acoustic transients: an interpretation of whole-nerve action potentials. *J. Acoust. Soc. Am. 34:* 1438-1459, 1962.

Wilson, P. and Ramsden, R.T. Immediate effects of tobramycin on the human cochlea and correlation with serum tobramycin levels. *Brit. Med. J. 1:* 259-261, 1977.

Yoshie, N. and Ohashi, T. Abnormal adaptation of human cochlear nerve action potential responses: clinical observations by non-surgical recording. *Rev. Laryngol. Otol. Rhinol.,* Bord. Suppl. *92:* 673-690, 1971.

CM IN CLINICAL DIAGNOSIS

Stanley Zerlin and Ralph F. Naunton

University of Chicago

INTRODUCTION

The cochlear microphonic has been the subject of scrutiny for some 45 years and its intimate relation to the hair cell well established. With the recent rise of transtympanic recording in humans, a resurgence of interest in the CM has taken place; the superior signal-to-noise ratio achieved by this technique has led to a re-examination of the CM's potentialities. A number of quite recent studies have sought to establish a basis for the measurement of CM in humans and for assessment of its clinical utility. (Hoke, 1976a, 1976b; Aran and Charlet de Sauvage, 1976, Heike, 1976).

The present study is a preliminary attempt to relate qualitatively changes in CM amplitude to changes in hearing sensitivity.

METHODS

In our practice of transtympanic ECoG, the sound stimuli are alternately reversed in polarity and responses recorded on magnetic tape; our stimuli are third-octave clicks; these have been described (Zerlin and Naunton, 1975).

On playback, the recorded material is octave-band filtered around the microphonic frequency. The computer is instructed to sum on separate traces only responses to the same stimulus polarity; this results in two traces each containing one of the polarities of CM. (A schematized illustration of the recording technique is given in Figure 2 of the paper "Recording and Analyzing Techniques", ibid.)

Figure 1 illustrates the results of the summing process in the two top traces (CM_1 and CM_2). One of the CM waveforms is then inverted by the computer and added to the other; this process of algebraic addition is illustrated in the lowest trace of Figure 1. CM amplitude, now doubled, is taken as the maximum peak-to-peak excursion of the resulting CM envelope.

Contamination by artifacts

Before continuing, we must first settle a technical issue of considerable importance. In ECoG recording the thin transtympanic needle on the promontory

ISBN 0-12-514960-3

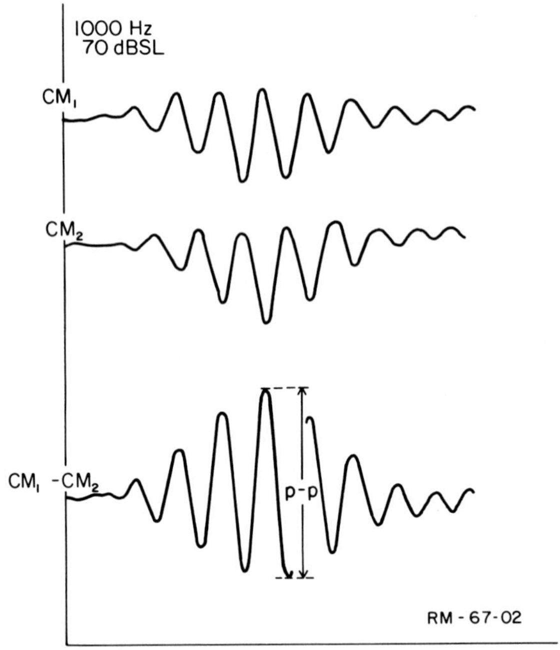

Fig. 1. Top two traces: the result of summing separately the two polarities of a recorded microphonic to third-octave click. This is an example of AP contamination of the CM as indicated by the asymmetry of the waveforms. Lowest Trace: Result after trace CM_2 has been inverted and combined with trace CM_1. CM amplitude (designated peak-to-peak) had been doubled.

is held in place at the near end by a rubber band. We cannot, a priori, discount the possibility that intense sound waves delivered to the ear may vibrate the electrode at the stimulus frequency, introducing artifacts that resemble the cochlear microphonic.

We have taken the following steps to evaluate the possibility of artifact contamination in our recordings. We routinely place a ¼ inch monitor microphone at the ear-canal entrance and record its output on one channel of the magnetic tape used to record the ECoG responses. Wideband clicks at high intensity are then used to stimulate the ear. On playback, the acoustic output of the microphone channel is summed along with the summed response of the ECoG channel. Illustrative results for one subject are shown in Figure 2.

Both polarities of the acoustic waveform are seen in the two lower traces; the presumed CM responses appear in the two upper traces. It may be seen that the click onset at the ear-canal entrance precedes the onset of the CM by 0.2 msec. (The 0.2 msec time difference comprises the acoustic travel time in the ear canal and the mechanical transit time across the middle ear structures.) Additional tests have shown that if the promontory response were indeed artifactual, that is the result of electrode vibration, the time lag between the two sets of waveforms would disappear. In other words, mechanical vibration of the electrode, perhaps resulting in a varying resistance at the point of contact, produces an electrical onset that is simultaneous with the acoustic onset.

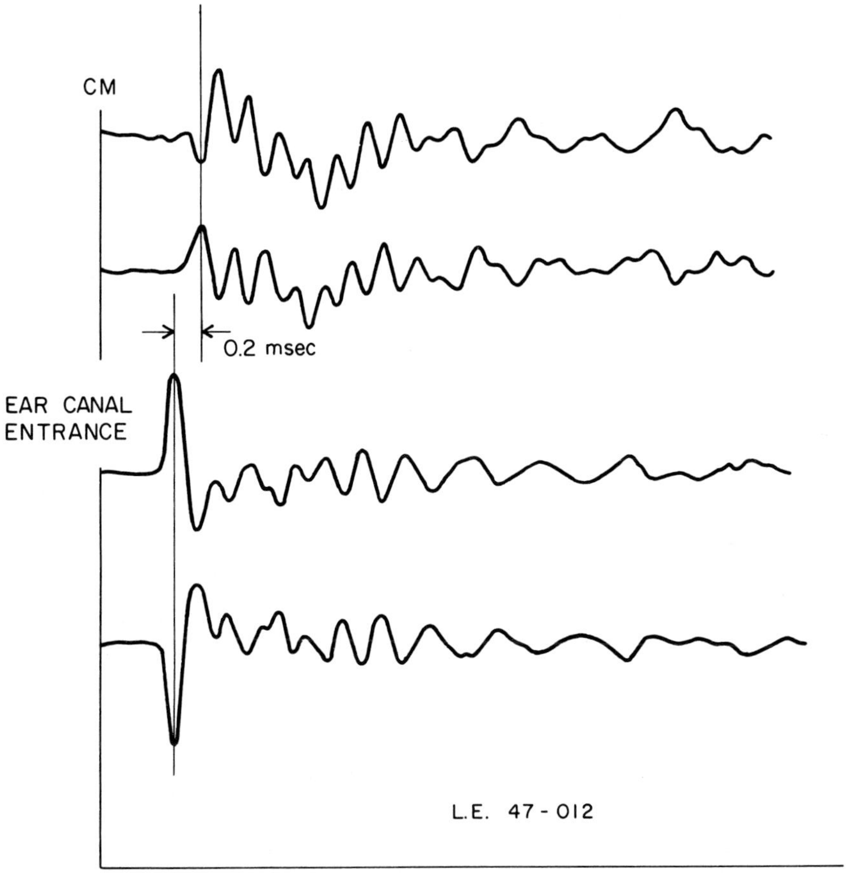

Fig. 2. Comparison of the time relation between the arrival of a click at the entrance of the ear canal (two lower traces) and the click CM recorded at the promontory (two upper traces). The acoustic click precedes the CM by 0.2 msec. See text for further explanation.

RESULTS

These techniques were used to study the cochlear microphonic in four cases of impaired hearing seen in our laboratory. Each individual was seen on two separate occasions, all four cases showing significant changes in hearing from test to retest. Two exhibited an increase and two showed a decrease in auditory sensitivity. The CM comparisons presented here are limited to comparisons of the same ear using the same frequencies and stimulus levels.

To establish the relevance of the CM to the hearing process we begin by comparing the CM amplitudes with their corresponding AP amplitudes; in Figure 3 is seen results for Case #1, a case of sudden hearing loss showing improvement between test and the retest occurring about a week later. (Puretone audiometric

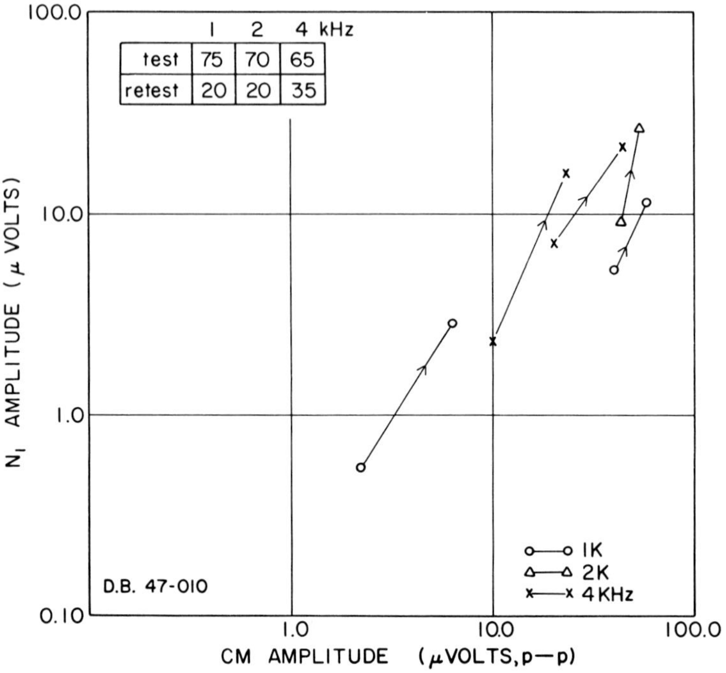

Fig. 3. Test-retest relations between CM and AP amplitudes for a young adult exhibiting sudden hearing loss with subsequent recovery. Audiometric threshold findings at test and retest shown in the insert at upper left. Click frequencies indicated by the legend at lower right. Symbols connected by lines indicate the test-retest results for a given condition of frequency and sensation level, arrowheads point from test toward retest. All results shown are for 70 and 90 dB SL re normal. Note that both CM and AP amplitudes increase with improvement in hearing sensitivity.

results for 1, 2, and 4 kHz are shown in the insert near the top left of the figure.) Each data point represents the CM amplitude and corresponding AP amplitude for a given condition of frequency and level. Test-retest results for that same condition are joined by a line, the arrowhead indicating the direction from test to retest; click frequency is given in the legend at the lower right. Throughout, test-retest comparisons are at levels of 70 and 90 dB SL re normal. Omission of some levels in the series of figures to follow are simply in the interests of clear graphic presentation. The main point to be noted in Figure 3 is that both CM and AP amplitude increase as hearing sensitivity improves between test and retest.

A potential problem may exist in interpreting the CM - AP data at 1000 Hz: it is often difficult to separate out CM from AP components at 1000 Hz because of the similarity in frequency composition of the two components. Thus, growth in CM amplitude at 1000 Hz could conceivably be attributable to growth in the AP only, or perhaps to both CM and AP.

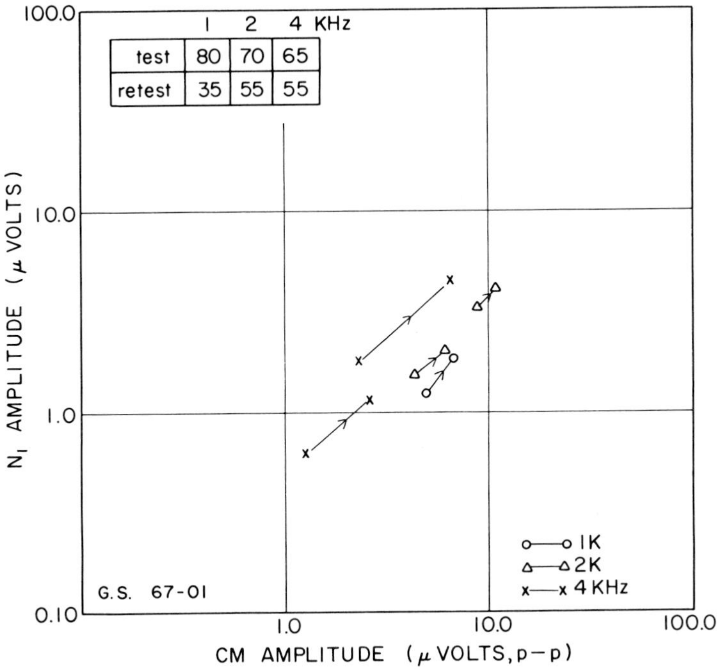

Fig. 4. Relations between CM and AP amplitude for an adult with sudden hearing loss and subsequent recovery. Same as Figure 3. Note that CM and AP amplitudes increase with improvement in hearing sensitivity.

Fortunately, as the frequency of CM increases beyond 1000 Hz, the spectral composition of the CM departs from that of the AP and we can be reasonably confident that the filtered CM at 2 and 4 kHz includes little or no contribution by the AP.

A second case of sudden deafness with subsequent improvement is seen in Figure 4. (The audiometric results are shown at the upper left). Again, increases in both CM and AP amplitudes are seen accompanying the improved sensitivity.

Effects of Electrode Resistance

Consideration of another technical point is required before continuing the analysis: it is well known that the resistance at the electrode-tissue interface can influence the amplitude of the recorded signal, the higher the resistance, the poorer the recorded amplitude. A question then naturally arises: might not the test-retest relations shown here, increased CM amplitudes accompanying larger AP amplitudes on retest, be simply the result of reduced electrode resistances during retest?

That objection is considered in Figure 5; here are shown the relations

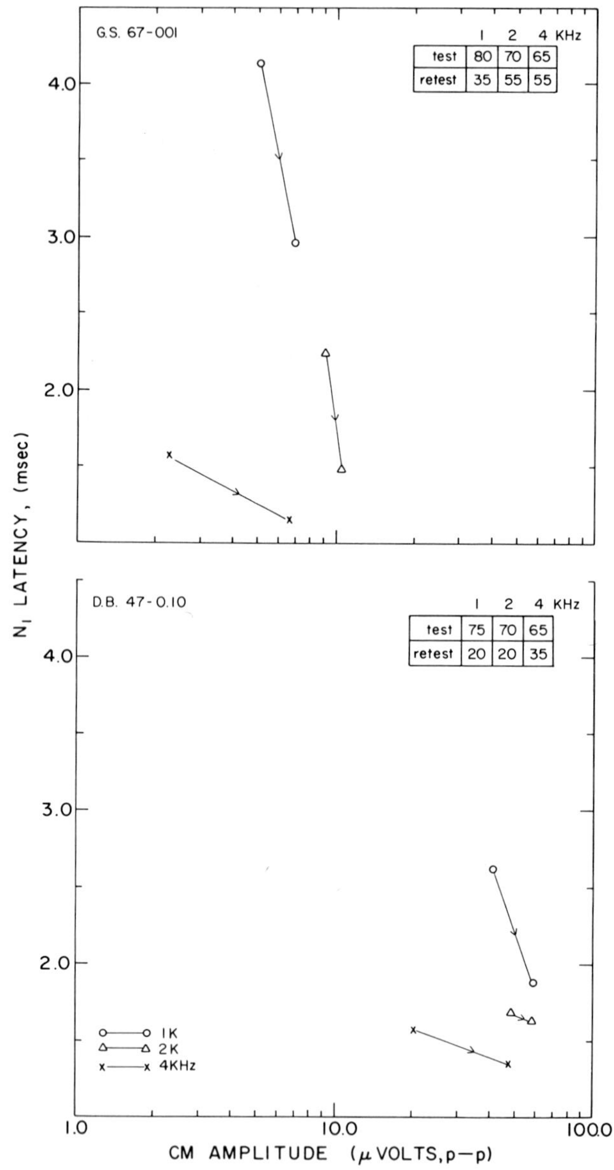

Fig. 5. Relations between CM amplitude and N_1 latency for the two cases showing improved hearing sensitivity from test to retest. (Figures 3 and 4). Note that N_1 latency decreases as CM amplitude increases. See text for relevant discussion.

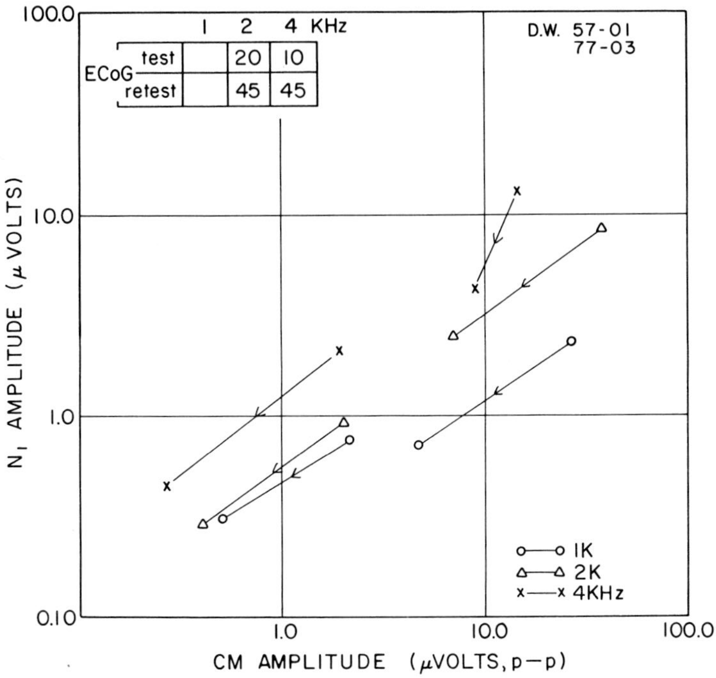

Fig. 6. Relation between CM and AP amplitude for a child with multiple involvements. Same as Figure 3. Note that, as hearing sensitivity declines, CM and AP amplitudes decrease.

between CM amplitude and N_1 latency for the two cases just presented. Here, an increase in CM amplitude and a decrease in N_1 latency is seen. Since N_1 latency would not be affected by changes in electrode resistance, we conclude that our measurements of amplitude reflect real changes in the peripheral system. We turn now to two additional cases showing decreased sensitivity at the time of retest.

Figure 6 shows results for a child, age four years at the time of the original test and re-evaluated two years later. The child was premature, had perinatal episodes of anoxia, and convulsions at an early age. Behavioral test results had initially been inconclusive and ECoG testing was therefore advised. The later test was performed when a subsequent followup was required since the hearing status was again in doubt and conventional testing had again been inconclusive. In this case only, the threshold findings seen in the upper left are the result of ECoG determination. Results at 1000 Hz are not included because of difficulties encountered in estimating ECoG threshold at that frequency. It is clear, at both frequencies and levels, that CM and AP amplitudes have decreased markedly from test to retest.

The results for a 41-year-old patient with Menière's disease are shown in Figure 7. Here the entries at 1, 2, and 4 kHz are again conventional audiometric

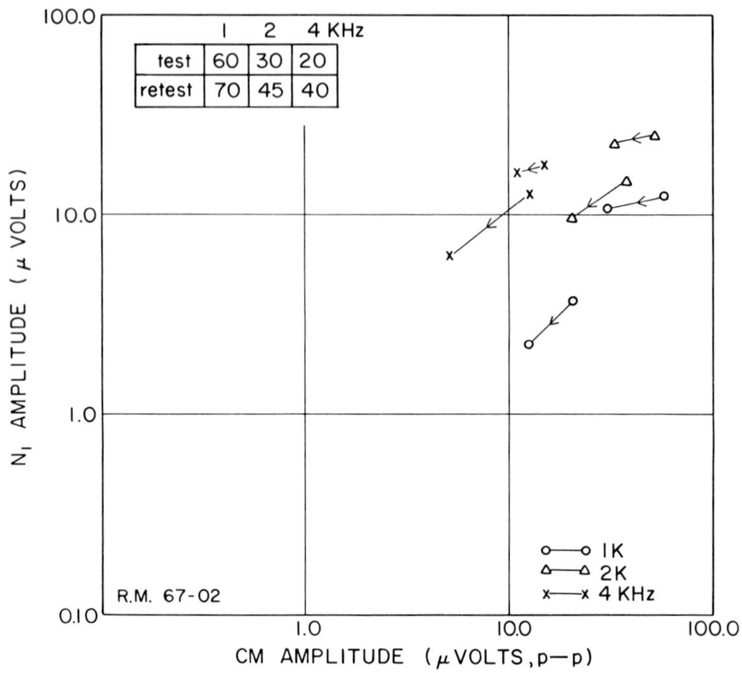

Fig. 7. Relation between CM and AP amplitude for an adult with Meniere's disease. Same as Figure 3. Note that, as hearing sensitivity declines CM and AP amplitudes decrease.

thresholds. Again, for all frequencies and levels, both the CM and the AP show concomitant reductions in amplitude.

Figure 8 illustrates for these two last cases the changes in the N_1 latency that accompany the CM amplitude changes. For both, it is clear that reductions in CM amplitude are related to increases in N_1 latency, again precluding changes in electrode resistance as a possible influence on response amplitude.

DISCUSSION

A number of clinical cases have shown consistent changes among CM amplitude, AP amplitude and AP latency. As auditory sensitivity increases from test to retest, we have seen CM amplitude increase, AP amplitude increase, and AP latency decrease.

As auditory sensitivity decreases, CM amplitude decreases, AP amplitude also decreases and AP latency increases. The relationships are, at this point, qualitative, indicating only the direction of change.

For present purposes, it is not necessary to ask whether the CM is an essential part of the excitatory process or an epiphenomenon instead. The microphonic is known to be intimately related to hair cell function and is a measure of hair cell

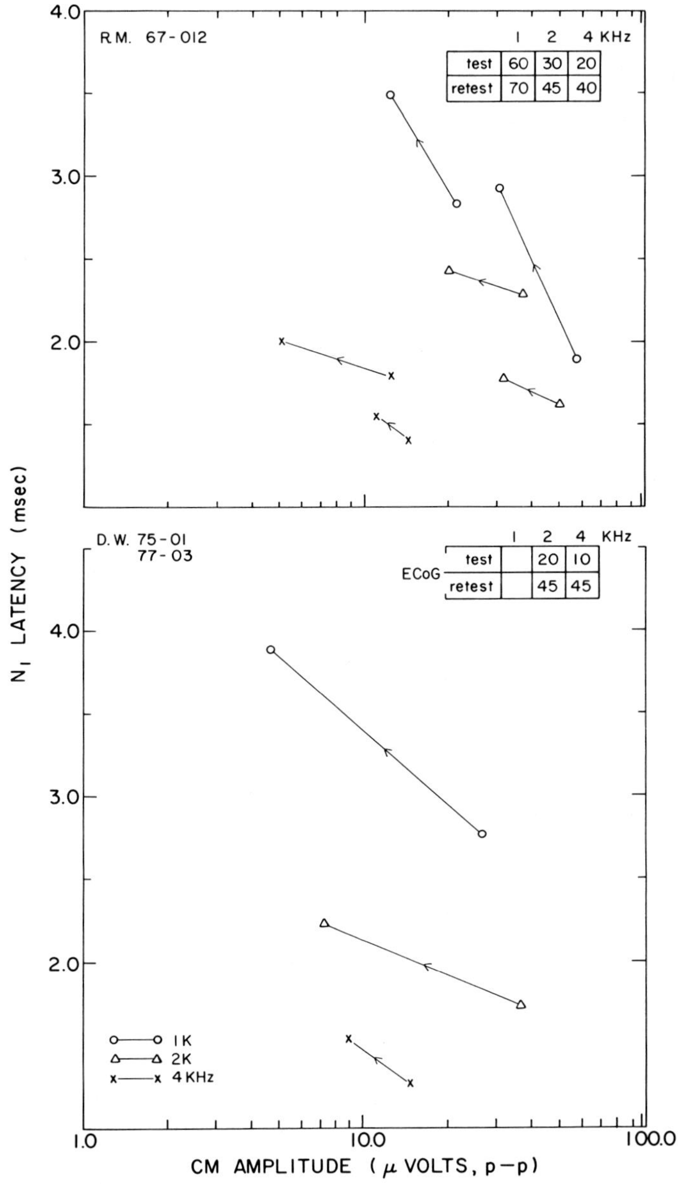

Fig. 8. Relation between CM amplitude and N_1 latency for the two cases showing decreased hearing sensitivity from test to retest (Figures 6 and 7). Note that N_1 latency increases as CM amplitude decreases. See text for relevant discussion.

viability. How good a measure it is of course depends upon the recording technique: differential electrodes sample electrical activity from a quite limited region of hair cells normal to the electrodes, while promontory electrode, such as used in the present study, will record CM most heavily weighted by the segment of basal hair cells nearest the electrode. Additionally, what the electrode "sees" might be further complicated by phase - interactive effects between nearby and more remote regions.

Those caveats notwithstanding, we have demonstrated quite measurable changes in CM amplitude with changes in hearing state, indicating that hair cell activity is related to changes in hearing sensitivity. We have also been able to demonstrate, in retro-cochlear tumors, changes in AP amplitude with changes in click repetition rate; in these cases, CM remained of constant amplitude (unpublished data).

It follows that the techniques of CM extraction outlined here may permit more adequate distinctions to be made between the sensory and the neural components of hearing disorders.

Acknowledgements

This work was supported by DHEW/PHS/NIH grant 5-P50-NS-03358-15.

REFERENCES

Aran, J.-M. and Charlet de Sauvage, R. Clinical value of cochlear microphonic recordings. In: *Electrocochleography,* edited by R.J. Ruben, C. Elberling and G. Salomon. Baltimore: University Park Press, 1976, p. 55-65.

Heike, D. Problems in the interpretation of cochlear microphonic responses. In: *2nd International ERA Symposium,* Milan, 1976, p. 15-25.

Hoke, M. Cochlear microphonics in man and its probable importance in objective audiometry. In: *Electrocochleography,* edited by R.J. Ruben, C. Elberling and G. Salomon. Baltimore: University Park Press, 1976a, p. 41-54.

Hoke, M. Cochlear microphonics: physiological basis and recording technique. In: *2nd International ERA Symposium,* Milan, 1976b, p. 3-14.

Zerlin, S. and Naunton, R.F. Physical and auditory specifications of third octave clicks. *Audiology 14:* 135-143, 1975.

ECoG DIAGNOSIS

ROUND TABLE DISCUSSION

Moderator: F. Blair Simmons

Discussants: J.-M. Aran
H. A. Beagley
J. J. Eggermont
R. F. Naunton
S. Zerlin

Simmons: Would each of you, starting with Dr. Eggermont, give a one-minute capsule of the instrumentation that you use, and including parts and serial numbers if you would like to, and very briefly your reason for picking that kind of system as opposed to some other.

Eggermont: The system we use is not commercially available as a whole. It is built up out of equipment we think is useful in a general setting. We use a Data-Lab DL micro 4 as an averaging system. We have a home-built stimulus generating system including tone burst generator, power amplifier. We use an exponential horn type of loudspeaker (Vitavox GP1), and it is possible with such a system to have very high outputs up to about 115 dB SPL for tones. We use the Princeton Applied Research #113 amplifier and a safety input stage to be sure that accidental damage to the input transistors will not lead to some minor shock. We are not using a commercial type of evoked response equipment.

Beagley: We originally started off with equipment assembled in the lab and used it for a number of years, starting with the V-potential and switching over later to ECoG, and subsequently the last year or two have used commercial equipment, the Amplaid-Medelec system which is very flexible. You can do all the auditory electrophysiological tests you would wish as well as myography, if you just choose the right switches.

There is a tremendous array of possibilities in this system. We use it mostly for ECoG, also brain stem responses. To do this we usually switch the filter setting from 3 Hz - 3 kHz, as used for ECoG, to another setting of 250 Hz - 3 kHz for brain stem responses. You can also alter the sweep time and filter settings to do the V potential. And there are good commercial systems available these days.

ISBN 0-12-514960-3

I must say I am very envious of the system Dr. Eggermont has for producing acoustic stimuli. In fact, we are in the process of copying it and using microprocessors so we can do this numerically. This will give us very good control of stimuli. There is nothing quite like it available commercially at the moment. However the commercial equipment of today is very satisfactory on the whole; for example, and you can do sums and differences simply by moving a switch that will allow you to separate AP and CM during ECoG.

Aran: We have been using different equipment.

Simmons: If you had your choice of all possible systems?

Aran: It depends. It is not so simple. I want to say that most of the data we presented in our papers up to now for human ECoG were obtained with very simple equipment, based mainly on the Princeton Applied Research 100- point averager, which was very convenient for this purpose. Then we got some more sophisticated equipment based on the Histomat S minicomputer. For a few years, I have not been performing electrocochleography myself. The electrocochleograms are made by ENT residents. They used the Amplaid-Medelec equipment, and now they use a smaller and simpler apparatus which is made by a factory in Bordeaux, Racia, and which is the simplest we could design. If I were to do electrocochleography myself again, I would like to use the equipment I dispose of in my experiments, which has to be flexible to allow recordings of either cortical responses or cochleography.

Zerlin: Ours is also a non-commercial setup. I will deal with the sound system first. We use the third octave clicks commercially available backed by a heavy power amplifier. We use a horn driver speaker so we can get to levels of essentially 110 dB SPL if we need it on occasion.

The computer is a Digital equipment, 8L for those of you who like to think about the near-past. We programmed it. It does come with available averaging programs, but it is also very helpful to have someone around who can revise the program for you to get the few bells and whistles that are not provided, such as some of the things we have been talking about: for example to extract both polarities of the microphonic, and that kind of thing.

The preamplifiers we use are also Princeton Applied Research, also safetied with a few resistors at the input to prevent possible damage. It is getting to the point now where some of the modern hardware averagers have incorporated many of the features we put in ourselves for our own satisfaction, so it is not necessary to go the non-commercial route. One can get these things commercially these days, and gain a lot of versatility. We do brain stem testing too, using the same equipment. For this purpose we use shielded earphones, of course. Some are commercially available. We have built our own as well.

Naunton: Stan Zerlin and I work together and are using the same equipment. He omitted mention of one key item, the tape recorder; this enables us to record our test results and to go over them at our leisure later. The other item critical to me as the surgeon, is Stan Zerlin.

Simmons: I have a few prepared questions. I am not sure whether I want to ask this first one or not, after last night's heated discussion, but the Chair will consider statements about the superiority of brain stem responses *out of order* for this particular session.

Anyway, I think this question is worth asking: When is electrocochleography most appropriately used to estimate hearing in children? I assume none of you use it in preference to brain stem potentials or behavioral hearing tests as a routine. Having failed with those two methods, what in general are your decision criteria when to go to cochleography?

Naunton: I indicated in my presentation of yesterday those situations where we would want to use ECoG. First, the infant where there is good reason to suspect a hearing impairment of significant degree, and where it is important to get information about the magnitude of a hearing impairment as early as possible. Second, the older child in whom, for whatever reason, it is proving impossible to get conventional test results.

Simmons: Having failed brain stem audiometry or what-have-you as other tests, when would you consider cochleography for diagnosis of hearing loss? What are the criteria?

Aran: I would say we do it on different occasions, first of all in children where we cannot derive information by any other means.

Simmons: Routine test?

Aran: Not as a routine test. For instance we do cochleography on only about 12% of the children seen in the Audiology Department.

Beagley: Of course one will only use any form of electrophysiologic testing if simple clinical testing is unsuccessful. Simple clinical testing with rattles and squeakers, and so on, can be achieved within a few minutes by a skilled clinician. You do have the occasional untestable child, with multiple handicaps, blindness, various forms of hyperactivity, and so on. For these you may have to resort to some sort of electrophysiological test. We started with the V potential, but dropped it in favor of the test (ECoG) which was developed by my colleague, Dr. Aran, which really cut through the whole problem. You can now diagnose the most difficult child by means of an ECoG, if necessary under anesthesia, -in fact, generally under anesthesia, because for this type of child we find that anesthesia is essential.

As far as brain stem audiometry is concerned I came into this via cochleography, and I am slightly out of step with some of the opinion, perhaps; but what we do is, wherever there is an ECoG carried out on a child which shows any AP response at all, we also do a brain stem response under the same anesthesia (Beagley Discussion Fig. 1). The idea is to get a long-term comparison a year or so after the test with the idea that perhaps we may change our technique. The brain stem may eventually become our first choice, but not just yet.

There is one situation in which I think you can't possibly contemplate brain stem testing, and that is the athetotic cerebral-palsied child. You have to use anesthesia of some sort. Under Ketamine anesthesia muscular movement will smudge a brain stem trace out of recognition; far better to put in a transtympanic needle electrode and really get the information you need. I think you can say we are slowly but very deliberately moving toward brain stem audiometry, but it is also my opinion that ECoG will not be completely displaced from its present important position.

Eggermont: You can use less invasive types of electric response audiometry, and if you don't get results you can go to electrocochleography. We are faced with the problem that the ENT department asks me to deliver an audiogram of a child, and I mean not just an estimate of threshold. At the moment the only way to measure an audiogram in two ears in a child within reasonable time, that is, within one session, two hours or so, is with electrocochleography. That is mainly because of the problem of signal-to-noise ratio. You need many more averages for brain stem responses.

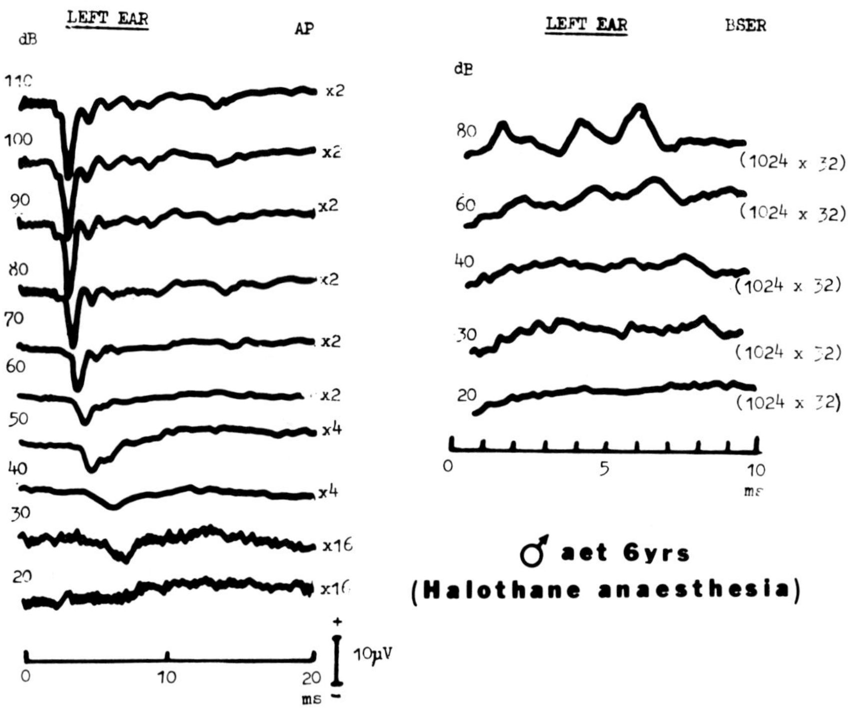

Beagley Discussion Fig. 1. This shows the ECoG (left) and the BSER (right) recorded on the same subject, under general anesthesia, at the same session.

If you have a very young child and you want only an indication that this child has a threshold around 30, 60 or 75 dB or so, I would take brain stem and click stimuli to get an idea of what is going on. If the child of 2 or 3 years old doesn't develop speech, and you want to know what his audiogram is, at the moment I would choose electrocochleography.

The number of children referred to our department is in line with what Dr. Aran said—about 9 to 10 per cent, in those cases we use electrocochleography. It all depends on whether you want to do the audiogram in one session for the child. Then you need electrocochleography. If you say you don't want to use invasive technique but you want to use brain stem potentials, I think you need three or four sessions to get complete audiograms on both ears.

Aran: If I were in charge of physiological testing in children now, when objective audiometry were needed, I would systematically use electrocochleography for thresholds and study of peripheral function, and then brain stem (at least at a high level of stimulation) because in some children cochleography alone is not enough; you might find good peripheral responses but with no hearing, due to brain stem or central disorders. BER should be a systematic procedure in such cases.

Simmons: I have another prepared question which anyone may speak to. I think this panel was intended to be on clinical application.

Other than childhood hearing loss, what other types of hearing loss would you consider as appropriate for clinical development in the sense of research for aid in diagnosis. We have heard, I think, a rather impressive talk on acoustic neuroma. I wonder what the thoughts of the panel are on acoustic neuroma in their own experience. In what other conditions is this a diagnostic technique?

Naunton: May I make an initial comment on this? My attitude where tumor diagnosis is concerned has in the past been that we already have so many ways of making this diagnosis that I wonder whether we need another. Moreover, the type of tumor that is small and limited to the internal meatus is probably rare. Remember, I qualified this by saying that this has hitherto been my approach. However, as I listened to some of the papers that have been presented here, I wonder whether the reason the small tumors are diagnosed so rarely may be the fact that we are not using ECoG to go after them. It may well be that ECoG is of great value in the diagnosis of the small tumors that are difficult to diagnose by other more conventional means short of myelography.

Eggermont: I started to comment why we use electrocochleography for clinical diagnostic tests. It may turn out to be something like Menière's disease. It may turn out to be something not that specific, although you cannot say Menière's disease is specific. It can turn out to be an acoustic neuroma. In our opinion one should always combine electrocochleography and brain stem. Our results with acoustic neuromas so far are that the only consistent finding is that the brain stem response is abnormal. It doesn't point to anything specific; it just says, "Refer this patient to the neurologist and see what he can do".

Cochleography has the advantage that you know what the tumor is doing on the periphery, on the auditory nerve and on the cochlea, and you can compare electrocochleographic findings, as Dr. Beagley said in his paper. That is quite valuable in indicating there might be something present, but I think the ultimate diagnosis for any neurosurgeon would be a myelogram. If he doesn't see there is a tumor he won't operate. That is quite obvious.

We try to use ECoG also in finding an index for chance of recovery from sudden deafness. We have found until now that, when there are normal summating potentials present in ECoG, there is a very good chance that within 2 or 3 months the hearing will return to normal in sudden deafness. When there are no summating potentials present you cannot say that the hearing will not return to an appreciable level, but it is likely that it will not be better than 40 dB in the higher frequencies.

Simmons: I would like to turn the audience loose on the panel and entertain questions from the floor.

Davis: I would like to put a question to the panel for the benefit of those who are considering equipment for ECoG. Do you recommend high pass masking as one of the adjuncts, or do you consider that clicks or tone pips are reasonable substitutes? To me, one of the most impressive generalizations from the slides shown this morning is the close agreement between results with filtered clicks and with derived potentials from high-pass masking.

Eggermont: May I comment on that? I think it depends on what you want. If you want an audiogram, I think the appropriately filtered click or a tone burst which is appropriately shaped is quite reliable. We carried out a study in 100 patients (Spoor, A. and Eggermont, J.J. Electrocochleography as a method for objective audiogram determination. In: *Hearing and Davis,* edited by S.K. Hirsh, D.H. Eldredge, I.J. Hirsh and S.R. Silverman. St. Louis: Washington University Press. 1976, p. 411-418) in whom we had a subjective audiogram and compared it with the thresholds from 500 Hz up to 8 kHz. Correlation coefficients were always high, at least 0.9. In general for 1, 2 and 3 kHz the slope was 1, indicating there was no bias across the threshold densities. At 500 Hz we had a little more problem when we had low subjective threshold levels. At 500 Hz we were always about 10 to 15 dB less sensitive than the audiogram indicated, while at high threshold elevations, 60 dB or so, we tended to be more sensitive than the subjective audiogram, resulting in a slope of about 0.7 for the regression line.

In our group were included a lot of patients with dominantly low frequency hearing loss, and in those cases one overestimates the hearing at low frequencies using this technique because you have the patient's contribution of the more normal basal turn. The point that one has less sensitivity at low levels is mainly due to the fact that the AP is not so well synchronized way out in the apical turn, and you just lose amplitude and detectability. A filtered click or tone burst is quite appropriate.

For neurological purposes I think the click is the obvious thing to use, especially in brain stem recordings.

High pass noise masking is quite a nice toy to play with, and using high pass noise masking of wide band clicks you get the same type of results as with tone bursts.

Simmons: Would anyone on the panel disagree with that? Any other questions?

Thomas: I would like to ask the panel a simplistic question that is fairly practical: Where do you do the ECoG? Do you do them in the clinic or, since as indicated in most of the papers you are using general anesthetics, do you do it in other facilities such as the operating room where support facilities are available to you?

Naunton: We work in a sound-treated, custom-made booth, with support facilities built in (oxygen and vacuum). We tried to do the test in the operating room, largely because it is easier to work there and more children would be available for us for calibration purposes. However, operating rooms are commonly very noisy, electrically, and we ran into severe problems for that reason.

Thomas: What support facilities do you have other than oxygen and vacuum?

Naunton: Nothing, except the equipment that the anesthesiologist wheels in on the standard anesthesiology cart.

Eggermont: I think ECoG is basically a clinical procedure and therefore should be carried out in a room where you have adequate facilities. We use a large soundproof room 6 x 6 meters, and it is fully equipped with anesthesiology equipment.

During the whole test you need an anesthesiologist of course, even, in my opinion, if you use a type of sedation or something like that. You need to have somebody who is adequately capable of supervising the child. I am a physicist, so I cannot decide if a child is doing well; so I am really hesitant to do a brain stem under sedation, because the policy of some departments (at least ours) is that if a child is under sedation it is difficult to get adequate supervision. On the other hand, if you apply anesthesia, you get the best care you can have, so I think in our situation it is even more safe than using sedation.

Thomas: Are your rooms electrically shielded?

Simmons: Let's finish this question first.

Beagley: Perhaps we can encompass the last question as well. In our hospital we have a specially built area which has a pair of IAC booths, the largest 3 x 4 meters (internally), which is about the minimum you need for ECoG under anesthesia. Intrinsically, an IAC booth is moderately well screened, being made of steel and grounded. We don't go to the extreme of using thick copper, but we do take advantage sometimes of the steel lining, and occasionally we throw the external isolator switch if we are in difficulties with electrical interference; this works well. That is probably all you need in the clinical situation. If you need more than that you are getting into the realm of experimental neurophysiology shielding, which is not called for.

In the IAC booth mentioned we have adequate space for proper anesthetic facilities, suction, gases, oxygen and so forth. If you have a skilled anesthesiologist whose job it is to apply himself to the whole problem you should have no difficulties. You don't want people alternating with one another; the anesthesiologist should be a member of the team. We have a very skilled anesthesiologist who makes it part of his job all the time to deal with these cases. In this way we seem to have avoided difficulties. We have a recovery area for three children adjacent to the booths. This system, which I think is the minimum that you should have, works very satisfactorily.

Aran: It is interesting that we all use approximately the same set-up: a soundproof room, anesthesiologists, and so on.

Simmons: All except the panel chairman. I think it is a matter really of logistics, but we find it very difficult to get an anesthesiologist down to the operating room. We find it is hard to do in the operating room. It is a matter of hunting around. We take a high-quality 2-channel audiocasette tape recorder and oscilloscope monitor plus a couple of portable amplifiers, and that is the system. We do our analysis basically off line and find no problem in doing it in that other fashion, either.

Naunton: An additional item we use is a television monitor so we can observe the child during the test. We also provide the anesthesiologist with ear-muffs, not because we really think his or her ears are in danger, but because it makes them feel much better.

Unidentified voice from the audience: I presently have a 10-month-old in my clinic where brain stem testing indicated moderate hearing loss; and I am wondering what the next step should be. The parents report that the child was unable to go under anesthesia in the past. I wonder if you have come across that problem?

Eggermont: The only comment I might make is that we never do electro-cochleography before a child is 6 to 9 months old. Before that time I think it is easier to do brain stem without sedation, I do not think it is a necessity to have a detailed audiogram before a child is 1-½ years old. You must have a reasonable indication of the amount of hearing loss. So, I would more or less suggest to repeat brain stem audiometry. The problem with electrocochleography is actually the anesthesia. You must basically have a healthy child to do an anesthesiology procedure for diagnostic reasons. It is not for treatment but for diagnosis, and that makes it a little more difficult. I am sorry that I cannot give you any distinctive answer.

Beagley: Although electrocochleography is for diagnosis and not for treatment, it is often necessary to give an anesthetic to sort the problem out, and this you must do. Concerning the child who was reported as creating an emergency under anesthesia, you must look carefully into that. What if the child develops acute appendicitis or similar problems? Are you going to say, "Don't operate on him because he once gave trouble under anesthetic"? It is best to check up first. If the anesthesiologist is faced with a problem of this kind, he has to sort the matter out in a calm fashion. If there really is a contraindication it must be pretty rare; but if there is, that's it. I think on many occasions the matter can be approached a second time with perfect safety, especially if forewarned. Forewarned is forearmed in this situation.

Rapin: Why, in the child described as premature, is it necessary to do cochleography? I think one can get the information one needs to decide if a particular child needs amplification on the basis of the brain stem data plus, if one wants to know about the low frequencies, one can quite easily obtain this information from the late potentials. We find we can test most of the very severely handicapped children referred to us with sedation, without the need for an anesthetic, without the need for an anesthesiologist, and with no problem. We simply have the mother stay with the infant and we monitor his EEG.

Simmons: I must warn you if this gets to be a brain stem session I am going to stop the questions in midair.

Starr: Who can do electrocochleography? Do you have to be an otorhinolaryngologist? Can you be a general physician, skilled neurophysiologist, or a technician? What is the medicolegal implication of inserting an electrode through the tympanic membrane?

Naunton: In this country it would have to be, as the phrase goes, "a physician licensed to practice medicine in all its branches"; in other words, not necessarily a specialist.

Eggermont: In our clinic the ENT specialist places the needle and waits until the first response appears, to be sure it is in the right position.

Berlin: I would like to ask a question of the panel pertinent to high frequency hearing losses and the latency of N_1. Most of the literature, in our experience, indicates that as long as the loss is not total the N_1 latency usually remains quite normal. There has been some literature in brain stem studies suggesting that the N_5 latency and N_1 latency will be shifted in high frequency hearing losses among children or a presumed high frequency loss among neonates.

Then there is the question of N_5 latency shifts in the presence of tumors vs a high frequency hearing loss. Will the panel address itself to the question of latency shifts and when they occur in electrocochleography? Maybe this afternoon we will be able to raise the question in BSER.

Aran: It is difficult to discuss latency shifts while using the clicks, because latency depends on the area of the basilar membrane which contributes to the response to the click. If you want to study latency you have to use filtered clicks or pips or high pass masking. Then you know more precisely where you are on the basilar membrane. With a click it is very difficult. You can be confused by conduction loss or high frequency hearing loss. Using high frequency pips there should be no problem.

Wiederhold: Does anybody have any information on whether these shape changes you see in the transtympanically recorded N_1 in different pathological situations can be seen from ear canal recordings?

Eggermont: I think sometimes you see them in brain stem recording. If you record from the ear canal the summating potential is attenuated with respect to the AP. That may change shape in Menière's disease, for instance, but as far as I know even in brain stem recordings in acoustic tumors, you see the widening of the first peak instead of the normal diphasic type of thing. I think it is not strictly related to the place of the recording.

Thornton: I would like to ask the panel for their results and their opinions regarding differential diagnosis with acoustic neuromata. In your paper, Harry, you showed several clear-cut results. You seemed to be implying that these were consistent with the idea of a monophasic unit response with acoustic neuromata. I would like to ask how often the panel thinks this actually occurs.

With regard to your point about computerized tomography in comparing the accuracy of your results. As you know, Andrew Morrison in London has been working up a series, and he has reported tumors up to 3 cm that have been missed by computerized tomography. I would like any evidence the panel has on data like that, on the sizes of tumors that have been missed, and how electrocochleography really relates to other diagnostic techniques with this pathology.

Beagley: Practically all of these cases that I discussed were Andrew Morrison's, and it is true that CT does sometimes miss a tumor as big as 3 cm. In fact I have heard of a 4 cm one being missed. It is a fairly new technique. The problem of course is that if you have a tumor within the internal meatus, you shouldn't expect too much from CT, but is is a very valuable and remarkable technological achievement and has transformed neurological diagnosis.

As far as the monophasic widened response is concerned, I am sure that is at the root of the AP changes of the early neuromas. The experimental evidence is in favor of this (Beagley, H.A., Legouix, J.P., Teas, D.C. and Redmond, M.C. Electrocochleographic changes in acoustic neuroma: some experimental findings. *Clinical Otolaryngology 2:* 213-219, 1977). When a tumor is present one would like to be able to demonstrate this monophasic response in all cases. We put our hopes in Eggermont's method of successive high-pass masking.

The problem is, that it is sometimes a little difficult to achieve because "Nature's experiments" often present a mixed picture. You don't always get a very clear change due to a specific lesion. There are usually several things happening at once. I certainly like to have high-pass masking available in the hopes of being able to confirm the monophasic responses, which should be very helpful in differentiating acoustic neuroma from unilateral Menière's disease. But there are many other cases of neuroma where the destruction and damage has gone beyond the stage of the simple monophasic response, in which case you have to consider the other criteria.

Marcus: I am bothered by the thought that in using electrocochleography alone in children, and especially in those who are markedly retarded or who have some other kind of brain problem, the peripheral organ may be found to be normal but the hearing apparatus as such would be nonfunctional. I saw a movie by Dr. Viet some time ago, of a newborn with cerebral agenesis, subsequently shown at post mortem, who gave all the auditory responses one would suspect. Of course this child had no brain to use it with.

Beagley: Dr. Marcus, I wonder just what difficulty this causes in dealing with children who have not developed speech. Apart from the case you mention of cerebral agenesis, which is an extreme situation, I agree that confirming peripheral hearing may not be the end of your difficulties. The child may still have a central lesion preventing the development of speech. But the reverse situation is quite definite - no peripheral hearing means no input, and therefore deafness. Electrocochleography will allow the clinician to direct his rehabilitative efforts in the appropriate direction.

Marcus: The situation of these children, whether or not they are institutionalized, is that some appear to function as deaf children. To say that normal electrophysiologic responses represent normal auditory may cause considerable confusion for otologist, neurologists, audiologist, teachers of the deaf, and parents, because it does not resolve the clinical problem. The relationship of neuronal activity in the auditory apparatus to observed auditory behavior remains unclear. We should avoid reporting results of electrocochleography that equate the findings with conventional audiometry.

Beagley: I agree.

Naunton: Our uniform practice in reporting ECoGs, if we have no other information available than the ECoG, is to stress the fact that we are only talking about the peripheral organ and the first-order neuron.

Simmons: I have a question pertinent to individuals who may be getting into the business of cochleography. After having established equipment and run it on experimental animals, what would the panel consider important in setting up standards as to what is normal and what is abnormal? What kind of a normal hearing population (if that is the appropriate way to start) would be a bare minimum, and what kinds of variation can they expect?

Eggermont: I will tell you how we started. It depends on whether you have volunteers from a normal population. We didn't have volunteers, so we had to wait for several years until we had a reasonably large normal group. We had a few test cases to start with. They were children having middle ear problems and in which ventilation tubes had to be placed. That was a surgical procedure, before the insertion of the ventilation tube we placed the needle, and measured the threshold. We generally had a behavioral threshold that was quite reliable, so we could make our calibrations.

It depends from clinic to clinic, we see a lot of children where these tubes are placed and it takes a few weeks to get a reasonable population of mild-to-moderate hearing losses so that one can test the equipment. It will be different for other groups. It just depends on the situation. It is preferable to start with a group of normal hearing volunteers. You can also ask them, "Do you still hear this sound," or something like that to have a comparison of ECoG and subjective thresholds.

Beagley: A good solution would be to use a "population" of people with dry tympanic perforations which are often available around an ENT hospital. These people have hearing, but with conductive losses of varying degrees, and perhaps you can start off with these. The other group from which I got a lot of information was the group of patients with an acoustic neuroma in one ear where the opposite ear is used as a control, and it was in most cases pretty normal. Of course the use of normal volunteers would be perfect, but that is not always feasible.

Zerlin: One comment concerning stimuli. The fact that we all tend to use somewhat the same stimuli gives us quite comparable results. I think we all use stimuli that rise to maximum in 2, 3 or 4 cycles. As far as I can see from the data, there is little discrepancy in the latency of the responses we get. You can always use the microphonic as the starting point if you want to.

Simmons: I would like to put forth a suggestion that a normal volunteer population is quite easy to get without paying, simply by asking the clinicians themselves and other people involved in hearing testing in the facility to volunteer their own ears for this innocuous technique.

Naunton: I would go along with that, except that I would have awful trouble passing that needle through my drum, and I would not let anybody else do it.

Moore: In our clinical experience we have had a number of normal hearing subjects who do not give the classical brain stem response. Has any member of the panel tested individuals by ECoG and failed to obtain an N_1 response where hearing was normal?

Eggermont: In our group of reasonably normal hearing people we studied a large group of Menière's patients and I think you can consider them as representative for normals; we never found absence of AP. There may be differences in amplitude up to a factor of 20, maybe. In some cases, I don't know what the reason is, they just show 1μV output at 90 dB HL, but you might also run into an occasion with 50 microvolts at the same point. Maybe different states of the middle ear mucosa cause different types of shunt resistance from the promontory to the ear lobe or mastoid. I don't have experience with brain stem in that regard. In cochleography I have never seen a normal case without a response. We found sometimes thresholds in normal populations elevated by about 25 dB, which is actually a little bit too high, but that is the case where you have very small amplitudes.

Unidentified voice from the audience: Apart from pathology, can you factor out an effective age?

Zerlin: We have begun some quasi-systematic studies on that, as shown by the slides we presented on latency norms, and it is merely qualitative. We have been unable to show any systematic latency difference in our age span. We have data from children a few months old up to 10 or 12 years of age, and at this point I don't see anything systematic over that range.

Witter: Have you been able to differentiate in any of your recordings the inner hair cell versus outer hair cell loss with any of the–

Zerlin: Come back next year.

Simmons: I have one final question which I would like some numbers on rather than opinions. In terms of small children who do not have a previous audiogram, unable to get an audiogram–and this is the reason for cochleography–let's say a one-year-old child–when you do obtain an audiogram at age 3, and so on, what is your approximate hit rate in terms of predicting what that threshold will be?

Eggermont: We carried out a long-term study in which we compared the cochleogram obtained at age 6 months to 1-½ years. It depended on the type of audiogram. We were quite accurate in the case where there was a severe hearing loss, more than 80 dB. Then the cochleogram was always confirmed by the subjective audiogram later on. When there was a hearing loss at 60 dB cochleographically, in all but four cases out of fifty it was accurate. In those four cases the subjective audiogram was much better than the cochleogram. The only consistent finding was that all these children had a hearing loss due to kernicterus. They showed definitely reliable subjective audiograms later on.

When we retested one of those children after obtaining the subjective audiogram we got the same results as before. It just didn't work in this case. In the mild types of hearing loss we were sometimes overestimating the audiogram by ECoG, but I think we were about 90 per cent correct that it was within 15 dB of the ultimate audiogram. In the adults we had varying differences up to 30 dB, but 95% was within 20 dB.

Beagley: I would say broadly that is the case. The biggest surprise that I had was in a case in which there was a reverse J-shaped audiogram; a tremendous high tone drop at 1000 Hz from about 20 dB down to over 90 dB, and I got no response from the wide-band click in this case, and diagnosed considerable hearing loss. The child was fitted with an aid and this proved to be quite a sensible thing to have done. The next time we saw him, in a few months' time, he was beginning to speak quite a lot. This surprised me, so much so we repeated the cochleogram; once again I could see only a small, minimal response to wide-band click. We followed him up and eventually got the audiogram I spoke of.

I think this is the sort of case where you are going to have difficulties. Judicious use of filtered clicks will probably keep you on the right track. The problem, of course, is not that you may incorrectly diagnose hearing loss, - that is a relatively innocuous thing to do. The really bad thing is to *miss* a hearing loss and declare that the child is not deaf. I think it is desperately unfortunate to say a child hears normally, and later to find that he has, in fact, a substantial hearing loss. A lot of valuable rehabilitation time will have been wasted.

Deuel: Has anyone had the opportunity to use ECoG on comatose patients? If so, is there any difference between findings in comatose patients and what you would expect in normal awake, or normal but anesthetized patients?

Simmons: I gather not.

McCormick: Has anyone done studies with these techniques, either brain stem or the end organ, in stroke patients?

Simmons: We drew another negative.

Naunton: Early in our experience with BSER testing we tested three patients, all of whom had had strokes; latencies were normal in all three. We were not, at that point, as skilled in doing brain stem testing as we are now.

Berlin: We did two patients by BSER who had normal cochleograms but abnormal BSER's. The question was directed to relative procedures. A patient like that would appear to be without auditory function by brain stem recording, but with clear-cut auditory function from electrocochleography; the behavioral audiogram went along with the brain stem, not the cochleography. The patient made no behavioral response to sound.

INNER EAR PROSTHESES

Moderator: *Nelson Y. S. Kiang*

THE ACOUSTIC GANGLION IN PROFOUND SENSORINEURAL DEAFNESS

John R. Lindsay and Raul Hinojosa

University of Chicago

The guidelines recommended for the evaluation of cochlear implantation in man in the published proceedings of the first International Conference on electrical stimulation of the acoustic nerve are intended apparently to prevent a false positive interpretation of the effect of the implant. The possibility that a negative response to stimulation with the implant may be falsely interpreted because of absence of viable ganglion cells and nerves in the cochlea is also an essential consideration. The degree of degeneration and its distribution within the cochlea which may be predicted on the basis of known pathological states may influence both the method of implantation and the probability of sufficient neural elements surviving to permit useful stimulation. A review of the pathological state of the acoustic ganglion and nerve in those cases of profound deafness that have been examined in the various laboratories therefore becomes of primary significance in the selection of cases for evaluation of cochlear implants.

The observations on the state of the spiral ganglion to be described here, were made in a series of selected cases; the cases were chosen to demonstrate the condition of the acoustic ganglion in the presence of deafness that had been shown to be profound in both ears to the degree indicated by hearing tests for the duration of one or more years.

Cases of congenital deafness in the young and in children in whom normal speech had not developed are considered unsuitable for evaluation of cochlear implantation at the present stage of investigation. However, since the heredo-degenerative Scheibe type of degeneration may *eventually* warrant consideration for an implant one such adult case is included in this series.

The cases chosen for demonstration of ganglion degeneration include also the following disorders: bacterial labyrinthitis, viral labyrinthitis, head trauma, drug ototoxicity, presbycusis, otosclerosis, the Kearns-Sayre Syndrome and one adult case with the Scheibe type of degeneration.

METHOD

The organ of Corti was reconstructed in each case presented according to the method of Guild (1921, 1931) as modified by Schucknecht (1953). The recon-

ISBN 0-12-514960-3

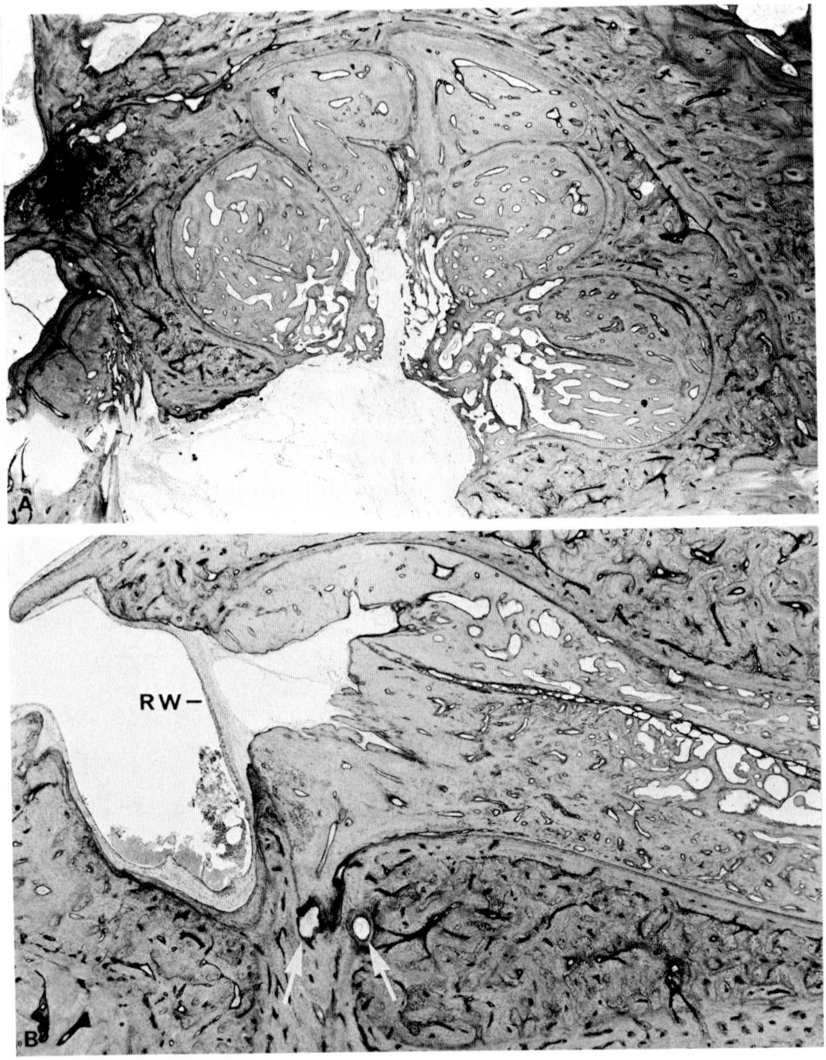

Fig. 1. Case M.K. Age 43 years. Bacterial labyrinthitis, meningogenic. Left ear.
A. All soft tissue of the cochlea has been destroyed by the inflammatory process and has been replaced by bone. Hematoxylineosin stain. x11.
B. The basal coil is almost filled by new bone down to the round window membrane (RW). The cochlear aqueduct and the channel for the inferior cochlear vein (arrows) are not ossified. Hematoxylineosin stain. x17.

struction of the organ of Corti was made in histological preparations of human temporal bones consisting of horizontal sections cut at 20μ with every tenth section stained with hematoxylin-eosin.

The method used for the reconstruction of the spiral ganglion was a modification (Otte, 1968) of that described by Guild (1931) and Schuknecht (1953). The organ of Corti of the basal turn was the reference point to reconstruct the basal turn of the spiral ganglion. The distance between the organ of Corti and the internal and external borders of the spiral ganglion itself were measured. The borders of the Rosenthal's canal were not used in this case. The second and third turns of the spiral ganglion were measured from the borders of the spiral ganglion of the first turn and not from the organ of Corti.

All ganglion cells which showed a nucleolus were counted in each tenth section. A correction factor of 0.95 was used for doubly counted nucleoli. The number of cells in each section was then recorded in the outline of the spiral ganglion in their corresponding place.

The spiral ganglion was divided into 6 areas. Each area corresponded to 5 mm on the outline of the organ of Corti with the exception of the last area which corresponds to the rest of the length of the organ of Corti after 25 mm. The numbers of ganglion cells counted in each 5 mm area were added and multiplied by 10 to obtain the total number of ganglion cells in that particular area. A similar procedure was used to obtain the total number of ganglion cells in each of 5 normal human temporal bones used as controls, the average of these normal bones being used a base for comparison in each case studied.

Bacterial Labyrinthitis

Profound bilateral deafness due to labyrinthitis of bacterial origin was most commonly due to the meningoccus in the pre-antibiotic era. Survivors of meningococcal meningitis were frequently deafened by extension of the infection into both labyrinths. Observations of fatal cases which terminated in the acute stages of bacterial meningitis indicate that extension of infection from the meninges to the inner ear had occurred both through the modiolus and the cochlear aqueduct (Perlman and Lindsay, 1939; Matz et al., 1968); hence, extensive invasion of the acoustic ganglion was a common characteristic in these early stages of meningogenic invasion. When examined in the late or healed stage of bacterial labyrinthitis the degree of destruction of inner ear structures has varied from total loss with replacement by bone (Fig. 1a, 1b) to incomplete degeneration of the acoustic ganglion and partial obliteration of labyrinthine spaces by fibrosis and new bone (Fig. 2b and 2c). A common characteristic of healed cases of bacterial labyrinthitis has been the deposition of new bone in the scala tympani adjoining the round window membrane with varying degrees of obstruction of the lower turn of the basal coil (Suga and Lindsay, 1977).

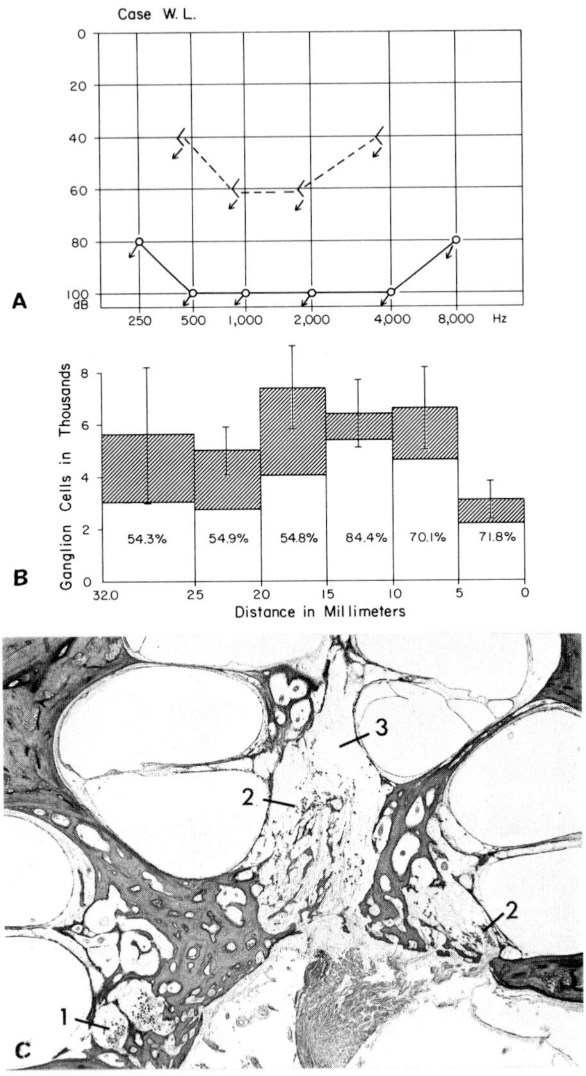

Fig. 2. Case W.L. Age 52 years. Bacterial labyrinthitis, meningogenic. Right ear.
A. Audiogram shows no response for air or bone conducted sound. The frequencies on the audiogram correspond to the positions indicated immediately below on the histogram.
B. The histogram represents the ganglion cells counted in each six 5mm areas along the organ of Corti from the base to the apex of the cochlea.

The normal average of ganglion cells counted in each 5mm area is represented by the height of the etched area plus the clear area at its base. The average normal number of ganglion cells is expressed in thousands along the left margin. The standard deviation in each area is indicated by the vertical marker in each section. The number of surviving ganglion cells is indicated

Viral Meningogenic Labyrinthitis

Profound deafness has occasionally occurred as a complication of meningo-encephalitis due to viral infection. Either unilateral or bilateral profound deafness has been produced. The type of virus has not always been identified. Evaluation of the effect of the virus on the acoustic ganglion requires a sufficient time interval to allow for degeneration. A characteristic of meningogenic invasion by the virus appears to be the development of an endolymphatic hydrops along with degeneration of the acoustic ganglion due to its direct exposure to the invading infection (Cohn et al., 1970) (Figs. 3b and 3c).

The possibilities of adequate stimulation of the auditory system by means of a cochlear implant in this type of deafness is likely to be limited because of this form of degeneration.

Viral Endolymphatic Labyrinthitis

Viral labyrinthitis, limited primarily and mainly to the endolymphatic system, has been observed to cause degenerative or destructive changes primarily in the endolymphatic system, along with a tendency to reduction in volume of endolymph in the cochlear duct and saccule. The ganglion cells, as observed in certain instances (Lindsay et al., 1960) after a time lapse of over one year, tend to show a variable but moderate reduction in numbers mainly in the basal coil. There has been progressively less reduction, approaching a normal quota, in the upper middle and apical coils (Figs, 4b and 4c). Formation of new bone in the perilymphatic space bordering the round window has not been characteristic of this type of infection.

A cochlear implant that would permit stimulation of ganglion cells in the middle and apical coils might be suitable for trial in such instances.

Head Trauma

Profound bilateral deafness has resulted from severe head trauma in certain instances without demonstrable fracture of the temporal bone (Lindsay and Zajtchuk, 1970) either by X-ray or post-mortem examination. Diffuse extensive hemorrhage into the inner ear has been observed in this type of case in which the injury had been fatal. Unilateral total deafness has usually been found after trans-

in percentage by the clear area at the base of each 5mm section. The basal coil is represented approximately by the three 5mm areas from right to left. The middle coil by the fourth and fifth 5mm areas and the apical coil by the last area on the left.

C. Mid-modiolar section showing the ganglion cells in upper basal (1) middle (2) and lower apical (3) coils. Hematoxylin-eosin. x17.

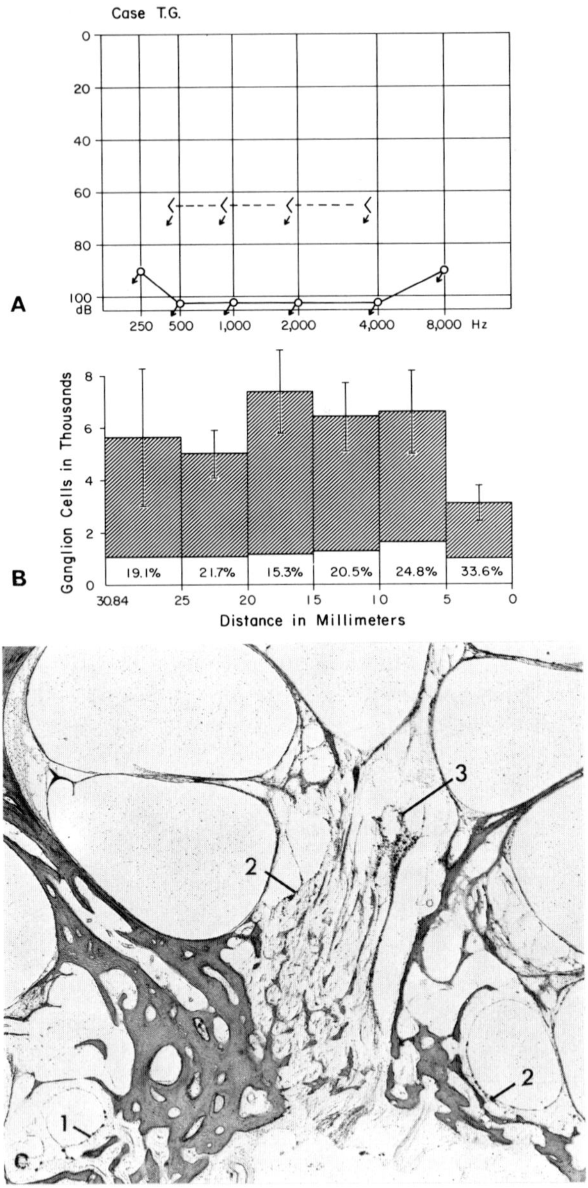

Fig. 3. Case T.G. Age 73 years. Viral labyrinthitis, meningogenic. Right ear.

A. The audiogram shows no response for air or bone conducted sound.

B. The percentage of ganglion cells remaining is indicated in each of the 5mm regions along the organ of Corti.

C. Mid-modiolar section showing the ganglion cells in upper basal (1), middle (2), and lower apical (3) coils. Hematoxylin-eosin. x24.

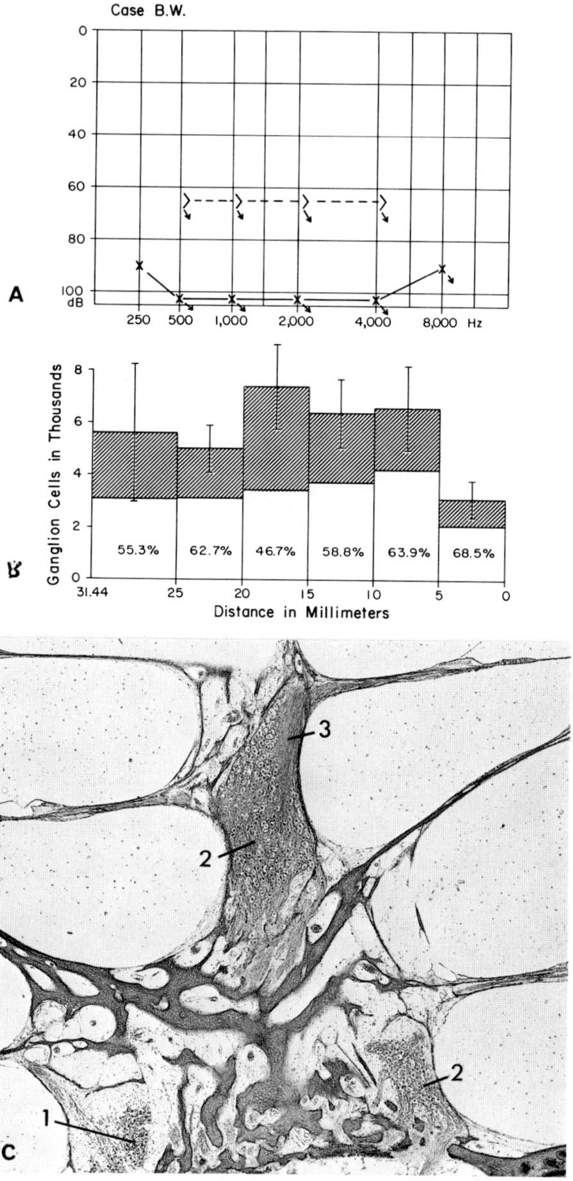

Fig. 4. Case B.W. Age 6 years. Viral endolymphatic labyrinthitis. Left ear.

A. The audiogram shows response at 90 dB at 250 Hz.

B. The ganglion cells counted show a relatively high percentage of ganglion cells remaining in all regions of the cochlea.

C. Mid-modiolar section showing the ganglion cells in upper basal (1) middle (2) and lower apical (3) coils. Hematoxylin-eosin. x24.

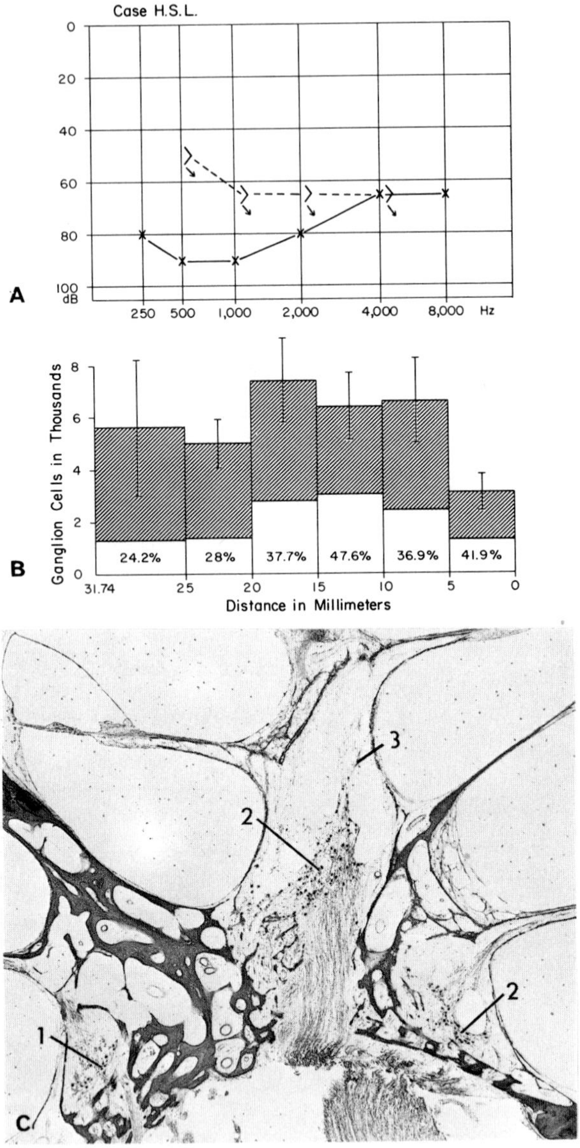

Fig. 5. Case H.S.L. Age 80 years. Head trauma. Left ear.

A. The audiogram shows no response above the 80 dB level in the speech range.

B. The percentage of ganglion cells shows fairly close correspondence to the audiogram

C. Mid-modiolar section showing the ganglion cells in upper basal (1) middle (2) and lower apical (3) coils. Hematoxylin-eosin.

verse fracture of the temporal bone when the fracture gap has opened sufficiently to be made visible on examination by X-ray. A combination of unilateral profound deafness due to demonstrable transverse fracture with sub-total deafness in the opposite ear without demonstrable fracture has sometimes occurred. In such instances partial recovery may occur in the ear in which the deafness had been incomplete and was presumably due to hemorrhage. In the absence of any recovery of hearing in either ear the question of the condition of the spiral ganglion may be worthy of consideration.

Transverse fractures of the temporal bone usually have been observed to create an open fistulous tract, from the middle ear into the inner ear, lined by middle ear epithelium. Any middle ear infection may then extend directly into the remaining labyrinthine spaces usually with extension directly to the meninges. Clinically, a complete labyrinthectomy may be required in certain instances as a preventative of rapidly developing meningitis, the hazard to life consequent upon middle ear infection being the primary consideration in such cases.

The state of the acoustic ganglion in a case of bilateral profound deafness without a transverse fracture of the pyramid is demonstrated by Figures 5a, 5b, and 5c. In this instance the degeneration of the ganglion corresponds fairly closely to the degeneration of the sensory elements.

Deafness Due to Ototoxic Drugs

The degeneration of spiral ganglion cells due to ingestion of an ototoxic drug in animal experiments has been found to require several weeks to reach full development. Most human inner ears deafened by ototoxic drugs have been examined in the acute stages of infection before degeneration of the ganglion has fully developed.

One instance in which the subject survived for 20 months after development of deafness following ingestion of an ototoxic drug is demonstrated in Figures 6a, 6b, and 6c. Deafness was moderate for tones in the lower speech range, but profound or sub-total for frequencies above 1000 Hz. Degeneration of the organ of Corti was total throughout the lower three-fourths of the basal coil, extending to a lesser degree up into the lower middle coil. The ganglion cells were greatly depleted in the lower two-thirds of the basal coil, slightly decreased in the lower middle and to a lesser extent in the upper coil. The stria vascularis was present in all coils. Degeneration of the ganglion cells was fairly marked in those areas with total loss of the organ of Corti (Fig. 6b). The specific antibiotic used in this case could not be established.

Presbycusis

Progressive sensorineural hearing impairment, beginning in middle life or later, forms the most common type of impairment to be observed in late adult years. Evidence of an autosomal dominant type of heredity with variable expressivity can frequently be traced in these cases. Profound bilateral deafness for all

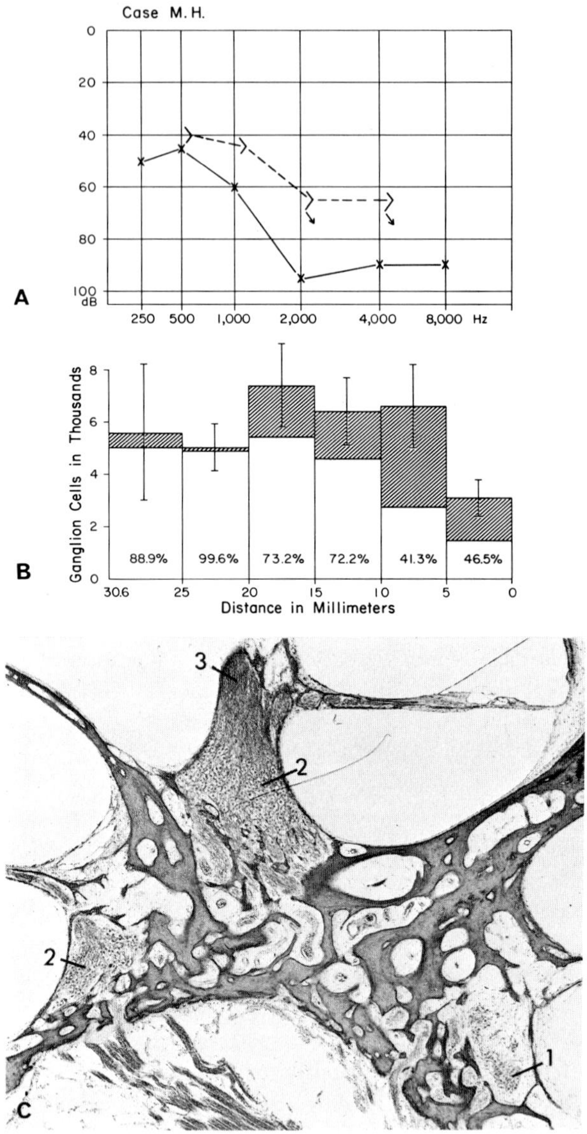

Fig. 6. Case M.H. Age 10 years. Left ear. Hearing level recorded after ingestion of ototoxic drug following surgery. Death 20 months later.

A. The audiogram shows profound deafness for tones 2000 Hz and up. Moderately severe deafness for lower tones.

B. The histogram shows loss of ganglion cells corresponding to the loss of hearing for high tones. The organ of Corti was totally absent in the lower three fourths of the basal coil.

C. Mid-modiolar section showing the ganglion cells in upper basal (1) middle (2) and lower apical (3) coils. Hematoxylin-eosin. x26.

speech frequencies has been observed in this group in a relatively small percentage, usually in those surviving well beyond the average age of termination.

Several detailed studies, including the state of the ganglion cells, have been reported. The most consistent pathological finding in a series of cases reported from this laboratory (Suga and Lindsay, 1976) has been the degree and extent of degeneration of the acoustic ganglion (Figs. 7a, 7b, 7c). The state of degeneration of the ganglion that must be anticipated in profound deafness of this type has tended to be proportionate to the degree of impairment of hearing but not to the same advanced stage.

Otosclerosis

Although otosclerosis varies greatly in the extent of its development in adult life, two general types may be distinguished on the basis of its distribution within the otic capsule (Lindsay, 1973). In one type the otosclerosis is limited to a focus at one or more of the areas of predilection which are at the windows and, less frequently, at the internal meatus. In some instances this type may, in the advanced decades of life become associated with progressive degeneration of the acoustic ganglion, more or less diffuse in all coils (Figs. 8a, 8b and 8c). The degeneration of the ganglion corresponds closely to that observed in the type of presbycusis characterized by threshold loss for all tones (Suga and Lindsay, 1976). Whether the degeneration of the ganglion associated with this type of otosclerosis has any etiologic relationship to otosclerosis is uncertain.

The second and more active type of otosclerosis is that which shows multiple foci in both cochlear and vestibular parts of the otic capsule. Fixation of the stapes with impairment of sound conduction occurs in the early stages of this type; but with expansion of the multiple foci in the cochlear capsule and promontory the otosclerotic process tends to fuse and to occupy the major portion of the endochondral and endosteal layers of the cochlear capsule and promontory (Figs. 9a, 9b, and 9c). Sensorineural impairment of hearing becomes superimposed on impairment of conduction of sound. Degeneration of the spiral ganglion progresses from the basal region to the upper coils along with degeneration of the saccular macula in late decades of life in this type.

In five ears with this type of advanced otosclerosis the scala tympani in the round window region was filled by new bone (labyrinthitis ossificans) into which the otosclerotic process has shown beginning invasion (Fig. 10). The state of the spiral ganglion has varied in the three cases of this advanced type in our collection. One case showed extreme degeneration of ganglion cells in the basal and lower middle coils, the other two showing extreme ganglion degeneration in all coils of the cochlea along with degenerative changes in the saccule. One case showed marked constriction of vascular spaces by new bone in the modiolus along with extreme thickening of the walls of arteries in the fundus of the meatus. An impressive feature of far advanced and diffuse otosclerosis in the cochlear capsule in this latter case has been a generalized diffuse encroachment of the otosclerotic walls of

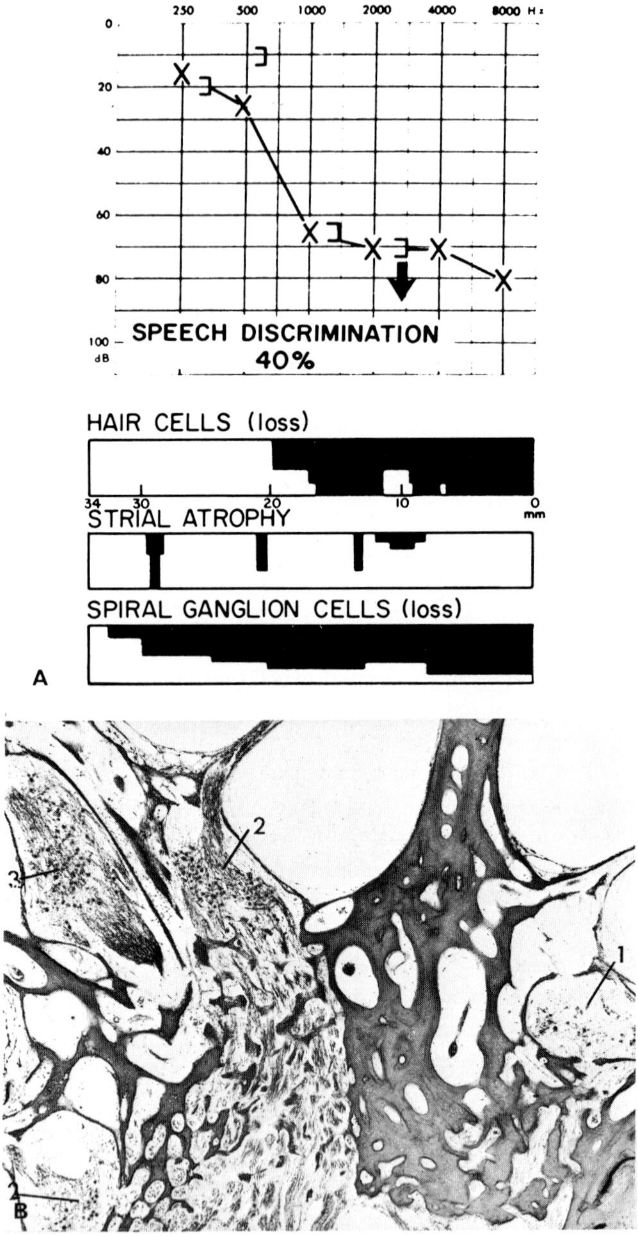

Fig. 7. Case J.S. Age 76 years. Presbycusis. Left ear.
A. Audiogram and hair cell loss (Published by Suga, F. and Lindsay, J.R. 1976). Severe hearing impairment at the 1000 Hz and above. Corresponding ganglion cell loss is indicated.
B. Mid-modiolar section showing the ganglion cells in upper basal (1) middle (2) and lower apical (3) coils. Hematoxylin-eosin. x25.

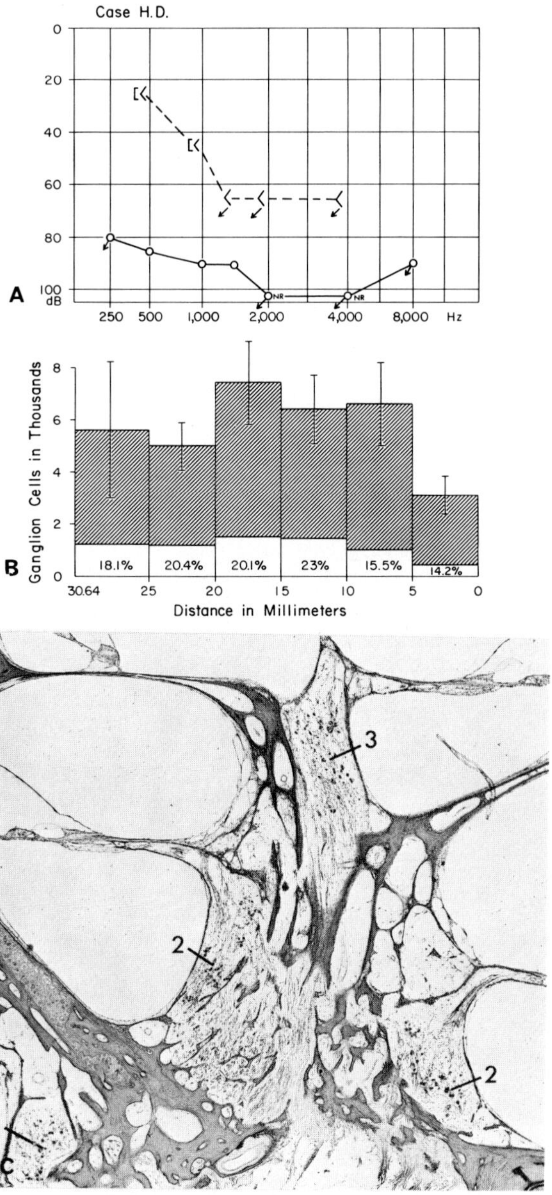

Fig. 8. Case H.D. Age 92 years. Otosclerosis with fixation of the stapedial footplate. Right ear.

A. This figure represents the audiogram made following stapedectomy 10 years before death. Deafness was reported to have become profound in the final years.

B. The acoustic ganglion showed an extreme degree of diffuse degeneration throughout all areas as demonstrated by the histogram. The otosclerosis in this case was limited to the region of the stapes and small area of the round window margin.

C. Mid-modiolar section illustrating the diffuse degeneration of the ganglion throughout its entire extent. Upper basal (1) middle (2) and apical (3) coils. Hematoxylin-eosin. x24.

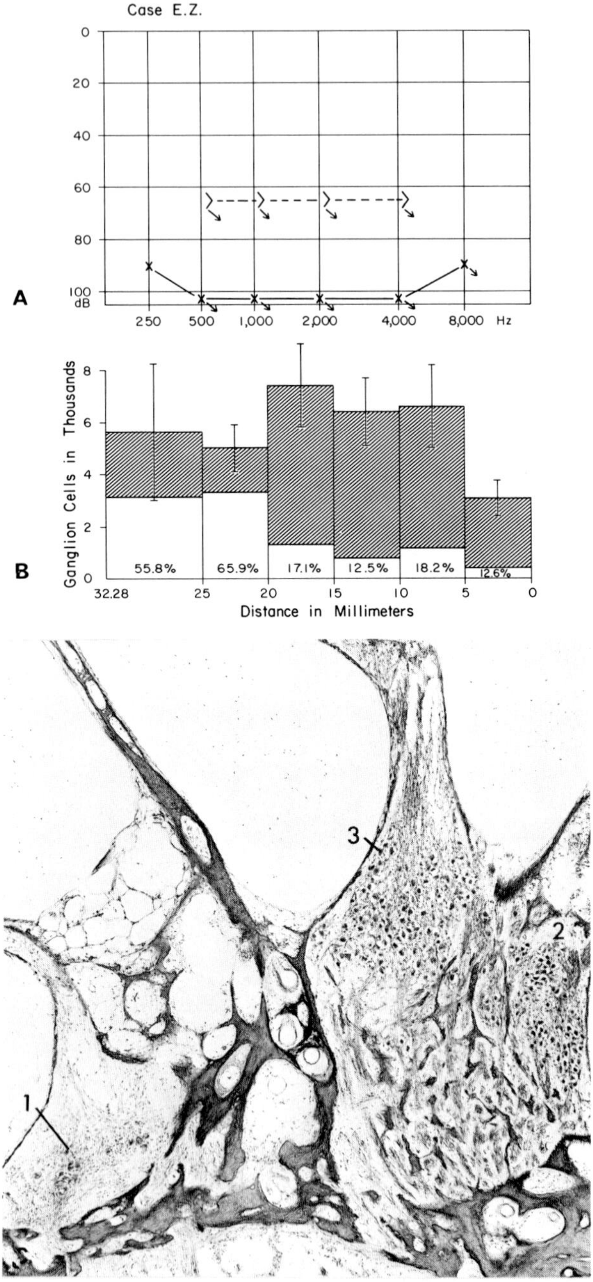
Case E.Z.
A
0
20
40
60
80
100
dB
250
500
1,000
2,000
4,000
8,000 Hz
B
Ganglion Cells in Thousands
8
6
4
2
0
55.8%
65.9%
17.1%
12.5%
18.2%
12.6%
32.28
25
20
15
10
5
0
Distance in Millimeters
1
2
3

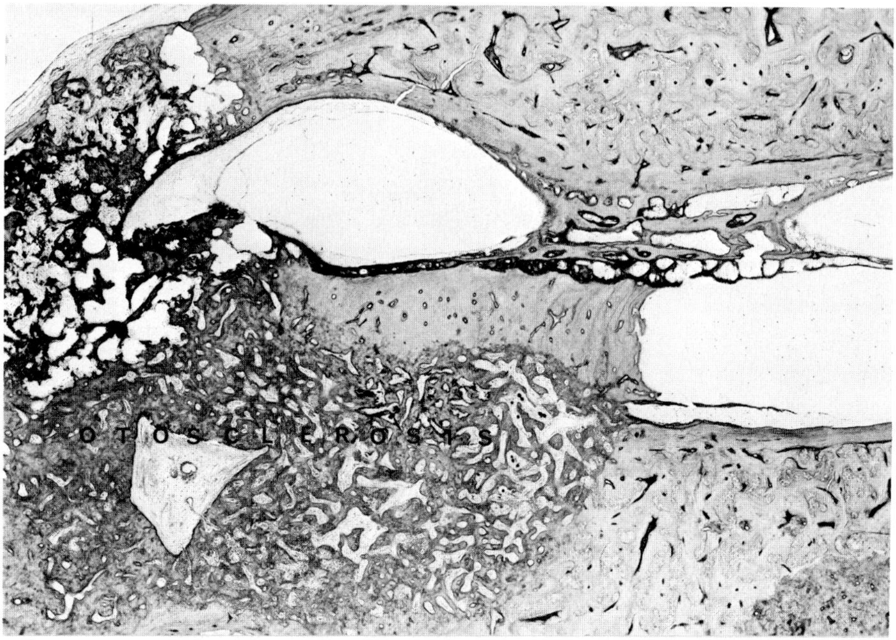

10

Fig. 10. Case E.Z. Age 60 years. Section through the lower half of the basal turn of the cochlea and the round window region. Extensive otosclerosis occupies the round window region. New bone (labyrinthitis ossificans) occupies the scala tympani and obstructs the round window completely. The otosclerotic process has invaded extensively into this new bone. Labyrinthitis ossificans of this type has occured in 5 ears as a complication of otosclerosis in the U of C collection. Hematoxylin-eosin. x17.

Fig. 9. Case E.Z. Age 60 years. Advanced Otosclerosis diffusely distributed throughout the cochlear capsule and canal regions. Left ear.

A. Audiogram showing profound deafness for all tones. Response obtained at 250 Hz only.

B. The histogram illustrates the severe reduction of acoustic ganglion cells in the basal and lower middle coils with a moderately severe reduction in the upper middle and apical coils.

C. Photomicrograph showing the lower middle (1) upper middle (2) and apical (3) coils. Hematoxylin-eosin. x39.

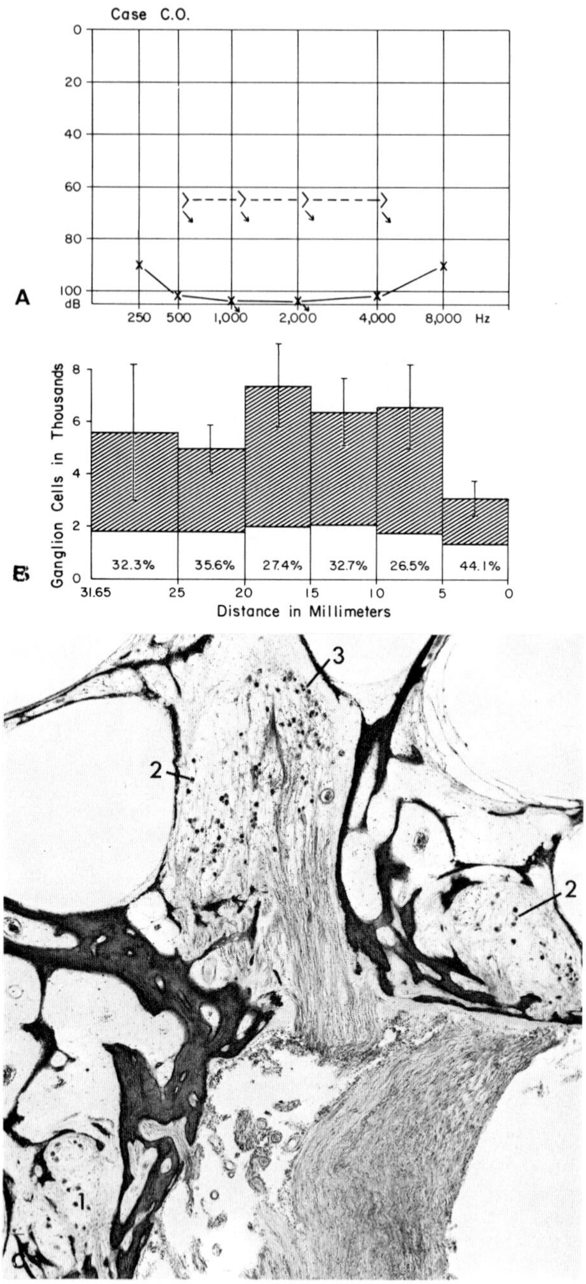

Fig. 11. Case C.O. 19 years. Kearns-Sayre Syndrome. Left ear.

A. The audiogram shows profound hearing loss.

B. Histogram shows a severe degree of degeneration throughout the entire acoustic ganglion.

C. The picture shows the severe degeneration diffusely distributed in the acoustic ganglion. Upper basal (1) middle (2) and lower apical (3) coils. Hematoxylin-eosin. x34.

the middle and upper coils of the cochlea on the cochlear spaces, with distortion and fractures of the cochlear partitions.

The variety and severity of the pathological changes in the cochlear structures, including the spiral ganglion, in these far advanced cases of the diffuse type of otosclerosis appear seriously to reduce the possibility of useful implantation.

The Kearns-Sayre Syndrome

Sensorineural deafness of varying degrees has occurred in many of the reported cases of this syndrome (Lindsay and Hinojosa, 1976). The deafness may progress to the profound stage in some instances. In one case which came to termination at the age of 19 years, the sensory cell system showed profound degenerative changes. The spiral ganglion cells and nerves were reduced in all coils of the cochlea as shown in Figure 11.

Deafness of the Heredo-degenerative Scheibe Type in the Adult

One case of profound deafness, present since infancy, but of undetermined cause, came to termination in late adult life and is presented. The essential pathological finding was a cochleo-saccular or Scheibe type of degeneration. The degeneration of sensory structures within the cochlear duct and saccule was extreme, along with hydrops of the cochlear duct. The ganglion cell count also showed a reduction in numbers as shown in Figures 12b and 12c.

Residual hearing, as tested in later years, had been limited to frequencies below 1000 Hz at the 80 dB level in one ear; there was no demonstrable residual hearing in the opposite ear.

DISCUSSION

The temporal bones from eleven cases with either total or severe sensorineural deafness were studied under light microscopy to determine the rate of survival of acoustic ganglion cells expressed as a percentage of the average normal. The cases included eight etiologic types; three represented types of slowly progressive deafness, while five represented deafnesses of acute or rapid onset with known duration. The duration of the deafness had been a minimum of 20 months, in the case of ingestion of an ototoxic drug, and 3 years in the case of bilateral deafness due to mumps. Three cases also with an acute onset were of many years duration.

Inasmuch as a primary objective was to obtain information on the possible suitability for effective electrical stimulation of the ganglion by means of a cochlear implant the corresponding state of the sensory cells and the organ of Corti was not included routinely in the descriptions. The state of survival of the sensory cells and organ of Corti varied widely in the cases demonstrated. The greatest variation in survival rate of ganglion cells has been observed in cases of bacterial labyrinthitis.

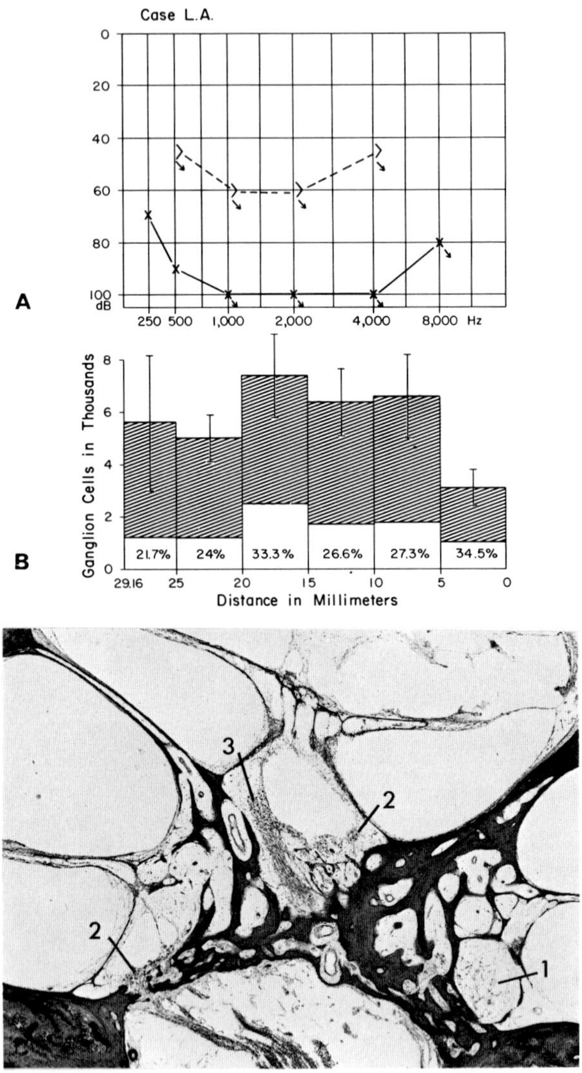

Fig. 12. Case L.A. Age 73 years.

A. Patient profoundly deaf since infancy.

B. The histogram shows relatively severe degeneration of the acoustic ganglion throughout the cochlea.

C. The picture shows the remnants of the acoustic ganglion supplying the upper basal (1) middle (2) and lower apical (3) coils. Hematoxylin-eosin. x21.

Cases M.K. and W.L. were chosen from among many to illustrate extremes of variation from total loss to a high percentage of surviving ganglion cells. Hair cells and pillar cells were rarely recognizable in the remnants of the organ of Corti.

Case T.G., believed to be of viral meningogenic origin with severe loss of ganglion cells, showed no recognizable remnants of the organ of Corti. Endolymphatic hydrops was also present.

Case B.W., representative of endolymphatic labyrinthitis, also demonstrated a relatively high survival rate of spiral ganglion cells. The organ of Corti appeared completely destroyed in the lower, middle and basal coils, except for the tectorial membrane which was rolled up, with some covering cells, and lying separately between the collapsed Reissner's and the basilar membranes.

Case M.H. with profound deafness for tones of 1000 Hz and above also showed total absence of the organ of Corti in the lower three-fourths of the basal coil. Treatment by an ototoxic drug had followed a tonsillectomy and adenoidectomy twenty months previously. Over 40% of the acoustic ganglion cells were found to be present in the lower two-thirds of the basal coil.

The case illustrated in Figure 8 is representative of a small group of otosclerotics who have profound deafness in the advanced decades of life, yet are found to have otosclerotic foci only at the windows. The degree and distribution of the degeneration of the acoustic ganglion in this group strongly suggests that the etiology is not related to the otosclerotic process, but represents a type of presbycusis.

SUMMARY

The cases of deafness presented here were selected to illustrate the degree to which the acoustic ganglion has degenerated in the presence of profound or total deafness. The series includes seven examples of acquired disease of the inner ear and one of probable congenital degeneration of uncertain etiology. The number of surviving ganglion cells in each 5 mm section of the cochlea has been expressed as a percentage of the normal average count corresponding to that section of the organ of Corti.

REFERENCES

Cohn, A.M., House, H.P. and Lindsay, J.R. Deafness in early childhood. *Laryngoscope 70:* 1665-1679, 1970.

Guild, S.R. A graphic reconstruction method for the study of the organ of Corti. *Anat. Rec. 22:* 141-157, 1921.

Guild, S.R., Crowe, S.J., Bunch, C.C. and Polvogt, L.M. Correlations of differences in the density of innervation of the organ of Corti with differences in the acuity of hearing, including evidence as to the location in the human cochlea of the receptors for certain tones. *Acta Otolaryngol. 15:* 269-308, 1931.

Lindsay, J.R. Histopathology of otosclerosis. *Arch. Otolaryngol. 97:* 24-29, 1973.

Lindsay, J.R. and Zajtchuk, J. Concussion of the inner ear. *Ann. Otol. Rhinol. Laryngol. 79:* 699-710, 1970.

Lindsay, J.R. and Hinojosa, R. Histopathologic features of the inner ear in the Kearns-Sayre Syndrome. *Arch. Otolaryngol. 102:* 747-752, 1976.

Lindsay, J.R., Davy, P.R. and Ward, P.H. Inner ear pathology in deafness due to mumps. *Ann. Otol. Rhinol. Laryngol. 69:* 918-935, 1960.

Matz, G.J., Lockhart, H.B. and Lindsay, J.R. Meningitis following stapedectomy. *Laryngoscope 78:* 251-261, 1968.

Otte, J. Estudio del ganglio espiral y su relación con la discriminación. *Rev. Otorrinolaringol. 28:* 89-99, 1968.

Perlman, H.B. and Lindsay, J.R. Relation of internal ear spaces to the meninges. *Arch. Otolaryngol. 29:* 12-23, 1939.

Schuknecht, H.F. Techniques for study of cochlear function and pathology in experimental animals. *Arch. Otolaryngol. 58:* 377-397, 1953.

Suga, F. and Lindsay, J.R. Histopathological observations of presbycusis. *Ann. Otol. Rhinol. Laryngol. 85:* 169-175, 1976.

Suga, F. and Lindsay, J.R. Labyrinthitis ossificans. *Ann. Otol. Rhinol. Laryngol. 86:* 17-30, 1977.

DISCUSSION

Simmons: I would like to know your feeling for what degree this select population represents an average sample of deaf ears in adults, with regard to neuron survival. I think with perhaps one exception I was impressed with the number of ears and the percentage of surviving neurons. According to what I have been taught, I believe the figure runs somewhere between 20 and 40 per cent total acquired deafness. Those are numbers bandied around by various people in terms of those who are likely to have a significant number of auditory nerve fibers remaining. Here I have looked at a group that would average close to 80 or 90 per cent. I am wondering if this is a select sample on the basis of these being ears which do survive, or whether this shows a more or less random sample of total acquired deafness.

Lindsay: As I mentioned, the three types that have most frequently in the past reached the laboratory with total deafness are those following a meningogenic labyrinthitis, and the next most frequent group would probably be those with otosclerosis. Presbycusis, however, is probably the most common type of deafness in late adult life, and yet the number of cases we have in the lab are quite large. We have probably sixty-odd cases at least. We couldn't find one case that had total deafness for all areas in that group. In other words, some people do develop total deafness for presbycusis, but usually it is only in those who live to a very advanced age. The other examples here are relatively infrequent in terms of numbers. Perhaps that answers the question.

Kiang: Would it be fair to say, Dr. Lindsay, that it is quite rare to find complete absence of ganglion cells in almost any temporal bone?

Lindsay: I should mention that I think we were all actually surprised to find the actual number of surviving ganglion cells in some of these conditions. If you just look at the specimen under the microscope you are likely to think the loss is much greater than it actually is. These have been counted very accurately, counting

Very few currently employed otologic procedures have been objectively evaluated. Consequently, carefully planned and executed studies of problem areas in otology should be instituted. A high priority study should include a critical examination of total resources available for ear research in relation to anticipated gains of cochlear implant procedures. Comparisons of the deployment of professional and financial resources should be compared with similar studies of treatment methods for other major otologic problems; such as chronic middle ear disease. Those responsible for setting priorities for expenditure of resources could then be guided by hard data. It makes little sense to invest in a mission impossible when achievable goals for some problems affecting a larger population are in sight. Considerations similar to these led to the following recommendation:

> *"Appropriate studies of the effectiveness of surgical treatment should be carried out for selected conditions, particularly those where uncertainty leads to professional disagreement."* (Bunker et al., 1977).

Appended to this recommendation should be clearly worded guidelines for clinical trials of surgical innovations, especially prostheses. Suggested training and educational background for both surgeons and surgical teams should accompany the guidelines. Prior to final sanction of a procedure or device for general use, recommendation number four below should have been accomplished.

Functional assessment techniques must be standardized and reporting methods improved in order to accomplish the first recommendation. Obtaining factual information from data routinely gathered in clinical settings has been a very difficult task in the past. Incomplete documentation in combination with lack of objective methodology has prevented the implementation of analytic methods for problem solving or controlled observation. The ability to conduct both carefully controlled clinical trials and epidemiological studies in otology also has been seriously hampered by presently employed local and national information systems. Separate outpatient and hospital record keeping systems prohibitively escalate information retrieval time and costs. Record keeping systems usually are not designed to expedite information retrieval and analysis. Data retrieval at arbitrary points in the course of progressive diseases cannot be corrected for the degree of functional impairment because staging data is not available for any otologic disorder except presbycusis. Consequently, much of the data obtained in this manner cannot be used for meaningful analysis of surgical end results. Attempts at prospective longitudinal studies will not be considered by most investigators under these circumstances.

Because most otologic disorders affect the quality and not the quantity of life, there is a need for methods of quantifying the functional status of patients, especially for those disease processes affecting the vestibular system. Fortunately, psychoacoustic and objective audiometric techniques are available for the assessment of many auditory functions.

To quote Bunker et al., (1977): *"We do not yet know enough about ran-*

domized trials and their consequences, their weaknesses, strengths, and costs compared with their alternatives. We still are not sure enough of when we should trust an observational study. We do not know how to combine epidemiology and observational and experimental information." Recommendation number two is concerned with improved methodology:

> *"Our grasp of the components of the cost benefit analysis and their interrelations, the values of the various data gathering techniques and our understanding of the ethics of data gathering must be improved by theoretical and empirical work and by continued discussion in the public forums."* (Bunker et al., 1977).

The legal issues, particularly regarding rights to privacy act as opposed to statutes, guaranteeing publication of federally funded research projects must also be clarified.

Continued evaluation of existing treatment methods and review of past developments for reasons for success or failure may provide valuable insights that would prevent past pitfalls from repetition and facilitate inductive reasoning. General policies and guidelines for the introduction of new medical and surgical methods could then be set forth in a manner analogous to the format required of all scientists who apply for grant support. Finally, physicians must begin training at the medical school level in the techniques required for the analytic methods described above. Recommendation number three is therefore as follows:

> *"These principles of cost-benefit evaluation should be included as an integral part of the medical school curriculum; and their application to the assessment of the efficacy of medical care should be incorporated into clinical practice and continuing medical education"* (Bunker et al., 1977).

The medical equivalent of a head-start program will be required in order to prepare physicians to perform, participate in, and evaluate these new techniques. Medical educational processes simply are not structured to prepare physicians for such a role in health care delivery.

The public understanding of the issues must be improved and their counsel sought for the final decision making process. A carefully proctored, organized, educational effort must be developed in order to accomplish this goal. In addition, the role of the physician as an adviser and decision maker must be clearly differentiated in order to avoid bias and advertising during discussions with the lay public. Recommendation four:

> *"Information on outcomes as well as costs of medical care should be routinely formulated in a manner suitable for presentation to the public"* (Bunker et al., 1977).

Research and development, delivery, and direct patient costs must be partitioned when possible.

COMMENT

If we have learned anything from the cochlear implant controversy, it is the fact that we have accomplished nothing by shouting at each other. As pointed out by Bunker et al., (1977), "*. . . the issue is not just that clinical data are inadequate, but rather that the fundamental biological questions upon which to base rational therapy remain to be answered*". In no other specialty of medicine does the nature of the problem compel the physician to have every aspect of the disease process so perfectly pinpointed in terms of accurate diagnosis relative to a proposed operation as it does in sensory systems. The cochlear implant does not fit the category of most otologic surgical procedures which were developed mostly to correct middle ear malfunctions. The kind of thinking and observation required for evaluation of conductive hearing losses cannot be applied without modification to sensorineural hearing problems. On the other hand, otologists should not ignore problems of the severely and completely deafened patient. While it may be more difficult to design and execute a good treatment strategy, this problem should be recognized as having a very narrow margin of good practice when compared to middle ear operations. We must now quantify those margins with carefully designed, prospective studies. For a completely postlingually deafened human, some hearing, no matter how primitive, is better than none providing a technique can be safely and economically delivered to him with a minimum of risk.

From a given patient's point of view, the cochlear implant may have enabled a continued existence in the hearing world. Such a patient could not be expected to view objectively an evaluation process for the cochlear implant. A prelingually deafened patient who was made more independent by the ability to detect environmental sounds would not be likely to minimize these minimal auditory benefits even though complete escape from a deaf subculture was not accomplished by cochlear implant.

From a broader perspective of resources available versus value or efficacy of a surgical procedure made with a view toward the most common unsolved problems in otology, it is questionable that current cochlear implants would stand an objective evaluation. This observer agrees with House et al., (1977) when he states: "*Let us not waste time; there is work to be done*", but we disagree on where dwindling resources should be expended. In the opinion of this participant in the Pittsburgh study, the thoughts of a leading authority and researcher of evoked electrical activity in the auditory system should be heeded now as they should have been nearly a decade ago (Simmons, 1969). Simmons has recently repeated his warning, "*If we do not proceed carefully (and speedily), we are likely to find ourselves in an otolaryngological version of the current apricot pit controversy. I would hate to see this happen again as it did in the early sixties. The fuss and furor of that period set implant research back at least a decade. It could happen again*" (Simmons, 1977).

SUMMARY

It is doubtful that present gaps in our basic knowledge of the auditory system will be filled in our lifetime by the efforts of many productive and capable, but arbitrarily constricted, scientists working in much the same manner as the many people from all walks of life who by simple trial and error made their contributions to fixed wing flight. Moreover, it is doubtful, under the presently organized structure of ear research support, that the concerted effort of available scientists can be efficiently organized in order to fully address even the most fundamental of the above problems. With the trend toward reduced federal funding, the potential level of financial support required to accomplish the development of a clinically cost-effective cochlear implant may not exist. The strong recommendation may therefore be made that the necessary organizational structure be established, the immediate and long term goals be articulated, and the required funds identified before embarking upon a project as ambitious as the development of a cochlear prosthesis. This recommendation can be accomplished expeditiously only after cost, risk, and benefit data, as outlined in this paper, have been accumulated and thoroughly studied by all concerned parties. The real value determination of the cochlear implant must await these developments.

In the meantime, accumulation of some information is better than ignoring the problem in hopes that a break-through will suddenly appear. Applied scientists should concentrate even more actively than in the past on the major unknowns in inner ear and auditory mechanisms in normal and diseased states. The cochlear implant device, as primitive and potentially damaging to the cochlea as it is, appears to provide a minimal auditory input. How this input method compares with vibrotactile devices in a controlled study is an example of an experiment that is presently feasible and should be performed. The relative value of the implant, however, lies in the stimulus that the controversy has given to the recognition of the problems of the completely deaf human. The limited accomplishments of research on deafness relative to developments in other areas of medicine, especially vision, reflects poorly upon those personally affected by and those concerned professionally with deafness.

Acknowledgements

This project was made possible by the findings of Contract #NO1-NS-5-2331 from the National Institute of Neurological and Communicative Disorders and Stroke.

I also wish to express my appreciation to Deborah FitzGerald and MaryAnn Czerniewski for their assistance in editing the manuscript.

REFERENCES

Bilger, R.C. Evaluation of subjects presently fitted with implanted auditory prostheses. *Ann. Otol. Rhinol. Laryngol.* Suppl. *38:* 1-176, 1977.

Black, F.O., Wall, C.III, O'Leary, D.P., Bilger, R.C. and Wolf, R.V. Galvanic disruption of vestibulospinal postural control of cochlear implant subjects. *Ann. Otol. Rhinol. Laryngol.*, submitted 1977.

Bunker, J.P., Barnes, B.A., Mosteller, F. *Costs, Risks, and Benefits of Surgery* New York: Oxford University Press, 1977.

Djourno, A. and Eyries, C. Prostheses auditive par excitation électrique a distance du nerf sensoriel a l'aide d'un bobinage inclus a demeure. *Presse Med. 35:* 14-17, 1957.

House, W.F., Norton, N., Berliner, K., Luckey, R., Miller, L. and Eisenberg, L. Letter to the editor. *Ann. Otol. Rhinol. Laryngol. 86:* 566-567, 1977.

House, W.F. and Urban, J. Long term results of electrode implantation and electrical stimulation of the cochlea in man. *Ann. Otol. Rhinol. Laryngol. 82:* 504-510, 1973.

Michelson, R.P., Merzenich, M.M., Petit, C.R. and Schlinder, R.A. A cochlear prosthesis; further clinical observations; preliminary results of physiological studies. *Laryngoscope 83:* 116-1122, 1973.

Simmons, F.B. Cochlear implants. *Arch Otolaryngol. 89:* 61-69, 1969.

Simmons, F.B. Letter to the editor. *Ann. Otol. Rhinol. Laryngol. 86:* 567, 1977.

Simmons, F.B., Epley, T.M., Lummis, R.C., Guttman, N., Frishkopf, L.S. and Harmon, L.D. Auditory nerve: electrical stimulation in man. *Science 148:* 104-106, 1965.

Wolf, R.V. and Bilger, R.C. Electroacoustic measures of present prostheses. *Ann. Otol. Rhinol. Laryngol.* Suppl. *38:* 61-69, 1977.

BRAINSTEM

Moderator: *Jerzy E. Rose*

PRIMARY AFFERENTS AND THE COCHLEAR NUCLEUS

Eileen S. Kane

University of Massachusetts

INTRODUCTION

The primary cochlear afferents and the cochlear nucleus they innervate, will be discussed in five major parts. First, the structural organization of the whole mammalian cochlear nucleus will be reviewed, as described in early microscopic studies. Then several schemas of morphological subdivisions will be introduced in order to discuss specific regions of the nucleus investigated by both light (LM) and electron (EM) microscopy in our laboratory. Third, the detailed arborizations of incoming afferent fibers and terminals from the ipsilateral cochlea that end within these limited zones will be examined. Fourth, several lines of experimental and developmental, morphological evidence confirming the pattern of primary afferent terminations in one unusual region will be considered. Fifth, electrophysiological findings in two regions will be reviewed in order to develop correlations between structural and functional results; such correlations are the major goals of our morphological work. Finally, possible clinical applications of these research endeavors will be presented.

ORGANIZATION OF THE COCHLEAR NUCLEUS IN MAMMALS

The cochlear nucleus of mammals lies at the dorsolateral border of the ponto-medullary junction and is innervated by the cochlear nerve from the ipsilateral cochlea. Held (1891) and Ramón y Cajal (1909) were among several early neuro-anatomists who subdivided this large nucleus on the basis of the branching patterns of all primary afferent axons, as seen in their reduced silver- and aniline dye-stained material and in Golgi-impregnated tissue. As illustrated by Lorente de No′(1933), each cochlear axon divides into an ascending branch and a descending branch each terminating in different zones of the ipsilateral cochlear nucleus only; Figure 1 is a schematized drawing of Lorente de Nó's findings. Ascending branches course forward to end as large end-bulbs of Held (Held, 1891; Ramón y Cajal, 1909) in the anteroventral region (AVCN; Fig. 1, ab) while descending branches arborize extensively in the posteroventral cochlear nucleus (PVCN) before coursing into the overlying dorsal cochlear nucleus (DCN) where they finally terminate (Fig. 1, ab). Accordingly, the three main divisions of the cochlear nucleus were designated as the

ISBN 0-12-514960-3

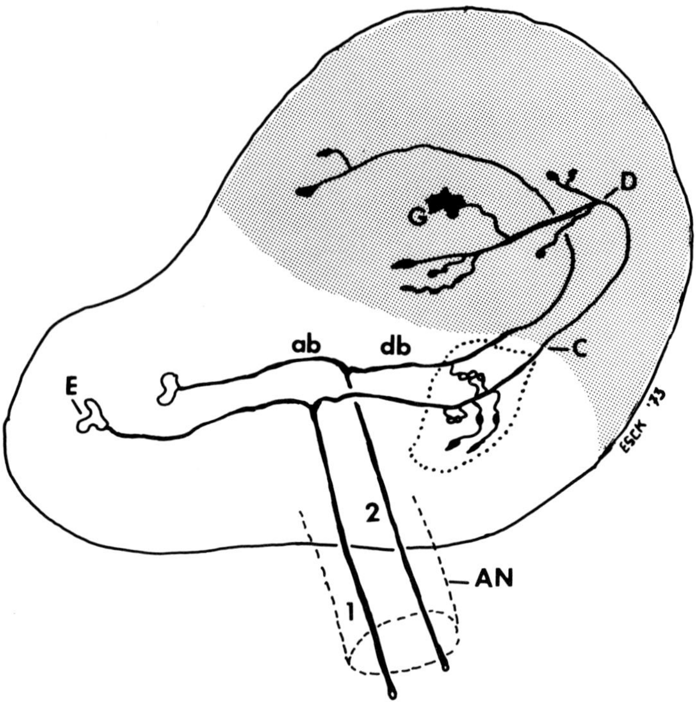

Fig. 1. Diagram of cochlear nucleus (from parasagittal section) showing typical division of primary afferent fibers (1, 2) into ascending (ab) and descending (db) branches plus arborizations of latter in OCA (within dotted line) and in DCN (stippled area, D). Ascending branches characteristically form end bulbs (E) within AVCN while descending branches form both small, large and very large, glomerular (G) endings in PVCN and DCN (Reprinted from Kane, 1974a).

three regions of distinct primary terminals (ie. AVCN, PVCN and DCN). A fourth major zone was the region of nerve root entry, the "interstitial nucleus".

While these four basic regions are useful for an overall view of the cochlear nucleus as a structure within the entire central auditory system, these subdivisions are too large to help make up the types of structural-functional correlations first suggested by Lorente de Nó (1933): *"The most urgent need of physiology is a knowledge of the minute structure of the central organs, with exact data on all the fibres that end upon any cell and on all cells upon which any fibre has synapses. Until this be known, the interpretation of physiological experiments will continue to be extremely difficult."*

In other words, it is the interaction between presynaptic and postsynaptic components of the nucleus that work together to produce specific, electrophysiologically recordable response patterns. Thus, any attempt to correlate structure with function must take cognizance of both elements. Accordingly, Lorente de Nó (1933) produced a schema of cochlear nucleus subdivisions based not only upon

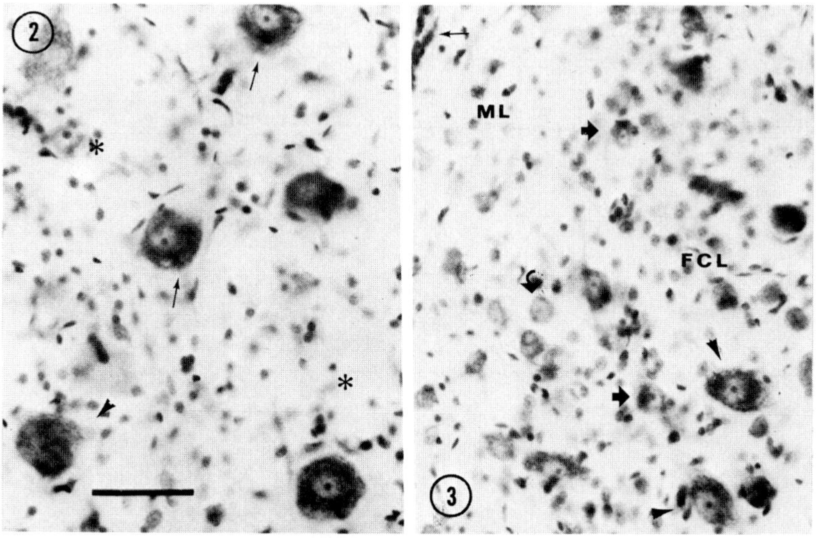

Fig. 2. Octopus cell area of posteroventral cochlear nucleus of adult cat in Nissl-stained section showing several large spherical octopus cell bodies (arrows), a thick basal dendrite (arrowhead) and large areas of neuropil (*). The OCA contains only one morphological type of neuron and is the focus of the present discussion. Bar = 50 μm for figures 2 and 3.

Fig. 3. Nissl-stained dorsal cochlear nucleus overlying OCA, containing outermost ependymal layer (arrow), molecular layer (ML), fusiform cell layer (FCL) and (not shown) deep DCN. The FCL, the second region subject to the LM and EM studies discussed here, contains large, elongate fusiform cells (arrowheads) as well as small cells (thick arrows) and granule cells (curved arrows).

the distribution of primary afferents (ie. presynaptic elements), but also upon specific, Golgi-impregnated neuronal types (ie. postsynaptic elements) within the complex, and upon the distribution of other-than-afferent axons on those same neurons. Lorente de Nó thereby described his schema of 13 cochlear nucleus subdivisions.

Osen (1969) published another system for subdividing cat cochlear nucleus as seen in Nissl- and Glees-stained brains. She defined several regions according to the distribution of nine neuronal types or postsynaptic elements only. Her schema was more simple, but still comparable to those of Ramón y Cajal (1909) and Lorente de Nó (1933). Thus, by the late 1960's, when our studies began, we already had schemas based upon presynaptic components only (Ramón y Cajal, 1909), postsynaptic elements only (Osen, 1969), and both elements (Lorente de Nó, 1933; Harrison and Warr, 1962; Harrison and Irving, 1966). Although combined data on

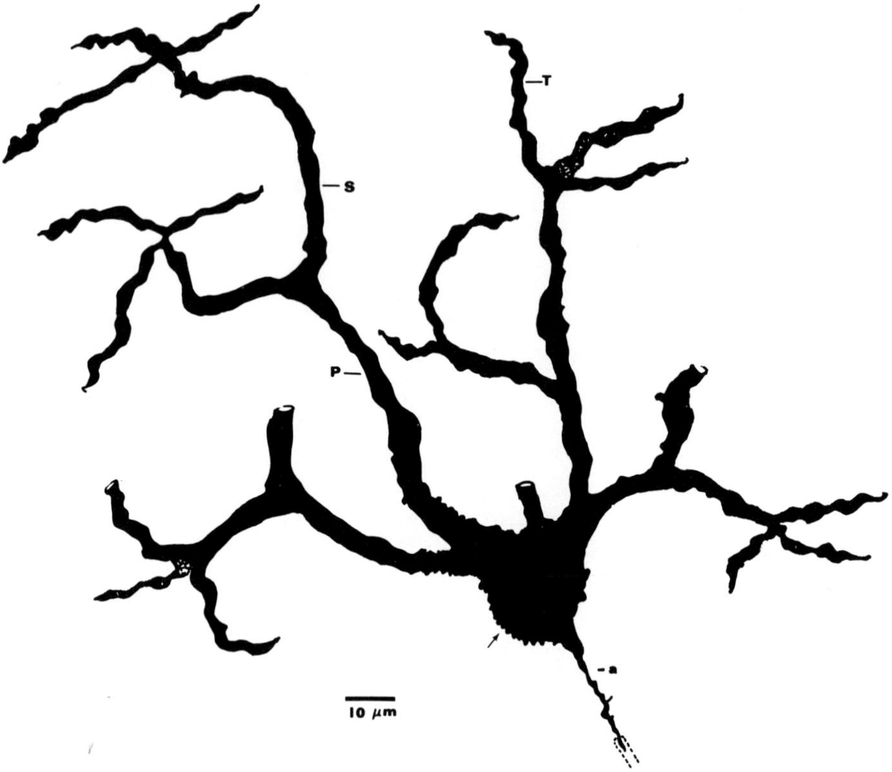

Fig. 4. Typical appearance of Golgi-impregnated, mature octopus neuron with large soma covered with spicules (arrow) long, straight primary (P) and secondary (S) dendrites, trifurcating tertiary (T) dendrites, and a thick initial axon segment (a). Camera lucida drawing.

cells and inputs was eventually necessary, the more limited schema of Osen (1969) provided a most interesting finding in that three different zones seemed each to contain a unique population of morphologically homogeneous neurons. These zones included two regions in AVCN and a group of packed octopus cells in PVCN.

Our subsequent studies of Nissl- and Protargol-stained cochlear nuclei demonstrated that Osen's octopus cell area (OCA) within the PVCN was the only region of a consistently homogeneous group of neurons (Kane, 1973). Octopus cells (Fig. 2) have large somata, diffuse Nissl substance and thick basal dendrites, extending into long primary dendritic shafts. After defining the three-dimensional boundaries of the Nissl-stained OCA, the region was studied in rapid Golgi impregnations of cat and kitten cochlear nuclei (Kane, 1973; Brawer, et al., 1974). These preparations revealed the OCA as a discrete central zone within caudal PVCN (PP of Kane, 1976) that contained only one morphological type of neuron (Fig. 4); the large soma is covered by projections or spicules while the large-diameter primary dendrites can

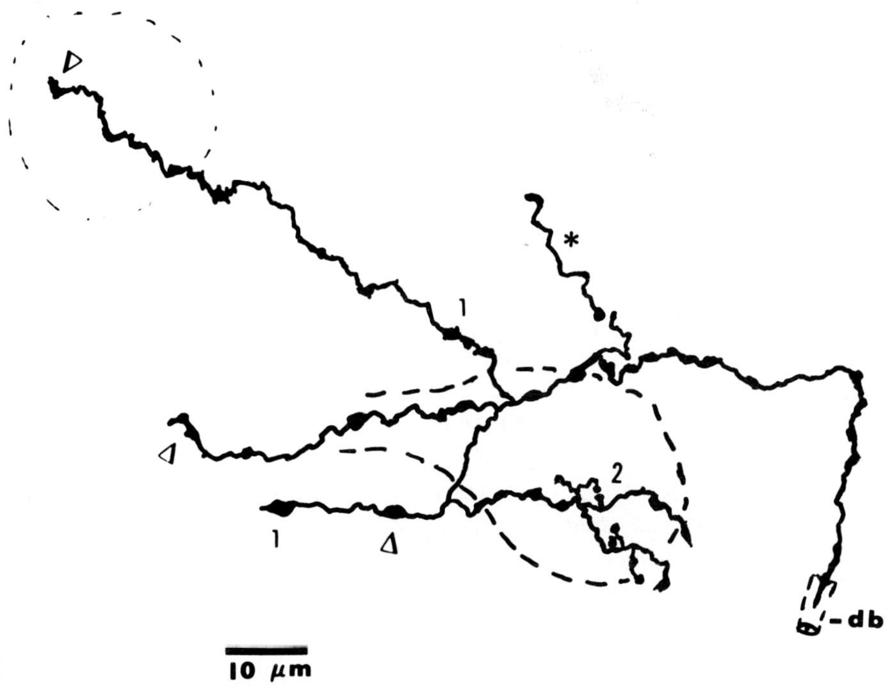

Fig. 5. Representative Golgi-impregnated, primary afferent descending branch (db) arborising over octopus cell soma and proximal dendrite (broken line outline). The myelinated axon (at db) branches into thick collaterals with large (Type 1) boutons (arrowheads) and into thin collaterals with small, clustered (Type 2) boutons. Tiny axons (*) of unknown origin can join the Type 2 clusters. Camera lucida drawing.

be traced into long shafts (without appendages) that bifurcate into thick secondary dendrites and then trifurcate, in an orthogonal plane, into tertiary or distal dendrites (Fig. 4).

At this point we may ask why such a zone of homogeneous neurons might be of particular interest to investigators of the auditory system. These neuronal populations are attractive candidates for making the type of structural-functional correlation suggested by Lorente de Nó (1933). If we assume that the morphology of a neuron reflects its function, then we would expect any region of one neuronal type to demonstrate only one function. Hence, by using a region of homogeneous neurons we immediately eliminate the postsynaptic variability in response to specific auditory stimuli. Furthermore, any observable variations in such responses (eg. extracellularly recorded unit response patterns to different auditory stimuli) would necessarily be attributed to differences in the presynaptic elements (Kiang et al., 1973: Morest et al., 1973). A large number of different inputs upon one cell type would complicate the association of one input with a single physiological effect. However, in the OCA we also found an unusually simple set of presynaptic components in the Golgi-impregnated cochlear nucleus and in electron micrographs (Kane, 1973). Thus, the presynaptic and postsynaptic structures are readily comparable to the physiology in the OCA.

AFFERENT INPUTS

As shown in Figure 5, octopus cells receive a distinct and predominant input from primary afferents. Those fibers end with two structurally different boutons on both octopus cell somata and proximal dendrites. Thick collaterals arise from the descending branches to produce large, elongate and tapered Type 1 boutons en passant and boutons terminaux (Fig. 5). Small, tightly clustered Type 2 boutons terminaux arise from thin collaterals to terminate also upon octopus cell somata and proximal dendrites. Thus, a single cochlear axon can provide two morphologically distinct endings associated with an octopus neuron (Kane, 1973).

By correlating the sizes (both range and average dimensions), shapes, and packing arrangement of Golgi-impregnated primary terminals with the several profiles of synaptic endings on octopus cells in electron micrographs, we concluded that Type 1 endings corresponded best to isolated terminals with heavily asymmetric complexes (Fig 6B) and that small Type 2 endings corresponded best to the small, packed profiles of endings with nearly symmetric complexes (Fig. 6D). Thus, on the basis of deduction from both LM and EM findings, we finally concluded that the OCA is an unusually simple zone where single cochlear axons can produce two cytologically distinct terminals upon the somata and most proximal dendrites of octopus neurons (Kane, 1973). Based on the assumption of functional capabilities reflected in structural differences, we would expect two distinct response patterns to the same auditory stimulus by units in the OCA. As discussed later, the electrophysiological studies of the OCA by Godfrey et al., (1975a) in fact demonstrated two such patterns of response to short tone bursts.

EXPERIMENTAL AND DEVELOPMENTAL CONFIRMATION

The synaptic organization of the OCA has been further substantiated in our laboratory by means of experimental, developmental and other types of normal microscopic techniques. For example, by surgically ablating the whole ipsilateral cochlea, we found that both the large, Type 1 synaptic endings and the small Type 2 synaptic endings degenerated. Calculations of the percentage of surface membrane covered by each of the endings before and after cochlear destruction were graphically illustrated (Kane, 1973) to show the sharp decline of both types of endings on somata and on basal dendrites after 2 and 4-day survivals. In addition, our more recent EM studies (Kane, 1977a) showed that, after large lesions of higher auditory nuclei eg. the superior olivary complex (SOC) and the inferior colliculus (IC), only Type 3 and Type 4 endings, on the distal octopus cell dendrites, degenerated (See Kane, 1977a, Figs. 6, 7, 10, 19). No degeneration was observed in either Type 1 or Type 2 endings after central lesions.

The presence of two cytologically distinct synaptic endings on octopus cells was further confirmed in an EM developmental study (Schwartz and Kane, 1977). This work demonstrated that both Type 1 and Type 2 endings develop over the same postnatal time interval to both attain a mature appearance at three weeks. Further, these studies showed that each of the two afferent endings terminate on a different postsynaptic type of projection on the octopus cell membrane. In immature kittens, Type 1 endings typically synapse on blunt spicules (Fig. 6A) while small Type 2 endings contact long, thin filopodia (Fig. 6B). Later in development, filopodia disappear and Type 2 endings contact a flat portion of membrane as in adults (Fig. 6D). Thus, there seems to be a simultaneous outgrowth and synaptogenesis of both types of endings that would be expected if they both arise from a single axonal source.

Our most recent studies have taken advantage of the normal anterograde transport of tritiated leucine (^{3}H-leu) in order to demonstrate the pattern of termination of primary afferents in autoradiographs (Kane, 1977b). Such autoradiographic preparations of the OCA, following an injection of 50μCi ^{3}H-leu into the ipsilateral cochlea, showed many scattered grains that are detectable with bright-field illumination (Fig. 7A). Such grains, which are much more easily seen with dark-field optics (Fig. 7C), were clustered around octopus cell somata and diffusely scattered in the surrounding neuropil of the experimental side, but were rarely found in the contralateral OCA (Fig. 7B). This pattern of grain distribution confirms our earlier Golgi and EM descriptions of abundant primary afferents on the cell bodies. However, this particular method shows the afferents in a physiologically normal way (Cowan and Cuénod, 1975).

The same methods of tissue preparation have also been applied to a second region of the cochlear nucleus, the dorsal cochlear nucleus (DCN) that lies over and around the PVCN. The DCN is a region of several neuronal types (Ramón y Cajal, 1909; Lorente de Nó, 1933; Brawer, et al., 1974) that we call "morphologically heterogeneous neurons" (Kane, 1974b). The several different neurons of the layered DCN (Fig. 3) receive different proportions of primary afferent terminals (Cohen et al., 1972). One distinctive DCN neuron, the fusiform cell (Fig. 3, thin arrow), receives direct and indirect cochlear inputs; the indirect input is carried via the axons of small (Fig. 3, curved arrows) and granule (Fig. 3, arrowhead) cells that also lie in the fusiform cell layer (FCL) of the DCN. In rapid Golgi impregnations of the DCN, large fusiform neurons extend an elaborate, appendage-covered dendritic tree into the so-called molecular layer (ML) and thick dendrites into the deep DCN (Kane, 1974b and Fig. 8).

The general distribution of primary afferents in classical histological preparations of the DCN was recently confirmed in autoradiographic studies after small, unilateral cochlear injections of tritiated leucine (^{3}H-leu), described above and elsewhere (Kane, 1977b). In these studies, the deep DCN was covered by the densest grains, the FCL by a moderate amount, and the ML by only sparse grains (ie. close

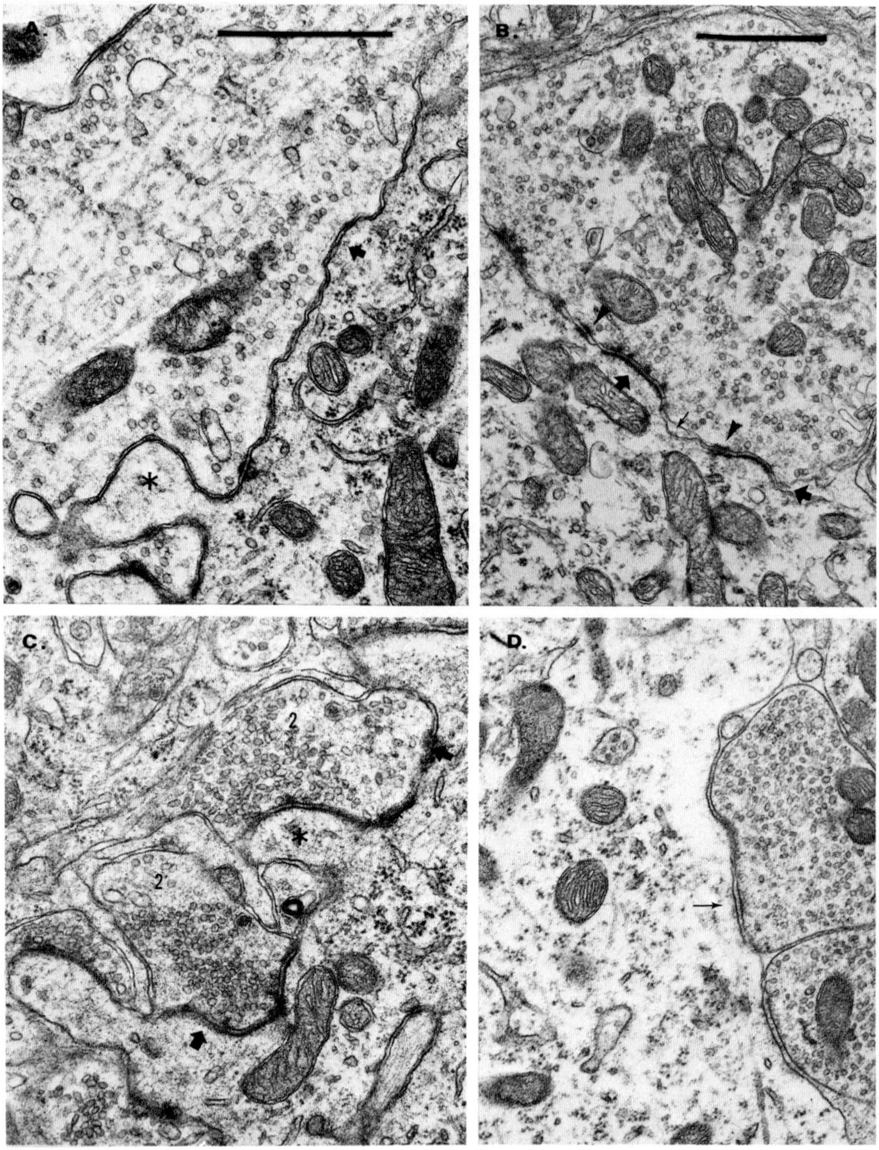

Fig. 6. EM's of immature and mature primary afferent OCA endings.

A. Portion of large, immature Type 1 terminal contacting octopus cell soma on spicules (*) and flat surface (thick arrow). This large ending also synapses on a large dendrite (upper left) and is nearly twice the length shown here. 7-day kitten. Bar = 1 μm for Figs. 6A and 6D. (Micrograph taken by A.M. Schwartz.)

B. Mature OCA Type 1 ending with typical large, round vesicles and several heavily asymmetric synaptic complexes (thick arrows) upon octopus cell soma. Note puncta adhaerentia to background) as shown in Figure 7D. Grains were consistently found over giant and small cell somata and neuropil of deep DCN, fusiform cell and small cell somata and neuropil of the FCL and neuropil of the ML (Fig. 7D). This grain distribution mirrors that of stained or impregnated primary afferent fibers and terminals in the DCN.

ELECTROPHYSIOLOGICAL STUDIES: ATTEMPTS AT STRUCTURAL-FUNCTIONAL CORRELATIONS

The distinct synaptic organizations of the OCA and the overlying DCN of the cochlear nucleus can be matched by the distinct extracellularly recorded response patterns to electrophysiological tone bursts (and other auditory stimuli) from single units in those regions. Many of these recordings resulted from the work of Godfrey et al., (1975a, and b).

In the OCA, Godfrey et al., (1975a) found two very similar but distinguishable response patterns to short tone bursts, as seen in histogram data. These "on" type PST histograms both have short latencies and large bursts of initial activity. The O_I unit (Godfrey et al., 1975a) has no other activity during a 50 msec tone delivery; the unit is silent or turns off. The O_L unit, however, has irregular residual activity following the initial onset response. Since there are two distinct primary terminals upon octopus cells and since there are two distinct response patterns, it seemed logical to associate the morphology with the electrophysiology. For example, the Type 1 endings might be the source of the initial onset response of both O units while the Type 2 endings might produce the later, irregular small spikes (the O_L pattern); in that case, the O_I response would result from an octopus cell covered by relatively more Type 1 than Type 2 endings.

Similar types of recording in the DCN (Godfrey et al., 1975b) revealed three major PST histogram patterns--the so-called pauser, build-up and chopper units. Our microscopic studies revealed direct inputs from primary afferents to fusiform cells, indirect primary inputs to fusiform cells via small cells, and indirect primary inputs via granule cells as shown in our Golgi-EM correlations (Kane, 1974b). Hence, we proposed a matching between fusiform cells (with their inputs) and the three response patterns based on the predominant type of input to that cell or unit, as

(arrowheads) and enlarged subsynaptic spaces (thin arrows). Adult cat. Bar = about 1 μm for Figs. 6B and 6C.
Immature OCA Type 2 (2) endings typically contacting long, thin somatic process (*) or "filopodium" plus flat somatic membrane (thick arrows). 7-day kitten. (Micrograph taken by A.M. Schwartz.)
Mature OCA Type 2 endings tightly apposed and both contacting flat somatic membrane only with grazed synapse (arrow). Note the pleomorphic vesicles, dense matrix and consistent width of the cleft beneath these endings. Long somatic filopodia have disappeared as Type 2 postsynaptic sites. Adult cat.

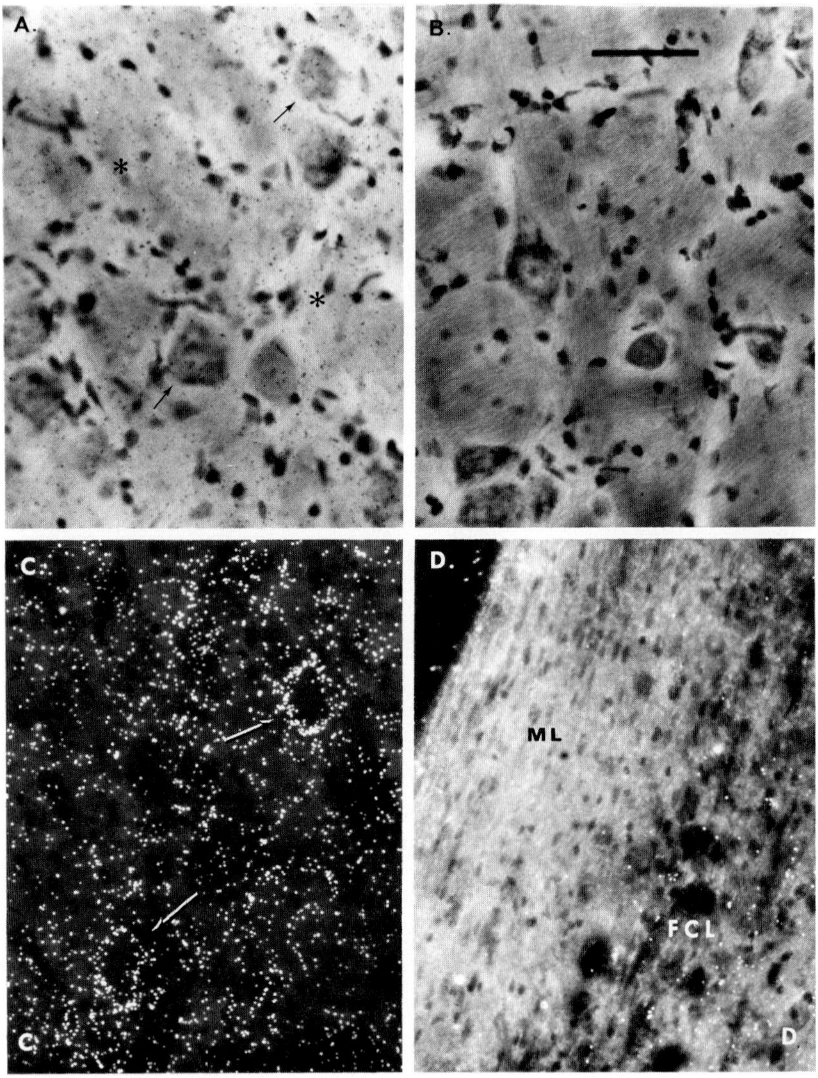

Fig. 7. Photomicrographs of autoradiographs following unilateral cochlear injection of ^{3}H-leu (50 μCi) and 24-hour survival. Bar = 50 μm for Figs. A to D.

A. Bright-field photo of experimental OCA (ipsilateral to injection) showing dense granules throughout neuropil (*), but particularly over octopus cell somata (arrows).

B. Bright-field photo of control OCA (contralateral to injection) showing lack of any visible grains over somata or neuropil.

C. Dark-field photo of experimental OCA for better visualization of grain localization around somata (arrows) compared to scattered grains in surrounding neuropil.

D. Dark-field photo of experimental DCN, showing dense labelling over deep DCN (D) with progressively sparser grains over FCL and ML.

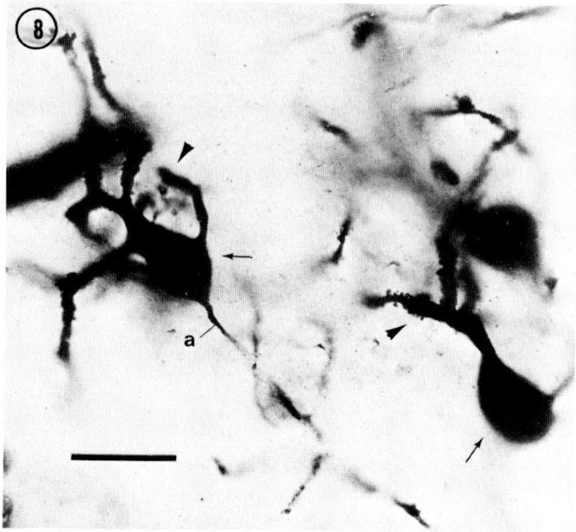

Fig. 8. Golgi impregnation of adult cat DCN showing two fusiform neurons (arrows) with elongate somata, elaborate apical dendritic trees (arrowheads), and axons (a) in focus. Bar = 50 μm.

follows: (1) Neurons with pauser patterns probably have a large direct input (source of initial large spike) and substantial indirect inputs (sources of later increasing response train); (2) neurons with build-up patterns probably have less direct primary input (ie. no initial large burst) but substantial indirect primary input; and (3) neurons with chopper patterns may have an unusually large granule cell input (possible source of apparent, intermittent inhibition of those units). Since that study, no investigation, including any from our group, has continued this matching via the essential identification and quantitation of all inputs to fusiform cells. Until this is done, we cannot verify our speculative correlation between structure and function. Nonetheless, the eventual matching of the synaptic organization and the electrophysiology in the FCL of the dorsal cochlear nucleus as well as in the OCA is a real possibility.

FUTURE CLINICAL POSSIBILITIES

Lorente de Nó's call for complete morphological studies for understanding function seems well underway for the two cochlear nucleus regions just discussed. However, you may well ask what significance such research endeavors may have to clinicians in the field of Otolaryngology.

If we are able to delineate the complete inputs to octopus neurons, for example, and if we can assign a physiological role to those inputs and to the octopus cell (eg. responding quickly to unilateral inputs of a specific frequency range and sound intensity) then we may be able to develop precise hearing tests associated with certain units or regions of units. If such tests can detect the human's ability to hear just that known range at a given intensity then we could localize an abnormality of that auditory function to a specific zone of the cochlear nucleus. Furthermore, if a hearing loss involves a loss of presynaptic input, for example, we may be able to eventually treat the disorder by administering the missing neurotransmitter (or its precursor or synthetic enzyme), as is the case with Parkinson's disease. Clearly such diagnoses and treatments are for the future.

Acknowledgements

The author is grateful for the advice and encouragement of many colleagues including Drs. César Fernández, Jay M. Goldberg, Nelson Y.G. Kiang, D. Kent Morest and Sam L. Clark. Ann Marie Schwartz, Anna Lysakowski, John Conlee, Bev Brown, Chris Habib and Elsie Larson were all important in the completion of this manuscript. This work has been supported by the University of Chicago, the University of Massachusetts Medical School, The Deafness Research Foundation and USPHS Grants #NS-12071 and NS-00290.

REFERENCES

Brawer, J.R., Morest, D.K. and Kane, E.C. The neuronal architecture of the cochlear nucleus of the cat. *J. Comp. Neurol. 155:* 251-300, 1974.

Cohen, E.S., Brawer, J.R. and Morest, D.K. Projections of the cochlea to the dorsal cochlear nucleus in the cat. *Exper. Neurol. 35:* 470-479, 1972.

Cowan, W.M. and Cuénod, M. (Eds.) *The Use of Axonal Transport for studies of Neuronal Connectivity.* New York: Elsevier Scientific Publishing Co., 1975.

Godfrey, D.A., Kiang, N.Y.S. and Norris, B.E. Single unit activity in the posteroventral cochlear nucleus of the cat. *J. Comp. Neurol. 162:* 247-268, 1975a.

Godfrey, D.A., Kiang, N.Y.S. and Norris, B.E. Single unit activity in dorsal cochlear nucleus of the cat. *J. Comp. Neurol. 162:* 269-284, 1975b.

Harrison, J.M. and Irving, R. The organization of the posterior ventral cochlear nucleus in the rat. *J. Comp. Neurol. 126:* 391-402, 1966.

Harrison, J.M. and Warr, W.B. A study of the cochlear nuclei and ascending pathways of the medulla. *J. Comp. Neurol. 119:* 341-380, 1962.

Held, H. Die centralen Bahnen des Nervus acusticus bei der Katze. *Arch. Anat. Physiol., Anat. Abt.:* 271-291, 1891.

Kane, E.C. Octopus cells in the cochlear nucleus of the cat: heterotypic neurons. *Internat. J. Neurosci. 5:* 251-279, 1973.

Kane, E.C. Patterns of degeneration in the caudal cochlear nucleus of the cat. *Anat. Rec. 179:* 67-92, 1974a.

Kane, E.C. Synaptic organization in the dorsal cochlear nucleus of the cat: a light and electron microscope study. *J. Comp. Neurol. 155:* 301-330, 1974b.

Kane, E.C. Descending projections to specific regions of cat cochlear nucleus: a light microscopic study. *Exper. Neurol. 52:* 372-388, 1976.

Kane, E.C. Descending inputs to the octopus cell area of the cat cochlear nucleus: an electron microscopic study. *J. Comp. Neurol. 173:* 337-354, 1977a.

Kane, E.C. Autoradiographic evidence of primary projections to the caudal cochlear nucleus in cats. Manuscript submitted, 1977b.

Kiang, N.Y.S., Morest, D.K., Godfrey, D.A., Guinan, J.J.Jr. and Kane, E.C. Stimulus coding at caudal levels of the cat's auditory nervous system: I. Response characteristics of single units. In: *Basic Mechanisms in Hearing,* edited by A. Møller. New York: Academic Press, 1973, p. 455-478.

Lorente de Nó, R. Anatomy of the eighth nerve. III. General plan of structure of the primary cochlear nuclei. *Laryngoscope 43:* 327-350, 1933.

Morest, D.K., Kiang, N.Y.S., Kane, E.C., Guinan, J.J.Jr. and Godrey, D.A. Stimulus coding at caudal levels of the cat's auditory nervous system: II. Patterns of synaptic organization. In: *Basic Mechanisms in Hearing,* edited by A. Møller. New York: Academic Press, 1973, p. 479-509.

Olsen, K.K. Cytoarchitecture of the cochlear nuclei in the cat. *J. Comp. Neurol. 136:* 453-484, 1969.

Ramón y Cajal, S. *L'Histologie du Systéme Nerveux de L'homme et des Vertébrés. Vol 1,* 1909. Reprinted by Instituto Ramón y Cajal, 1952, p. 754-838.

Schwartz, A.M. and Kane, E.C. Development of the octopus cell area in the cat ventral cochlear nucleus. *Amer. J. Anat. 148:* 1-18, 1977.

DISCUSSION

Davis: I would like to congratulate Dr. Kane and point out what I believe is the tremendous importance of this particular work and other work of this type for those of us who are concerned with responses from brain stem and higher in the nervous system. Most of us have grown up with very simplified working models of the functional anatomy of the central nervous system and we draw very simple diagrams of the auditory tract, from the cochlea up to the cortex. Dr. Kane's fundamental point is that already in the cochlear nucleus there is subdivision, anatomical branching of the dendrites, different groupings of cells on which they terminate, and different physiological functions related to them.

Our problem is going to be to learn to *think at least in triplicate* from now on. I will point out, when it comes to the brain stem responses, that we will be dealing with one particular functional group, namely, the timekeepers. They are "On units" that simply respond once, very regularly and reliably, to each incoming volley. I would like to ask Dr. Kane whether there is in the cochlear nucleus a synaptic arrangement of this kind, the envelopes of Held, which seem very well adapted for this one-to-one type of transmission. These are not on the octopus cells, are they?

Kane: Thank you. No, the end-bulbs of Held are classically defined as being in the rostral region of AVCN (Held, 1893; Ramón y Cajal, 1909). The end-bulbs are much larger than the large OCA endings I showed you, and they would, in fact, be a site for very secure synaptic contact, if I may use that phrase. People are, in fact, doing the same kinds of studies (ie. understanding complete synaptic organization) of that zone (AVCN) too. Again, I think it is important to emphasize that there are other than primary inputs to that region too, which have to be taken into consideration.

Warr: Do you have any evidence, Eileen, that the cochlear nerve may provide synaptic contacts which are both excitatory and inhibitory? Maybe you could explain the state of the art now in recognizing excitatory and inhibitory endings.

Kane: I have no evidence that these endings are excitatory versus inhibitory. It seems, from the work that I have read and studied and talked about (see Kiang et al., 1973), most of them seem to be excitatory. For those of you who are not familiar with the "state of the art", the two types of endings I showed you are classically associated with excitation versus inhibition in other regions of the brain, particularly the cortex (Bodian, 1966; Eccles, 1969), but I think we have enough studies now of nice correlations between cytology and electrophysiology that demonstrate that that correlation between, say, large round vesicles and excitation need not hold true (Sotelo, 1971). Maybe Dr. Kiang might want to comment further on it at this stage.

Kiang: In my opinion the discussions here are too simple to do justice to the complexity of the system. Dr. Davis said that you have to learn to think of this at least in triplicate. I would like to emphasize the phrase "at least". The auditory nervous system consists of a great many different kinds of cells along with their processes and endings. Just to find out the response characteristics of each element is going to take considerable work to say nothing about measuring the effective voltage developed at the gross electrodes from such activity.

Huang: Dr. Kane, from your morphological studies can you identify elements responsible for secure synaptic transmission? For example, the calyxes of Held would ensure secure synaptic transmission; on the other hand, the octopus cells would seem to me to have very secure synapses, judging from their highly repeatable discharge patterns but they have drastically different morphological features.

Kane: For one thing, the response pattern in the two region (AVCN and OCA) is somewhat different (Godfrey et al., 1975). As Dr. Kiang mentioned, the "on" unit is only one kind of response pattern one can look at. There are many others (Godfrey, 1971). If one has evoked responses or uses other stimuli you get an entirely different picture. From the morphological point of view, the end-bulbs of Held are endings with several sites of synaptic complexes, whereas with PVCN the endings are numerous and smaller (Kane, 1973). The number of actual contacts are about comparable to those in the AVCN. One would expect you would not get too many differences in terms of the effect of a lot of these afferent endings impinging on octopus cells as opposed to one large one encompassing the entire surface. Of course, there will be temporal factors.

Bodian, D. Synaptic types on spinal motorneurons: an electron microscope study. *Bull. Johns Hopkins Hosp, 119:* 16-45, 1966.

Eccles, J.C. *The Inhibitory Pathways of the Central Nervous System.* Liverpool: Liverpool University Press, 1969.

Godfrey, D.A. Localization of single units in the cochlear nucleus of the cat. Ph.D. thesis, Harvard University, 1971.

Godfrey, D.A., Kiang, N.Y.S. and Norris, B.E. Single unit activity in the posteroventral cochlear nucleus of the cat. *J. Comp. Neurol. 162:* 247-268, 1975.

Held, H. Die centrale Gehörleitung, *Arch. Anat. Physiol. Abteil.* 201-248, 1893.

Kane, E.C. Octopus cells in the cochlear nucleus of the cat: Heterotypic synapses upon homeotypic neurons. *Internat. J. Neurosci. 5:* 251-279, 1973.

Kiang, N.Y.S., Morest, D.K. Godfrey, D.A., Guinan, J.J. and Kane, E.C. Stimulus coding at caudal levels of the cat's auditory nervous system. I. Response characteristics of single units. In: *Basic Mechanisms in Hearing,* edited by A. Møller. New York: Plenum Press, 1973, p. 455-478.

Ramón y Cajal, S. *L'Histologie du Système Nerveux de L'Homme et des Vertébrés.* Reprinted by Consejo Superior de Investigaciones Cientificos. Madrid: Instituto Ramón y Cajal, 1952.

Sotelo, C. General features of the synaptic organization in the central nervous system. In: *Chemistry and Brain Development*, edited by R. Paoletti and A.N. Davison. New York: Plenum Press, 1971, p. 239-280.

THE AUDITORY SYSTEM OF THE BRAIN STEM

John M. Harrison

Boston University

It is the purpose of this paper to describe the ascending connections of the auditory system of the brain stem as revealed by anatomical methods. Emphasis will be placed upon the cellular details of connections between the various nuclei of the ascending system.

COCHLEAR NUCLEUS AND SUPERIOR OLIVARY COMPLEX

The central auditory system arises from nerve cells in the dorsal and ventral cochlear nuclei, the axons of these neurons innervating the superior olivary complex and the inferior colliculus. The details of the cochlear nuclei have been described elsewhere in this volume (see also Brawer, et al., 1974).

The superior olivary complex is shown schematically in Figure 1. The major ascending nuclei are the medial and lateral superior olivary nuclei, and the medial and lateral nuclei of the trapezoid body. The periolivary cell groups which surround the ascending nuclei are concerned principally with the descending system (Adams and Warr, 1976; Harrison and Howe, 1974b) and they will not be further considered here. The region of the ventral cochlear nucleus which contains the round cells (Osen, 1969; Harrison and Irving, 1966a) innervates the medial and lateral superior olivary nuclei (Warr, 1966, Stotler, 1953; van Noort, 1969; Strominger and Strominger, 1971; Harrison and Irving, 1966a; Goldberg and Brown, 1968; Borg, 1973a; West and Harrison, 1973; Barnes, et al., 1943; Powell and Cowan, 1962). While it is not certain that it is the round cells which innervate the two olivary nuclei, it has been suggested that the larger round cells at the most anterior end of the ventral cochlear nucleus innervate the medial superior olive and that the small spherical cells innervate the lateral superior olive.

This suggestion is based on several considerations. Large spherical cells are not prominent or are absent in those species in which the medial superior olivary nucleus is either small or absent, while the small spherical cells are always present (Harrison and Howe, 1974a; Osen, 1969, 1970). Studies of the innervation of the cochlear nucleus by the cochlea have been interpreted as showing that only the middle and apical parts of the cochlea are connected with the anterior part of the ventral cochlear nucleus, thus limiting the region of the large spherical cells to low and intermediate frequencies. The region of the small spherical cells is connected

ISBN 0-12-514960-3

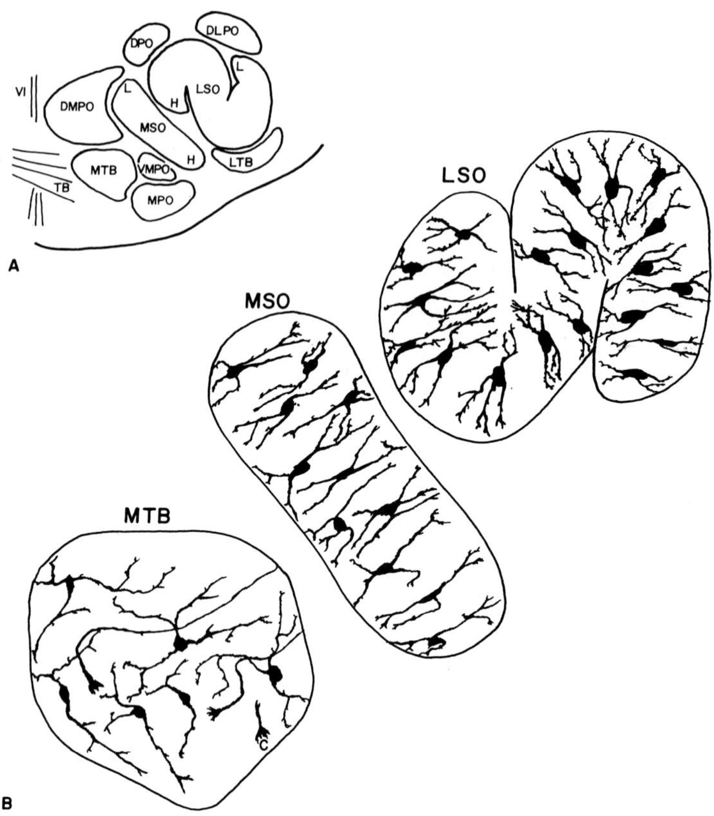

Fig. 1. A. Major nuclear groups of the superior olivary complex. The lateral and medial superior olive and the medial and lateral nuclei of the trapezoid body are the ascending nuclei. The other nuclei are associated with the descending system. B. The arrangement of principal cells in the major ascending nuclei as shown by Ramon y Cajal, 1952. C, calyx of Held: DLPO, dorsolateral periolivary cell group: DMPO, dorsomedial periolivary cell group: DPO, dorsal periolivary cell group: H-L, high-low frequency representation: LTB, lateral nucleus of the trapezoid body: LSO, lateral superior olive: MPO, medial periolivary nucleus: MSO, medial superior olivary nucleus: MTB, medial nucleus of the trapezoid body: TB, trapezoid body: VMPO, ventromedial periolivary cell group.

to the full length of the cochlea (Moskowitz and Liu, 1972; Webster, 1971; Osen, 1970). Physiological studies have indicated that low and intermediate frequencies are predominently represented in the medial superior olivary nucleus (Guinan, et al., 1972).

The details of the innervation of the medial superior olivary nucleus were first shown by Stotler (1953) (Fig. 2). The cells of the medial superior olive are fusiform with a laterally and medially directed dendrite. The dendrites are covered with a large number of small synaptic endings as shown in the top of the figure.

Destruction of the anterior ventral cochlear nucleus on one side leads to the degeneration of synaptic endings, bilaterally, on the dendrites on the same side of the cell as the damaged cochlear nucleus. The cells are thus binaurally innervated. Electronmicroscopic study of the cells of the medial superior olivary nucleus confirms that the great majority of the terminals are of cochlear nucleus origin (Perkins, 1973; Clark, 1969). Warr (1966) placed small lesions in the anterior ventral cochlear nucleus and found that more dorsal parts of the cochlear nucleus projected to more ventral parts of the medial olive and the more ventral parts of the nucleus project to the more dorsal parts of the medial olive, indicating topographic projection from the cochlear nucleus.

The medial nucleus of the trapezoid body is innervated from the globular (bushy) cells located in the middle part of the ventral cochlear nucleus of the opposite side. The axons of the globular cells which run in the trapezoid body end

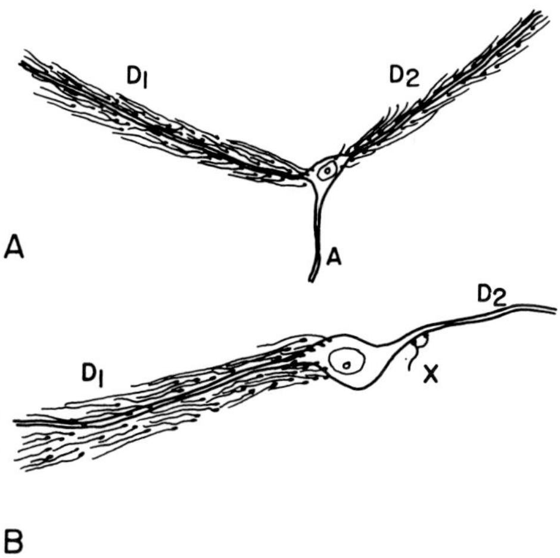

Fig. 2. Innervation of cells of the medial superior olive after Stotler, 1953. A. Normal appearance of cell of the medial superior olive. B. Appearance after destruction of cochlear nucleus of the right side. A few endings remain, as shown at X. D1 and D2 are the medial and lateral dendrites of the cells.

on the principal cells of the medial nucleus with a single calyx of Held (Harrison and Warr, 1962; Harrison and Irving, 1964, 1966a; Tolbert and Morest, 1977; Jean-Baptiste and Morest, 1975).

Like the medial superior olive, the lateral superior olivary nucleus is also bilaterally innervated (Harrison and Feldman, 1970). The spherical cell area of the anterior ventral cochlear nucleus innervates the ipsilateral lateral superior olive (Warr, 1966; Stotler, 1953; Harrison and Irving, 1966a). Warr's (1966) data also indicate that this innervation is topographic, the ventromedial portion of the "S" being innervated from the more dorsal part of the cochlear nucleus, and the lateral part of the "S" being innervated from more ventral parts of the cochlear nucleus. The contralateral innervation of lateral superior olive reaches it from the cochlear nucleus via the medial nucleus of the trapezoid body of the same side (Harrison and Warr, 1962; Rasmussen, 1965; van Noort, 1969; Browner and Webster, 1975).

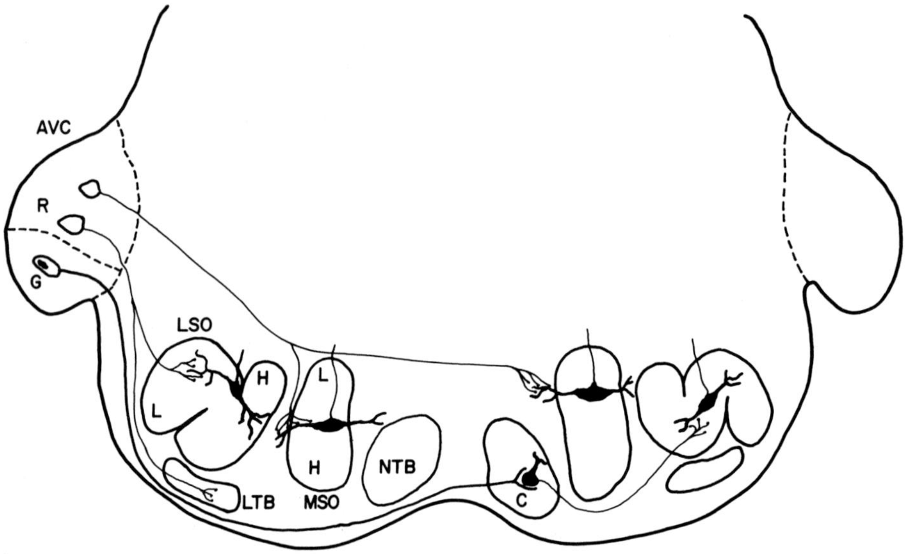

Fig. 3. Summary of ascending connections to the superior olivary complex. AVC, anterior ventral cochlear nucleus: C, chalice of Held: G, globular cell region: H, L, high and low frequencies: LSO, lateral superior olive: LTB, lateral nucleus of the trapezoid body: MSO, medial superior olive: NTB, medial nucleus of the trapezoid body: R, round cell region.

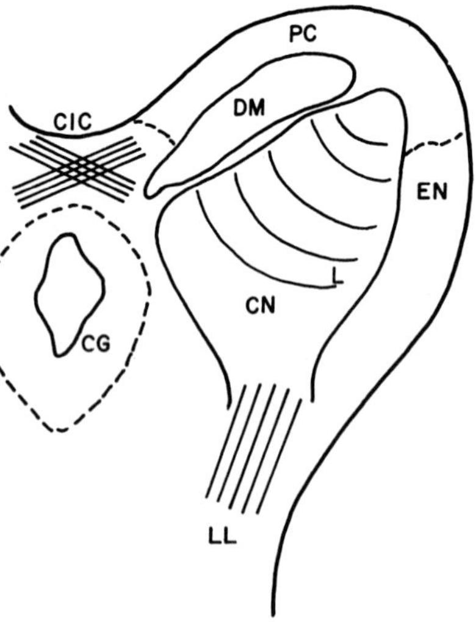

Fig. 4. Major divisions of the inferior colliculus, schematic transverse section. CG, central grey: CIC commissure of inferior colliculus: CN, central nucleus: DM, dorsomedial nucleus: EN, external nuclei: L, orientation of laminae: LL, lateral lemniscus: PC, pericentral nucleus.

These connections are summarized in Figure 3. The bilateral innervation of the medial and lateral superior olivary nuclei has attracted considerable attention because of the implications of this mode of innervation for localization in azimuth (Erulkar, 1972).

The lateral nucleus of the trapezoid body is innervated from the anterior ventral cochlear nucleus of the same side, but the details of innervation are not well understood (Harrison and Irving, 1966a, 1966b; Warr, 1966).

The anatomical and behavioral investigation of the two middle ear reflexes indicates that the Vth and VIIth motor nuclei receive axons from cells located in the region of the medial superior olivary nucleus, although the cells of origin have not been identified (Borg, 1973b; Browner and Webster, 1975). It is assumed that these connections are part of the reflex paths from the cochlea to the two muscles.

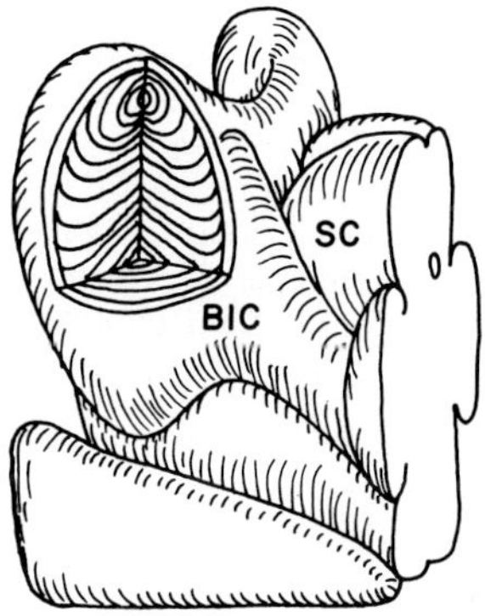

Fig. 5. Schematic representation of the laminae of the central nucleus of the inferior colliculus reconstructed from Golgi preparations. Redrawn from Rockel and Jones, 1973a. BIC, brachium of inferior colliculus: SC, superior colliculus.

INFERIOR COLLICULUS

The major subdivisions of the inferior colliculus are shown in Figure 4. The colliculus consists of a central cell mass, the central nucleus, and a surrounding capsule of nerve cells forming the pericentral (dorsal and caudal cortex) and external nuclei (lateral zone). The dorsomedial part of the central nucleus (the dorsomedial nucleus) is differentiated from the central nucleus (Geniec and Morest, 1971; Rockel and Jones, 1973a). The central is the major ascending nucleus, receiving the ascending axons from the lateral lemiscus (Goldberg and Moore, 1967; Rockel and Jones, 1973a, 1973b; Morest, 1964). The dorsomedial and pericentral nuclei are innervated from the auditory cortex and form part of the descending system (Rockel and Jones, 1973b, van Noort, 1969; Diamond, et al., 1969; Forbes and Moskowitz, 1974; Martin, 1969; Martin and Megirian, 1972; Harting and Martin, 1970; Casseday, et al., 1976). The external nucleus is innervated from the efferent axons of the central nucleus and also from the gracile and cuneate nuclei (Moore and Goldberg, 1961, 1963, 1965; Jones and Rockel, 1971; Jones and Powell, 1971; Powell and Hatton, 1969; Rasmussen, 1961; Tarlov and Moore, 1966; van Noort, 1969; Schroeder and Jane, 1976).

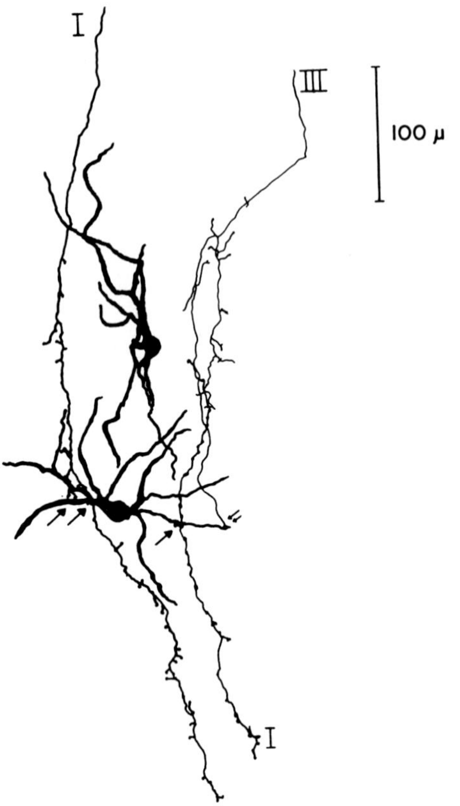

Fig. 6. Type I and III axons in the central nucleus of the inferior colliculus. Type I are the ascending axons from the lateral lemniscus. They make contact with the proximal dendrites of principal cells (large arrows) and the dendrites of the small multipolar cells (not shown). Type III axons (origin unknown) contact the more distal parts of the dendrites (small arrows) of principal cells and make climbing contact with the dendrites of the small multipolar cells (not shown). Both axon types run in the laminae. Redrawn from Rockel and Jones, 1973a.

The central nucleus consists of principal cells and small and large stellate (multipolar) cells. The principle cells have been tentatively divided into two classes on the basis of the orientation of their dendrites (bitufted and fusiform principal cells) (Rockel and Jones, 1973a). It was first shown by Morest (1964) that the cell bodies and dendritic fields of the principal cells were arranged into layers or laminae within the central nucleus. The ascending axons from the lateral lemniscus ascend through the central nucleus along these laminae. The arrangement of the laminae in the cat as worked out by Rockel and Jones (1973a) is shown in Figure 5. FitzPatrick (1975) has shown an analagous arrangement in the monkey. It is assumed that these laminae form the basis of the topographical projection of lower nuclei upon the central nucleus.

The central nucleus has been found to have three major classes of axons (Rockel and Jones, 1973a, 1973c). Type I, the ascending axons, enter the central nucleus from the lateral lemniscus and ascend in the laminae (Fig. 6). These axons are of large diameter (5μ to 8μ diameter), beaded (en passent synaptic regions), and have short side branches ending in terminal enlargements. These enlargements make contact with the spines on the basal dendrites of the principal cells. The en passent synaptic regions contact the more distal dendrites of the multipolar cells.

As will be shown, ascending lemniscal axons arise from a number of different sources (and nerve cell types) and it is surprising that only one type of ascending axon has been identified in the central nucleus. Type IV axons (Figure 7) arise from the principal cells and are thought to be the efferent axons of the central nucleus, running in the brachium of the inferior colliculus (Morest, 1964; Rockel and Jones, 1973a). These axons give rise to a number of collaterals after leaving the cell body, the collaterals ramifying in the vicinity of the parent cell.

Type III axons, which are of intermediate thickness, also run in the laminae (Fig. 6). These axons make contact via fine sprays of endings with the more distal parts of the dendrites of the principal cells. Type III axons also form climbing contacts along the dendrites of the multipolar cells. The origin of these axons is not known.

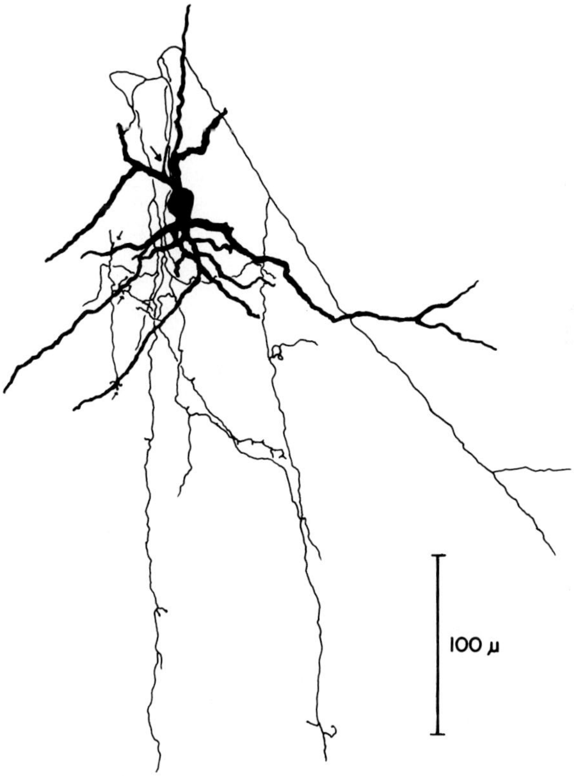

Fig. 7. Type IV axon, central nucleus of inferior colliculus. The axon arises (large arrow) from a principal cell. The collaterals apparently make contact (small arrow) with the dendrites of the parent cell. Redrawn from Rockel and Jones, 1973a.

Ascending axons to the central nucleus arise from three major sources, the cochlear nuclei, the superior olivary complex and the nuclei of the lateral lemniscus.

The central nucleus is innervated from both the dorsal and ventral cochlear nuclei (Figure 8). The fusiform cells of the dorsal cochlear nucleus give rise to axons which run to the central nucleus of the opposite side via the dorsal acoustic stria. These same axons, or axons from other cells in the dorsal cochlear nucleus, innervate the ventral and dorsal nuclei of the lateral lemniscus of the opposite side (von Monokow, 1891; Warr, 1969; van Noort, 1969; Strominger, 1973; Osen, 1972; Fernandez and Karapas, 1967; Goldberg and Brown, 1968; Adams and Warr, 1976).

The spherical cell regions of the anterior ventral cochlear nucleus which innervate the medial and lateral superior olivary nuclei also send axons to the contralateral central nucleus and the ventral and dorsal nuclei of the lateral

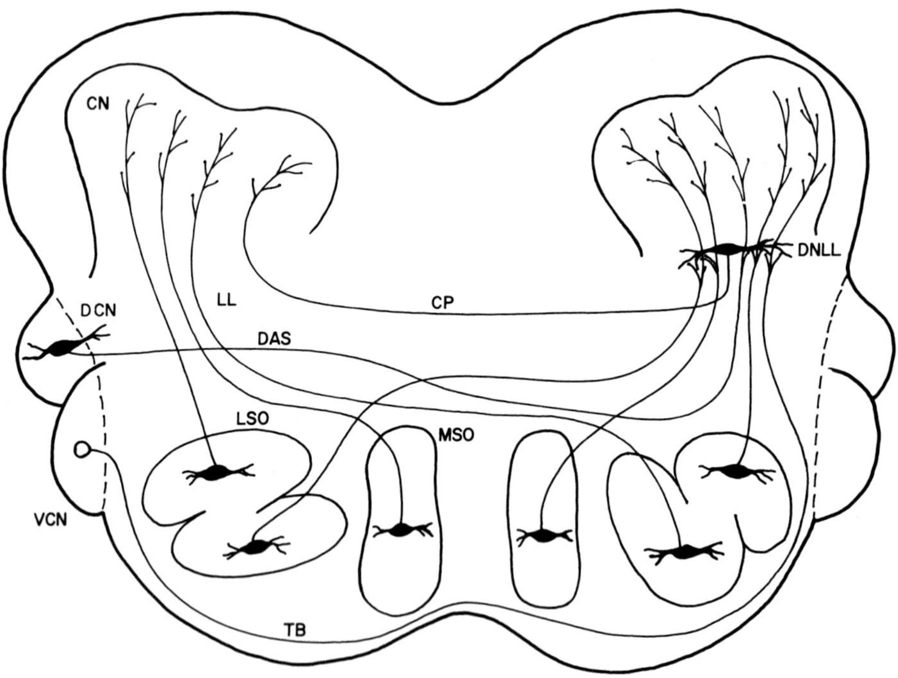

Fig. 8. Summary of the projection of the cochlear nuclei and superior olivary complex on the central nucleus of the inferior colliculus. CN, central nucleus: CP, commissure of Probst: DAS, dorsal acoustic stria: DCN, dorsal cochlear nucleus: DNLL, dorsal nucleus of lateral lemniscus: LL, lateral lemniscus: LSO, lateral superior olive: MSO, medial superior olive: TB, trapezoid body: VCN, ventral cochlear nucleus.

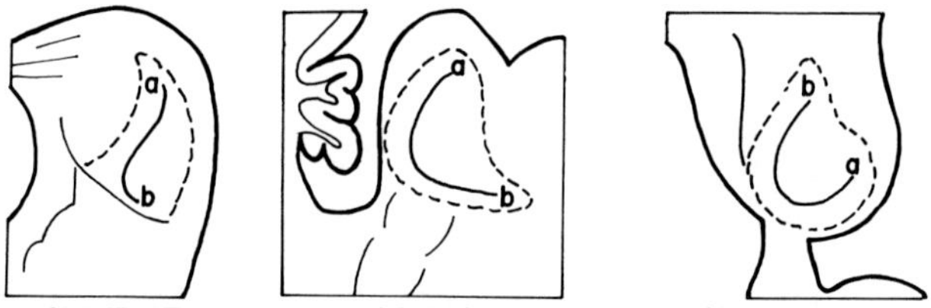

Fig. 9. Projection of the cochlear nuclei on the central nucleus of the inferior colliculus, based on Osen, 1972. a and b, projection of apical and basal ends of the cochlea.

lemniscus (Warr, 1966; Harrison and Irving, 1966a; Goldberg and Brown, 1968; Strominger and Strominger, 1971; van Noort, 1969). Warr's (1966) observations suggest the medial and lateral superior olivary nuclei receive collaterals of axons which continue to higher levels. Other data indicate that the spherical cells of the ventral cochlear nucleus innervate the contralateral central nucleus (Brusno-Bechtold and Thompson, 1976). These two sets of observations suggest that the superior olivary complex and the central nucleus of the inferior colliculus are innervated from the same nerve cells.

Lesions of the globular cell area of the ventral cochlear nucleus also produce degeneration in the contralateral central nucleus and the nuclei of the lateral lemniscus, but the cells of origin have not been identified (Warr, 1972).

Some experimenters report ipsilateral as well as contralateral innervation of the central nucleus by the cochlear nuclei. When such innervation is noted it is always reported as being less than the contralateral innervation.

It has been assumed that the laminar arrangement of the central nucleus is the basis of the tonotopic projection that has been reported in physiological experiments (FitzPatrick, 1975; Merzenich and Reid, 1974). It is, however, difficult to discover the nature of the topographical projection of the cochlear nuclei upon the central nucleus because of the nature of the projection of the cochlea on the cochlea nuclei (van Noort, 1969). Ideally, thin sheet-like lesions would have to be made in the cochlear nuclei to produce isofrequency bundles of degenerating axons. In spite of the difficulties, Osen (1972) has indicated that there is a topographical projection of the cochlear nuclei on the central nucleus. Small lesions were made in the anterior ventral cochlear nucleus and the dorsal cochlear nucleus and the resulting degeneration was mapped in transverse, sagittal and horizontal planes in each animal. The results are shown in Figure 9. The anatomical projection is in agreement with the functional maps to the extent that both indicate that frequency increases with increases in depth from the dorsal edge of the central nucleus.

Some experimenters have reported degeneration at higher levels than the inferior colliculus following lesions of the cochlear nuclei. Warr (1966), Strominger

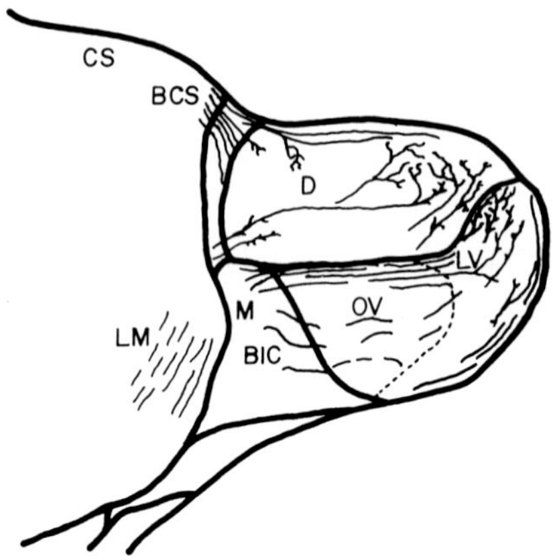

Fig. 10. Schematic transverse section of medial geniculate body showing major divisions, after Morest, 1964. BCS, brachium of superior colliculus: BIC, brachium of inferior colliculus: CS, superior colliculus: D, dorsal division: LV and OV, ventral division: LM, medial lemniscus: M, medial division.

(1973) and Strominger and Strominger (1971) reported degeneration in the brachium of the inferior colliculus or the medial division of the medial geniculate body. These data, however, were conservatively interpreted as not violating the general view that all ascending axons do not penetrate beyond the inferior colliculus. Recently, however, Strominger, et al., (1977) have reported considerable degeneration in the magnocellular (medial) and principal (ventral part) divisions of the medial geniculate body in the chimpanzee following destruction of the cochlear nuclei of one side. The authors consider these data to show that lemniscal axons penetrate beyond the colliculus in chimpanzee, and suggest that apes and humans may possess a different organization of this part of the auditory system from that found in other forms.

The projection of the medial and lateral superior olivary nuclei to the central nucleus is shown schematically in Figure 8. The medial superior olive projects to the central nucleus of the same side, while the lateral superior olive projects to the central nucleus of both sides (Stotler, 1953; van Noort, 1969; Browner and Webster, 1975; Brusno-Bechtold and Thompson, 1976). Whether this projection is topographical is not known.

Lesions of the lateral lemniscus which include the dorsal nucleus of the lemniscus produce degeneration in the commissure of Probst (1902) and the contralateral central nucleus (Goldberg and Moore, 1967; Casseday, et al., 1976) (Figure 8). The degeneration produced by high lemniscal lesions is confined to the central nucleus (with slight penetration to the dorsomedial nucleus) and to type I synaptic terminals (Goldberg and Moore, 1967; Jones and Rockel, 1973; Jones and Rockel, 1971; Rokel and Jones, 1973c). The distribution of degeneration in the central nucleus following high lemniscal lesions is the same as that following destruction of the various sources of the lateral lemniscus.

ASCENDING CONNECTIONS OF THE MEDIAL GENICULATE BODY

The medial geniculate body consists of ventral, medial and dorsal divisions; the ventral is the principal ascending division (Figure 10). The ventral division, composed of ovoid and lateral parts, is composed of principal cells and Golgi type II nerve cells. The cell bodies and tufted dendrites of the principal cells were shown by Morest (1964, 1966), to be arranged into layers or laminae as shown schematically in Figure 11. The afferent axons from the inferior colliculus enter and ascend in the laminae. The afferent axons give rise to dense multivesicular synaptic terminals which are part of the complex synaptic nests found in the ventral division (Morest, 1975; Majorossy and Kiss, 1976a, 1976b; Majorossy and Rethelyi, 1968; Jones and Rockel, 1971). The arrangement as worked out by Morest is shown in Figure 12, together with the direction of synaptic action. The multivesicular terminals arise from the afferent axons, pale terminals are terminal dendritic processes of the Golgi type II cells.

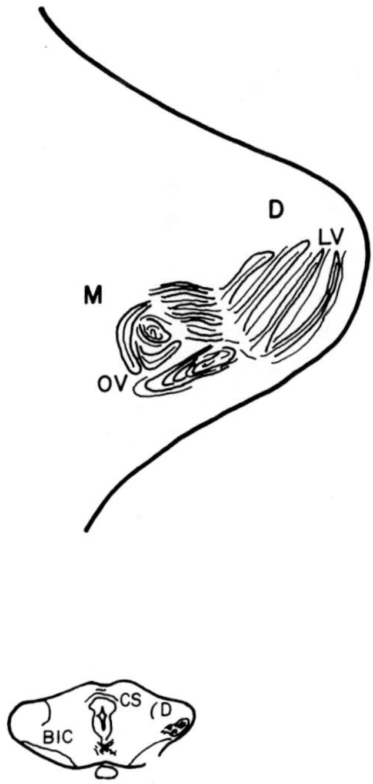

Fig. 11. Schematic transverse section of the medial geniculate body showing the general arrangement of the laminae, after Morest, 1965. Inset shows position of ventral division. BIC, brachium of inferior colliculus: CS, superior colliculus: D, dorsal division of medial geniculate body: LV, lateral part of ventral division: M, medial division of medial geniculate body: OV, ovoid part of ventral division.

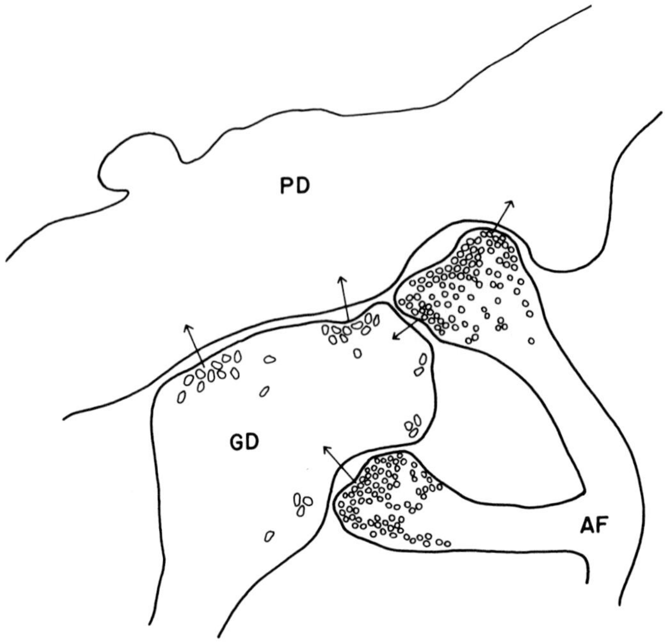

Fig. 12. Schematic illustration of a synaptic nest in the ventral division of the medial geniculate body, after Morest, 1975. The corticogeniculate axons (AF) terminate on the dendrites of the principal cells (PD) and Golgi type II cells. The endings contain many round vesicles and the synaptic contacts are asymmetrical. The dendrites of the Golgi type II cells (GD) make contact with the dendrites of the principal cells. The vesicles are larger and flattened. Arrows indicate the presumed direction of synaptic action.

The medial (magnocellular) division of the medial geniculate body contains nerve cells with both radiate and tufted arrangements of dendrites. This division also receives afferent axons from the inferior colliculus, but the details of its innervation have not been extensively explored (Morest, 1964, 1966).

Lesions of the central nucleus of the inferior colliculus produce degeneration in the ipsilateral and contralateral ventral divisions of the geniculate body. Ipsilaterally, degeneration can be followed through the damaged central nucleus to the brachium of the inferior colliculus. Some axons are given off to the external nucleus (Figure 13). Axons terminate in the interstitial nucleus of the brachium and the parabrachial area. The majority of axons terminate in the ventral division of the medial geniculate body (Powell and Hatton, 1969; Casseday, et al., 1976; Moore and Goldberg, 1963, 1966; Moore and Tarlov, 1963; Carey and Webster, 1971; Tarlov and Moore, 1966; Woolard and Hartman, 1940; Rasmussen, 1961; van Noort, 1969). As already indicated, it is the dark multi-vesicular endings which degenerate following such lesions. Small lesions placed in the central nucleus have not revealed a clear topographical projection of the nucleus on the medial

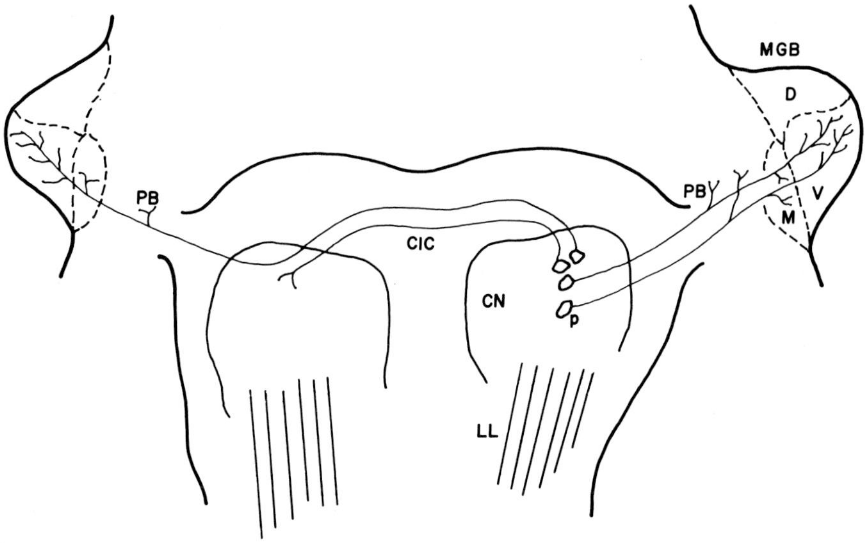

Fig. 13. Summary of the efferent connections of the central nucleus of the inferior colliculus, schematic transverse section. CIC, commissure of inferior colliculus: CN, central nucleus: D, dorsal division of the MGB: LL, lateral lemniscus: M, medial division of the MGB: MGB, medial geniculate body: PB, parabrachial region: p, principal cells.

geniculate body (Casseday, et al., 1976). The axons of the principal cells of the ventral division project to the auditory cortex. All the foregoing experiments also reported that some brachium axons gave rise to terminal endings in the medial divisions of the geniculate.

Prominent connections to the superior colliculus from the inferior colliculus are not reported. Powell and Hatton (1969) and Moore and Goldberg (1963, 1965) report some evidence of innervation of the deeper layers on the posterior superior colliculus. Other workers, however, do not mention such connections (Casseday, et al., 1976, for example).

Contralaterally, degeneration runs through the commissure of the inferior colliculus, some terminal degeneration being found in the contralateral central nucleus, to the brachium. Axons pass from here to the medial and ventral divisions of the geniculate in smaller numbers than on the ipsilateral side. Innervation of the dorsal division of the medial geniculate body was not reported in any of the aforementioned experiments.

REFERENCES

Adams, J. and Warr, B. Origins of axons in the cat's acoustic striae determined by injection of HRP into several tracts. *J. Comp. Neurol. 170:* 107-122, 1976.

Barnes, W.T., Magoun, H.W., and Ranson, S.W. Ascending auditory pathways in the brain stem of the monkey. *J. Comp. Neurol. 79:* 129-152, 1943.

Borg, E. Neuroanatomical study of the brain stem auditory system of the rabbit. Part I. Ascending connections. *Acta Morphol. Neerl. Scand. 11:* 31-48, 1973a.

Borg, E. On the neural organization of the acoustic middle ear reflex. A physiological and anatomical study. *Brain Res. 49:* 101-123, 1973b.

Brawer, J.R., Morest, D.K. and Kane, E.C. The neuronal architecture of the cochlear nucleus of the cat. *J. Comp. Neurol. 155:* 251-300, 1974.

Browner, R.H. and Webster, D.B. Projections of the trapezoid body on the superior olivary complex of the kangaroo rat. *Brain Behav. Evol. 11:* 322-354, 1975.

Brusno-Bechtold, J.K. and Thompson, G.C. Auditory hindbrain projections to the inferior colliculus as demonstrated by HRP in the cat. *Anat. Rec. 184:* 365, 1976.

Carey, C.L. and Webster, D.B. The projection of the inferior colliculus in the kangaroo rat. *Anat. Rec. 169:* 289, 1971.

Casseday, J.H., Diamond, I.T. and Harting, J.K. Auditory pathways to the cortex in *Tupaia glis. J. Comp. Neurol. 166:* 303-340, 1976.

Clark, G.M. The ultrastructure of endings in the medial superior olivary nucleus in the cat. *Brain Res. 14:* 293-305, 1969.

Diamond, I.T., Jones, E.G. and Powell, T.P.S. Projection of the auditory cortex upon the diencephalon and brain stem in the cat. *Brain Res. 15:* 305-340, 1969.

Erulkar, S.D. Comparative aspects of spatial localization of sound. *Physiol. Rev. 52:* 277-360, 1972.

Fernández, C. and Karapas, F. The course and termination of the stria of Monakow and Held in the cat. *J. Comp. Neurol. 131:* 371-386, 1967.

FitzPatrick, K.A. Cellular architecture and topographic organization of the inferior colliculus in the squirrel monkey. *J. Comp. Neurol. 164:* 185-208, 1975.

Forbes, B.F. and Moskowitz, N. Projection of the auditory responsive cortex in the squirrel monkey. *Brain Res. 67:* 239-254, 1974.

Geniec, P. and Morest, D.K. The neuronal architecture of the human posterior colliculus. *Acta Otolaryngol.* Suppl. *295:* 1-33, 1971.

Goldberg, J.M. and Brown, P.B. Functional organization of the dog superior olivary complex: an anatomical and electrophysiological study. *J. Neurophysiol. 31:* 639-656, 1968.

Goldberg, J.M. and Moore, R.Y. Ascending projection of the lateral lemniscus in cat and monkey. *J. Comp. Neurol. 129:* 143-155, 1967.

Guinan, J., Guinan, S. and Norris. B. Single auditory units in the superior olivary complex. I: responses to sound and classification based on physiological properties. *Internat. J. Neurosci. 4:* 101-120, 1972.

Harrison, J.M. and Feldman, M.L. Anatomical aspects of the cochlear nucleus and superior olivary complex. In: *Contributions to Sensory Physiology. Vol 4,* edited by W.D. Neff. New York: Academic Press, 1970, p. 95-142.

Harrison, J.M. and Howe, M.E. Anatomy of the afferent auditory system of mammals. In: *Handbook of Sensory Physiology. Vol. V/1,* edited by W.D. Keidel and W.D. Neff. Heidleberg: Springer-Verlag, 1974a, p. 282-336.

Harrison, J.M. and Howe, M.E. Anatomy of the descending auditory system (Mammals). In: *Handbook of Sensory Physiology, Vol. V/1,* edited by W.D. Keidel and W.D. Neff. Heidleberg: Springer-Verlag, 1974b, p. 363-388.

Harrison, J.M. and Irving, R. Nucleus of the trapezoid body; dual afferent innervation. *Science 143:* 473-474, 1964.

Harrison, J.M. and Irving, R. Ascending connections of the anterior ventral cochlear nucleus in the rat. *J. Comp. Neurol. 126:* 51-64, 1966a.

Harrison, J.M. and Irving, R. Organization of the posterior ventral cochlear nucleus in the rat. *J. Comp. Neurol. 126:* 391-403, 1966b.

Harrison, J.M. and Warr, B. The cochlear nucleus and ascending auditory pathways of the medulla. *J. Comp. Neurol. 119:* 341-380, 1962.

Harting, J.K. and Martin, G.F. Neocortical projection to the mesencephalon of the armadillo. *Brain Res. 17:* 447-462, 1970.

Jean-Baptiste, M. and Morest, D.K. Transneuronal changes in synaptic endings and nucleus chromatin in the trapezoid body following cochlear ablation in the cat. *J. Comp. Neurol. 162:* 111-134, 1975.

Jones, E.G. and Powell, T.P.S. An analysis of the posterior group of thalamic nuclei on the basis of its afferent connections. *J. Comp. Neurol. 143:* 185-216, 1971.

Jones, E.G. and Rockel, A.J. Observations on complex vesicles, neurofilamentous hyperplasia and electron density during terminal degeneration in the inferior colliculus. *J. Comp. Neurol. 147:* 93-118, 1973.

Jones, E.G. and Rockel, A.J. The synaptic organization in the medial geniculate body of afferent fibers ascending from the inferior colliculus. *Z. Zellforsch. Mikrosk. Anat. 113:* 44-66, 1971.

Majorossy, A. and Kiss, A. Specific pattern of neuron arrangement and of synaptic articulation in the medial geniculate body. *Exp. Brain Res. 26:* 1-17, 1976a.

Majorossy, A. and Kiss, A. Types of interneurons and their participation in the neuronal networks of the medial geniculate body. *Exp. Brain Res. 26:* 19-37, 1976b.

Majorossy, K. and Rethelyi, M. Synaptic architecture in the medial geniculate body (ventral division). *Exp. Brain Res. 6:* 306-323, 1968.

Martin, G.H. Efferent tectal pathways of the opossum *(Didelphis virginiana). Comp. Neurol. 135:* 209-224, 1969.

Martin, G.H. and Merigirian, D. Corticobulbar projections of the marsupial phalanger. *J. Comp. Neurol. 144:* 165-192, 1972.

Merzenich, M. and Reid, M.D. Representation of the cochlea within the inferior colliculus of the cat. *Brain Res. 77:* 397-415, 1974.

Moore, R.Y. and Goldberg, J.M. Midbrain auditory connections in the cat. *Anat. Rec. 139:* 256, 1961.

Moore, R.Y., and Goldberg, J.M. Ascending projection of the inferior colliculus in the cat. *J. Comp. Neurol. 121:* 109-135, 1963.

Moore, R.Y. and Goldberg, J.M. Ascending connections of the inferior colliculus in the macque monkey. *Anat. Rec. 129:* 389-390, 1965.

Moore, R.Y. and Tarlov, E.C. Ascending projections of the inferior colliculus of the rabbit. *Anat. Rec. 145:* 262, 1963.

Monakow, C. von. Striae acousticae und untere Schleife. *Arch. Psychiat. Nervenkr. 22:* 1-26, 1891.

Morest, D.K. The laminar structure of the inferior colliculus of the cat. *Anat. Rec. 148:* 314, 1964.

Morest, D.K. The cortical structure of the inferior quadrigeminal lamina of the cat. *Anat. Rec. 154:* 389-390, 1966.

Morest, D.K. Synaptic relations of Golgi type II cells in the medial geniculate body of the cat. *J. Comp. Neurol. 162:* 157-194, 1975.

Moskowitz, N. and Liu, J.-C. Central projection of the spiral ganglion of the squirrel monkey. *J. Comp. Neurol. 144:* 335-344, 1972.

Osen, K.K. Cytoarchitecture of the cochlear nuclei in the cat. *J. Comp. Neurol. 136:* 453-483, 1969.

Osen, K.K. Course and termination of the primary afferents in the cochlear nucleus of the cat. *Arch. Ital. Biol. 108:* 21-61, 1970.

Osen, K.K. Projection of the cochlear nucleus in the inferior colliculus in the cat. *J. Comp. Neurol. 144:* 355-372, 1972.

Perkins, R.E. An electronmicroscopic study of the synaptic organization of the medial superior olivary nucleus of normal and experimental chinchillas. *J. Comp. Neurol. 148:* 387-416, 1973.

Powell, T.P.S. and Cowan, W.M. An experimental study of the projection of the cochlea. *J. Anat. 96:* 269-284, 1962.

Powell, W.E. and Hatten, J.B. Projections of the inferior colliculus in the cat. *J. Comp. Neurol. 136:* 183-192, 1969.

Probst, M. Experimentelle untersuchunger über die Anatomie und Physiologie der Leitungsbahnen der Gehirnstammes. *Arch. Anat. Physiol.* Suppl. *47:* 254, 1902.

Rasmussen, G.L. Distribution of fibers from the inferior colliculus. *Anat. Rec. 139:* 266, 1961.

Rasmussen, G.L. Efferent connections of the cochlear nucleus. In: *Sensori-neural Hearing Processes and Disorders,* edited by A.B. Graham. Boston: Little Brown, 1965, p. 61-76.

Rockel, A.J. and Jones, E.G. The neuronal organization of the inferior colliculus of the cat. I. The central nucleus. *J. Comp. Neurol. 147:* 11-60, 1973a.

Rockel, A.J. and Jones, E.G. The neuronal organization of the inferior colliculus of the cat. II. The pericentral nucleus. *J. Comp. Neurol. 149:* 301-334, 1973b.

Rockel, A.J. and Jones, E.G. Observations on the fine structure of the cochlear nucleus of the cat. *J. Comp. Neurol. 147:* 61-92, 1973c.

Stotler, W.A. An experimental study of the cells and connections of the superior olivary complex of the cat. *J. Comp. Neurol. 98:* 401-432, 1953.

Schroeder, D.M. and Jane, J.A. The intercolliculus area of the inferior colliculus. *Brain Behav. Evol. 13:* 125-141, 1976.

Strominger, N.L. The origin, course and distribution of the dorsal and intermediate acoustic stria in the monkey. *J. Comp. Neurol. 147:* 209-234, 1973.

Strominger, N.L., Nelson, L.R. and Dougherty, W.J. Second order auditory pathways in the chimpanzee. *J. Comp. Neurol. 172:* 349-366, 1977.

Strominger, N.L. and Strominger, A.I. Ascending brain stem projection of the anterior ventral cochlear nucleus in the monkey. *J. Comp. Neurol. 143:* 217-241, 1971.

Tarlov, E.C. and Moore, R.Y. The tecto-thalamic connections in the brain of the rabbit. *J. Comp. Neurol. 126:* 403-414, 1966.

Tolbert, L.P. and Morest, D.K. Combined Golgi, HRP and electronmicroscopic study of bushy cells in the cochlear nucleus. *Neurol. Abstr. 3:* 12, 1977.

van Noort, J. *The Structure and Connections of the Inferior Colliculus.* Netherlands: A. vanGorcum, 1969.

Warr, B. Fiber degeneration following lesions in the posterior ventral cochlear nucleus of the cat. *Exp. Neurol. 14:* 453-474, 1966.

Warr, B. Fiber degeneration following lesions in the anterior ventral cochlear nucleus of the cat. *Exp. Neurol. 23:* 140-155, 1969.

Warr, B. Fiber degeneration following lesions in the multipolar and globular cell areas in the ventral cochlear nucleus of the cat. *Brain Res. 40:* 247-270, 1972.

Webster, D.B. Projection of the cochlea to cochlear nucleus in Merriam's kangaroo rat. *J. Comp. Neurol. 143:* 323-341, 1971.

West, C. and Harrison, J.M. Transneuronal cell atrophy in the congenitally deaf white cat. *J. Comp. Neurol. 151:* 377-398, 1973.

Woolard, H.H. (the late) and Hartman, J.A. The connexions of the inferior colliculus and the dorsal nucleus of the lateral lemniscus. *J. Anat. 74:* 441-458, 1940.

DISCUSSION

Galambos: I would expand on Dr. Davis' point about a special neuronal pathway responsible for the brain stem evoked response. Some of us working on this system hypothesize a group of very precisely timed neurons, presumably a large axon rapidly conducting system, with extremely secure synapses, to explain the extraordinarily regular sequence of electrical events that make up the brain stem response.

Dr. Davis started this system for us in the cochlear nucleus and you have carried it via very large axons to the trapezoid nucleus of the superior olive. Where else does this end-bulb of Held system go? Where does the trapezoid nucleus project, and what are the terminals of its axons there?

Harrison: It projects to a lateral superior olive of the same size and its terminals are small. In other words, once you leave the level of the complex you don't find any of these large things any more.

Galambos: There are none in the nucleus of the lateral lemniscus?

Harrison: No. You have lost them there. One time we showed some large endings, but in general as you ascend the system they vanish.

Galambos: Our chairman has demonstrated physiologically that there are some extremely precise timing units in the anterior ventral cochlear nucleus, (Rose, J.E., Galambos, R. and Hughes, J.R. Microelectrode studies of the cochlear nucleus of the cat. *Johns Hopkins Med. J. 104:* 211-251, 1959) and in the inferior colliculus (Hind, J.E., Goldberg, J.M., Greenwood, D.D. and Rose, J.E. Some discharge characteristics of single neurons in the inferior colliculus of the cat. II. Timing of the discharges and observations on binaural stimulation. *J. Neurophysiol. 26:* 321-341, 1963). Precise timers also exist in the accessory superior olive (Galambos, R., Schwartzkopff, J. and Rupert, A. Microelectrode study of superior olivary nuclei. *Am. J. Physiol. 197:* 527-536, 1959).

Harrison: Don't forget that the pathway which Nelson was talking about earlier is not actually part of the ascending system, so you have to bear that in mind.

Galambos: What I am asking for is a special subdivision of the afferent system, up to the level of the inferior colliculus at least in which the moment of stimulus onset is exactly preserved. Presumably it consists of secure synapses and large fibers. Can you or any of the other anatomists here give us a notion of what this pathway might be?

Harrison: What you do find is that in the major ascending nuclei which I have talked about, the endings, whether they be small or large--you won't necessarily find large endings which you can point to as being very secure in this sense, but I think you can point to the fact that the vast majority of endings in the major ascending system are in fact ascending endings; so you don't have a lot of endings from other places coming in which might muddy things up.

I think one could say you have a very large number of small endings, all of which arise from a few axons, rather than one big one that might in fact act to approximate the same thing, if that will satisfy you. I think that is probably how you have to look at it.

Thornton: If I may follow Bob Galambos' point, we are getting very precise timing results in brain stem recordings, and it leads me to worry that what you described as the major pathway–in other words, the pathways that are major from the anatomical point of view–the pathways that are perhaps major in the signal processing aspects of the physiology of the system–may not be the pathways that are important in generating evoked responses in the brain stem potentials.

In other words, it may be that all that is required for an evoked potential is good synchrony, and the pathways that provide this may, in terms of anatomy and processing, be very much minor pathways within your frames of reference. Would you comment on that?

Harrison: Well, first of all I would not lightly dismiss these. These are physically large compared to other ascending pathways. I don't want to go into behavioral lesion studies. Here you start breaking down the various kinds of auditory control behavior. They are in fact doing something with respect to the way in which animals respond to auditory stimuli. You can't dismiss them as perhaps not being important in that sense. They are in fact doing something.

I assume you assume that the things you look at are of equal significance as they have something to do with what organisms people or animals are hearing. So, I think in this sense you have to relate the two, and I don't see how you can dismiss the possibility that they are related.

Thornton: I don't want to give the wrong impression. What I am saying is really the opposite. The major pathways are clearly important in the processing functions of hearing. What may be responsible for our responses may just reflect detection within the auditory system and may not be important in the hearing processes.

Harrison: I see; yes.

Kane: I would like to emphasize that some of the things Dr. Harrison pointed out as being "major pathways" in the auditory system include many things that we are looking at as being important in our overall concept of "hearing processes". For instance, MNTB is very important. We know it is involved in local circuitry. I think it is important to recognize that we have identified where those axons do, in fact go; they don't ascend. So if you are looking for a direct line, obviously you want to go to other "major" cells that are going directly up the lateral lemniscus. I think that search is a completely different problem than what was being described by Dr. Harrison and what he defined as "major".

Warr: I have looked for the large fiber pathway, including the calyx of Held, in the medial nucleus of the trapezoid body in the brain stem of man, and I am not the only one who has failed to find them. I am not the only one who has even failed to find very large axons in the trapezoid body of man. If Dr. Galambos absolutely desperately needs a large axon, perhaps he should return to the cat.

Harrison: I take it you read Strom's thing on the identification of the units of the spheroid complex in man. Do you remember that recent paper of his? He makes exactly the same point. I wasn't going to make comparative points, but he does raise it. If you look at the chimpanzee, he does find at least in the chimp that there is a median nucleus trapezoid body.

Brownell: Dr. Harrison did show us a fiber pathway that could play an important role in mediating brain stem evoked response. In his drawings it orginated in the anterior-ventral cochlear nucleus, traveled in the trapezoid body and sent collaterals to nuclei in the superior olivary complex and lateral lemniscus, finally terminating in the inferior colliculus. While the fibers in this pathway are not as large as those Dr. Warr has just discussed, in the cat their diameters fall between 3-5μm. Such diameters are quite respectable for the central nervous system and would indicate fairly high conduction velocities (approximately 20 m/sec). Futhermore, these fibers have precise temporal response characteristics (Brownell, *Brain Res. 94:* 413-433, 1975). Such relatively rapidly conducting fibers with precisely timed discharge characteristics may be part of the pathway that Dr. Galambos requires.

Diamond: Mike has intentionally avoided mentioning pathways that bypass the inferior colliculus: one terminates in the dorsal nucleus of the medial geniculate and then projects to auditory cortex. There are other paths, for example, from the pericentral division of the inferior colliculus to the caudal division of the median geniculate body which, in turn, projects to the temporal area. So, there are multiple paths which Mike has deliberately omitted for the purpose of dealing with the complexity of what you might call the main lemniscal path.

Warr: I personally am not convinced that the large spherical cells which are so plentiful in the cochlear nucleus and which form a major part at least of the input to the superior olive and lateral lemniscus, actually continue all the way to the inferior colliculus, and I think the only way to find this out definitely is to use the new horseradish peroxidase method.

Harrison: That is where my information came from. There is such a paper in which you put horseradish peroxidase in the inferior colliculus.

Warr: Some of them do light up, Mike; some of them don't. It is the low-frequency ones that apparently don't. So, I think we may have a mixed story here. Dr. Joe Adams at the NIH is working on this very problem. I would be more comfortable thinking of the olivary complex as being a very major source of a synchronous ascending input to the colliculus.

Kiang: The discussions that have taken place here in the last few minutes have been at an intolerably superficial level. The real system is so much more complicated that it doesn't make any sense, at this time, to speculate at a detailed level about which group of fibers is likely to be a candidate for this or that bump in the electric response. If the subject is to be treated seriously is should be done in depth and not at this level of casual banter.

Rose: I want to make a comment in regard to the question asked by Dr. Galambos. The neuron need not be phase-locked to have a very precise timing. I do not see the necessity for existence of a large-diameter pathway, and certainly we cannot say that there are important and unimportant pathways. There are only pathways about which we know something and pathways we know nothing about.

LOWER AUDITORY BRAIN STEM STRUCTURES OF THE CAT

Chiyeko Tsuchitani

University of Texas Health Science Center

As proposed by Lorente de Nó in 1933, the anatomical description of cell morphology, synaptology and connectivity is essential to the interpretation of physiological data. This paper is a brief review of recent developments in the anatomy and physiology of lower auditory brainstem structures.

The brain stem nuclei which are considered part of the auditory system are illustrated in Figure 1. All auditory nerve fibers enter the cochlear nuclear complex, bifurcate and terminate within the complex. The axons of cochlear nuclear neurons project to other brain stem nuclei, including the superior olivary complex, the nuclei of the lateral lemniscus and the inferior colliculus. Early anatomists considered the cochlear nuclei to be "relay" nuclei that routed auditory information into two separate pathways: the central auditory path and the auditory reflex path (Ramón y Cajal, 1899). The superior olivary complex and the nuclei of the lateral lemniscus were considered acoustic reflex nuclei that did not contribute to the central auditory path. The inferior colliculus was regarded as the brain stem structure that relayed auditory information to higher auditory centers in the thalamus. More recent anatomical and physiological studies have demonstrated that the organization of the auditory system is more complex than this early conceptualization.

THE COCHLEAR NUCLEAR COMPLEX

Although the complexity of the anatomical structure of the cochlear nuclear complex (CNC) has been recognized since the nineteenth century, it is only in recent years that the organization of the CNC has been described in some detail. Harrison and co-workers (Feldman and Harrison, 1969; Harrison and Irving, 1965, 1966a, 1966b; Harrison and Warr, 1962) described the organization of the rat CNC utilizing a variety of staining techniques. Osen (1969a, 1969b, 1970a, 1970b) has provided a detailed description of the cell types, their distribution and their afferent terminals as derived from Nissl-stained and silver-impregnated cat CNC. Computerized maps of Nissl-stained and Golgi-treated cat CNC (Kiang et al., 1975) have resulted from the work of Brawer et al., (1974). Figures 2 and 3 are representational drawings of the findings of these and other studies (Kane, 1973; Lorente de Nó, 1976, Ramón y Cajal, 1899) of the cat CNC.

ISBN 0-12-514960-3

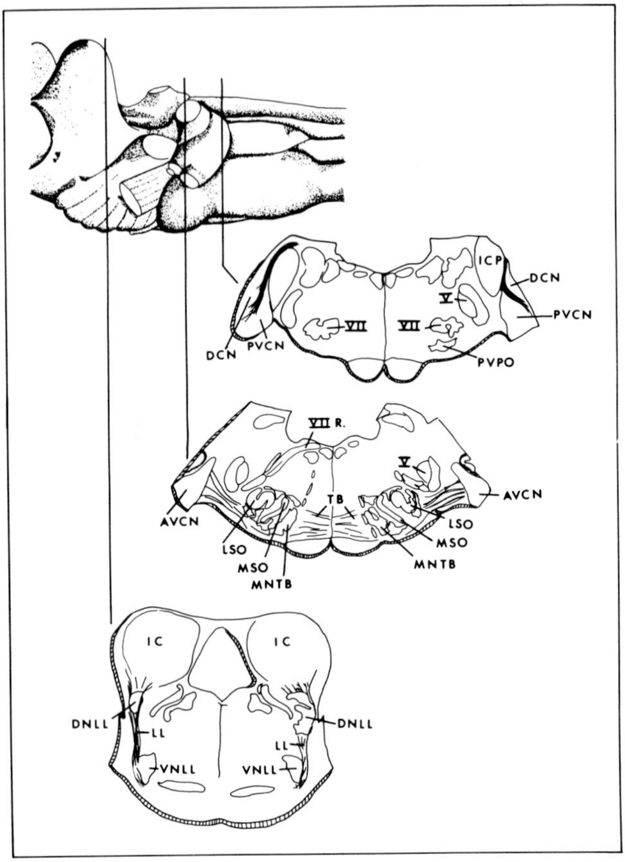

Fig. 1. Auditory brain stem structures in transverse sections of the cat brain. The approximate level of each section is indicated on the drawing (upper left) of the cat brain stem in lateral view. Components of the cochlear nuclear complex include the anteroventral (AVCN), posteroventral (PVCN) and dorsal (DCN) cochlear nuclei. Cell groups of the superior olivary complex included in this figure are the posteroventral periolivary nucleus (PVPO), the lateral superior olive (LSO), the medial superior olive (MSO), and the medial nucleus of the trapezoid body (MNTB). The dorsal (DNLL) and ventral (VNLL) nuclei of the lateral leminiscus (LL) and the inferior colliculus (IC) are located rostral to the superior olivary complex. Other abbreviations: ICP, inferior cerebellar peduncle; TB, trapezoid body; V, spinal nucleus and tract of the trigeminal nerve; VII, facial nucleus; VII R, facial nerve root.

The cat CNC (Fig. 2) consists of a dorsal cochlear nucleus (DCN) and a ventral cochlear nucleus (VCN). The entering auditory nerve root subdivides the VCN into the anteroventral cochlear nucleus (AVCN) and the posteroventral cochlear nucleus (PVCN). Upon entering the CNC each auditory nerve fiber bifurcates and sends an ascending branch into the AVCN and a descending branch into the PVCN and DCN (Fig. 4).

In the Nissl-stained AVCN (Fig. 2) five types of neurons are commonly observed: the spherical cell with a round cell body containing a centrally located

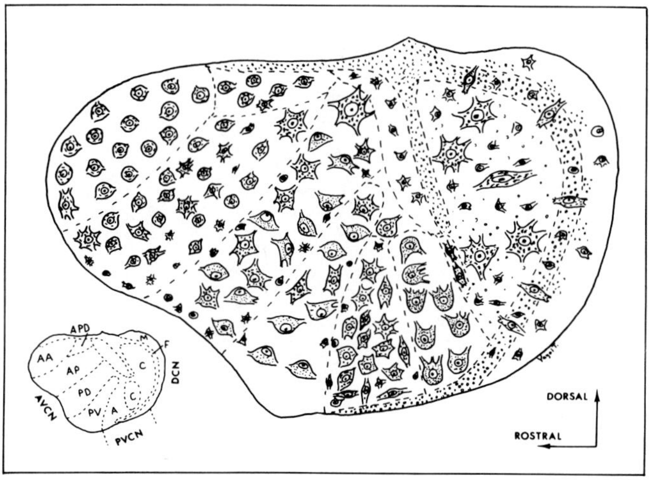

Fig. 2. A representational drawing of the types of neurons observed in a sagittal section of the Nissl-stained cat cochlear nuclear complex (After Osen, 1969a). The cells are drawn larger than their actual size. See the text for a description of the subdivisions of the cochlear nuclear complex.

nucleus and a concentric ring of coarse Nissl granules; the multipolar cell with a round or oval cell body that contains a centrally or eccentrically located nucleus and clumped or dispersed Nissl substance; the globular cell with oval cell body, eccentrically placed nucleus and dispersed Nissl granules; the small cells with small somata of a variety of shapes and Nissl patterns; and the giant multipolar cell with a disc-shaped cell body, large nucleus and coarse Nissl granules (Osen, 1969b). In the rostral AVCN the spherical cells predominate, with the slightly oval-shaped small spherical cells located caudal to the large spherical cells. Few multipolar cells occur in the large spherical cell area (AA-AVCN of Brawer et al., 1974) and in dorsal regions of the small spherical cell area (APD-AVCN). Multipolar cells make up to one-third the neural population of the ventral small spherical cell area (AP-AVCN). In more caudal areas of the AVCN few spherical cells occur and multipolar and globular cells predominate. The cells in the area of the bifurcation of the auditory nerve fibers, the globular cell area (PV-AVCN), are less densely packed than in the multipolar cell area (PD-AVCN) rostral to it. Small cells occur infrequently in the rostral AVCN and are found primarily along the margins of the other subdivisions of the AVCN and in the small cell cap area overlying the caudal AVCN. A few giant cells are located dorsally within central areas (AP and PD) of the AVCN.

Neurons in the Nissl-stained PVCN are predominantly of the multipolar and small cell type, and typically have oval or elongate cell bodies. Within the rostral PVCN adjacent to the auditory nerve root (A-PVCN), the multipolar cells are smaller and more densely packed than the cells in the AVCN. The multipolar cells in central areas of caudal PVCN (C-PVCN) have a distinctive dendritic pattern that gives them the appearance of an octopus (Osen, 1969b). These octopus cells are

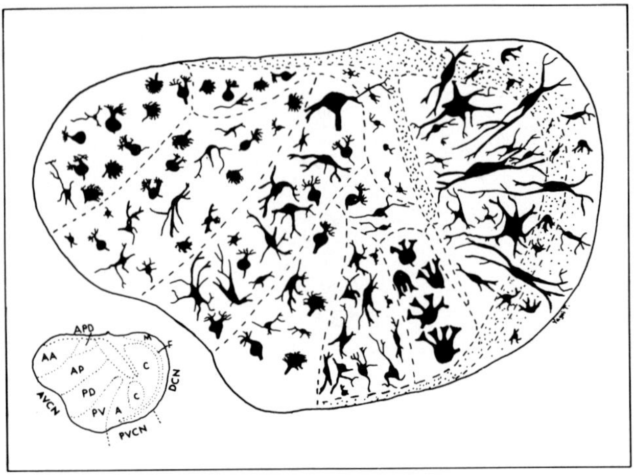

Fig. 3. A representational drawing of the cell types observed in a sagittal section of the Golgi-treated cat cochlear nuclear complex (Drawn after Brawer et al., 1974).

larger than the multipolar cells located within most of the surrounding areas of the PVCN. Small cells are distributed in all areas of the PVCN, but are few in number in the octopus cell area.

The DCN appears laminated in Nissl-stained sections and consists of an outer granular or ependymal layer, a molecular layer, a pyramidal or fusiform cell layer, and a central or polymorph layer. The molecular layer (M-DCN) is the outermost neural layer that contains both small neurons and granular cells. The fusiform cell

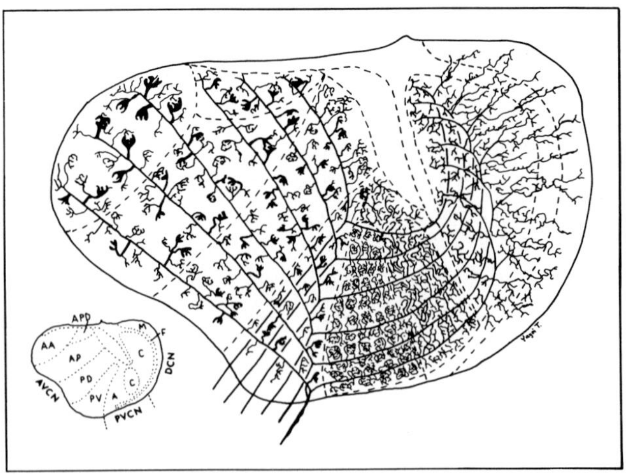

Fig. 4. A representational drawing of the terminal plexus of the Golgi-treated cat cochlear nuclear complex. (Drawn after Ramón y Cajal, 1899; Lorente de Nó, 1933 and Cohen et al., 1972).

layer (F-DCN) consists of large spindle-shaped fusiform cells, small cells with round or oval cell bodies and numerous granular cells. The central layer (C-DCN) consists of giant multipolar cells and small cells, with round or oval cell bodies, and granular cells.

In the Golgi-treated cat AVCN (Fig. 3) only four types of neurons can be distinguished: the bushy cell with round or oval cell body and short dendrites; the stellate cell with multiple thin dendrites radiating from a round or oval cell body; the small stellate cell; and the giant multipolar cell with large, thick dendrites (Brawer et al., 1974; Lorente de Nó, 1976). The bushy cells correspond to the spherical cells of the rostral AVCN (Brawer and Morest, 1975) and to the globular cells of the caudal AVCN (Tolbert and Morest, 1977). The stellate cells are similar in shape and size to the Nissl-stained multipolar cells. The small stellate cells correspond to the small cells and the giant multipolar cells to the giant cells of the Nissl-stained AVCN. The cell types observed in Golgi-treated PVCN are of a greater variety than those observed in the Nissl-stained PVCN (Brawer et al., 1974). Brawer et al. (1974) subdivide the multipolar cells into separate groups on the basis of cell body shape and dendritic pattern. Multipolar neurons in the A-PVCN are subdivided into stellate cells, small stellate cells and small elongate cells with bipolar dendritic orientation. The C-PVCN is more confined than Osen's octopus cell area, and is an area consisting almost exclusively of octopus cells. The P-PVCN (collectively the D-PVCN and V-PVCN of Brawer et al., (1974)) surrounds the C-PVCN and contains a variety of multipolar cell types with different dendritic patterns; ie., large and small stellate cells, large and small elongate cells, bushy multipolar cells with short thick dendrites and antenniform cells with long thin dendrites that radiate from the cell body at right angles to one another. The three remaining PVCN subdivisions of Brawer et al. (1974) are small in size and will not be described in this review. In Golgi-treated DCN, granular cells and a variety of small cells occur in all neural layers, with fusiform cells in the F-DCN and three types of giant cells in the C-DCN (Fig. 8).

The terminal plexus in the various subdivisions of the CNC differ with respect to neuropil density and terminal types (Fig. 4). In the AVCN spherical and globular cells make synaptic contact with large primary afferent terminals in the form of endbulbs of Held and with small boutons (Held, 1893; Ramón y Cajal, 1899; Brawer and Morest, 1975; Lorente de Nó, 1976). The endbulbs arise from thick collateral fibers and form enlarged endings that wrap around the cell soma. A single process of an endbulb of Held reportedly can make up to 14 synaptic contacts with the cell soma (Lenn and Reese, 1966). The endbulbs are larger and more complex in shape rostrally (Ramón y Cajal, 1899; Brawer and Morest, 1975). In most cases each spherical cell in AA-AVCN receives one large endbulb of Held which covers half of the surface area of the cell soma (Lorente de Nó, 1976). The spherical cells in areas caudal to the AA-AVCN and the globular cells may receive two or more endbulbs of Held as well as numerous bouton terminals (Ramón y Cajal, 1899; Lorente de Nó, 1976). Bouton endings formed by axon collaterals and by collaterals arising from the endbulbs terminate on the somata and dendrites of the spherical and globular cells. The multipolar cells in the AVCN are surrounded by pericellular baskets of afferent terminal fibers that form bouton terminals and terminals en passant which end primarily upon their dendrites (McDonald and Rasmussen, 1971). The cell bodies of AVCN small and giant cells are reported to be surrounded by pericellular nests of afferent terminal fibers (Lorente de Nó, 1976). The afferent terminals form a fine and diffuse terminal plexus in the rostral AVCN and in the PV-AVCN and a coarser and denser terminal plexus in the PD-AVCN (Brawer and Morest, 1975).

The collaterals of descending auditory nerve branches produce dense pericellular networks of coarse terminal fibers in the rostral PVCN (Lorente de Nó, 1933). Large numbers of terminal boutons form somatic and dendritic contacts on the multipolar cells of A-PVCN (Osen, 1970b). In the octopus cell area the neuropil is also dense but diffuse, and large terminals en passant and small boutons cover most of the surface area of the cell body and dendritic trunks of the octopus cells (Kane, 1973, 1976a).

The descending branches of auditory nerve fibers do not appear to be equally distributed within the DCN (Lorente de Nó, 1933; Osen, 1970b; Cohen et al., 1972). The greatest concentration of afferent terminal fibers appears in the central DCN, where they form a loose neuropil of thick terminal fibers. The terminals form somatic and dendritic contacts with all types of neurons in the C-DCN (Kane, 1974b). Most of the collateral fibers entering the fusiform cell layer terminate there, and few fibers enter the molecular layer of the DCN. Bouton endings, terminals en passant, and irregular-shaped "mossy" endings are formed in the fusiform cell layer and molecular layer. Afferent terminals make contact with fusiform cell soma and dendritic trunks and with small and granular cells within the F-DCN and M-DCN.

Transection of the auditory nerve results in primary afferent terminal degeneration that is greater in the AVCN and PVCN than in the DCN. The endbulbs of Held and many of the bouton terminals in the rostral AVCN degenerate following auditory nerve section (Osen, 1970b). The remaining nonprimary fibers form pericellular nests of thin to medium-sized fibers that end as coarse terminals or fine bouton endings (Cant and Morest, 1975). The non-primary terminal plexus stained for acetylcholinesterase (AChE) demonstrate a reactivity with long incubation times (Osen and Roth, 1969). In caudal AVCN the endbulbs of Held and most other terminals degenerate following auditory nerve section. The few endings that remain are small boutons (Rasmussen, 1967; Osen, 1970b), a few of which demonstrate AChE positive staining (Osen and Roth, 1969). In rostral PVCN only a few small terminals survive auditory nerve section, with even fewer terminals remaining in the caudal PVCN (Osen, 1970b; Kane, 1974a, 1976b, 1976c). The non-primary input to the DCN, which is also AChE-positive (Rasmussen, 1967; Osen and Roth, 1969; McDonald and Rasmussen, 1971), is so dense that it is difficult to detect loss of primary endings following auditory nerve section (Rasmussen 1967; Osen, 1970b).

The non-primary terminals of the CNC arise from a number of sources. Intranuclear connections have been observed between neurons in the DCN (Lorente de Nó, 1933; Kane, 1974b) and in the AVCN (Lorente de Nó, 1976). Internuclear paths between AVCN and DCN and between PVCN and DCN have also been demonstrated (Lorente de Nó, 1933; Rasmussen, 1967; Fernández and Karapas, 1967; Warr, 1969). Neurons of the superior olivary complex send descending axons to all areas of the CNC (Rasmussen, 1960, 1964, 1967; van Noort, 1969; Osen and Roth, 1969; Adams and Warr, 1976). The superior olivary efferents terminate

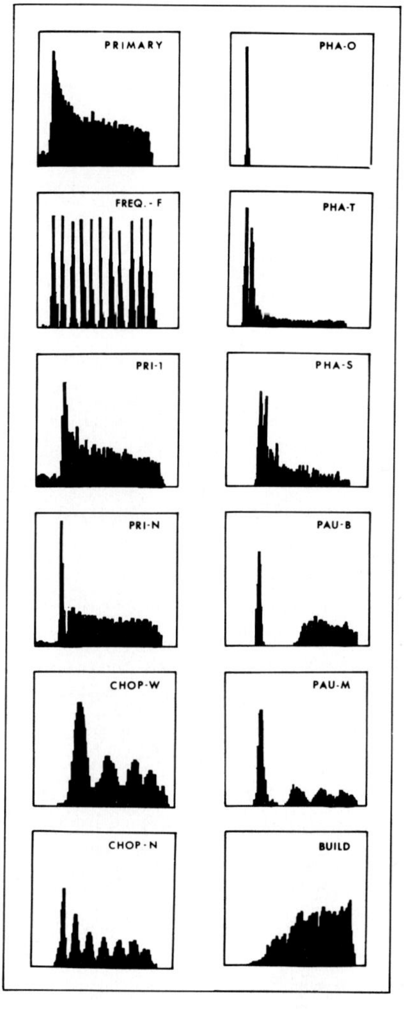

Fig. 5. Examples of the discharge patterns of auditory neurons to tone burst stimuli in the form of poststimulus time (PST) histograms. The PST histograms represent the temporal distribution of spikes after stimulus onset. Bin width of 0.2 msec and total analysis time of 40 msec.

bilaterally within the CNC, often with a greater density of efferent terminals in the contralateral cell groups (Kane, 1976b). The density of superior olivary efferent innervation is greater in central areas of DCN and in the rostral AVCN and decreases progressively in more caudal regions of the VCN (Kane, 1976b). Cells in the nuclei of the lateral lemniscus and the inferior colliculi provide efferent terminals to neurons in the DCN (Rasmussen, 1960, 1967; van Noort, 1969; Adams and Warr, 1976).

Electrophysiological studies of auditory nerve fibers indicate that the primary afferents typically produce one type of discharge pattern to short duration tone burst stimuli (Kiang et al., 1965b). The discharge pattern is characterized by an initial high rate of activity dropping gradually to a lower, more steady rate that is maintained for the duration of the stimulus (Primary in Fig. 5). When the stimulus is of sufficient intensity, the discharges of primary afferents are time-locked to a specific phase of low frequency sinusoids with an upper limit of phase-locking to a 5 kHz tone (Rose et al., 1967). The discharge patterns of primary units are synchronized with the sinusoidal stimulus and produce a frequency-following discharge pattern (Freq-F in Fig. 5).

Given the diversity of cell and terminal types within the CNC, it is not surprising that the discharge patterns of CNC units to short tone bursts are not uniform (Rose et al., 1959; Kiang et al., 1965a; Pfeiffer, 1966b; Mast, 1969). The primary-like patterns (Pri-1 and Pri-N, Fig. 5) of CNC units are similar to the discharge patterns of primary afferent fibers. The Pri-N pattern is a variation of the primary pattern that is characterized by a short period of reduced activity (the silent period) lasting less than 3 msec that follows the initial peak of activity. Often the instantaneous discharge rate of the Pri-N initial response is greater than that of the Pri-1 initial response. The CNC units that generate primary-like discharge patterns are also capable of generating frequency-following discharges to sinusoids with frequency up to 5 kHz (Bourk, 1976, 1977).

Chopper-type discharge patterns are produced by other CNC units (Chop-W and Chop-N, Fig. 5). These units emit spikes at very regular time intervals with the discharges time-locked to stimulus-onset. The time intervals between successive spikes in the chopper pattern increase and become less regular with increasing time after stimulus onset. Some units are capable of producing chopper patterns with very low rates of discharge (less than 50 spikes/sec) and with mean interspike intervals greater than 5 msec. The resulting chopper pattern is characterized by wide peaks of activity separated by long interpeak intervals (Chop-W). The discharge rates of other units producing chopper patterns may reach as high as 500 spikes/sec before the chopper-pattern becomes discernable (Chop-N). The Chop-N pattern is characterized by regular, narrow peaks of activity with short interpeak intervals. In some cases the chopper pattern is transient, and the discharge becomes irregular within 10 to 15 msec following stimulus onset. The CNC units producing chopper discharge patterns are only capable of producing frequency-following discharge to sinusoids with frequency less than 2 kHz (Bourk, 1976, 1977).

Other CNC units generate phasic or transient discharge to tone burst stimuli

(Pha-O, Pha-T and Pha-S in Fig. 5). These units emit a short burst of spikes to stimulus onset and then no spikes or a low level of discharge for the remainder of the stimulus duration. The Pha-O pattern is characterized by a short latency discharge of one spike, even to high level stimuli. The Pha-T pattern is similar to the Pha-O pattern, except that at moderate to high stimulus levels a low rate of discharge is produced for the duration of the stimulus. Units discharging with Pha-T patterns produce an increase in the number of spikes elicited with an increase in stimulus level, but require a large increase in level to produce a small increase in spike output. Most CNC units producing Pha-O and Pha-T discharges appear to be more widely tuned than other CNC units (Godfrey et al., 1975a). These units are capable of generating frequency-following responses to sinusoids with frequency up to 5 kHz. The discharge of CNC units producing Pha-S patterns is more sustained and is characterized by decreased output to increases in stimulus level beyond that eliciting the maximum discharge rate (Godfrey et al., 1975b). The

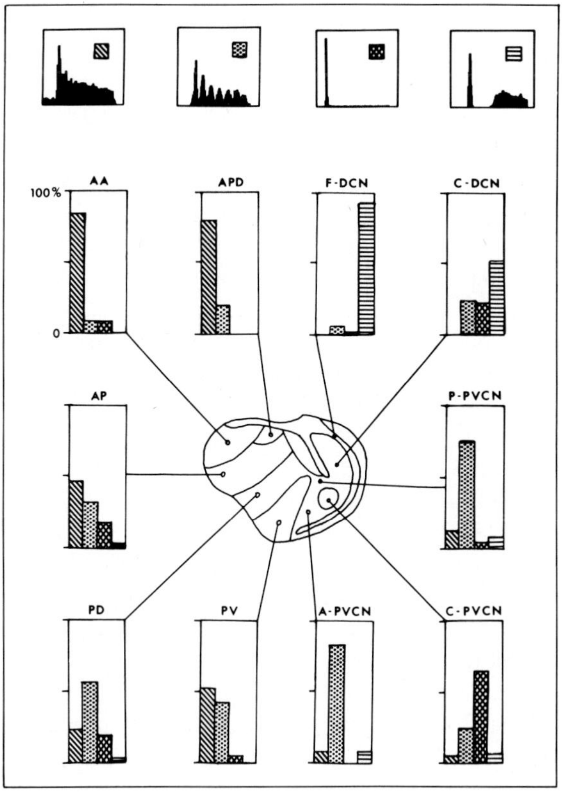

Fig. 6. The frequency distributions of discharge pattern types encountered within the different subdivisions of the cochlear nuclear complex. (Summarized from Bourk, 1976; Godfrey, 1971; Godfrey et al., 1975a, 1975b). The frequency histograms to the left are for the subdivisions of the AVCN. Discharge pattern types: diagonal lines, primary-like; dots, chopper-type; cross-hatch, phasic-type; and horizontal lines, pause or build-type.

initial responses of CNC units producing Pha-S discharges are often of longer latency and often are not as securely time-locked to stimulus onset as are the initial responses of CNC units producing Pha-O and Pha-T discharges.

The fourth class of discharge patterns produced by CNC units includes a collection of less frequently occuring types. The pause pattern (Pau-B and Pau-M, Fig. 5) is characterized by a silent period lasting 5 msec or more following the initial response to simulus onset. While the Pau-B pattern resembles the Pri-N pattern, the silent period lasts longer and the discharge following the silent period builds up more gradually to a steady rate in the Pau-B pattern. The CNC units generating Pau-M patterns appear to generate different types of patterns (eg., Build, Pau-B, Chop-W and Pau-M) under different stimulus conditions (Godfrey et al., 1975b). The build pattern (Build, Fig. 5) is characterized by a slow build up of activity to some level that is maintained for the duration of the stimulus.

Figure 6 summarizes the data describing the distribution of discharge pattern types in the PVCN and DCN as reported by Godfrey (Godfrey, 1971; Godfrey et al., 1975a, 1975b) and in the AVCN as reported by Bourk (1976). As first reported by Kiang et al., (1965a) the type of discharge pattern elicited from a CNC unit is related to the location of that unit in the CNC. Units producing primary-like discharges predominate in the rostral AVCN, occur with lower frequency in the remaining AVCN and occur infrequently in the PVCN and DCN. Units with chopper discharge patterns predominate in the A-PVCN and P-PVCN, occur with decreasing frequency in a rostral direction in the AVCN, and occur more frequently in the C-DCN than in the F-DCN. Units in the C-PVCN typically produce phasic discharge. The DCN is the only area in the CNC in which units generating pause and build discharge patterns outnumber those producing primary, chopper or phasic patterns.

The correlation between the distribution of discharge pattern types within the CNC and the distribution of different morphologically defined neurons has led Kiang and his associates (Kiang et al., 1973, Morest et al., 1973, Kane, 1973, 1974b; Kiang, 1975) to conclude that specific anatomically-defined neurons produce specific discharge patterns. It is assumed that the metal microelectrodes used by Godfrey (1971) and by Bourk (1976) did not record from the small and granular cells of the CNC. Units producing primary-like discharge patterns occur in areas of the VCN where spherical and globular cells are found (Fig. 7). As the proportion of spherical and globular cells decreases, the proportion of units producing primary-like discharge decreases. The spherical cells in the AA-AVCN have short, small dendrites and receive numerous terminal boutons and large endbulbs of Held, most commonly with a ratio of one endbulb per cell. Most units in the AA-AVCN produce Pri-1 discharges and the complex spike waveform illustrated in Figure 7. The spike is characterized by a positive presynaptic potential, believed to be generated by the large afferent terminal, that precedes the CNC unit postsynaptic potential by 0.5 msec. The Pri-1 pattern is believed to result from the secure transmission provided by the large area of synaptic contact between the endbulb and the spherical cell. This large area of synaptic contact insures the generation of a post-

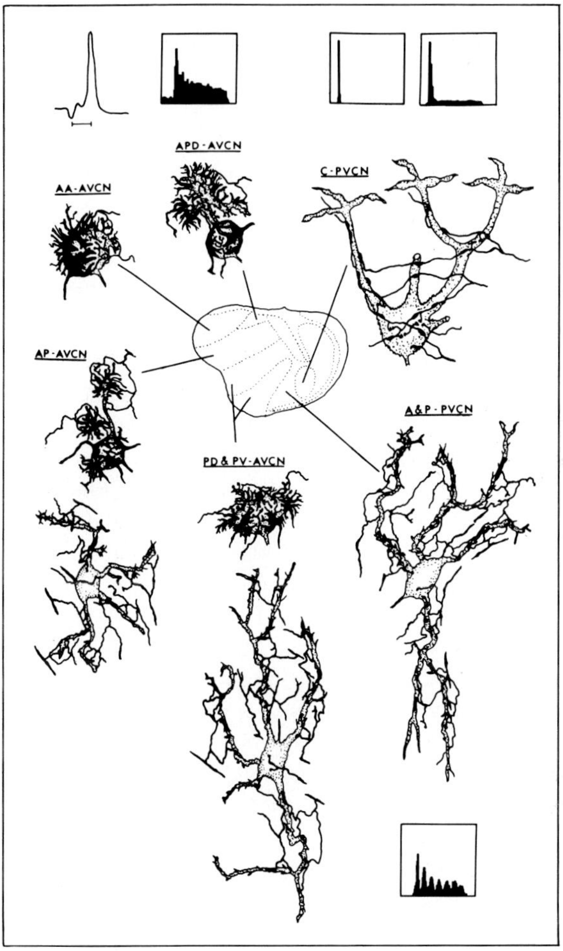

Fig. 7. Illustrated for the subdivisions of the cat ventral cochlear nucleus are their principal neuron types, their afferent terminals and the discharge patterns produced by the different neuron types. (Neurons and terminals drawn after Brawer et al., 1974; Brawer and Morest, 1975; Kane, 1973; Lorente de Nó, 1976). The bushy (spherical and globular) cells of the AVCN have short dendrites, receive endbulbs of Held and bouton terminals, and are believed to produce primary-like discharge patterns and complex spike waveform. The stellate or multipolar cells have longer, thin dendrites, receive afferent terminals that are smaller and more numerous than the endbulbs of Held and are believed to produce narrow chopper-type discharge patterns. The octopus cells with their thick, long dendrites and two morphologically different types of terminals are believed to produce phasic-type discharge patterns. Units producing pause or other types of discharges occur infrequently in the ventral cochlear nucleus and the morphology of the neurons producing these types of discharge patterns is not known. Spike waveform time scale is 0.5 msec, with negativity up.

synaptic spike with each incoming presynaptic auditory nerve potential (Pfeiffer, 1966a). As the size of the endbulbs of Held decreases in a caudal direction, so also does the proportion of the units producing Pri-1 discharge patterns decrease and the proportion of units producing Pri-N patterns increase (Bourk, 1976). The globular cells within the caudal AVCN receive two to four endbulbs of Held and numerous boutons, thus receiving auditory nerve input from a number of large and small sources. The integration of a small number of endbulb inputs and the more numerous bouton inputs by globular cells is believed to result in the PRI-N discharge pattern (Kiang, 1975).

The majority of the remaining units in the VCN produce either chopper or phasic discharge patterns. Most units within the A-PVCN and P-PVCN produce chopper patterns and are multipolar neurons (Fig. 7). These neurons have thin dendrites that extend some distance from their cell bodies. The neuron is surrounded by a pericellular basket of afferent terminals forming numerous terminal boutons. The regular firing pattern produced by these neurons has been ascribed to the temporal and spatial integration of numerous, small and irregularly-occuring auditory nerve inputs distributed over relatively large areas of the cell surface (Molnar and Pfeiffer, 1968). In the AVCN the units producing chopper patterns decrease rostrally as do the multipolar cells forming the neural population. The chopper patterns of units in the rostral AVCN and in the caudal PVCN appear to be more transient than those of units in more central areas of the VCN (Bourk, 1976; Godfrey, 1971).

Most units in the C-PVCN produce phasic discharges attributed to octopus cells with large dendrites that extend some distance from the cell somata (Fig. 7). Large terminals en passant and small bouton terminals of the descending branches of auditory nerve fibers cover over half of the surface area of the soma and dendritic trunks. The ultrastructural features of these two terminal types differ, suggesting that they may have different effects on the octopus cells (Kane, 1973). Kane (1973) has suggested that the larger terminals may be excitatory and the smaller ones inhibitory, and that their interaction results in the phasic discharge pattern produced by the octopus cells. Units producing pure phasic or onset discharges (Pha-O) occur only within the C-PVCN. Units producing Pha-T patterns occur in the C-PVCN and in other regions of the VCN. Although multipolar neurons with octopus-like dendritic patterns are observed in areas outside the C-PVCN (Lorente de Nó, 1933, 1976), it is not clear whether these neurons are similar in other respects to the octopus cells of C-PVCN.

The DCN differs from the VCN with respect to neural composition and types of discharge patterns observed (Fig. 8). Granular cells, small cells and large bipolar (fusiform) and multipolar (giant) neurons populate the DCN. Most fusiform and giant cells have large dendrites that extend great distances within the DCN. The primary afferent input to the DCN is minor compared to the input from neurons within the DCN, from the VCN and from other brain stem nuclei. The large cells in the F-DCN are fusiform cells that appear to produce build or pause type discharge patterns, with many of the pause patterns of the Pau-B type. Most large cells in the

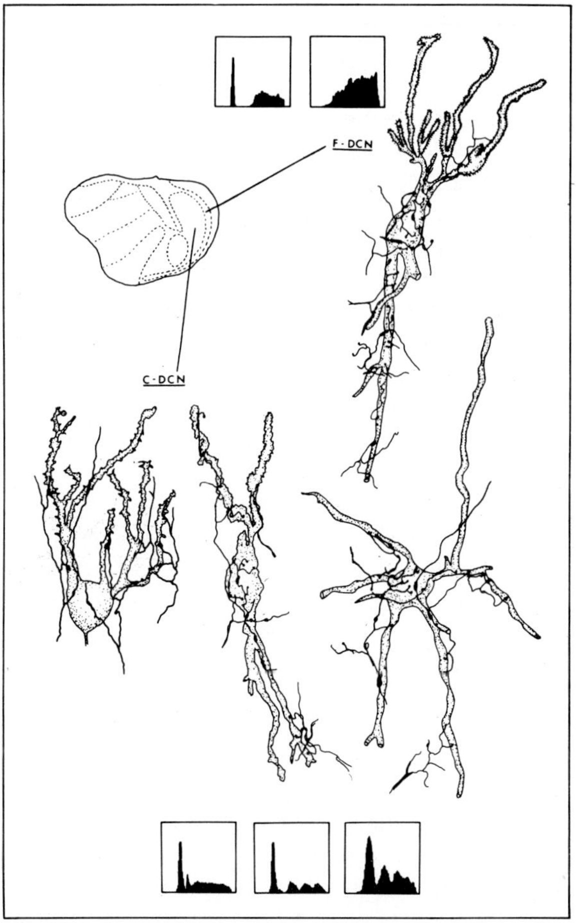

Fig. 8. Examples of the cat dorsal cochlear nuclear (DCN) neurons, their afferent terminals and the types of discharge produced by DCN units. (Neurons and terminals drawn after Brawer et al., 1974 and Kane, 1974b). Most of the fusiform cells in F-DCN appear to produce either pause-type or build-type discharges. The type of discharge pattern produced by each of the different C-DCN giant cells (from left to right; vertical giant cell, horizontal giant cell and radiate giant cell), is not known. Most units in the C-DCN produce discharge patterns unique to the C-DCN, Pha-S, Pau-M and Chop-W.

C-DCN are giant multipolar cells that produce Chop-W, Pau-M and Pha-S discharge patterns. As noted by Godfrey et al. (1975b), the greater complexity of the innervation of DCN neurons, the greater influence exerted by non-primary inputs on DCN units (Koerber et al., 1966), the binaural innervation of some DCN units (Mast, 1973) and the greater sensitivity of DCN units to anesthesia (Evans and Nelson, 1973, Mast 1973) make it difficult to speculate upon the effects of primary afferent inputs on DCN unit discharge patterns.

THE SUPERIOR OLIVARY COMPLEX

The CNC provides input to various cell groups in the superior olivary complex, in the nuclei of the lateral lemniscus and in the inferior colliculus (Held, 1893; Ramón y Cajal, 1899; Stotler, 1953; Fernández and Karapas, 1967; Harrison and Feldman, 1970; Warr, 1966, 1969, 1972; van Noort, 1969; Adams and Warr, 1976). The circuitry of the auditory brain stem nuclei is extremely complex with different subdivisions of the CNC supplying input to different cell groups in the brain stem. The exact site of termination of the axons of the different cell types within each CNC subdivision has been described for few cell types (Osen, 1970a; Tolbert and Morest, 1977). Thus in most cases the CNC input to other brain stem auditory structures must be specified in terms of the output of the subdivisions within the CNC rather than in terms of exact cell types. Anatomical and neurophysiological data of other auditory brain stem structures is not as complete as that for the CNC. Of the three auditory brain stem structures receiving CNC outputs most is known of the anatomy and physiology of the superior olivary complex.

The superior olivary complex (SOC) consists of a number of small nuclear masses located within the tegmentum of the pons. It has been described to contain at least twelve different nuclei in the cat (Warr, 1969, 1972). The two most distinctive nuclei, the lateral superior olive or S-segment and the medial superior olive or accessory olive, are surrounded by various smaller cell groups collectively called the periolivary nuclei and the nuclei of the trapezoid body (Fig. 9). Anatomical and/or neurophysiological data are available for only a limited number of these nuclei. Only those nuclei with sufficient discharge pattern data will be considered in this review.

The medial superior olive (MSO) is a crescent-shaped nucleus consisting of a plate of neurons approximately three to four cells thick. The lateral superior olive (LSO) is located lateral to the MSO and has a characteristic S shape in the cat. The medial nucleus of the trapezoid body (MNTB) lies within the fibers of the trapezoid body, medial to the MSO. In this review the dorsolateral periolivary nuclei (DLPO) are considered to consist of two cell groups located dorsal to the LSO, the dorsal and dorsolateral periolivary (DPO and DLPO) nuclei of Morest (1968).

Systematic studies of cell types in the Nissl-stained cat SOC have not been carried out and the following description (Fig. 9) is a summary from a number of sources. Most neurons in the MNTB, the principal cells of Morest (1968), resemble the globular cells of the caudal AVCN. They are medium-sized and appear round or oval-shaped with an eccentric nucleus and fine, diffuse, dark Nissl substance (Taber, 1961; Morest, 1968). The elongate neurons of the MNTB are slightly smaller than the principal neurons and have oval cell bodies that contain coarse Nissl substance and a centrally-placed nucleus (Morest, 1968). The MNTB stellate neurons are large multipolar cells scattered among the principal and elongate neurons of the MNTB. The nucleus of the stellate neuron is usually centrally placed and surrounded by large quantities of cell cytoplasm containing thin Nissl bodies arranged in a tigroid pattern (Morest, 1968). Multipolar cells in the MNTB are reactive to AChE and are

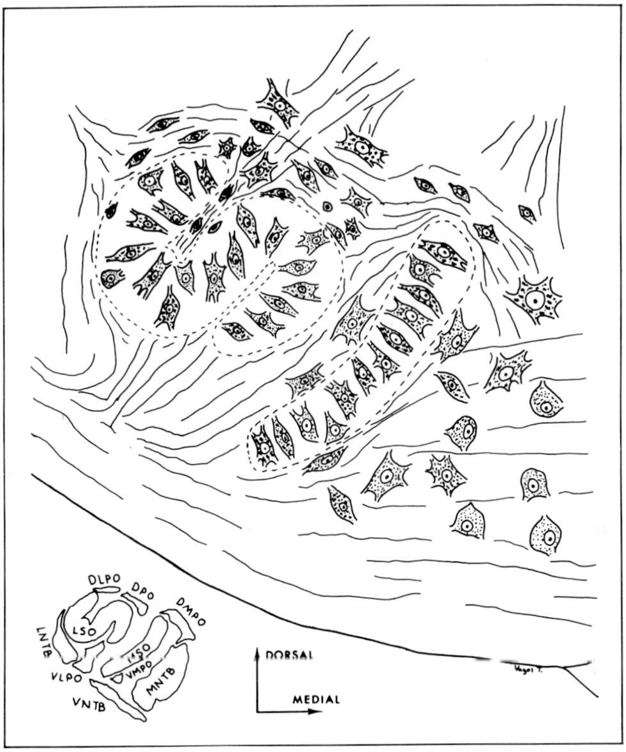

Fig. 9. A representational drawing of the neurons in the Nissl-stained cat superior olivary complex in transverse section. Abbreviations: DMPO, dorsomedial periolivary nucleus: DLPO, dorsolateral periolivary nucleus; DPO, dorsal periolivary nucleus; LNTB, lateral nucleus of the trapezoid body; LSO, lateral superior olive; MNTB, medial nucleus of the trapezoid body; MSO, medial superior olive; VMPO, ventromedial periolivary nucleus; VNTB, ventral nucleus of the trapezoid body; VLPO, ventrolateral periolivary nucleus.

believed to send their axons into the olivocochlear bundle (Osen and Roth, 1969; Warr, 1975). Neurons in the MSO are fusiform or multipolar in shape and contain a centered nucleus and fine-to-coarse Nissl substance. Marginal cells of the MSO are large, multipolar neurons located along the medial and lateral edges of the MSO. The LSO contains spindle-shaped, multipolar and round cells that are slightly smaller in diameter than those within the MSO. The LSO cell nucleus is often eccentrically placed, and the Nissl substance may be coarse and dark (Taber, 1961). Neurons in the DLPO vary in size and configuration but tend to be smaller than LSO neurons. Small spindle-shaped neurons around the LSO and DLPO and larger multipolar neurons in or around the DLPO and within the MNTB have been demonstrated to be reactive to AChE and to send their axons into the olivocochlear bundle (Osen and Roth, 1969; Warr, 1975).

The neuronal types observed in the Golgi-treated SOC (Fig. 10) have been

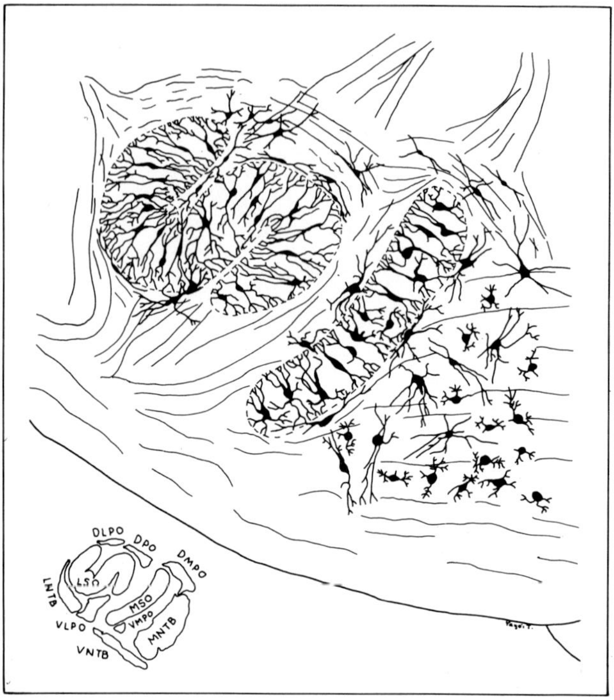

Fig. 10. A representational drawing of the neurons in the Golgi-treated cat superior olivary complex (Redrawn after Lavilla, 1898; Ramón y Cajal, 1899; Morest, 1968; Scheibel and Scheibel, 1974; Schwartz, 1977).

described in some detail for the MNTB (Ramón y Cajal, 1899; Morest, 1968) and the MSO (Lavilla, 1898; Ramón y Cajal, 1899; Scheibel and Scheibel, 1974; Schwartz, 1977), and in less detail for the LSO (Ramón y Cajal, 1899; Scheibel and Scheibel, 1974). The most frequently observed neurons in the MNTB, the principal cells (Fig. 12a), are round or oval in shape with two to four short, slender dendrites (Ramón y Cajal, 1899; Morest, 1968). The MNTB stellate neurons (Fig. 12b) are larger and multipolar in shape with a number of thick dendrites that radiate in various directions from the cell soma. The MNTB elongate neuron (Fig. 12c) has an oval or round cell body smaller than that of the principal cell and four or five long thin dendrites that usually extend in a dorsolateral to ventromedial direction. In transverse sections most MSO neurons appear to be fusiform or bipolar in shape (Fig. 10). The dendrites of most neurons extend toward the lateral and medial borders of the MSO with limited spread of dendrites in a dorsoventral direction. In sagittal sections through the MSO most neurons appear to be multipolar in shape (Fig. 13, cell on lower left) with dendrites that radiate from an irregular disc-shaped cell body in a rostrocaudal direction. Some of the neurons are bipolar with dendrites arising from the two poles of a spindle-shaped cell body (Fig. 13, cell on

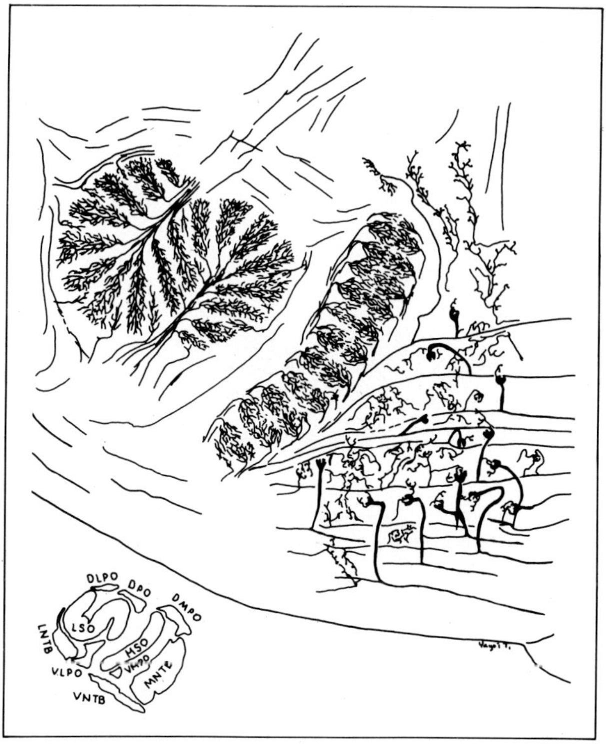

Fig. 11. A representational drawing of the terminal plexus of the Golgi-treated cat superior olivary complex (Redrawn after Ramón y Cajal, 1899; Morest, 1968).

lower right). Other MSO neurons are horizontally oriented and do not send dendrites across the width of the MSO to its medial and lateral borders (Fig. 11). The dendrites of these horizontal cells travel in a rostro-caudal direction and resemble peripheral and marginal MSO cells. Peripheral MSO neurons have cell bodies located within the MSO near its outer margins and produce dendrites that extend less than half the width of the MSO. The dendrites of most marginal MSO neurons spread along the border of the MSO with some entering into the MSO. The neurons of the LSO are similar to those in the MSO (Fig. 14), ie., many are multipolar with dendrites that spread longitudinally in a rostrocaudal direction (Ramón y Cajal, 1899; Scheibel and Scheibel, 1974).

The SOC receives bilateral inputs from the CNC. The axons from the CNC form different types of terminal plexus within the SOC (Fig. 11). The terminal plexus of the MNTB arises from the contralateral caudal AVCN (van Noort, 1969; Warr, 1972). It consists of pericellular nests of terminal fibers and of large endings, the calyces of Held that arise from thick axons of the trapezoid body (Held, 1893; Ramón y Cajal, 1899; Stotler, 1953; Morest, 1968). A single calyx arises from the axon of an AVCN globular cell (Tolbert and Morest, 1977) and envelops the soma

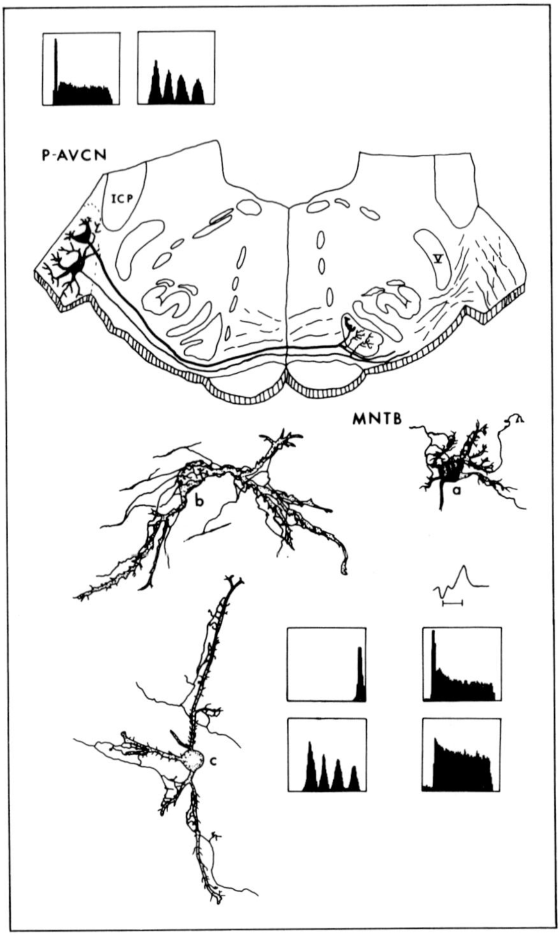

Fig. 12. Examples of the morphology and discharge patterns of three types of neurons in the medial nucleus of the trapezoid body (MNTB) and of their cochlear nuclear inputs. (MNTB neurons and terminals drawn after Morest, 1968). The discharge patterns of most neurons in the caudal AVCN (P-AVCN), which provides input to the MNTB, are predominantly primary-like and narrow chopper type (histograms at upper left). The AVCN globular cells supply input to the MNTB principal or globular cell (labeled a; in transverse section) which is also believed to produce primary-like discharge patterns. The MNTB principal cell has short dendrites, receives a single calyx of Held and bouton terminals and is believed to produce a complex spike waveform and primary-like discharge pattern. The MNTB stellate or multipolar cell (labeled b; in sagittal section) has long thick dendrites, makes somatic and dendritic synaptic contacts with numerous small terminals and may produce off-type discharges. The dendrites of the MNTB elongate cell (labeled c; in transverse section) are thin and long and receive small terminals from axon collaterals. Few elongate cells occur in the MNTB and few units producing wide chopper discharges are encountered in the MNTB. Spike waveform time scale is 0.5 msec., with negativity up.

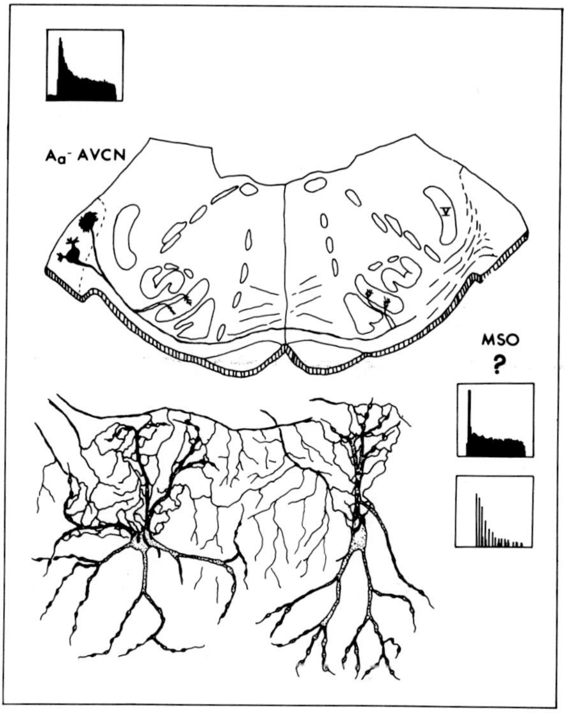

Fig. 13. Examples of the morphology and discharge patterns of medial superior olivary (MSO) neurons and their probable cochlear nuclear inputs (Aa-AVCN). (MSO neurons and terminals drawn after Ramón y Cajal, 1899; Scheibel and Scheibel, 1974; Schwartz, 1977). The most rostral AVCN (Aa-AVCN) consists predominantly of large spherical cells producing primary-like discharges (upper left). Axons of the Aa-AVCN neurons provide input to both the ipsilateral and contralateral MSO. Neurons in the MSO, when viewed sagitally, are predominantly of the multipolar type (lower left) with few bipolar types (lower right) and horizontal types (not illustrated). The lateral half of the MSO neuron is covered by the elongated and small round or oval terminals of ipsilateral AVCN axon collaterals. The only two examples available of possible MSO unit discharge pattern (Pri-N and Freq.-F)are illustrated in this figure.

of a principal neuron (Fig. 12a). The calyx contains numerous synaptic complexes that cover over half of the surface area of the cell soma (Lenn and Reese, 1966; Morest, 1973). The principal neuron receives a single calyx ending and numerous smaller endings on its soma and dendrites (Morest, 1968). Thin collateral fibers arise from the calyx, pass to nearby principal cells and terminate on the somata of these cells. The dendrites of the principal cells also receive small endings from other, medium-sized axons that provide dendritic terminals to MNTB stellate cells. Other, finer caliber axons produce extensive pericellular nests that envelop and terminate as small boutons on the somata and dendrites of MNTB stellate cells (Fig. 12b). Sparsely branched collaterals of axons passing through the MNTB and some collaterals arising from axons forming the pericellular nests around stellate cells and the calciform endings on principal cells end upon the dendrites of MNTB elongate cells (Fig. 12C).

The MSO receives bilateral projections from the rostral AVCN (Warr, 1966; van Noort, 1969) or, according to Osen (1970a), from the large spherical cell area of the AVCN. The axons from the ipsilateral AVCN enter the MSO along its lateral border (Fig. 13), while those from the contralateral AVCN enter along its medial border (Stotler, 1953; Warr, 1966; Lindsey, 1975). Upon entering the MSO the axons branch repeatedly (Fig. 11) to produce dense, flame-shaped terminal arbors (Lavilla, 1898; Ramón y Cajal, 1899; Scheibel and Scheibel, 1974). The terminal field of each axon extends longitudinally, overlapping the dendritic fields of the MSO neurons (Fig. 13). The terminal arbor of each axon is very dense and covers half of the surface area of an MSO neuron. Elongated, finger-like terminal processes (some as long as 20μm) that make multiple synaptic contacts and small, round or oval boutons form a dense layer of terminals covering the somata and dendrites of MSO neurons (Clark, 1969; Schwartz, 1972; Perkins, 1973; Lindsey, 1975).

The axons of neurons in the rostral AVCN or more specifically the small spherical cell area of AVCN (Osen, 1970a), provide a major ipsilateral input to the LSO (Warr, 1966, van Noort, 1969). A minor input arises from the contralateral caudal AVCN (Fig. 14) and terminates in the medial limb of the LSO (Warr, 1972). A second and larger source of input from the contralateral ear arises from the ipsilateral MNTB (Rasmussen, 1967; van Noort, 1969). The axons of the ipsilateral AVCN enter the LSO primarily through the hilar zones of the LSO (Fig. 11) and form terminal arbors that radiate like spokes in a wheel (Lavilla, 1898; Ramón y Cajal, 1899; Scheibel and Scheibel, 1974). As in the MSO each axonal terminal field extends rostrocaudally overlapping the dendritic fields of the LSO neurons (Fig. 14). The terminal fibers form a dense network that surrounds the cell bodies and dendrites of the LSO neurons. According to Stotler (1953), terminal boutons usually arise singly from a terminal fiber and end upon the body or dendrites of LSO neurons.

The DLPO receives input from the PVCN (Fig. 15). An ipsilateral input arises from the PVCN and travels by way of the intermediate acoustic stria of Held (van Noort, 1969; Warr, 1969; Adams and Warr, 1976) and the trapezoid body (Warr, 1969, 1972; van Noort, 1969) to the DLPO. The majority of fibers in the intermediate acoustic stria are reportedly the axons of the octopus cells of the C-PVCN (Osen, 1972). A smaller number of fibers in the intermediate acoustic stria arise from other neurons in the caudal PVCN and from neurons scattered through more rostral areas of PVCN (Adams and Warr, 1976). The afferent terminal fibers in the DLPO have not been described.

The discharge patterns of many SOC units are similar to those of CNC units (Guinan et al., 1972a). However, very few, if any, units producing pause or build type discharge are encountered in the SOC, and units producing discharge only to stimulus offset also appear within certain areas of the SOC.

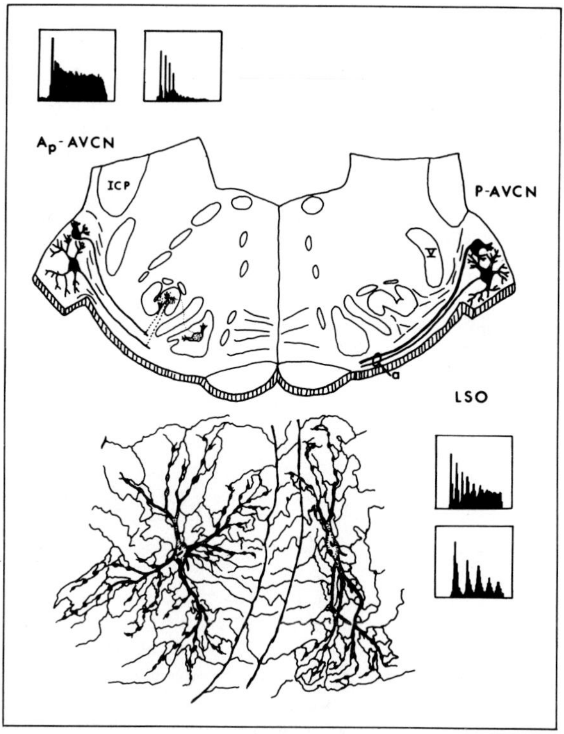

Fig. 14. Examples of the morphology and discharge patterns of lateral superior olivary neurons (LSO) and their probable cochlear nuclear input. (LSO neurons and their terminals redrawn after Ramón y Cajal, 1899 and Scheibel and Scheibel, 1974). The posterior part of the rostral AVCN (Ap-AVCN) contains both spherical and multipolar neurons with spherical neurons predominating. The majority of Ap-AVCN units produce primary-like discharges, with most of the remaining units producing chopper-type discharge patterns. The dotted lines from the axons of Ap-AVCN neurons indicate that the type or types of neurons and discharge patterns providing input to the LSO are unknown. A small contralateral input (labeled a) is provided to the medial limb of the LSO by neurons in the caudal AVCN (P-AVCN). A second major input from the contralateral ear is provided by neurons of the medial nucleus of the trapezoid body. Most LSO units appear multipolar in sagittal section (cell at lower left), with few appearing bipolar in shape (cell at lower right). Input to LSO neurons are provided by small terminals that synapse upon their somata and dendrites. Most LSO units produce transient Chop-N type discharge patterns (upper histogram at lower right), with few producing sustained chopper patterns.

MNTB units respond to stimulation of the contralateral ear with discharges of three general types (Guinan et al., 1972b): primary-like (78%), off-type (17%) and chopper type (3%) (Fig. 12). The MNTB units producing primary-like discharges also produce spike potentials of complex waveform similar to those produced by units in AA-AVCN. A positive presynaptic potential precedes the unit's post-

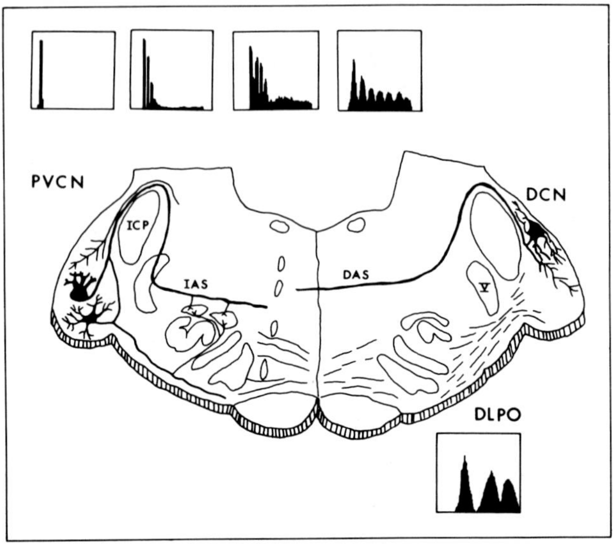

Fig. 15. Examples of the discharge patterns of dorsolateral periolivary (DLPO) units and of their probable afferent inputs. The octopus and multipolar cells of the postero-ventral cochlear nucleus (PVCN) provide input to the ipsilateral DLPO. The octopus cells that produce phasic type discharges (upper left) are suppressed by deep barbiturate anesthesia. The multipolar cells that produce chopper type discharges remain active to provide input to DLPO neurons. The morphology of DLPO neurons has not been described. Most DLPO units produce Chop-W type discharge patterns, often with a silent period between the first and second spike of the response. A contralateral input may arise from the dorsal cochlear nucleus (DCN).

synaptic potential by approximately 0.5 msec. (Li and Guinan, 1971). The MNTB principal neurons receive large calyx endings that provide a large area of synaptic contact that insures the generation of a postsynaptic spike potential with each incoming presynaptic potential. The calyx terminals in the MNTB arise from the thick axons of globular cells of the AVCN (Tolbert and Morest, 1977). The neural input to the MNTB principal neuron is most likely the primary-like output of units in the caudal AVCN. The MNTB units that produce other types of discharge patterns do not produce spike potentials of complex waveform, and are believed to be MNTB stellate cells or elongate cells. It has been suggested that because of similarities in the distribution of units producing off-type discharges and the distribution of MNTB stellate neurons that the stellate neurons may produce the off-type response (Guinan et al., 1972b). MNTB stellate neurons receive somatic and dendritic contacts from fine and medium-sized axons of caudal AVCN neurons. The multipolar cells of the caudal AVCN may produce chopper type discharges that serve as neural inputs to MNTB stellate neurons. Most of the few remaining MNTB units produce sustained chopper discharge patterns.

The cat MSO produces very large evoked potential fields to stimulation of either ear (Galambos et al., 1959; Tsuchitani and Boudreau, 1964; Guinan et al., 1972a). While the field potentials permit approximate localization of the MSO during an experiment, it is extremely difficult to isolate and record from individual units within the cat MSO (Guinan et al., 1967; Personal observations). Although much has been written about the role of MSO units in binaural localization of low frequency stimuli, it should be noted that most single unit studies of the MSO did not use adequate histological controls to localize units in the MSO (Guinan et al., 1967; Tsuchitani, 1977). It is in fact the case that very little is known about the response characteristics of cat MSO units. From the small amount of data available from units histologically confirmed to be located in the MSO (Guinan et al., 1972b) one may conclude that some MSO units are excited by stimulation of either ear and that most MSO units are most sensitive to tones of frequency less than 10 kHz. Of the two MSO units for which discharge pattern data is available, one produced a Pri-N discharge and one a frequency-following discharge (Fig. 13). MSO units probably receive primary-like input from AA-AVCN units through elongated terminals which are similar morphologically to the endbulbs and calyces of Held (Schwartz, 1972) and through small terminal boutons.

The majority of units within the LSO discharge with a chopper pattern to stimulation of the ipsilateral ear (Guinan et al., 1972b; Tsuchitani, 1977). Most of these LSO units produce Chop-N discharges in which the chopper pattern is very transient, often lasting less than 10 to 20 msec. The LSO ipsilateral input arises from the rostral AVCN where spherical cells producing primary-like discharges predominate. However, approximately 30% of the units in the small spherical cell area (APD and AP-AVCN) produce chopper type discharges. It is not known whether the LSO receives input exclusively from spherical cells or from both the spherical and multipolar cells of AVCN. The AVCN input to LSO cells arrives over numerous terminals that cover the surface of the cell soma and dendrites. Simultaneous stimulation of the two ears inhibits the discharges of LSO units most sensitive to stimulus frequencies above 1 kHz (Boudreau and Tsuchitani, 1970; Guinan et al., 1972b). The major source of input from the contralateral ear is provided by neurons in the MNTB. Although the majority of neurons within the MNTB are principal cells that produce primary-like discharges, the MNTB cell type projecting into the LSO is unknown. The contralateral input to the LSO reduces spike output and disrupts the chopper discharges to ipsilateral stimulation. The terminals of MNTB neurons on LSO neurons have not been described.

The discharges of units in the DLPO to stimulation of the ipsilateral ear are very regular at low rates of activity and produce Chop-W patterns (Tsuchitani, 1977). Frequently the interspike interval between the first two spikes of the response is longer than the succeeding interspike intervals (Fig. 15). The CNC input to the DLPO travels via the intermediate acoustic stria and trapezoid body from the ipsilateral PVCN. The axons of octopus cells, which produce phasic discharges, constitute the majority of fibers in the intermediate acoustic stria. The activity of phasically responding units in the caudal PVCN are suppressed during deep barbiturate anesthesia (Godfrey, 1971), the anesthetic state used in the study of the DLPO (Tsuchitani, 1977). Most units in the rostral PVCN appear to produce sustained Chop-N patterns even under deep anesthesia (Godfrey, 1971). Thus in deeply anesthetized cats the DLPO units receiving Chop-N type inputs appear to further integrate their inputs to produce a Chop-W output. The cell types and afferent terminal types of the DLPO have not been described in any detail. However there is anatomical and physiological evidence that different cell types exist within the DLPO. Some DLPO neurons are reactive to AChE and send their axons into the olivocochlear bundle to terminate in the cochlea (Osen and Roth, 1969; Warr, 1975). Other DLPO neurons are not reactive to AChE and send their axons back into the CNC (Warr, 1975; Adams and Warr, 1976). Some DLPO units are binaurally excited, while others appear to be excited by stimulation of the ipsilateral ear alone (Guinan et al., 1972b; Tsuchitani, 1977).

DISCUSSION

The anatomical complexity and the diversity of discharge patterns produced by lower auditory brain stem neurons indicate that selected features of the acoustic signal may be represented in the activity of different auditory neurons. While the specification of unit discharge pattern does not describe or represent all of the response properties of an auditory neuron, it does provide a basis for classification of single unit data that correlates with other response characteristics of the unit and with the morphological classification of neuron types. For example the AVCN units believed to provide input to the SOC nuclei involved in the processing of binaural information produce primary-like discharge patterns, with prepositive spike potentials and are capable of phase-locking to 5 kHz tones. In addition, many are spontaneously active, demonstrate relatively short latencies to click stimuli, are as narrowly tuned as auditory nerve fibers and are capable of producing increases in spike output to small and large increases in stimulus level (Kiang et al., 1965a; Kiang, 1975). Most units in the MNTB, which provides input to the LSO from the contralateral ear, have similar response properties. Most CNC units providing input to the superior olivary nuclei surrounding the MNTB, MSO and LSO produce narrow chopper or phasic discharge patterns. In turn, most of these superior olivary neurons project back to the cochlea and the CNC. The CNC units producing chopper discharges produce no spontaneous activity or low rates of spontaneous activity, respond with short to long latencies, are narrowly tuned and can signal stimulus level changes with changes in spike output (Kiang et al., 1965a; Kiang, 1975). Some of these units are also capable of producing greater maximum spike output than that produced by units discharging with primary-like patterns (Kiang, 1975). Neurons in the LSO, that compare interaural spectral differences and project to "higher" auditory nuclei, demonstrate similar response characteristics to stimulation of the ipsilateral ear. Some of the CNC units projecting to the dorsal cell groups of the SOC produce phasic discharge patterns and are more widely tuned at moderate to high stimulus levels. These CNC units respond with short latency and often are incapable of encoding stimulus level changes with changes in spike output. These neurons also appear to be more sensitive to anesthesia than other VCN units. Neurons with similar response characteristics are not observed in the SOC of deeply anesthetized cats. The outputs of most DCN cells bypass the SOC to project to the nuclei of the lateral lemniscus and the inferior colliculus. Most units in the DCN also demonstrate response characteristics that differ from those of VCN units. They produce pause, build, wide chopper or non-monotonic phasic discharge patterns. Many of the DCN units are spontaneously active in the absence of an auditory nerve input. The longest latencies produced by CNC units were produced by DCN units. DCN units are sensitive to anesthesia and some DCN units are responsive to binaural stimulation.

Although there have been significant advances in our understanding of the anatomical and physiological properties of auditory brainstem structures, much remains to be learned. In most cases the information available on the morphology, connections and physiology of the structures above the level of the CNC is insufficient for speculation as to their function. Further ultrastructural and histochemical studies will be required to specify the synaptic organization of all auditory neurons. The effects of the efferent input to auditory neurons have not been specified. Intracellular recording and dye-injection techniques should be utilized to verify the proposed relationships between cell morphology and discharge pattern. Furthermore a complete understanding of the function of auditory neurons may require the correlation of behavioral, clinical, psychophysical, as well as anatomical and physiological data.

Acknowledgements

The assistance of Sandra Flechsig and Larry Wasserman in preparing the illustrations is gratefully acknowledged. The patience of Jean Watkins in preparing the manuscript was especially helpful.

Supported in part by Public Health Service Grant 7 R01 NS 11218.

REFERENCES

Adams, J.C. and Warr, W.B. Origins of axons in the cat's acoustic striae determined by injection of horseradish peroxidase into severed tracts. *J. Comp. Neurol. 170:* 107-122, 1976.

Boudreau, J.C. and Tsuchitani, C. Cat superior olive S-segment cell discharge to tonal stimuli. In: *Contributions to Sensory Physiology, Vol. 4,* edited by W.D. Neff. New York: Academic Press, 1970, p. 143-213.

Bourk, T.R. Electrical responses of neural units in the anteroventral cochlear nucleus of the cat. Ph.D. Dissertation, Dept. E.E., MIT, 1976.

Bourk, T.R. Phase-locking in AVCN units of cat. *J. Acoust. Soc. Am. 61:* S59, 1977.

Brawer, J.R., Morest, D.K. and Kane, E.C. The neuronal architecture of the cochlear nucleus of the cat. *J. Comp. Neurol. 155:* 251-300, 1974.

Brawer, J.R. and Morest, D.K. Relations between auditory nerve endings and cell types in the cat's anteroventral cochlear nucleus seen with the Golgi method and Normarski optics. *J. Comp. Neurol. 160:* 491-506, 1975.

Cant, N.B. and Morest, D.K. Axonal types in the anteroventral cochlear nucleus (AVCN) of the cat: a Golgi study. *Neurosci. Abst. 1:* 36, 1975.

Clark, G.M. The ultrastructure of nerve endings in the medial superior olive of the cat. *Brain Res. 14:* 293-305, 1969.

Cohen, E.S., Brawer, J.R. and Morest, D.K. Projections of the cochlea to the dorsal cochlear nucleus in the cat. *Exper. Neurol. 35:* 470-479, 1972.

Evans, E.F. and Nelson, P.G. The responses of single neurones in the cochlear nucleus of the cat as a function of their location and the anesthetic state. *Exp. Brain Res. 17:* 402-427, 1973.

Feldman, M.L. and Harrison, J.M. The projection of the acoustic nerve to the ventral cochlear nucleus of the rat. A Golgi study. *J. Comp. Neurol. 137:* 267-294, 1969.

Fernández, C. and Karapas, F. The course and termination of the stria of Monakow and Held in the cat. *J. Comp. Neurol. 131:* 371-386, 1967.

Galambos, R., Schwartzkopff, J. and Rupert, A. Microelectrode study of superior olivary nuclei. *Amer. J. Physiol. 197:* 527-536, 1959.

Godfrey, D.A. Localization of single units in the cochlear nucleus of the cat: An attempt to correlate neuronal structure and function. Ph.D. Dissertation, Dept. of Physiology, Harvard University, 1971.

Godfrey, D.A., Kiang, N.Y.S. and Norris, B.E. Single unit activity in the posteroventral cochlear nucleus of the cat. *J. Comp. Neurol. 162:* 247-268, 1975a.

Godfrey, D.A., Kiang, N.Y.S. and Noris, B.E. Single unit activity in the dorsal cochlear nucleus of the cat. *J. Comp. Neurol. 162:* 269-284, 1975b.

Guinan, J.J., Guinan, S.S. and Norris, B.E. Single auditory units in the superior olivary complex. I. Responses to sound and classifications based on physiological properties. *Int. J. Neurosci. 4:* 101-120, 1972a.

Guinan, J.J., Norris, B.E. and Guinan, S.S. Single auditory units in the superior olivary complex. II: Locations of unit categories and tonotopic organization. *Int. J. Neurosci. 4:* 147-166, 1972b.

Guinan, J.J., Norris, B.E. and Swift, S.H. A paucity of unit responses in the accessory superior olive of barbiturate anesthetized cats. *J. Acoust. Soc. Am. 41:* 1585, 1967.

Harrison, J.M. and Feldman, M.L. Anatomical aspects of the cochlear nucleus and superior olivary complex. In: *Contributions to Sensory Physiology. Vol. 4,* edited by W.D. Neff. New York: Academic Press, 1970, p. 95-143.

Harrison, J.M. and Irving, R. The anterior ventral cochlear nucleus. *J. Comp. Neurol. 124:* 15-42, 1965.

Harrison, J.M. and Irving, R. Ascending connections of the anterior ventral cochlear nucleus in the rat. *J. Comp. Neurol. 126:* 51-64, 1966a.

Harrison, J.M. and Irving, R. The organization of the posterior ventral cochlear nucleus in the rat. *J. Comp. Neurol. 126:* 391-403, 1966b.

Harrison, J.M. and Warr, W.B. A study of the cochlear nuclei and ascending auditory pathways of the medulla. *J. Comp. Neurol. 119:* 341-380, 1962.

Held, H. Die centrale Gehorleitung, *Arch. f. Anat. u. Physiol. Anat. Abt. 17:* 201-248, 1893.

Kane, E.C. Octopus cells in the cochlear nucleus of the cat: heterotypic synapes upon homeotypic neurons. *Int. J. Neurosci. 5:* 251-279, 1973.

Kane, E.C. Patterns of degeneration in the caudal cochlear nucleus of the cat after cochlear ablation. *Anat. Rec. 179:* 67-92, 1974a.

Kane, E.C. Synaptic organization in the dorsal cochlear nucleus of the cat: a light and electron microscopic study. *J. Comp. Neurol. 155:* 301-330, 1974b.

Kane, E.S. Descending inputs to the octopus cell area of the cat cochlear nucleus: an electron microscopic study. *J. Comp. Neurol. 173:* 337-354, 1976a.

Kane, E.S. Descending projections to specific regions of cat cochlear nucleus: a light microscopic study. *Exper. Neurol. 52:* 372-388, 1976b.

Kane, E.C. Descending inputs to caudal cochlear nucleus in cats: a horseradish peroxidase (HRP) study. *Am. J. Anat. 146:* 433-441, 1976c.

Kiang, N.Y.S. Stimulus representation in discharge patterns of auditory neurons. In: *The Nervous System. 3: Human Communication and Its Disorders,* edited by D.B. Tower. New York: Raven Press, 1975, p. 81-96.

Kiang, N.Y.S., Godfrey, D.A., Norris, B.E. and Moxon, S.E. A block model of the cat cochlear nucleus. *J. Comp. Neurol. 162:* 221-246, 1975.

Kiang, N.Y.S., Morest, D.K., Godfrey, D.A., Guinan, J.J. and Kane, E.C. Stimulus coding at caudal levels of the cat's auditory nervous system: I. Response characteristics of single units. In: *Basic Mechanisms in Hearing,* edited by A.R. Møller. New York: Academic Press, 1973, p. 455-478.

Kiang, N.Y.S., Pfeiffer, R.R., Warr, W.B. and Backus, A.S.N. Stimulus coding in the cochlear nucleus. *Ann. Otol. Rhinol. Laryngol. 74:* 463-485, 1965a.

Kiang, N.Y.S., Watanabe, T., Thomas, E.C. and Clark, L.F. Discharge patterns of single fibers in the cat's auditory nerve. Cambridge: MIT Press, 1965b.

Koerber, K.C., Pfeiffer, R.R., Warr, W.B. and Kiang, N.Y.S. Spontaneous spike discharges from single units in the cochlear nucleus after destruction of the cochlea. *Exp. Neurol. 16:* 119-130, 1966.

Lavilla, I. Algunos detailles concernientes a la oliva superior y focos accesorios. *Rev. Trimes. Micrograf. 3:* 75-83, 1898.

Lenn, N.J. and Reese, T.S. The fine structure of nerve endings in the nucleus of the trapezoid body and the ventral cochlear nucleus. *Am. J. Anat. 118:* 375-389, 1966.

Li, R.Y.-S. and Guinan, J.J. Antidromic and orthodromic stimulation of neurons receiving calyces of Held. MIT Quart. Prog. Rpt. No. 100, 1971, p. 227-234.

Lindsey, B.G. Fine structure and distribution of axon terminals from the cochlear nucleus on neurons in the medial superior olivary nucleus of the cat. *J. Comp. Neurol. 160:* 81-104, 1975.

Lorente de Nó, R. Anatomy of the eighth nerve. III. General plan of structure of the primary cochlear nuclei. *Laryngoscope 43:* 327-350, 1933.

Lorente de Nó, R. Some unresolved problems concerning the cochlear nerve. *Ann. Otol. Rhinol. Laryngol.* Suppl. *34:* 1-28, 1976.

Luk, G.D., Morest, D.K. and McKenna, N.M. Origins of the crossed olivo-cochlear bundle shown by an acid phosphatase method in the cat. *Ann. Otol. Rhinol. Laryngol. 83:* 382-392, 1974.

Mast, T.E. Study of single units of the cochlear nucleus of the chinchilla. *J. Acoust. Soc. Am. 48:* 505-512, 1969.

Mast, T.E. Dorsal cochlear nucleus of the chinchilla: excitation by contralateral sound. *Brain Res. 62:* 61-70, 1973.

McDonald, D.M. and Rasmussen, G.L. Ultrastructural characteristics of synaptic endings in the cochlear nucleus having acetylcholinesterase activity. *Brain Res. 28:* 1-18, 1971.

Molnar, C.E. and Pfeiffer, R.R. Interpretation of spontaneous spike discharge patterns of neurons in the cochlear nucleus. *Proc. I.E.E.E. 56:* 993-1004, 1968.

Morest, D.J. The collateral system of the medial nucleus of the trapezoid body of the cat, its neuronal architecture and relation to the olivo-cochlear bundle. *Brain Res. 9:* 288-311, 1968.

Morest, D.K. Auditory neurons of the brain stem. *Adv. Oto-Rhino-Laryngol. 20:* 337-356, 1973.

Morest, D.K., Kiang, N.Y.S., Kane, E.C., Guinan, J.J. and Godfrey, D.A. Stimulus coding at caudal levels of the cat's auditory nervous system: II. Patterns of synaptic organization. In: *Basic Mechanisms in Hearing,* edited by A.R. Møller. New York: Academic Press, 1973, p. 479-510.

Osen, K.K. Cytoarchitecture of the cochlear nuclei in the cat. *J. Comp. Neurol. 136:* 453-484, 1969a.

Osen, K.K. The intrinsic organization of the cochlear nuclei in the cat. *Acta Otolaryngol. 67:* 352-359, 1969b.

Osen, K.K. Afferent and efferent connections of three well-defined cell types of the cat cochlear nuclei. In: *Excitatory Synaptic Mechanisms,* edited by P. Anderson and J.K.S. Jansen, Oslo: Universitetsforlaget, 1970a, p. 295-300.

Osen, K.K. Course and termination of the primary afferents in the cochlear nuclei of the cat. An experimental anatomical study. *Arch. Ital. Biol. 108:* 21-51, 1970b.

Osen, K.K. Projection of the cochlear nuclei on the inferior colliculus in the cat. *J. Comp. Neurol. 144:* 355-372, 1972.

Osen, K.K. and Roth, K. Histochemical localization of cholinesterases in the cochlear nuclei of the cat, with notes on the origin of acetylcholinesterase-positive afferents and the superior olive. *Brain Res. 16:* 165-185, 1969.

Perkins, R.E. An electron microscopic study of synaptic organization in the medial superior olive of normal and experimental chinchillas. *J. Comp. Neurol. 148:* 387-416, 1973.

Pfeiffer, R.R. Anteroventral cochlear nucleus: wave forms of extracellularly recorded spike potentials. *Science 154:* 667-668, 1966a.

Pfeiffer, R.R. Classification of response patterns of spike discharges for units in the cochlear nucleus: tone-burst stimulation. *Exp. Brain Res. 1:* 220-235, 1966b.

Ramón, y Cajal, S. The acoustic nerve: its cochlear branch or cochlear nerve. In: *Histologie due systeme Nervèux de l'Homme et des Vertébrés. Vol. I,* 1899, p. 774-838. English translation by Information Center for Hearing, Speech and Disorders of Human Communications, The John Hopkins Medical Institutions, PB 205-473, 1967.

Rasmussen, G.L. Efferent fibers of the cochlear nerve and cochlear nucleus. In: *Neural Mechanisms of the Auditory and Vestibular Systems,* edited by G.L. Rasmussen and W.F. Windle. Springfield: Charles C Thomas, 1960, p. 105-115.

Rasmussen, G.L. Anatomic relationships of the ascending and descending auditory systems. In: *Neurological Aspects of Auditory and Vestibular Disorders,* edited by W.S. Fields and B.R. Alford. Springfield: Charles C Thomas, 1964, p. 5-23.

Rasmussen, G.L. Efferent connections of the cochlear nucleus. In: *Sensorineural Hearing Processes and Disorders,* edited by A.B. Graham. Boston: Little Brown, 1967, p. 61-75.

Rose, J.E., Brugge, J.F., Anderson, D.J. and Hind, J.E. Phase-locked response to low-frequency tones in single auditory nerve fibers of the squirrel monkey. *J. Neurophysiol. 30:* 769-793, 1967.

Rose, J.E., Galambos, R. and Hughes, J.R. Microelectrode studies of the cochlear nuclei of the cat. *Bull. John Hopkins Hospital 104:* 211-251, 1959.

Scheibel, M.E. and Scheibel, A.B. Neuropil organization in the superior olive of the cat. *Exper. Neurol. 43:* 339-348, 1974.

Schwartz, I.R. Axonal endings in the cat medial superior olive: coated vesicles and intercellular substance. *Brain Res. 46:* 187-202, 1972.

Schwartz, I.R. Dendritic arrangements in the cat medial superior olive. *Neuroscience 2:* 81-101, 1977.

Stotler, W.A. An experimental study of the cells and connections of the superior olivary complex of the cat. *J. Comp. Neurol. 98:* 401-432, 1953.

Taber, E. The cytoarchitecture of the brain stem of the cat. I. Brain stem nuclei of cat. *J. Comp. Neurol. 116:* 27-70, 1961.

Tolbert, L.P. and Morest, D.K. Combined Golgi, horseradish peroxidase (HRP), and electron microscopic study of bushy cells in the cochlear nucleus. *Neurosci. Abst. 3:* 12, 1977.

Tsuchitani, C. and Boudreau, J.C. Wave activity in the superior olivary complex of the cat. *J. Neurophysiol. 27:* 814-827, 1964.

Tsuchitani, C. Functional organization of lateral cell groups of the cat superior olivary complex. *J. Neurophysol. 40:* 296-318, 1977.

van Noort, J. The Structure and Connections of the Inferior Colliculus. An Investigation of the Lower Auditory System. Van Gorcum, Assen, The Netherlands, 1969.

Warr, W.B. Fiber degeneration following lesions in the anterior ventral cochlear nucleus of the cat. *Exper. Neurol. 14:* 453-474, 1966.

Warr, W.B. Fiber degeneration following lesions in the posteroventral cochlear nucleus of the cat. *Exper. Neurol. 23:* 140-155, 1969.

Warr, W.B. Fiber degeneration following lesions in the multipolar and globular cell areas in the ventral cochlear nucleus of the cat. *Brain Res. 40:* 247-270, 1972.

Warr, W.B. Olivocochlear and vestibular efferent neurons of the feline brain stem: their location, morphology and number determined by retrograde axonal transport and acetylcholinesterase histochemistry. *J. Comp. Neurol. 161:* 159-182, 1975.

DISCUSSION

Trahiotis: Will you please describe two things: (1) generally the effects of kinds of levels of anesthesia on response patterns, and (2) the effects of binaural inputs?

Tsuchitani: These units were all stimulated monaurally. Most of the discharge patterns obtained in the cochlear nucleus and in the superior olivary complex were from animals under heavy anesthesia. The talk concentrated on monaural stimulus conditons to simplify the discussion of the role of neural discharge patterns in the input-output transfer functions of the ipsilateral or contralateral sound source by auditory units. Within the lateral superior olive units with CF above 1 kHz are excited by stimulation of the ipsilateral ear and inhibited by stimulation of the contralateral ear. In the DLPO, I find units are only excited by ipsilateral stimulation. Guinan reports he finds a number of binaurally excited units in the DLPO. In the MSO I think Guinan may have had ten units in which he could check this, and he found seven of the ten were binaurally excited.

Huang: I can appreciate your difficulty in recording single cells in areas around SOC due to large electrical fields. Is there any other brain stem area which may exhibit these fields?

Tsuchitani: There are fairly large fields within the nuclei of the lateral lemniscus also, but they are not as neat as we find within the MSO. Within the olfactory system (the prepyriform cortex) and hippocampus you will find these large dipole fields also. Within the auditory system the MSO is fairly unique in producing a dipole field.

BASIC AND CLINICAL ASPECTS OF BRAINSTEM RECORDING IN HUMANS

BRIEF FORMAL PRESENTATIONS AND ROUND TABLE DISCUSSION

Moderator: *Hallowell Davis*

The BER in the ICU
Galambos, Robert

Brainstem evoked potentials and auditory analysis of single cycle transients
Gerken, George M.

Recording procedures for brainstem potentials
Terkildsen, Knud, Osterhammel, P. and Huis in 't Veld, F.

Interpretation of cochlear nerve and brainstem evoked responses
Thornton, A. Roger D.

The generator of the auditory brainstem potentials as revealed by brainstem lesions in both man and cat
Starr, Arnold

INTRODUCTION TO FORMAL PRESENTATIONS

Davis: Folk, brain stem responses seem to have filtered somehow into the earlier discussions. I should, I suppose, now make a formal introduction of them to you by name and number.

The brain stem response (BSR) is usually recorded with one electrode on the vertex, but we have found that the forehead right here at the hair line does just as well. A reference electrode is on an earlobe or mastoid. BSR is a non-invasive way of getting at early electrical activity in response to acoustic signals. They are very small; they require the summing of perhaps 1000 or 2000 responses, but this can be done expeditiously because very rapid rates of repetition are quite permissible.

The key to the brain stem responses, which we will mention repeatedly, is synchronization. They depend on synchronized activity in the brain stem, and in the course of our discussion the question of just where in the brain stem the generators are located will finally emerge. The latency range we are dealing with is from about 1 or 2 msec to 10 or 12. A series of waves are spaced, curiously, almost exactly 1 msec apart. One of the best known names associated with the BSR is Jewett, who gave the first definitive description of them in the human and gave them numbers. (Jewett, D.L., and J.S. Williston. Auditory-evoked far fields averaged from the scalp of humans. *Brain 94:* 681-696, 1971).

I believe there have been at least ten different systems of numbering employed in the last couple of years, but I am proposing that we use today the Jewett nomenclature, in which wave I is a vertex-positive wave at about 1.5 to 2 msec, depending on the exact form of the stimulus. It is the auditory nerve in action. That is pretty well established. Wave II is variable, III is rather prominent, IV is highly variable, and Jewett's wave V, -that's our boy. It comes along with extraordinary precision, 4 msec after wave I; it is very robust and can be followed down to the behavioral threshold with certain stimuli. You will hear a lot about wave V. It is so robust and so sensitive that it can be used for screening newborn infants. This will be the topic that Dr. Galambos will deal with. We will lead off with this because it is a relatively simple procedure. I think he will emphasize also that it has considerable clinical value.

We will see in the later papers that we can also obtain a complete threshold audiogram. A quite different aspect will be the neurological implications of alterations in some of these waves.

Bob, will you take over and lead off these discussions?

THE BER IN THE ICU

Robert Galambos

University of California, San Diego

As our Chairman has stated, my task is to examine with you some of our data on the brain stem electric response (BER) infants. Figure 1 shows typical BERs obtained from normal babies, one a newborn (gestational age 40 wks), the other a baby estimated to be 6 or 7 weeks premature. At the time these recordings were made the babies were sleeping naturally after a feeding. Standard EEG electrodes had been attached to the vertex and the two mastoid regions, and an earphone, fixed in place over one ear with surgical tape, delivered clicks at 37 per sec to the ear lying beneath it. The electrophysiological responses to these clicks were extracted from the amplified EEG signal by a small averaging computer. Each BER tracing in Figure 1 displays such an average of 2000 responses to clicks at the intensity (re normal adult threshold) shown at the left. We always obtain two BERs at each intensity and superimpose them in the write-out; this allows the eye to estimate the reliability of the measurement.

The BERs consist of a sequence of waves labeled in the figure with Roman numerals. At high intensities waves I, III and V stand out prominently, and as intensity drops their amplitudes diminish and their latencies increase. Near threshold (see the 30 dB response from the premature) only wave V is identifiable. For making an audiologic diagnosis one establishes from such recordings first the weakest stimulus that produces a wave V, for this approximates the threshold, and second, the wave V latency obtained at each intensity (shown in the right column of the figure). The threshold for both babies shown in Figure 1 lies below 30 dB, and the wave V latency-intensity function is normal for the age.

In one of our studies we tested 220 healthy term newborns 7 hours to several days old (Schulman-Galambos and Galambos, 1978a). All but one yielded recordings like those in Figure 1. We attempted to establish the threshold in only 20 of them; all of these produced a wave V to a 20 dB click but not to a 10 dB click. It is evident, therefore, that the sensitivity of the peripheral auditory apparatus in a newborn is high, and that a normal baby should hear click stimuli (ie., process them at the cortical level) about as well at birth as he ever will.

We have been particularly interested in evaluating the BER as a neurological and audiological diagnostic tool in the population of premature babies one finds in an infant intensive care unit (ICU). Most of these infants are at high risk for sensory, motor and intellectual deficits associated with prematurity. We would like

ISBN 0-12-514960-3

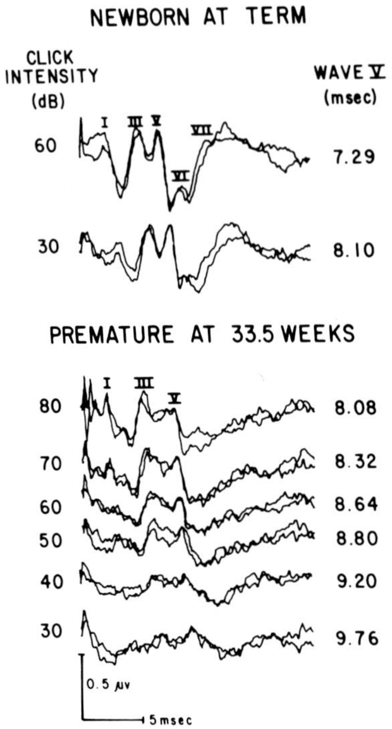

Fig. 1. See text.

to know how well the BER estimates the auditory threshold and the type of hearing loss (conductive vs sensory neural) on the one hand, and on the other, the degree to which the method can evaluate the functional capacities of the brain stem. I will deal here only with the audiological aspects of our studies. Before doing so, however, it will be useful to return to Figure 1 to consider what is known about the neural structures that give rise to the various waves in the BER, and to state some inferences to be drawn from these facts.

Wave I unquestionably reflects auditory nerve activity. If one experimentally establishes the latency of wave I at several intensities in adults (eg., Starr and Achor, 1975) and compares these values with similar measurements made on the N_1 wave in the electrocochleogram (eg., Eggermont, 1976), the agreement between the two turns out to be very close. From this one may conclude that the BER "sees" in its wave I the same phenomenon a transtympanic electrode reveals. In the BER the auditory nerve response is considerably smaller in size, but as Figure 1 shows it can readily be identified in many recordings.

The next BER wave to consider is wave V. Most authorities locate its generator somewhere in the region of the inferior colliculus. If this is correct the interval between I and V measures the time required for conduction of nerve impulses between the auditory nerve and the inferior colliculus. This brain stem conduction time is readily estimated in Figure 1; for the newborn it is about 4.5 msec, and for the premature 5.7 msec. In normal adults the I-V interval is 4 msec, as Starr and Achor first demonstrated, and this value (and hence the conduction time) is the same at all intensities (which is true for the responses in Figure 1 also). We can therefore conclude first, that impulse conduction in the brain stem auditory pathway speeds up with age, and second that whenever a wave V is visualized in the BER a wave I must have preceded it by a fixed time interval. This last is an important point, for it ties wave V closely to the N_1 response of the cochleogram; the BER wave V can be considered, as a first approximation, to be merely the N_1 of the cochleogram delayed by a fixed amount which depends on age. Theoretically any stimulus-induced change in N_1 could be faithfully reflected by a similar change in wave V. Drs. Eggermont and Don, among others, are presently testing the validity of this generalization, I believe.

Returning to our measurements on the ICU babies, we first established the rate at which wave V latency shortens with age. Consider Figure 1 again; in the newborn response to the 60 dB click wave V latency is 7.29 msec; for the premature it is 8.64 msec. This means that impulses aroused by the stimulus at the cochlea arrived at the inferior colliculus considerably earlier in the older baby, 1.35 msec earlier, in fact. In systematic studies of this problem we estimated the speeding-up to approximate 0.2-0.5 msec per week during this period of life (Schulman-Galambos and Galambos, 1975), and thereafter to proceed at a reduced rate for 12-18 months (Hecox and Galambos, 1974). Part of the postnatal decrease in conduction time appears to be due to an improvement in the ability of the cochlea to excite its auditory nerve and another part to myelination and/or increased synaptic efficiency in the brain stem tracts and nuclei (Hecox, 1975).

Our ICU studies have provided an opportunity to estimate the incidence of severe sensorineural hearing loss in this population. When we tested 75 babies at the time of their discharge we found four with losses greater than 60 dB in one or both ears (Schulman-Galambos and Galambos, 1977a). In a study just completed on 100 babies tested while in our ICU at Childrens Hospital in San Diego, Dr. Paul Despland has identified eight with losses greater than 40 dB in each ear. These two results suggest that the incidence of significant peripheral disease is very high in this group of infants, perhaps as high as 1:10 or 1:20. We presently test every infant at the time of discharge and recommend that others do so also; the results of this program will securely establish the incidence of hearing disorder in this group, and identify the infants who should be referred for audiological diagnosis and treatment.

In our hands the BER has proved to be a reliable and precise method for estimating threshold sensitivity in infancy. It is a simple test to perform, and it offers a non-invasive, objective way to evaluate the function of the peripheral auditory apparatus. Almost no infant is untestable, few if any healthy infants with normal hearing will be misdiagnosed as deaf, and only rarely will a hearing-impaired one be diagnosed as normal.

For those particularly interested in the use of the BER in hearing testing, two excellent reviews that discuss these matters can be consulted (Davis, 1976; Picton, et al., 1977). The publications from our laboratory include, in addition to those already cited, a complete summary of our experiences to date with the ICU population (Schulman-Galambos and Galambos, 1977b), the BER characterization of conductive and sensorineural hearing loss (Galambos and Hecox, 1977); a description of the effective stimulus (Hecox, et al., 1976); and the application of the BER method to a sample of 81 difficult-to-test pediatric patients (Mokotoff, et al., 1977).

REFERENCES

Davis, H. Principles of electric response audiometry. *Ann. Otol. Rhinol. Laryngol.* Suppl. *28:* 4-96, 1976.

Eggermont, J.J. Electrocochleography. In: *Handbook of Sensory Physiology. V/3. Clinical and Special Topics,* edited by W.D. Keitel and W.D. Neff. Berlin, Heidelberg, New York: Springer-Verlag, 1976, p. 625-705.

Galambos, R. and Hecox, K. Clinical applications of the human brain stem responses to auditory stimuli. In: *Proceedings of the Brussels Congress on Cerebral Evoked Potentials,* edited by J. Desmedt. Oxford: Oxford University Press, 1977.

Hecox, K. and R. Galambos. Brain stem auditory evoked responses in human infants and adults. *Arch. Otolaryngol. 99:* 30-33, 1974.

Hecox, K. Electrophysiological correlates of human auditory development. In: *Infant Perception: From Sensation to Cognition,* edited by L. Cohen and P. Salapatek. New York: Acedemic Press, 1975, p. 151-191.

Hecox, K., Squires, N. and Galambos, R. Brain stem auditory evoked responses in man: I. Effect of stimulus rise-fall time and duration. *J. Acoust. Soc. Am. 60:* 1187-1192, 1976.

Mokotoff, B., Schulman-Galambos, C. and Galambos, R. Brain stem auditory evoked responses in children. *Arch. Otolaryngol. 103:* 38-43, 1977.

Picton, T.W., Woods, D.L., Baribeau-Braun, J. and Healey, T.M.G. Evoked potential audiometry. *J. Otolaryngol. 6:* 90-119, 1977.

Schulman-Galambos, C. and Galambos, R. Brain stem auditory evoked responses in premature infants. *J. Speech Hear. Res. 18:* 456-465, 1975.

Schulman-Galambos, C. and Galambos, R. Brain stem evoked response audiometry in newborn hearing screening. *Arch. Otolaryngol.* 1978a, (In press).

Schulman-Galambos, C. and Galambos, R. Assessment of Hearing. In: *The Infant At-Risk,* edited by T. Field. 1978b, (In Press).

Starr, A. and Achor, J. Auditory brain stem responses in neurological disease. *Arch. Neurol. 32:* 761-768, 1975.

DISCUSSION

Davis: Dr. Galambos's work shows a very simple but very effective procedure for which the brain stems can be employed. We will now move toward something rather more analytic, something approaching the behavioral audiogram, and leading into audiology. For this, Dr. Gerken will take over for the next presentation.

BRAIN STEM EVOKED POTENTIALS AND AUDITORY ANALYSIS OF SINGLE CYCLE TRANSIENTS

George M. Gerken

University of Texas at Dallas

Many brief, transient sounds are easily discriminated by the human auditory system. For example, a difference is apparent between clicks that are generated by the presentation of single cycles of frequencies that differ by a factor of two or three. One dimension of this perceptual difference is that of tonality. I am assuming in this example that the clicks are produced by a type of earphone typically used in auditory research so that the acoustic clicks are one or two cycles of a damped sine wave.

Single cycles of 500, 1500, and 5000 Hz were used in the work described below. The initial portion of all acoustic signals was a rarefaction. The electrical signals applied to a TDH-49 phone and the resulting acoustic waveforms are shown in Figure 1.

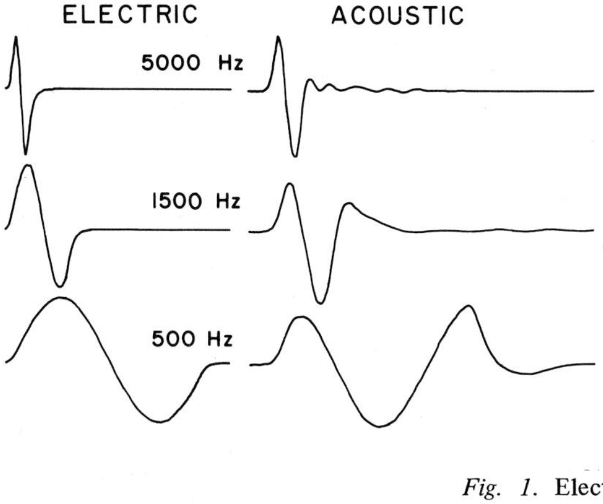

Fig. 1. Electrical signals applied to the phones and the resulting acoustic waveforms.

ISBN 0-12-514960-3

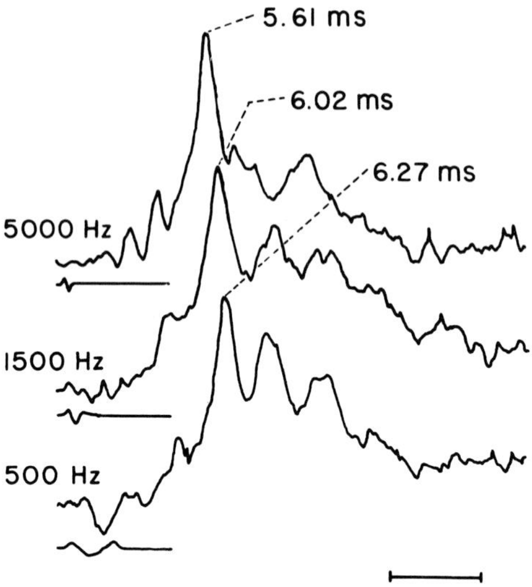

Fig. 2. Brainstem potentials (N= 2000) evoked by single cycle stimuli of 500, 1500, and 5000 Hz presented at 20 per second. Amplifier bandwidth for this and other figures was 0.3 Hz to 3.0 kHz and gain was 5 x 10^4. Stimuli were equated for peak-to-peak amplitude with zero decibel defined as the typical absolute behavioral threshold for the 500 Hz single cycle stimulus. Sensation level was 60 dB re the standardized 500 Hz reference. The short trace below each evoked potential is the acoustic stimulus. Latencies shown are from stimulus onset to wave V peak. Time marker is 5 msec.

The brainstem responses evoked by the single cycle stimuli are shown in Figure 2. The largest peak, wave V, is a prominent component in the response to all three stimuli. The main point to be gained from Figure 2 is that the latency between stimulus onset and the peak of wave V is related to stimulus frequency. Wave V latency is shortest for 5000 Hz (5.61 msec stimulus onset to peak of wave V), longer for 1500 Hz (6.02 msec), and still longer for 500 Hz (6.27 msec).

Derbyshire and Davis (1935) demonstrated that the rarefaction portion of the stimulus is the portion which initiates activity in the auditory nerve. In the present work the effective time of stimulation is thus assumed to occur at some point between onset of the initial wave, which was a rarefaction wave, and its peak. The range of possible latencies for wave V is then bounded by two measures: stimulus onset to wave V peak, and stimulus peak to wave V peak. Furthermore, time of stimulation presumably moves toward the stimulus peak as intensity is decreased.

Figure 3 shows the latency-intensity functions for wave V as produced by 500, 1500, and 5000 Hz single-cycle stimuli. For each frequency, the two latency measures are indicated. In contrasting the effects of stimulus frequency, it is appropriate to use only one or the other definition of latency but not both. Figure 3 was constructed as shown to argue for the almost complete separation of latency-intensity functions at the three frequencies.

The data for 500 Hz at 15 and 30 dB are not available because wave V abruptly disappears in the vicinity of 45 dB. The two prominent components following wave V shown in Figure 2 merge, however, into a single deflection that occurs at least down to 15 dB.

One interpretation of the results shown in Figure 3 is in terms of traveling wave delay on the basilar membrane (Teas et al., 1962; Tonndorf, 1960). At any

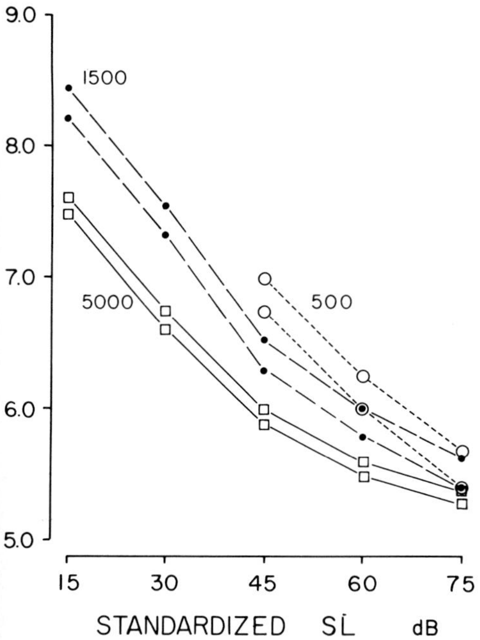

Fig. 3. Wave V latency-intensity functions for single cycle stimuli of 500, 1500, and 5000 Hz. For each frequency, the longer latency is the time from stimulus-onset to wave V peak and the shorter latency is the interval from stimulus peak to wave V peak.

given intensity level, the evoked potential latency should be shortest for the 5000 Hz stimulus, longest for 500 Hz, and of an intermediate value for the 1500 Hz stimulus. The partial convergence of the three latency-intensity curves at the 75 dB intensity level, however, might be taken to indicate that the 500 and 1500 Hz stimuli were activating high frequency neurons and thereby generating shorter latencies. The convergence then could be explained in terms of stimulating the tails of high frequency neurons (Kiang and Moxon, 1974). The abrupt termination of the latency-intensity function for 500 Hz as intensity is decreased supports this interpretation since a relatively intense stimulus is needed to stimulate the tails at frequencies well removed from best frequency.

The hypothesis that the separations of the latency-intensity functions of Figure 3 are entirely attributable to stimulation of the tails of high frequency neurons was evaluated in the following experiment. Two bands of noise were selected on the basis of perceptual observations for maximal masking of the 1500 Hz and 5000 Hz single-cycle stimuli. For the 1500 Hz stimulus, the noise band was centered on 1000 Hz and extended from 550 Hz to 1800 Hz. For the 5000 Hz stimulus, the noise band was centered on 2500 Hz and extended from 1800 to 3500 Hz. The filter used has 76 dB per octave skirts.

In the evoked potential portion of the experiment, the maximum intensity was determined for each single cycle stimulus which just failed to produce an averaged evoked potential in the presence of the corresponding masking noise. For example, the lack of response to the 1500 Hz stimulus in the presence of the 550 to 1800 Hz band of noise is shown in Figure 4, top left. With the same intensity of

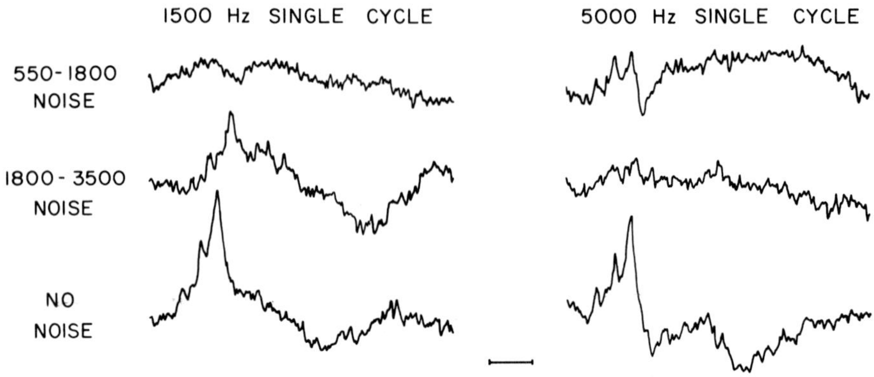

Fig. 4. Double dissociation of masking effects. Left column: stimulus was a single cycle of 1500 Hz at 30 dB SL. Right Column: stimulus was a single cycle of 5000 Hz at 24 dB SL. Top row: masking noise band of 550 to 1800 Hz at 84 dB SPL. Middle row: masking noise band of 1800 to 3500 Hz at 84 dB SPL. Bottom row: no masking noise. N=4000 and time marker is 5 msec.

the 1500 Hz stimulus, it may be seen that an evoked potential was obtained in the presence of the 1800-3500 Hz band of noise (Fig. 4, middle left). In the same manner, the absence of response to the 5000 Hz single cycle stimulus in the presence of the 1800 to 3500 Hz band of noise is shown in Figure 4 (middle right). A response was obtained, however, with the same intensity of the 5000 Hz stimulus in the presence of the 550-1800 Hz noise band. This double dissociation of masking effects indicates that the single cycle stimuli activate different regions of the basilar membrane.

The responses to the 1500 and 5000 Hz stimuli without masking noise are shown in Figure 4, bottom left and right, respectively. Since these responses are larger than the evoked potentials obtained in the presence of a masking noise, it would seem that the regions of the basilar membrane activated by the two stimuli overlap.

Transient stimuli are subjected to frequency analysis by the cochlea (Teas et al., 1962) and the consequences of this analysis may be observed in the brainstem evoked potentials. On the basis of the masking experiment, it can be concluded that at least a portion of the differences among the latency-intensity functions of Figure 3 can be attributed to traveling wave delay in the cochlea. Clinical testing to relate auditory pathology with the latency-intensity functions for the single cycle stimuli is suggested by these findings.

REFERENCES

Derbyshire, A.J. and Davis, H. The action potentials of the auditory nerve. *Am. J. Physiol. 113:* 476-504, 1935.

Kiang, N.Y.S. and Moxon, E.C. Tails of tuning curves of auditory-nerve fibers. *J. Acoust. Soc. Am. 55:* 620-630, 1974.

Teas, D.C., Eldredge, D.H. and Davis, H. Cochlear responses to acoustic transients: an interpretation of whole-nerve action potentials. *J. Acoust. Soc. Am. 34:* 1438-1459, 1962.

Tonndorf, J. Response of cochlear models to aperiodic signals and to random noises. *J. Acoust. Soc. Am. 32:* 1344-1355, 1960.

Acknowledgement

I am indebted to Thomas M. Helfer and Irvin J. Gerling for their assistance in these experiments. This work was supported in part by the Fikes, Fleischmann, Jonsson, Moody, and Sloan Foundations.

DISCUSSION

Davis: Thank you, Dr. Gerken. You have introduced the important dimension of frequency. It is a temptation to get into a debate now on the basis of this information, on the relative merits of the click, the single cycle, the tone pip and the tone burst; and concerning their various degrees of frequency specificity. We will reserve that for the final discussion if we have time for it.

In the interest of equal time for all, I will call on Dr. Terkildsen now. I am not sure which part of his manuscript he is going to present. You tell them, and I will listen.

RECORDING PROCEDURES FOR BRAIN STEM POTENTIALS

Knud Terkildsen, P. Osterhammel and F. Huis in 't Veld

University Hospital, Copenhagen

Just a few years ago the brain stem potentials were thought of as an interesting phenomenon from a scientific point of view, but generally were not expected to be useful for clinical work because of the very small amplitude of the response.

We have devoted a good deal of our efforts to optimize the recording procedure in order to overcome this difficulty and improve the signal-to-noise situation. Electrode placement is an important problem and very early we found that responses could be recovered all over the scalp; but the main place of activity was the vertex (C_Z). We also came to the conclusion that our purpose would be served best by having a relatively neutral site of reference, which could be the side of the neck (Terkildsen, et al., 1974). Figure 1 illustrates this point. These responses from five different test subjects were obtained by means of a reference electrode on the thorax; they are essentially monopolar recordings from a number of selected positions on the head. It is evident that the sequence of waves is most prominent at the vertex and that the neck is almost neutral. The most common mode of recording is to place the reference electrode at the ear which is stimulated (ear lobe or mastoid). Figure 2 shows what influence this will have on the response pattern. The upper tracing is from the vertex and the lower one from the mastoid, both obtained simultaneously in the same recording situation. N_1 in the AP complex appears as a negative deviation at the mastoid and a positive deviation at the vertex. In both tracings there follows a somewhat more pronounced swing in the opposite direction. This period of complete phase reversal is suddenly interrupted at 2.6 msec, where a small negative-going swing at the mastoid turns positive, while at the vertex there is one continuous, uninterrupted deviation in the positive direction. From there on the two recordings are essentially in the same phase. In a differential mode of recording between these two positions the N_1 becomes enhanced, but the later part of the response will be distorted and the Jewett V wave in particular tends to be diminished. Furthermore, the contamination will confuse any detailed analysis of individual waves.

In essence the brain stem potentials are on-responses, but still it is possible to obtain a reasonably good frequency specificity with tone-bursts, that have rise-times with 2-4 waves up (Terkildsen et al., 1977). Figure 3 shows objective recordings from a normal hearing child. At 2 and 4 kHz the rise-time was 1 msec and at 1 kHz 2 msec. As it might be expected, the threshold sensitivity is poorer in the low

ISBN 0-12-514960-3

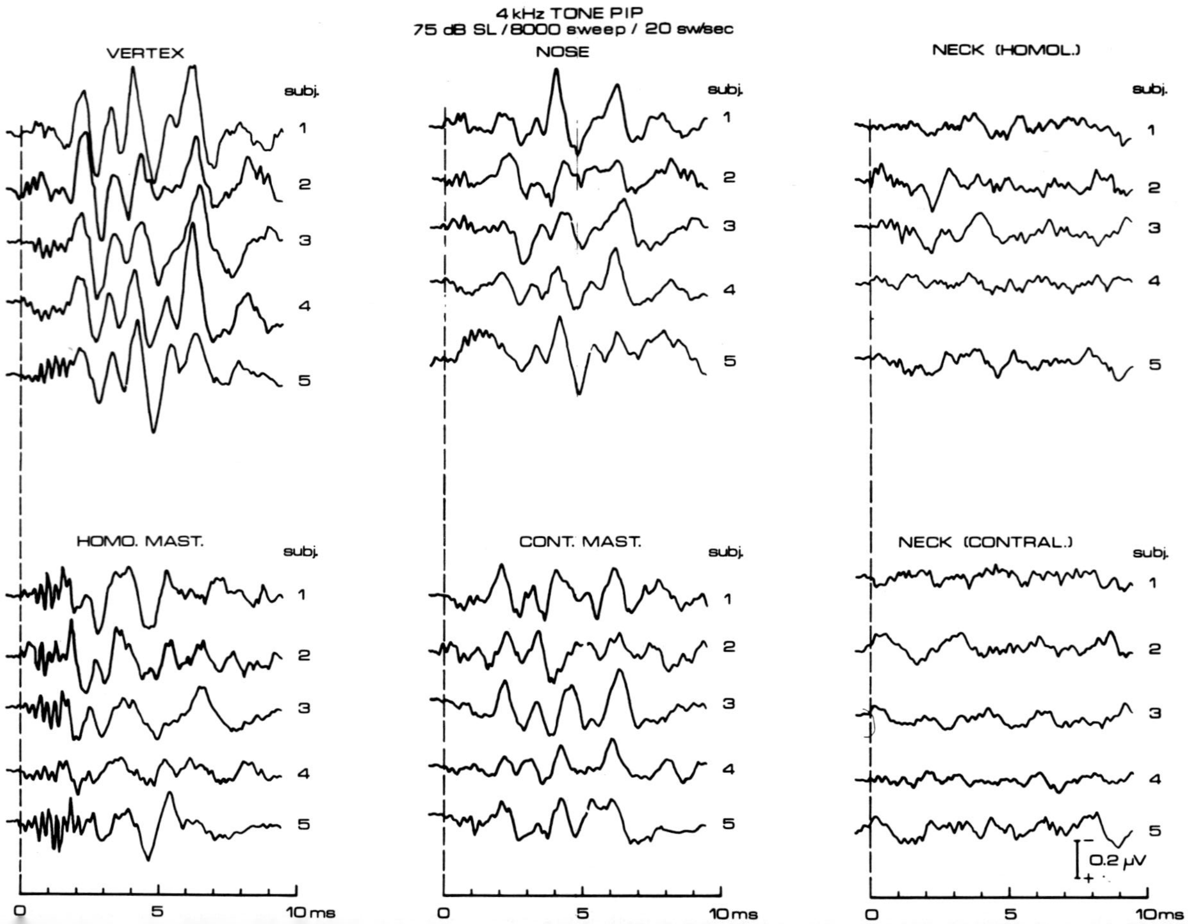

4 kHz TONE PIP
75 dB SL / 8000 sweep / 20 sw/sec
VERTEX
NOSE
NECK (HOMOL.)
HOMO. MAST.
CONT. MAST.
NECK (CONTRAL.)
subj.
1
2
3
4
5
0.2 μV
0
5
10 ms

Fig. 1. Recordings from 5 normal subjects at 6 selected electrode positions (Vertex, homolateral mastoid, tip of the nose, contralateral mastoid, homolateral side of the neck and contralateral side of the neck). Reference, thorax. Stimulus level, and sweep time as indicated. (Terkildsen et al, *Scand. Audiol.*, 1974).

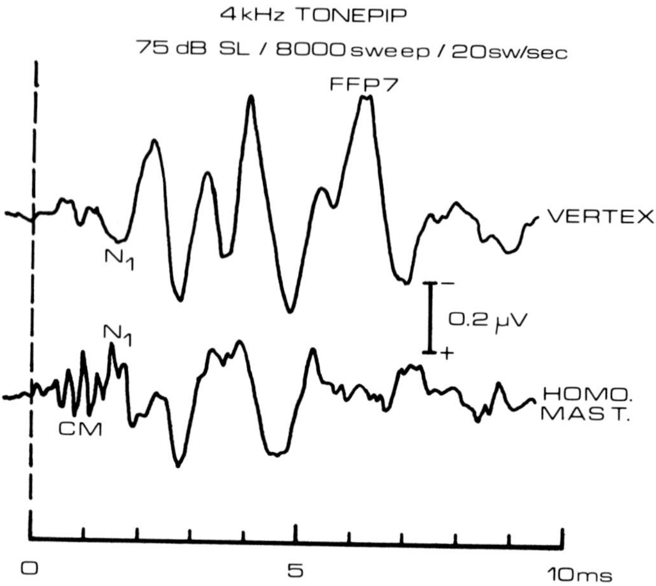

Fig. 2. Simultaneous recordings from Vertex and homolateral mastoid. Reference, thorax. Stimulus level, and sweep time as indicated. FFP_7, the 7 msec far field potential. (Terkildsen et al, 1977).

frequencies, and at present the low frequencies remain a problem in any objective evaluation of hearing by means of the early electrophysiological responses. The 500 Hz frequency-following response (FFR) is of some help, but masking experiments and clinical experience have demonstrated that it is generated over a rather wide area of the basilar membrane that extends from the 500 Hz tonotopic point down almost to the middle of the cochlea. It has been suggested that progressive masking, beginning from the high frequencies, might improve the situation but our experience has been that masking may have very peculiar effects on the vertex recorded FFR. The upper right part of Figure 4 demonstrates a rather dramatic change in the FFR caused by a 1.5 kHz masker. At a very low masking level the later part of the response disappears almost completely; when the masking is increased the response recovers but undergoes complete phase reversal. To the lower right is a simultaneous recording from the mastoid; quite clearly there is no such effect to be observed at this electrode position.

Figure 5 shows results from a severely hard of hearing child. There is good agreement between the objective and the subjective thresholds in the higher frequencies. The threshold for the 500 Hz FFR is somewhat poorer, but there can be no doubt that it indicates the presence of relatively good function in the apical part of the cochlea. At the same time the results would prove that the 500 Hz FFR cannot just be a repetitive Jewett V wave configuration.

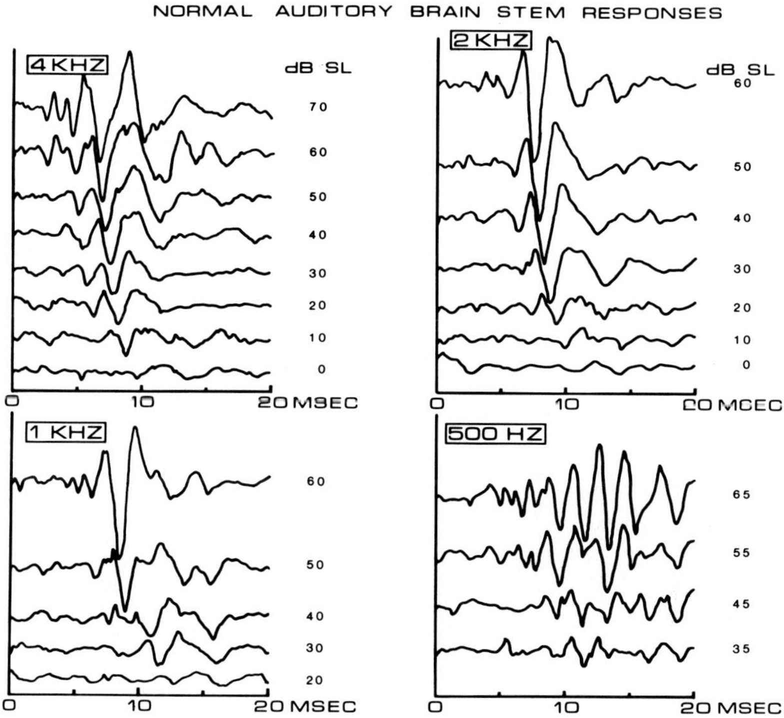

Fig. 3. Response patterns from a 2 year old, normal hearing, psychotic child. Sedation 60 mg Nembutal rectally. Active electrode at the Vertex, reference consisted of 2 linked electrodes attached to either side of the neck. 500 Hz stimulus: rise-decay times 2 msec, plateau 6 msec; 1 kHz stimulus: rise-decay times 2 msec, plateau 1 msec; 2 and 4 kHz stimuli: rise-decay times 1 msec, plateau 1 msec.

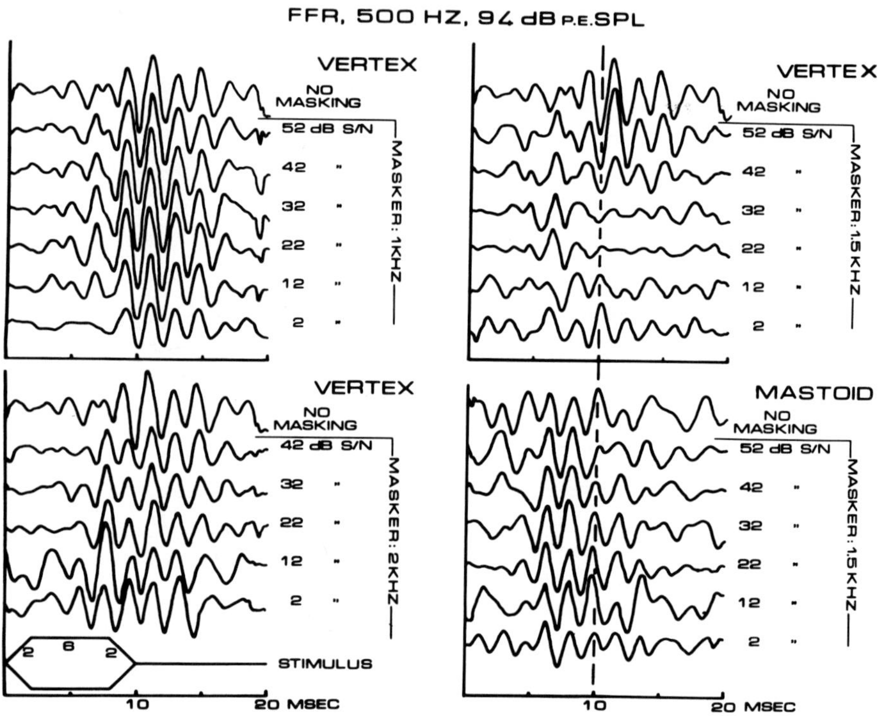

Fig. 4. Progressive masking of the 500 Hz FFR. Stimulus rise-decay times 2 msec, plateau 6 msec. Stimulus intensity and S/N ratios as indicated. (Left) Vertex recorded responses in the presence of continuous 300 Hz wide noise bands at center frequencies of 1 and 2 kHz. (Right) Results with the use of a noise band centered at 1.5 kHz. Uppermost, the Vertex response and below that the mastoid-derived activity. Both were obtained in the same recording situation via two parallel channels, and with a neutral point of reference. (Terkildsen et al, *Scand. Audiol.* 6, 1977).

Lately we have experimented with simultaneous recording of the brain stem responses and the middle latency response. For this purpose we have used a 50 msec recording window and a bandpass that extends from 22 Hz to 1 kHz. In Figure 6 we used abrupt-rising 2 kHz stimuli with very different durations. The onset generates a brain stem and a middle latency response that is completely independent of stimulus duration, even a one half sine wave will suffice. There is also very clearly an offset brain stem response. It diminishes for the short stimulus durations but can still be traced when the duration is only 3 msec. In Figure 7 we used a recording window of 150 msec and a 4 kHz stimulus. In the upper tracing the stimulus lasted only 2 msec and in the lower tracing it covered half of the recording period, 75 msec. The off-response is completely identical with the on-response. Thus the middle latency response has the same characteristics as the brain stem responses and the slow cortical responses; they are on-off responses; but the recovery time increases gradually with the latency of the response.

Figure 8 shows the response to stimuli with rise-times of 10 msec. The 4 kHz stimulus yields a Jewett V wave even at low stimulus levels and this wave appears to be just as sensitive as the middle latency response with regard to the threshold sensitivity. With the 500 Hz stimulus the situation is reversed and we may have here a means of improving our diagnostic capability at the low frequencies.

SUMMARY

Recording Procedures for the Brain Stem Potentials

The brain stem response amplitude is so small that recording technique is critical. The most active electrode position is the vertex. At the mastoid the activity relates to the vertex response in such a manner that a differential recording between these two points will enhance the N_1 of the AP while the later part of the response tends to be diminished and more difficult to interpret in physiological terms. It is possible to obtain a reasonable degree of frequency selectivity during objective hearing testing by means of stimuli with rise times of 2-4 waves. The sensitivity in the low frequencies is relatively poor. Here the 500 Hz FFR may be helpful in patients suffering from a high-tone loss. Simultaneous recordings of the brain stem and the middle latency responses clearly show that they both are on-off responses in the same manner as the slow cortical response, but the recovery time increases with the latency of the responses. With long rise-times the middle latency response exhibits a fair sensitivity with regard to the subjective threshold in the low frequencies and may be the best choice for audiometric testing in this part of the audiometric range.

Acknowledgements

This work was partially supported by the Danish Medical Research Council.

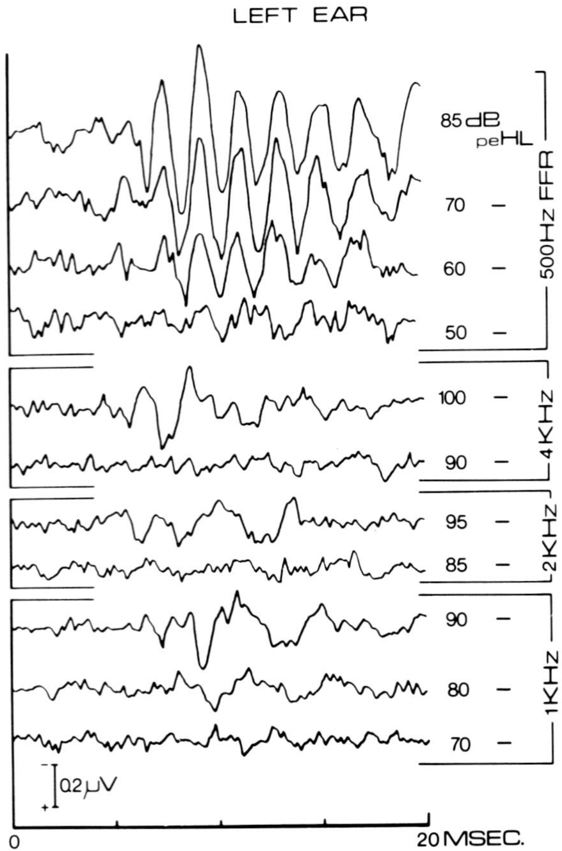

LEFT EAR
85 dB peHL
70
60
50
500Hz FFR
100
90
4KHz
95
85
2KHz
90
80
70
1KHz
0.2 μV
0
20 MSEC.

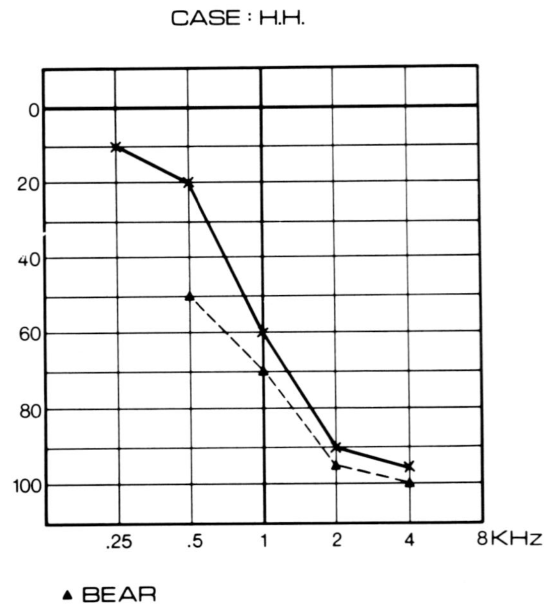

CASE : H.H.
0
20
40
60
80
100
.25
.5
1
2
4
8KHz
▲ BEAR

Fig. 5. Response patterns from a 3.5 year old child with congenital sensorineural hearing impairment. Sedation, recording, and stimuli as in Figure 3. Except for the 500 Hz FFR, only those responses that were obtained around the threshold are shown.

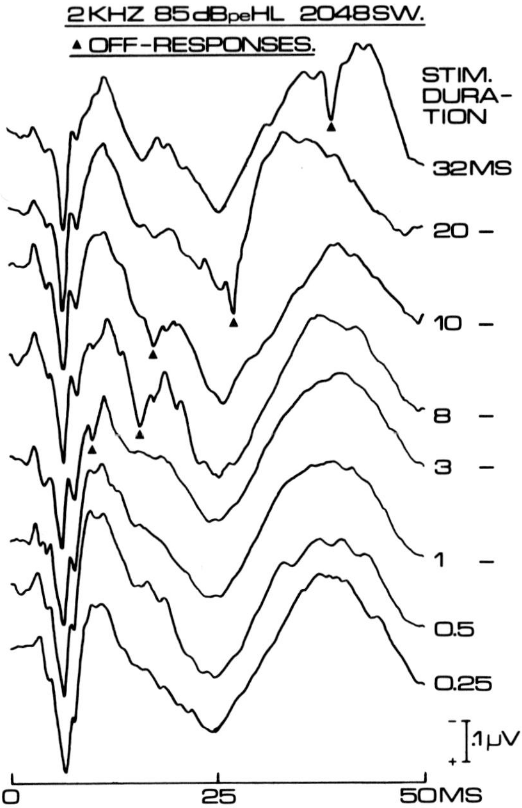

Fig. 6. Brain stem and middle latency responses obtained simultaneously. Bandpass of the recording: 22Hz-1 kHz. Active electrode at the Vertex, reference on the neck. Activity at the Vertex recorded with negativity up. 2 kHz stimuli with abrupt rise-decay and durations as indicated for each tracing. The filled triangles point to the Jewett5 wave in the off-set response.

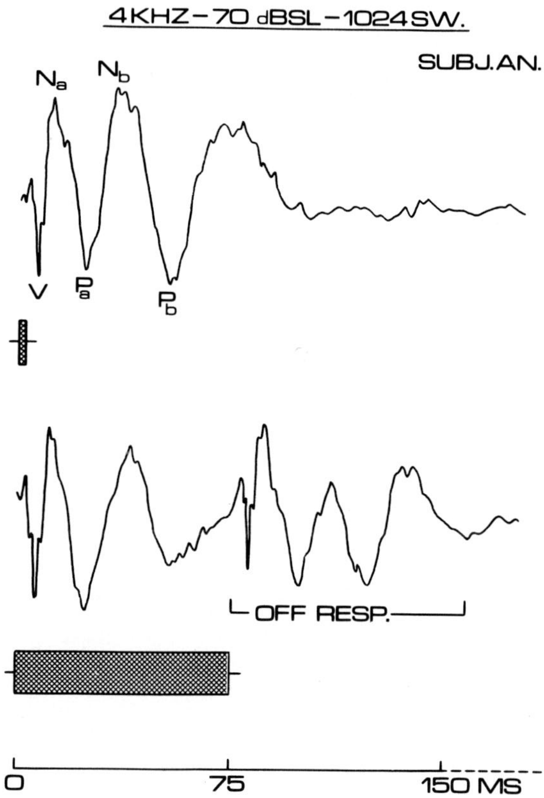

Fig. 7. Recording as in figure 6 except for a longer window of recording. Stimuli were 4 kHz tone pulses with abrupt rise-decay. In the upper tracing the duration was 2 msec. In the lower tracing the stimulus lasted 75 msec and here the off-set of the tone generates a response that almost duplicates the on-set response.

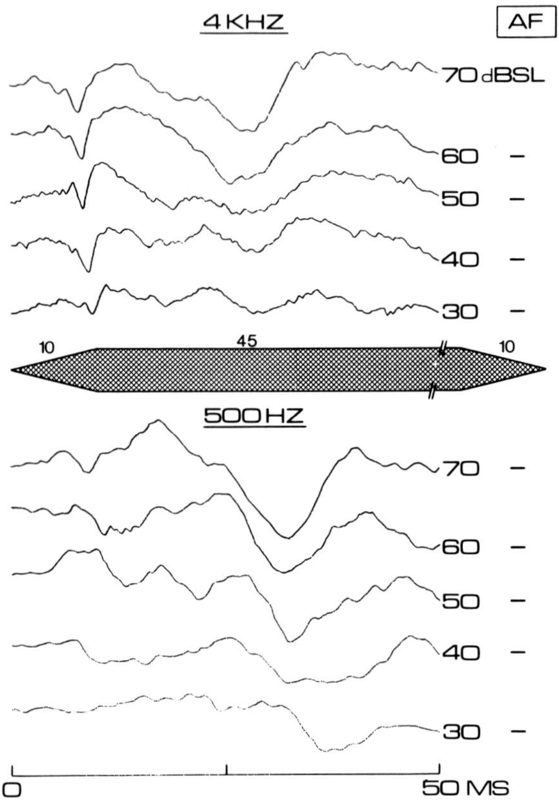

Fig. 8. Recording as in figure 6. Stimuli as indicated with rise-decay times of 10 msec. The 4 kHz stimulus generates a pattern where the Jewett$_5$ wave is at least as detectable as the middle latency response at low presentation levels. With a 500 Hz stimulus the sensitivity of the middle latency response is definitely superior.

REFERENCES

Terkildsen, K., Osterhammel, P. and Huis in't Veld, F. Far field electrocochleography, electrode positions. *Scand. Audiol. 3:* 123-129, 1974.

Terkildsen, K., Osterhammel, P. and Huis in't Veld, F. The frequency selectivity of the 500 Hz frequency following response. *Scand. Audiol. 6:* 35-42, 1977.

DISCUSSION

Davis: I want to emphasize two of the points Dr. Terkildsen made. One is that this is a practical method but it does require sedation for children. The other is that the method is only called for when behavioral audiometry does not work.

Another point is that frequency is really in the picture now, but the method does not give an equally good end-point at all frequencies. Excellent at 8000, excellent at 4000, very good at 2000, quite usable at 1000, and still very murky at 500 Hz. We are still working on this in various ways, and Dr. Terkildsen has illustrated a very promising approach by using the middle frequency response as well as the Jewett 5.

We now move to the second part of this round table discussion: an entirely different approach, looking at what the brain stem responses have to tell us not about the ear but about the brain stem. This is the neurological application of this technique. We will be going back to very simple stimuli: raw clicks. We don't care now about the frequency aspects. Dr. Thornton will tell us something about the anatomy and the relation of the responses to the anatomy in normal and pathological conditions.

Evoked Electrical Activity in the Auditory Nervous System

INTERPRETATION OF COCHLEAR NERVE AND BRAIN STEM EVOKED RESPONSES

A. Roger D. Thornton

Southampton University

INTRODUCTION

In 1967 Sohmer and Feinmesser described recordings of the cochlear nerve response and a series of later neurogenic responses. Although up to seven components of this short latency complex can be recorded (Jewett and Williston, 1971; Picton et al., 1974) there are five main components which can be found most consistently (Thornton, 1976a) and which are shown in Figure 1. The work of Lev and Sohmer (1972) and of Buchwald and Huang (1975) has led to the generating sites of the five main responses being identified as follows: N_1 from the cochlear nerve, N_2 from the cochlear nucleus, N_3 from the superior olivary complex, N_4 from the nuclei of the lateral lemniscus and N_5 from the inferior colliculus. The ability to obtain an "electrophysiological map" of the brainstem has clear application to both audiological and neurological problems.

The $N_4P_4N_5$ complex (Jewett V, FFP7) can be used to estimate auditory thresholds as it is robust against stimulus rate (Hyde et al., 1976) and the effects of masking (Parker and Thornton, 1978a); it shows little adaptation (Thornton and Coleman, 1975) and can be detected at stimulus levels close to audiometric threshold (Lev and Sohmer, 1972).

Neurological and audiological disorders in which it is useful to locate the site of a lesion require the measurement of all responses in the complex. The basic measurement methods and properties of the cochlear and brainstem evoked responses (CBER) have been detailed elsewhere (Thornton 1975a; Thornton, 1975b) and an approximate clinical baseline, shown in Figure 2, has been proposed. Here, data from normal subjects have been used to estimate the 90% confidence limits for amplitude and latency values at various stimulus levels. These are presented on a plot of peak-to-peak amplitude by latency and form five ellipses, one for each response. The values obtained from a patient's record are plotted on the same graph and assessed. The example given in Figure 2 shows that the N_1 response is of an abnormally small amplitude but that the brainstem responses (with binaural stimulation) were normal. These data, combined with the fact that

ISBN 0-12-514960-3

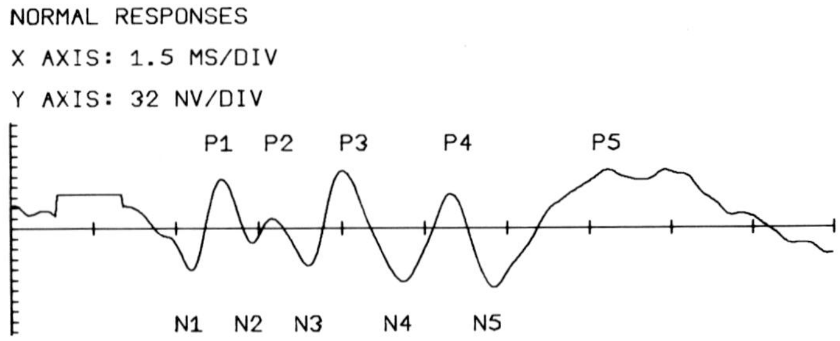

Fig. 1. Cochlear and brain stem responses from a normal subject showing the five main responses.

cochlear microphonics of normal shape and equal amplitude had been obtained from each side, led to a conclusion of a right sided cochlear nerve lesion. At operation this proved to be a cochleovestibular Schwannoma (acoustic neuroma). Findings such as these are the most common results encountered with acoustic neuromata (Thornton, 1976b).

There have been various clinical studies showing the diagnostic information that can be obtained from CBER recordings (Thornton, 1975c; Starr and Hamilton, 1976; Thornton and Hawkes, 1976; Terkildsen et al., 1977) and from such data

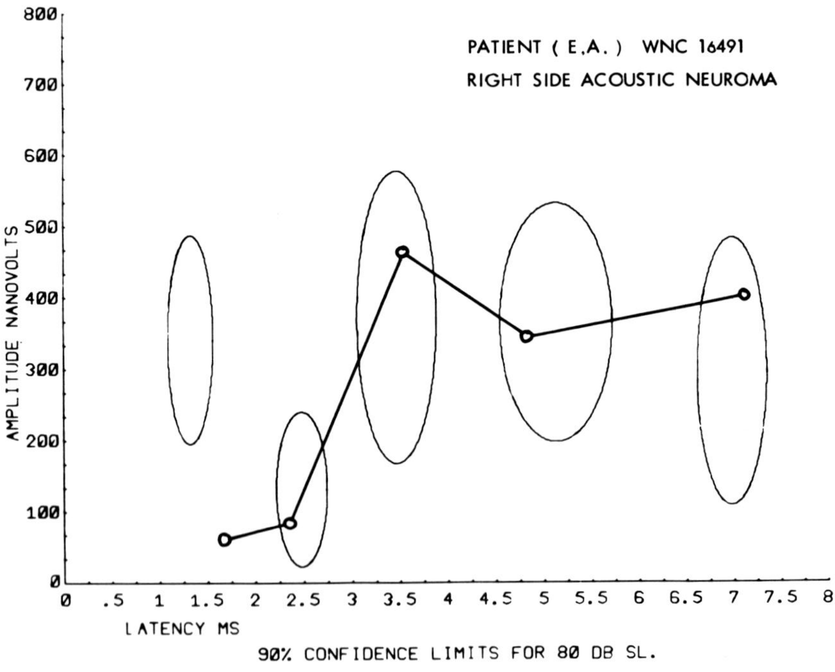

Fig. 2. Peak-to-peak amplitudes and latency values obtained from the right side with binaural stimulation from a patient with a right-sided acoustic neuroma which had not involved the brain stem. The data are compared to the 90% confidence limits for normal subjects..

there has been no clear counter example to contradict the locations of the brainstem generating sites described earlier.

Two specific aspects of CBER work will be discussed here. These are both concerned with the concepts and interpretations involved in CBER records and may be described as "The crossover problem" and "Derived brainstem responses".

THE CROSSOVER PROBLEM

Jewett and Williston (1971) have pointed out that these neurogenic responses are obtained by recording far field volume-conducted potentials. This involves a particular problem when bilateral recordings are made. The records obtained from the contralateral side could be due to at least three possible mechanisms or some combination of these mechanisms:

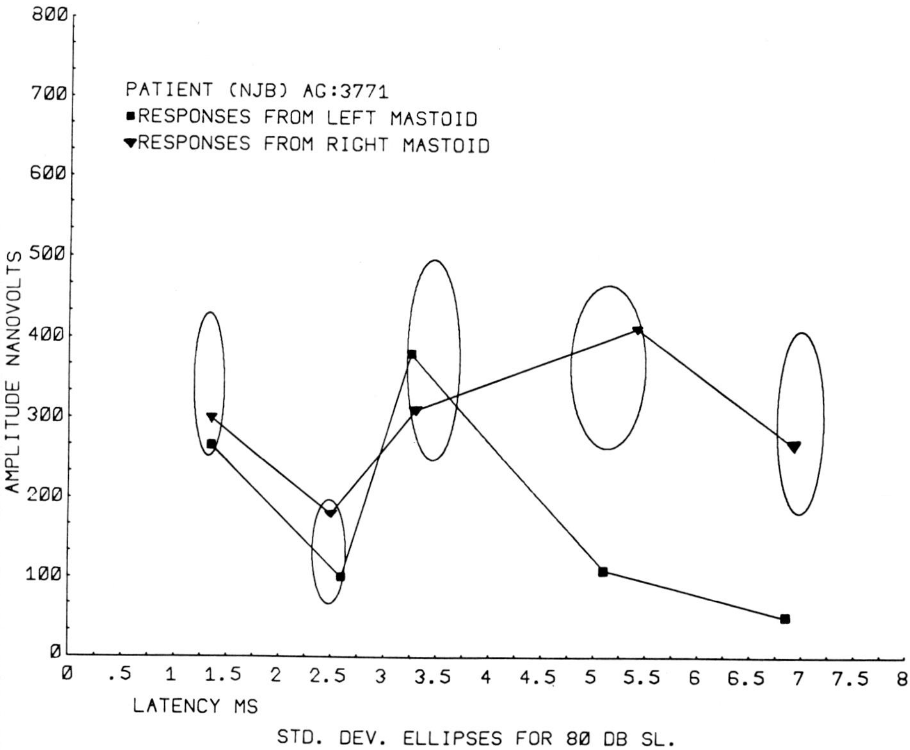

Fig. 3. Response values obtained from simultaneous left and right recordings from a patient with a suspected midbrain lesion.

Common Reference Activity

The responses N_2 to N_5 could represent predominantly at the reference electrode and thus be common to records obtained from each side when separate active electrodes and a common reference electrode are used.

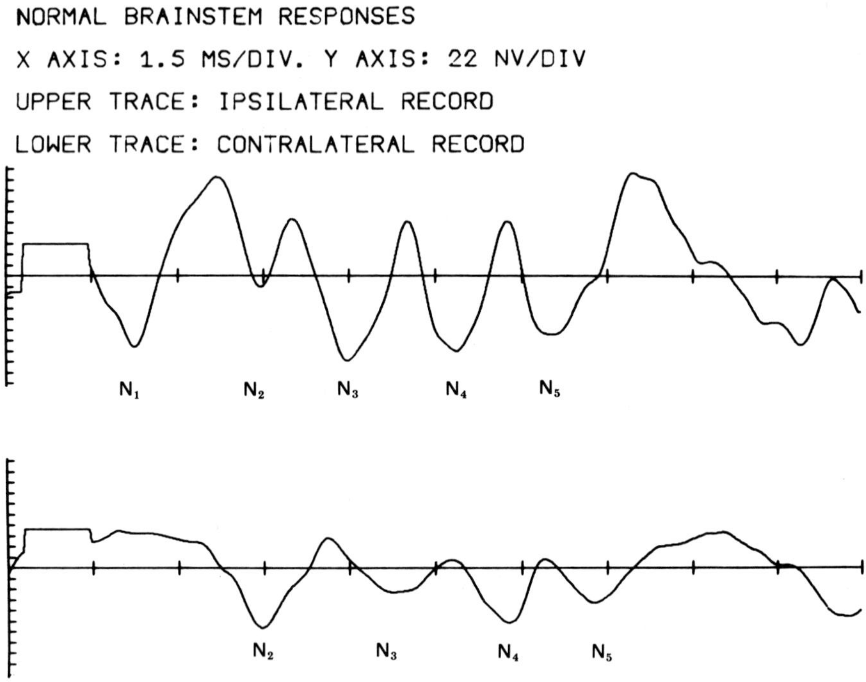

Fig. 4. Ipsilateral and contralateral recordings from a normal subject.

Electrical Crossover

The responses recorded on the contralateral side could predominantly be due to the activity of the ipsilateral brainstem nuclei which has been electrically transmitted across the head as a far field volume-conducted signal.

Neurological Crossover

Because of the neural pathways that traverse the brainstem the contralateral nuclei could receive neural signals and act as the generators predominantly responsible for the responses recorded on the contralateral side.

In practice, it is probable that all three of these mechanisms contribute to the responses that are measured but, for purposes of clinical interpretation, it is of importance to try to determine if the situation may be approximately described by one of the mechanisms.

Figure 3 shows results taken from a patient with a suspected midbrain lesion which gave values on the right side which were all within the normal range as given by the 90% confidence limits from the normal study. The recordings from the left side showed normal values for responses N_1, N_2 and N_3, but reduced amplitudes for responses N_4 and N_5. If the common reference activity or electrical crossover mechanisms predominated it would not have been possible to obtain such a difference between left and right sides for the responses N_4 and N_5, whereas these

TABLE I. Ipsilateral and Contralateral Latency Variances ms²
Where the F ratio between the ipsilateral and contralateral variances is significant the level of significance has been indicated on the larger variance as follows: * <10%, ** <5%, *** <1% level of significance.

	STIMULUS LEVEL dB SL					
	70		80		90	
PEAK	IPSI	CONTRA	IPSI	CONTRA	IPSI	CONTRA
P_1	.032	** .069	.022	** .059	.027	** .070
N_2	.033	.033	.025	** .058	.045	.036
P_2	.043	*** .119	.054	** .120	.043	*** .122
N_3	.044	*** .325	.062	*** .313	.036	*** .299
P_3	.049	*** .273	.034	*** .321	.038	*** .462
N_4	.087	*** .315	.126	.129	.114	.186
P_4	.049	*** .137	.054	.085	.037	*** .153
N_5	.034	*** .165	.049	** .114	.037	*** .183
P_5	.017	*** .161	.018	*** .311	.043	*** .207

results are consistent with the neurological crossover model. The results obtained from several patients with known disorders have all confirmed this conclusion.

In addition there are more quantitative data from experiments involving bilateral recording and monaural stimulation of normally hearing subjects. The method and techniques are described elsewhere (Thornton, 1975d) and a representative set of records is shown in Figure 4. The ipsilateral record shows the full set of 10 peaks, N_1 to P_5, whereas the contralateral record shows no N_1 response, a possible but not clearly defined P_1, but then contains peaks equivalent to N_2 through to P_5. The differences in results expected from the various models of the crossover mechanisms may be highlighted by considering three analyses of the data. These are the latency variance, the behavior of the difference in latency (LD) between corresponding peaks in ipsilateral and contralateral peaks and, finally, the correlations over stimulus levels for latency values within and between ipsilateral and contralateral records.

For both the common reference activity and the electrical crossover models, the contralateral records are obtained by electrical transmission of the ipsilateral responses. There should be no additional variance of the latency values due to this process and hence the latency variances of corresponding peaks from each side

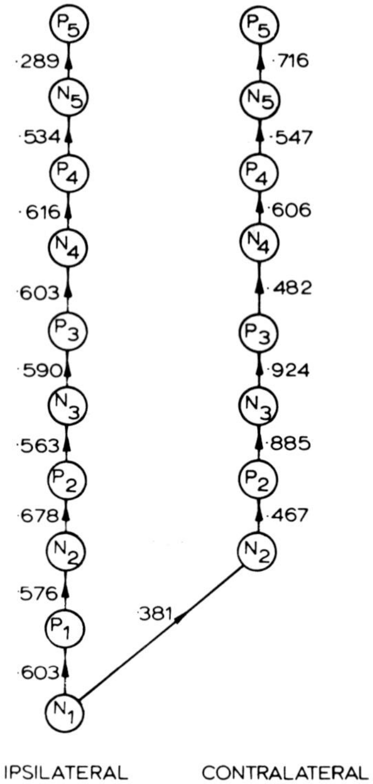

Fig. 5. Schematic relationship between response peaks based on latency correlation (see text for full explanation).

should be equal. Clearly, over stimulus levels, the corresponding peaks from both sides should be highly, positively correlated. For the common reference activity model, there should be no latency difference (LD) between corresponding peaks from each side; whereas with the electrical crossover model any LD value should represent the electrical transmission time across the head and should give LD values that are independent of stimulus level.

For the neurological crossover model, the LD value is due to the time taken for the signal to travel along a neural crossover pathway. In this case, the LD value could well be different at different stimulus levels. Furthermore, the increased distance of neural pathway traversed by the signals that generate the contralateral responses could produce a larger latency variance for these responses compared to the ipsilateral ones. Therefore, for corresponding peaks, the latency variance of the contralateral responses is expected to be greater than or equal to that of the ipsilateral responses. Finally, from the arguments given above, it is clear that the latency values of corresponding peaks need not be well correlated.

The results of the latency variance analysis are shown in Table I. The contralateral variance is greater than, or equal to the ipsilateral variance in all but one of the 27 measurements. In 22 of these cases the contralateral variance is significantly greater than the ipsilateral value.

The change in LD value with stimulus level is summarized in Table II. The change in LD was tested with a two-tailed t-test and 9 of the 16 measures show significant changes. This is too great a proportion to represent a chance finding and, overall, there is a significant change in LD with stimulus level.

The crosscorrelation coefficients between corresponding peaks showed only one significant positive correlation (N_4, $p < .05$). There was one significant negative correlation (P_2, $p < .1$) and the other peaks were not significantly correlated.

All of these results agree with the neurological crossover model and strongly disagree with the alternative models. Therefore, these findings, together with pathological results, have led to the conclusion that, for clinical purposes, it is reasonable to regard the responses recorded from one side as being due predominantly to the activity of nuclei of that side.

TABLE II. Statistical Significance of Amount of Change in the Difference between Contralateral and Ipsilateral Latencies with Change in Stimulus Level.

Entries are the percentage level of significance given by a two-tailed *t* test. Non-significant changes are indicated by (-).

CHANGE IN LEVEL	RESPONSE PEAK							
	N_2	P_2	N_3	P_3	N_4	P_4	N_5	P_5
70 dB to 80 dB	<5	<5	<5	<1	-	-	<10	-
80 dB to 90 dB	<5	<10	<10	-	-	-	-	<5

The schematic relationship for the ipsilateral and contralateral response peaks can be derived from the latency correlation matrices for the ipsilateral and for the contralateral data and from the cross correlation matrix between ipsilateral and contralateral. For each peak the maximum correlation coefficient is selected from the correlations given by the three preceding peaks on the same side and from those given by the corresponding peak together with the three preceding peaks on the other side. A line is then drawn from the peak showing maximum correlation to the peak being considered and the correlation value is marked alongside. The details are shown in Figure 5 and it can be seen that the contralateral N_2 response correlates maximally with the ipsilateral N_1 response. However, for all the other responses the peaks maximally correlate with the preceding peaks on the same side. This is another indication that the recordings taken from one side are predominantly due to the responses from the brainstem nuclei on that side.

These findings have provided the basis of clinical interpretation of CBER at Southampton and, to date, no clear counterexamples have been found to disprove this approach. There are many unresolved difficulties associated with the concept of a neurological crossover mechanism, not the least of which is that there is no clear anatomical evidence of a pathway consistent with the generation of the contralateral N_2 response.

DERIVED BRAINSTEM RESPONSES

The derived response concept and technique was initiated by Teas et al., in 1962 when it was applied to recordings taken from the guinea pig cochlea. Eggermont and Odenthal (1974) and Elberling (1974) applied the method to the whole-nerve AP from the cochlear nerve. Essentially, the procedure comprises stimulation with a short duration sound delivered with high-pass filtered white noise from, say, f_1 Hz. The resultant averaged AP is stored and the procedure is repeated with the high-pass filter set to a lower frequency, say, f_2 Hz. Subtracting the second AP from the first produces the derived AP from the frequency band f_2 to f_1.

The power of this technique is that it enables frequency-specific responses to be obtained and the basic nature of the components of the compound response to be studied. The application of this method to the brainstem responses has been developed over several years at Southampton and preliminary results concerning the validity of such application were presented at the European Symposium on the Neurophysiology of Hearing held in Bordeaux in 1976. What follows is a brief summary of four main studies on this topic.

The Validity of the Method

For various reasons (Parker and Thornton, 1978a) it was considered that the derived response technique need not necessarily be valid when applied to the surface-recorded CBER. An experiment was performed to obtain direct, non-derived responses and derived responses which, if the technique is valid, should be equal. No overall significant differences were found between these two response categories leading to the conclusion that the derived response concept is valid in its application to CBER.

Derived Response Characteristics

Derived CBER responses were obtained for five frequency bands and at three stimulus levels. At the same time the effect of maintaining a constant masker level for all stimulus levels was compared to a constant signal-to-noise ratio condition for each stimulus (Parker and Thornton, 1978b). Figure 6 shows the various high-pass masked responses and their derived responses for one subject. The derived responses show clearly the shorter latency components only in the high frequency bands whereas the later components are represented, with increasing latency, down to the lowest frequencies. The mean values, shown as mean waveforms, from six subjects are presented in Figure 7 for constant masker level and constant signal-to-noise conditions. Both conditions show similar features. The unmasked, or compound CBER, is a complex summation of many components. Particularly for the later waves, several components are in antiphase with those from other derived bands. Thus, elimination of a component, dependent upon the one selected, could

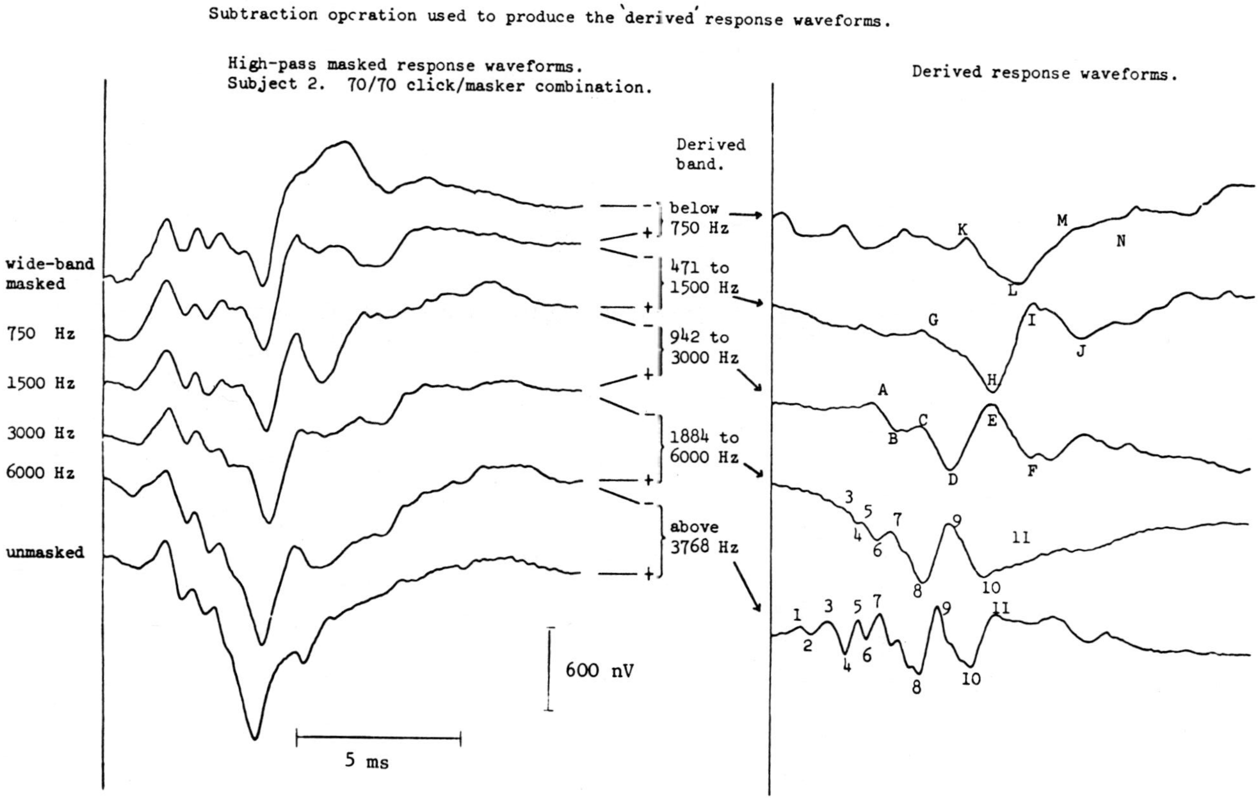

Fig. 6. High-pass filtered responses and the derived responses obtained by subtraction.

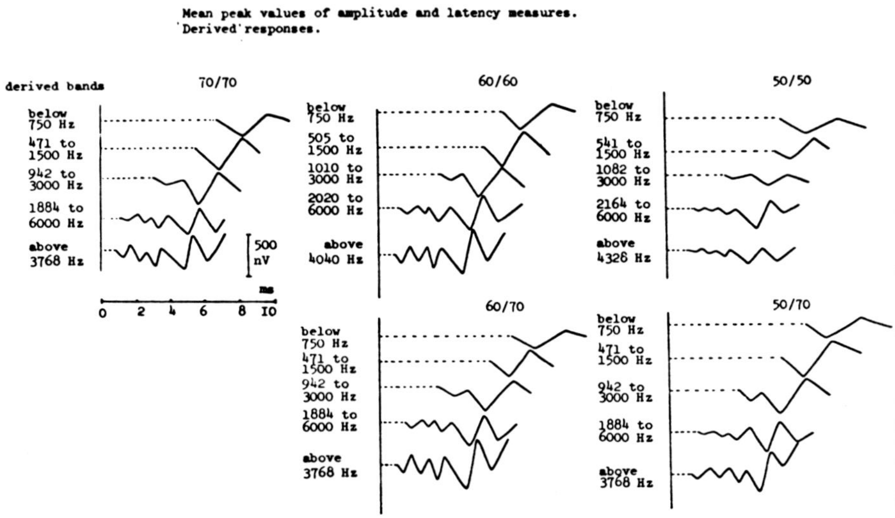

Fig. 7. Mean values of derived responses for the constant signal-to-noise condition (70/70, 60/60, 50/50) and for the fixed masker level condition (70/70, 70/60, 70/50).

cause an increase or a decrease in amplitude and in latency values of the compound CBER. This implies that a disorder which affects only a localized frequency region could cause an abnormally large response in the unmasked CBER. Such occurrences are liable to be rare but one case of a proven brainstem lesion associated with an abnormally large response has been seen at this Institute.

Analyses of the input/output functions for the different masker conditions show that less complex interactions occur with the constant masker level technique which, because of its simplicity, might be preferred in clinical application.

All of the results underline the highly complex nature of the unmasked CBER.

Frequency-specificity of the Derived Responses

The frequency specificity of the derived responses was explored by using a filtered noise masker presented with the click stimulus. The derived responses in five frequency bands were obtained for each of three different masking noise conditions. The results showed that, when the derived band was centered on the masker band, the derived response was markedly altered for that band but not for adjacent

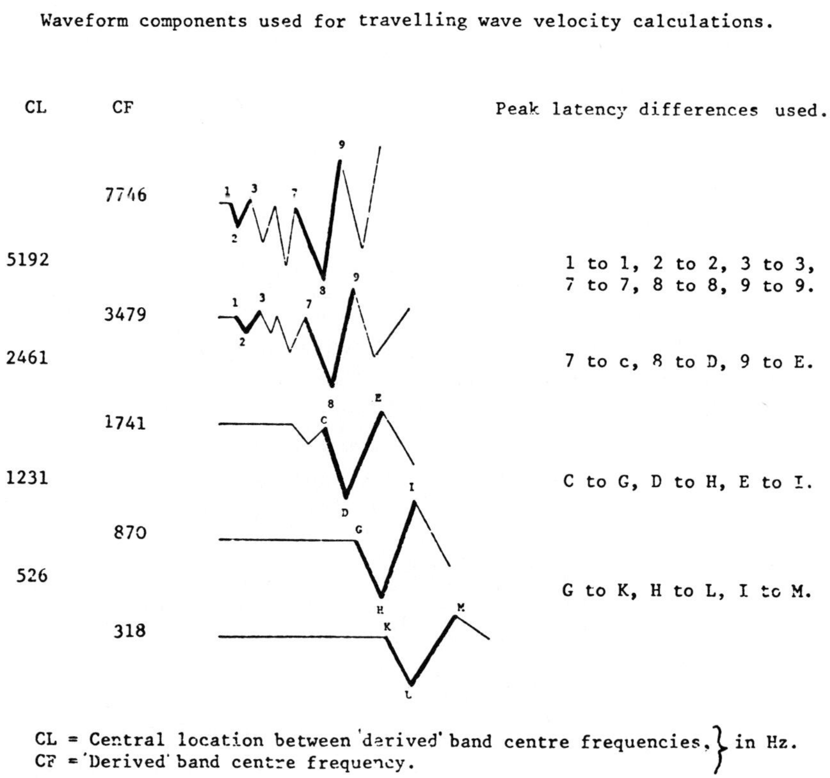

Fig. 8. Derived response components (thick lines) used in the estimation of cochlear traveling wave velocity. CF is the center frequency of the derived band and CL is the central location frequency for the velocity estimate taken from latency differences between adjacent bands.

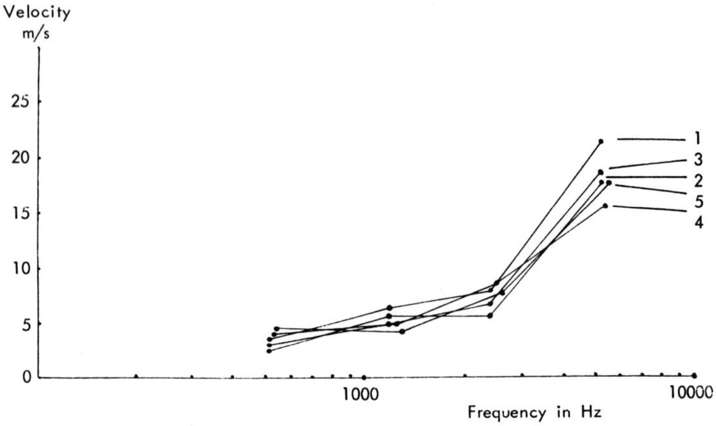

Fig. 9. Traveling wave velocity estimates for the five click/masker level combinations (70/70, 70/60, 70/50, 60/60 and 50/50).

bands. In the absence of experimental data, the width of the derived bands had been taken as the largest value given by the physical parameters of the high-pass masker used to obtain the band. This experiment showed that the derived bands were considerably narrower than this figure and the results enabled more realistic bandwidths to be calculated (Parker and Thornton, 1978c).

Cochlear Traveling Wave Velocity

Various measurements of the traveling wave velocity have been made. Békésy (1960) used cochlear models. Zerlin (1969) used psychoacoustic techniques. Electrophysiological estimates have been obtained by Teas et al. (1962) using the cochlear microphonic, by Elberling (1974) and Eggermont and Odenthal (1974) using the latency of the cochlear nerve AP and masking techniques. The same technique could be applied to the derived CBER (Parker and Thornton, 1978d) and Figure 8 shows the early and late components used in the calculation. Where traveling wave velocities could be calculated from the early components and the late components, the results were very similar and could be averaged. Figure 9 shows the traveling wave velocities calculated for each of the five stimulus/masker intensity conditions. There were no significant differences between these estimates and the data were combined to give an overall velocity estimate which is compared to the results obtained from other studies in Figure 10. It is clear that there is good agreement between the AP, psychoacoustic and CBER estimates of the cochlear traveling wave velocity.

Such a finding produces the concept that the neural elements, which are germane to the production of an evoked potential, are arranged such that the projections from regions of the cochlea initiating events in the brainstem maintain their relative frequency and propagation parameters constant. Thus, in this context, the

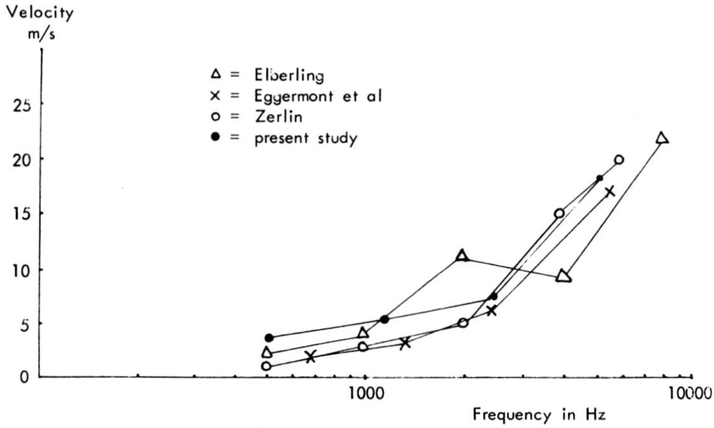

Fig. 10. Mean traveling wave velocities obtained from this study compared with other estimates.

brainstem evoked potentials could be regarded as the result of a linear system which maintains the temporal relationships between the various frequency regions whose input is supplied by the cochlear events.

The results obtained with the derived brainstem responses are in good agreement with those from recent studies by Don and Eggermont (1978).

Acknowledgements

The author gratefully acknowledges the contributions of Dr. D.J. Parker, whose doctoral researches produced the derived response studies, Dr. C. Elberling and Dr. J.J. Eggermont for helpful discussions on derived response concepts.

The work was supported by the Medical Research Council, Grant No. 970/512C.

REFERENCES

Békésy, G.von, *Experiments in hearing.* New York: McGraw Hill, 1960, p. 403-534.

Buchwald, J.S. and Huang, C.-M. Far-field acoustic response: origins in the cat. *Science 189:* 382-384, 1975.

Don, M. and Eggermont, J.J. Analysis of the click-evoked brain stem potentials in man using high-pass noise masking. *J. Acoust. Soc. Am.* (In press, 1978).

Eggermont, J.J. and Odenthal, D.W. Frequency selective masking in electrocochleography. *Rev. Laryngol. Otol. Rhinol.,* Bord. *95:* 489-496, 1974.

Elberling, C. Action potentials along the cochlear partition recorded from the ear canal in man. *Scand. Audiol. 3:* 13-19, 1974.

Hyde, M.L., Stephens, S.D.G. and Thornton, A.R.D. Stimulus repetition rate and the early brain stem responses. *Brit. J. Audiol. 10:* 41-46, 1976.

Jewett, D.L. and Williston, J.S. Auditory-evoked far fields averaged from the scalp of humans. *Brain 94:* 681-696, 1971.

Lev, A. and Sohmer, H. Sources of averaged neural responses recorded in animal and human subjects during cochlear audiometry (electrocochleogram). *Arch. Klin. Exp. Ohren Nasen Kehlkoptheikd. 201:* 79-90, 1972.

Parker, D.J. and Thornton, A.R.D. The validity of the derived cochlear nerve and brain stem evoked responses of the human auditory system. *Scand. Audiol.* (In press, 1978a).

Parker, D.J. and Thornton, A.R.D. Frequency specific components of the cochlear nerve and brain stem evoked responses of the human auditory system. *Scand. Audiol.* (In press, 1978b).

Parker, D.J. and Thornton, A.R.D. Derived cochlear nerve and brain stem evoked responses of the human auditory system: the effect of masking in the derived band. *Scand. Audiol.* (In press, 1978c).

Parker, D.J. and Thornton, A.R.D. Cochlear traveling wave velocities calculated from the derived components of the cochlear nerve and brain stem evoked responses of the human auditory system. *Scand. Audiol.* **(In press, 1978d).**

Picton, T.W., Hillyard, S.A., Krausz, H.I. and Galambos, R. Human auditory evoked potentials. I: evaluation of components. *Electroencephalogr. Clin. Neurophysiol. 36:* 179-190, 1974.

Sohmer, H. and Feinmesser, M. Cochlear action potentials recorded from the external ear in man. *Ann. Otol. Rhinol. Laryngol. 76:* 427-435, 1967.

Starr, A. and Hamilton, A.E. Correlation between confirmed sites of neurological lesions and abnormalities of far-field auditory brain stem responses. *Electroencephalogr. Clin. Neurophysiol. 41:* 595-608, 1976.

Teas, D.C, Eldredge, D.H. and Davis, H. Cochlear responses to acoustic transients. An interpretation of whole-nerve action potentials. *J. Acoust. Soc. Am. 34:* 1438-1459, 1962.

Terkildsen, K., Huis in't Veld, F. and Osterhammel, P. Auditory brain stem responses in the diagnosis of cerebellopontine angle tumors. *Scand. Audiol. 6:* 43-47, 1977.

Thornton, A.R.D. The measurement of surface-recorded electrocochleographic responses. *Scand. Audiol. 4:* 51-58, 1975a.

Thornton, A.R.D. Statistical properties of surface-recorded electrocochleographic responses. *Scand. Audiol. 4:* 91-102, 1975b.

Thornton, A.R.D. The diagnostic potential of surface recorded electrocochleography. *Brit. J. Audiol. 9:* 7-13, 1975c.

Thornton, A.R.D. Bilaterally recorded early acoustic responses. *Scand. Audiol. 4:* 173-181, 1975d.

Thornton, A.R.D. and Coleman, M.J. The adaptation of cochlear and brain stem auditory evoked potentials in humans. *Electroencephalogr. Clin. Neurophysiol. 39:* 399-406, 1975.

Thornton, A.R.D. Electrophysiological studies of the auditory system. *Audiology 15:* 23-38, 1976a.

Thornton, A.R.D. Surface-recorded electrocochleographic findings in cases of acoustic neuromata. In: *Sondersforchungsbereich 88, Teratologische Forshung und Rehabilitation Mehrfachbehinderter. Vol. I,* edited by M. Hoke and G. von Bally. University of Münster, 1976b, p. 211-219.

Thornton, A.R.D. and Hawkes, C.H. Neurological applications of surface-recorded electrocochleography. *J. Neurol. Neurosurg. Physchiatry 39:* 586-592, 1976.

Zerlin, S. Traveling wave velocity in the human cochlea. *J. Acoust. Soc. Am. 46:* 1011-1015, 1969.

DISCUSSION

Davis: Thank you, Dr. Thornton. You have raised many good points that we might discuss, but time is short, and I will call immediately on Dr. Starr to tell us where these responses come from and what they can be used for by neurologists.

THE GENERATORS OF THE AUDITORY BRAINSTEM POTENTIALS AS REVEALED BY BRAINSTEM LESIONS IN BOTH MAN AND CAT

Arnold Starr and J. Achor

University of California, Irvine

The measurement of auditory brainstem potentials provides the clinician with a noninvasive method of examining the physiological function of the central nervous system in patients with disorders of sensory or neurological functions. The test is of particular value because the potentials are independent of level of arousal or attention which may frequently be impaired in clinical situations. We have examined many patients comatose as a result of overdoses of medication; their brainstem potentials are in all respects similar to those obtained from normal waking subjects (Starr and Achor, 1975).

Auditory brainstem potentials are relatively easy to record; the equipment is compact and can be brought to the bedside to test the patient who is ill. This is a particularly important attribute of the test because if the patient is healthy and free to come to the laboratory there may be little need for evoked potential measurement. Furthermore, one can obtain quantitative measures of brainstem function to complement the clinical evaluation which is qualitative and requires both experience and skill to be reproducible.

We would like to present some of our clinical material derived from patients who have subsequently expired, correlating changes in auditory brainstem potentials with the anatomical distribution of the pathological process. This material is primarily derived from recent publications by Starr and Hamilton (1976) and by Stockard and Rossiter (1977).

In our hospital laboratory we record between the vertex and the ipsilateral ear receiving the click stimulus. We only test monaurally at click rates of 10/sec to insure the definition of all of the components of the brainstem potentials.

Figure 1 is a comparison of a normal auditory brainstem potential with that obtained from a patient with a lesion of the VIIIth nerve. The patient, with an acoustic neuroma, has a wave I and wave II but the other brainstem components are

ISBN 0-12-514960-3

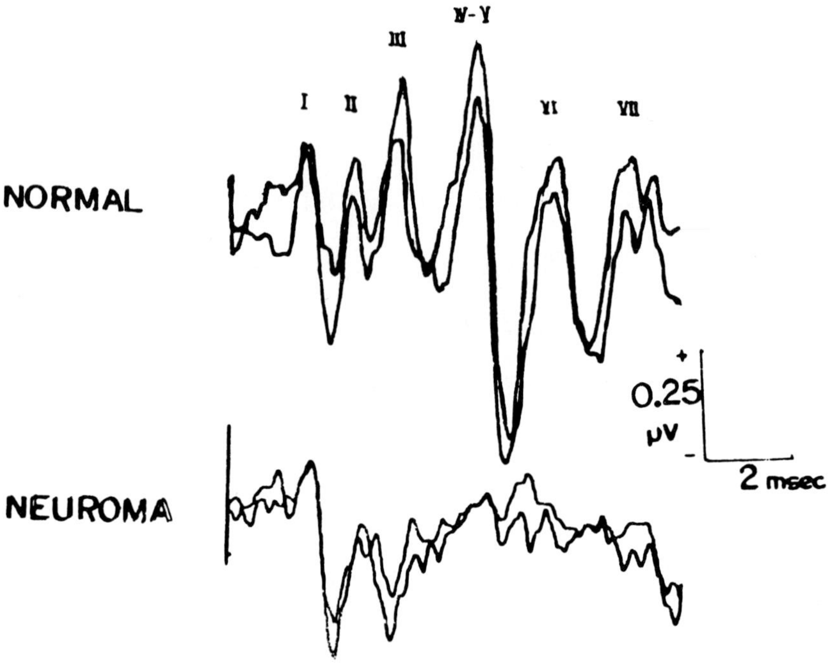

Fig. 1. Auditory brainstem potentials recorded from a normal subject and from a patient with a confirmed acoustic neuroma. Note the loss of components after wave II in the neuroma. The potentials were recorded between vertex and the mastoid ipsilateral to the ear receiving 65dB HL click presented at 10/sec. Two thousand clicks comprise each average and duplicate averages were obtained. Positivity at vertex electrode is displayed as an upward deflection. The amplifier band pass was 0.1 to 3 kHz. All these parameters were identical in the subsequent figures except where noted otherwise.

difficult to define. There may be another wave at the end of the trace with a latency of 9 msec that could be wave V. This would result in a central conduction time difference between waves I and V of about 8.0 msec whereas the normal value is up to 4.3 msec. In other patients who have suffered "brain death" wave I is the only component that can be detected (Fig. 2). Thus wave I and maybe wave II are generated external to the brainstem by the VIIIth nerve.

Figure 3 is from a patient with tuberous sclerosis, a condition associated with both mental retardation and the development of brain tumors. The distribution of the tumor shown in Figure 3 involved the left cochlear nucleus and the left inferior colliculus. Stimulating the left ear (L) evoked a wave I, followed by a large negative deflection, but no other component. This result supports the earlier conclusion that wave I originates extrinsic to brainstem in the eighth nerve and that lesions at the entry zone of the VIIIth nerve to the brainstem will affect the detection of the subsequent components. When the right ear (R) was stimulated all of the components were present but the amplitude of the IV-V complex was considerably less than

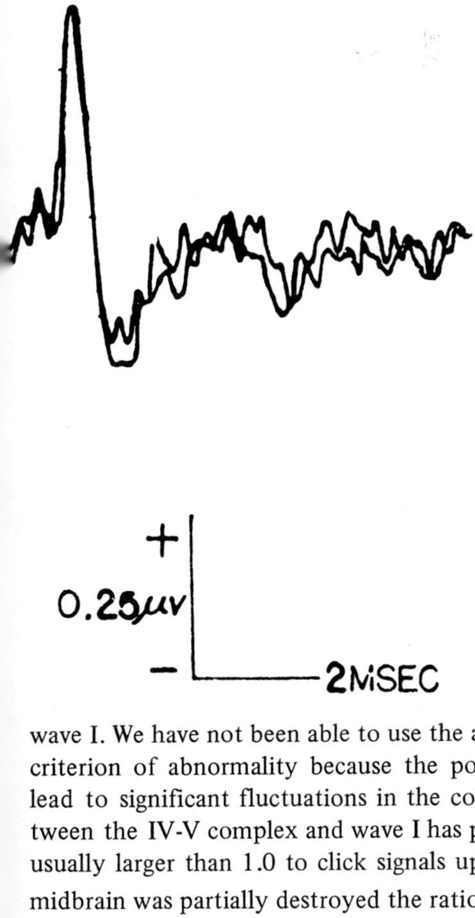

Fig. 2. Auditory brainstem potentials recorded from a patient with cerebral death. Note the presence of wave I in the record. (From Starr and Hamilton, 1976).

wave I. We have not been able to use the absolute amplitude of the components as a criterion of abnormality because the poor signal/noise ratio of the potential can lead to significant fluctuations in the components. However, the relative ratio between the IV-V complex and wave I has proved to be of use. In normals this ratio is usually larger than 1.0 to click signals up to 65dB SL. In this patient in whom the midbrain was partially destroyed the ratio was only about 0.5.

Figure 4 is from a patient with a tumor that originated in the pineal gland and destroyed the midbrain while preserving the pons and cochlear nucleus. Waves I, II, III are preserved but the IV-V complex is absent. Waves I and II are of exceptionally large amplitude raising the possibility that there are descending influences from the midbrain that can affect the amplitude of these first few components via efferent inhibitory pathways. However a definite conclusion from this patient is that waves IV-V require the integrity of function of the midbrain for their detection.

The abnormalities of the auditory brainstem potentials from these cases are very dramatic but the patients were also quite ill. In most clinical situations individual components will not be lost. We have found that a useful measure in clinical situations is that of alterations in latency between the various components. We routinely measure the latency difference between waves I and V as an index of central conduction time. In our laboratory the central conduction time is 3.9 msec ± 0.2 msec. Thus if the central conduction time is 4.4 msec it exceeds by 2 SD our "normal values" and indicates an abnormality in the central auditory pathway (Starr,

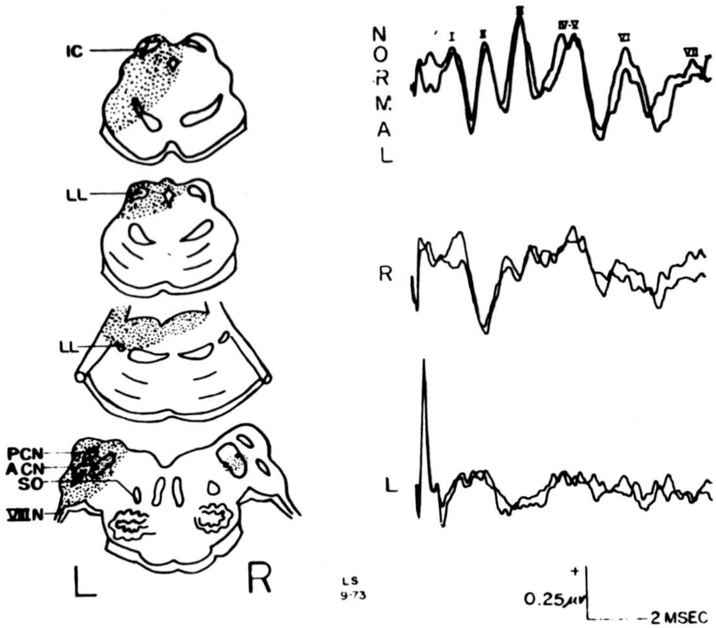

Fig. 3. Distribution of pathology (stippled areas on left) and the auditory brainstem potentials from a normal and a patient who died with tuberous sclerosis. R and L refer to stimulation of the right (R) and left (L) ears. (From Starr and Hamilton, 1976).

1977). This measure of central conduction time is independent of hearing levels. If, for example, a patient has a hearing loss of 30dB, the central conduction time should still be less than 4.4 msec. Other clinical laboratories have also reported a figure of 4.3-4.4 msec as being the upper limit of normal in central conduction times between waves I and V (Stockard et al. 1977, Gilroy et al. 1977).

Figure 5 is from a patient (A) and a normal control (B). The first component is aligned in the two tracings. Note that wave IV is slightly shifted, but wave V is definitely shifted almost 0.5 msec. This patient had hydrocephalus with increased pressure within the fourth ventricle due to a rare parasitic inflammation.

Drs. Gambin and Holstein working at the University of California, Irvine, have used the measure of central conduction time to help define brainstem alterations in multiple sclerosis. The abnormality of central conduction time can occur from stimulation of just one ear. In a series of patients with multiple sclerosis, they examined the time difference between adjacent waves, i.e. I and II, II and III, III and IV, IV and V as well as between I and V. This is a fine grained analysis of central conduction time but allows definition as to where along the pathway the lesions may be. In their series of patients with multiple sclerosis who had clinical signs of brainstem involvement, central conduction times were abnormal in approximately 90% of the tests. However, in those patients without clinical signs of brain-

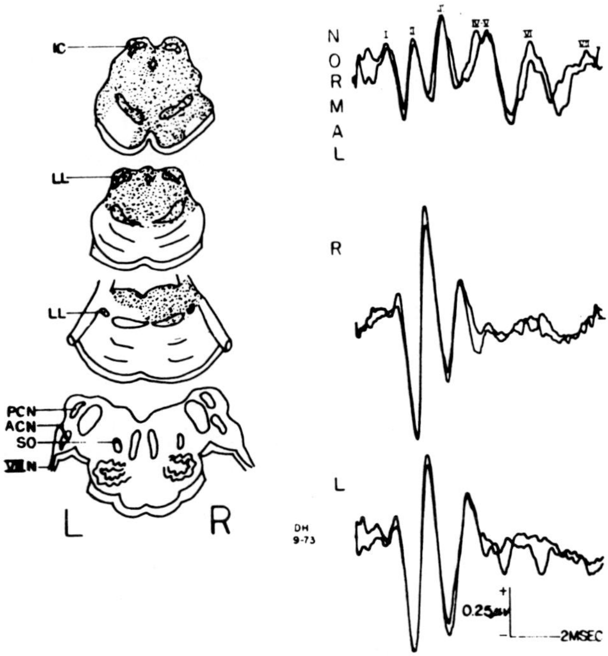

Fig. 4. Auditory brainstem potentials from a patient who died with a pinealoma that compressed the midbrain (stippled areas on left). (From Starr and Hamilton, 1976).

stem disturbance only 50% had abnormalities of central conduction times. It is obvious that auditory brainstem potentials can provide significant information for the clinician dealing with multiple sclerosis.

Additional information is needed as to the precise generators of the auditory brainstem components and to the effects of various types of pathological processes on their morphology, latency and amplitude. We have used two techniques in cats to help define the locus of the generators of the auditory brainstem potentials. We have made detailed recordings of click-evoked potentials from within brainstem structures to define the spatial and temporal distribution of the potential fields and then relate these fields to the components of the auditory brainstem potentials recorded from the scalp. The second method utilized discrete electrolytic lesions of portions of the auditory pathway to determine their effects on the scalp-derived brainstem evoked potentials.

Figure 6 contains the auditory brainstem potentials recorded from both man and cat. The potentials are remarkably similar except that the components are ten fold higher in amplitude and temporally compressed in the cat. P4 in the cat is believed to correspond to the IV-V complex in man.

Figure 7 contains the click-evoked potentials as recorded from various subcortical sites in the auditory brainstem pathway of the cat. At each site there is a sequence of potentials that lasts for many milliseconds following a click signal. Thus at the time of the occurence of each scalp component of the ABR there are many separate sites in the brainstem that are active, complicating the assumption that a particular scalp component is the result of activity in just a single auditory brainstem site. Our data would suggest that certain of the scalp-derived components reflect activity originating in at least six auditory brainstem sites.

The effects of discrete brainstem lesions on auditory brainstem potentials in the cat provides additional evidence contradicting the simple assignment of generator sites. Figures 8 and 9 show the effects of a discrete lesion in the ventral cochlear nucleus of a cat on the auditory brainstem potentials recorded from the scalp. The

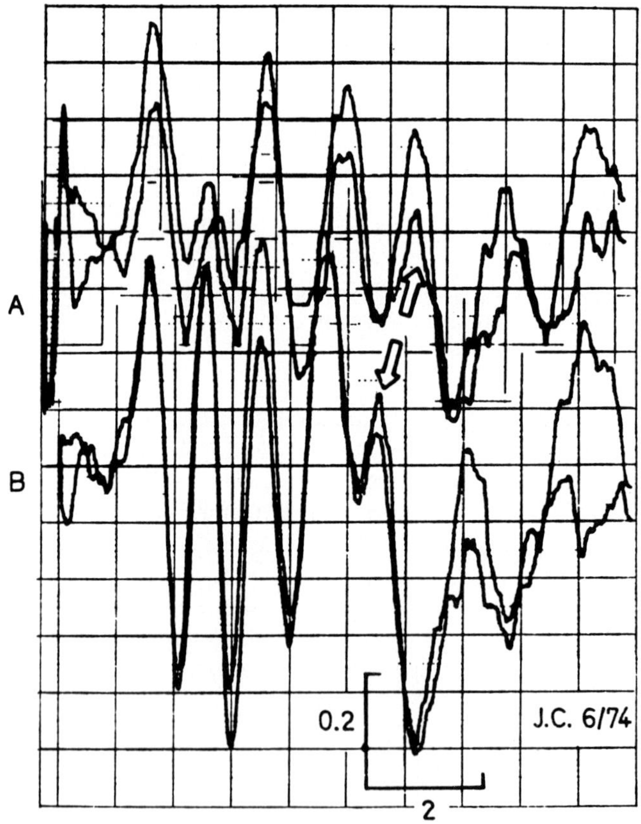

Fig. 5. Auditory brainstem potentials from a normal subject (A) and a patient (B) with increased pressure within the IV ventricle from a parasitic cyst. Wave I has been aligned to show the shift of wave V (arrows) indicating a prolonged central conduction time. Calibration is in μV and msec. (From Starr, 1977).

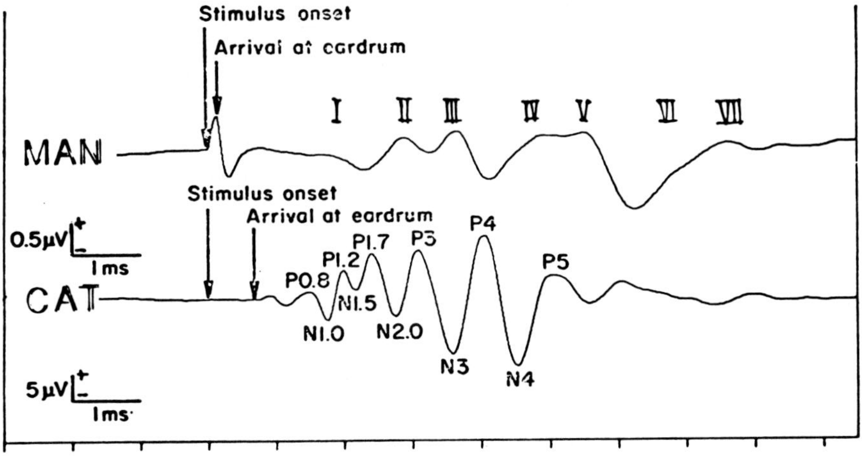

Fig. 6. Auditory Brainstem Responses obtained from man (upper trace) and cat (lower trace). The components in man have been labelled with Roman numerals and in the cat by the letters P and N to designate peaks and troughs, respectively, and with a number representing the approximate latency of the components under "typical" experimental conditions. The latency values were obtained at a click rate of 25/sec at 65dB (re: normal adult human threshold) and represent the latency from the time of arrival of the stimulus at the eardrum. Except for the first few components of the ABR of the cat, the latency values have been rounded to the nearest whole number. In the upper trace a stimulus artifact is present at the onset of the stimulus. The arrival of the stimulus at the eardrum in man was computed on the basis of the distance from the transducer to the eardrum, whereas in the cat the latency was empirically determined using the output voltage of a sound level meter positioned at the central end of a hollow ear bar in the absence of the cat. The recordings in both examples were made between the vertex and a reference site on the neck. Wave VI is poorly defined in this subject.

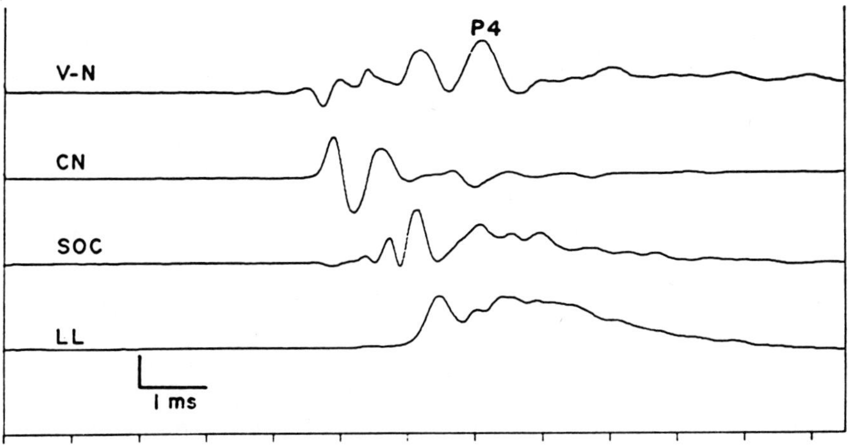

Fig. 7. Microstructure of evoked potentials from the auditory pathway of the cat. From top to bottom: The far field auditory brainstem potential recorded between vertex-neck (V-N), and depth recordings in cochlear nucleus (CN), superior olivary complex (SOC), lateral lemniscus (LL). The amplitude calibration is 10 μV for the vertex-neck recording and 500 μV for the depth recordings.

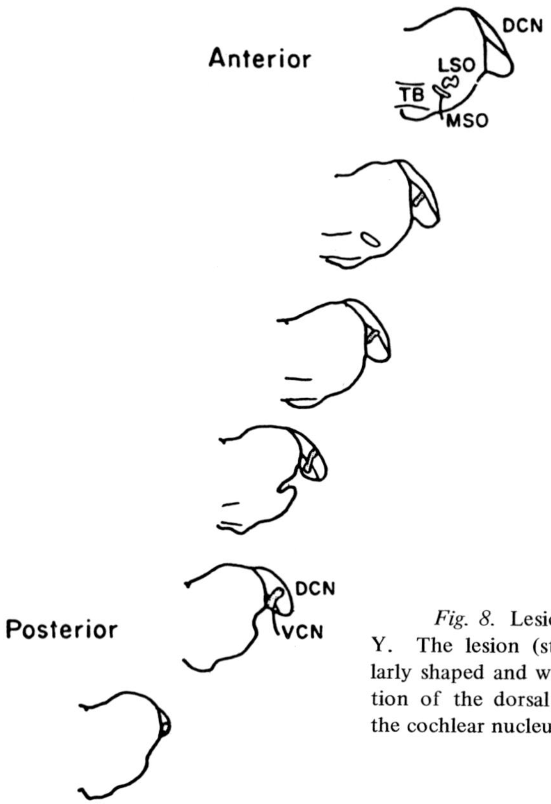

Fig. 8. Lesion reconstruction for cat Y. The lesion (stippled area) was irregularly shaped and was positioned at the junction of the dorsal and ventral divisions of the cochlear nucleus.

potentials recorded prior to the lesion are represented by the thin trace while the thick trace represents the potentials recorded after the lesion. Note that following the lesion the amplitude of all of the components from P3 on were attenuated without any change in their latency. Thus a discrete lesion of one particular nucleus can affect many components of the scalp-derived auditory brainstem potential. In contrast we have found that lesions in certain other areas of the auditory pathway may be without any influence on the scalp-derived auditory brainstem potentials. The sites identified with the lesion technique as not contributing to the far-field auditory brainstem potential include the inferior colliculus, the lateral lemniscus, and the dorsal cochlear nucleus.

The results of these experiments require us to reconsider the issue of the identity of the generators of the auditory brainstem potentials. The correlations observed in the clinical material between the site of lesion and abnormality of the auditory brainstem potential are clear and reliable. However it is important to remember that the lesions in patients are large and have widespread effects on brainstem function due to pressure or vascular changes. In contrast, the experimental lesions in cats are quite small and may have more widely differing pathophysiological ef-

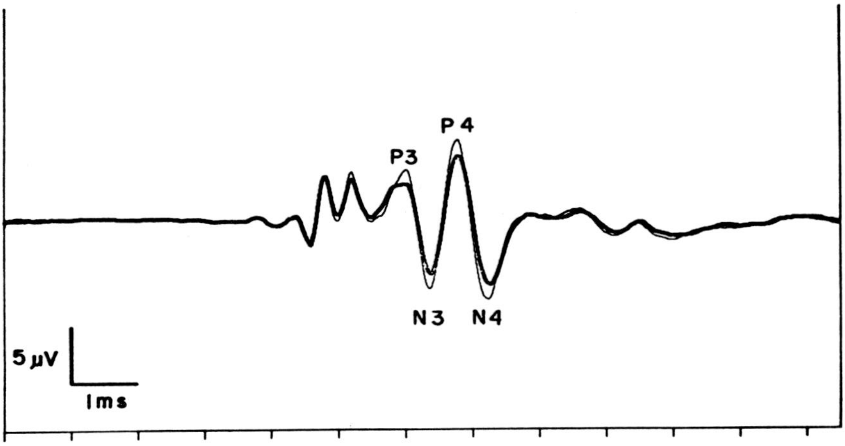

Fig. 9. Effects of lesion in the cochlear nucleus on the scalp-derived auditory brainstem potentials to ipsilateral stimulation in cat Y. The light trace is the potential recorded prior to the lesion and the dark trace is the potential recorded after the lesion. The lesion produced significant amplitude reductions to ipsilateral stimulation for P3 (25%), N3 (20%), P4 (19%) and N4 (19%).

fects on the brainstem than the lesions observed in patients. For instance, the animal studies were all done on anesthetized cats and we observed only the acute effects of the electrolytic lesions. The patients were generally comatose and had pathological processes that had been present many weeks. We subscribe to the position that there is clinical value in assigning the various components of the scalp-derived auditory brainstem potential to particular portions of the auditory pathway, and that changes in these components suggest a localizing lesion in that part of the brainstem. The experimental data from the cats, however, indicate that the clinical data is incomplete. It seems that only portions of the auditory pathway contribute to the far-field auditory brainstem evoked potentials, and that the major effect of disruption of the pathway is a reduction in amplitude without any change in latency. The paradox is enhanced since, in the clinical situation, latency change rather than amplitude change is the principal measure of abnormality encountered. The unresolved issues are prominent. Their solution should result in more accurate application of evoked potential measures to clinical neurology.

REFERENCES

Gilroy, J., Lynn, G.E., Ristow, G.E. and Pellerin, R.J. Auditory evoked brain stem potentials in a case of "Locked-in" syndrome. *Arch. Neurol. 34*:492-495, 1977.

Starr, A. Clinical relevance of brain stem auditory evoked potentials in brain stem disorders in man. In: *Auditory Evoked Potentials in Man: Psychopharmacology Correlates of Evoked Potentials,* edited by J.E. Desmedt, Volume 2. Brussels, 1977.

Starr, A. and Achor, J. Auditory brainstem responses in neurological disease. *Arch. Neurol. 32*: 761-768, 1975.

Starr, A. and Hamilton, A. Correlation between confirmed sites of neurological lesions of far-field auditory brainstem responses. *Electroenceph. Clin. Neurophysiol. 41*:595-608, 1976.

Stockard, J.J. and Rossiter, V.S. Clinical and pathological correlates of brain stem auditory response abnormalities. *Neurology 27*:316-325, 1977.

Stockard, J.J., Stockard, J.E. and Sharbrough, F.W. Detection and localization of occult lesions with brainstem auditory responses. *Mayo Clin. Proc. 52*:761-769, 1977.

Evoked Electrical Activity in the Auditory Nervous System

BASIC AND CLINICAL ASPECTS OF BRAIN STEM RECORDING IN HUMANS

A ROUND TABLE DISCUSSION

Moderator: Hallowell Davis

Scheduled Discussants: R. Galambos
J.M. Gerken
A. Starr
K. Terkildsen
A.R.D. Thornton

Davis: First of all, I have been strict in timekeeping and have cut off practically every one of the speakers. I am now going to go down the line and ask each one if he has any special afterthoughts that he would like to mention, or a pertinent question for some other member of the panel.

Bob, I think you have a generalization of some sort you want to make.

Galambos: I have spoken a lot about the virtues of the cochleogram and the brain stem response as techniques for assessing auditory status. I have been pressing the matter for the last two days, I hope not too obnoxiously, because I believe this is an extremely important question to resolve. Let us compare them on the dimensions of cost, benefit and risk.

As for cost, there can be little question that the brain stem response is usually much cheaper to obtain. Now risk. I was taught as a medical student that you never do anything to a patient that you don't have to do. To obtain a cochleogram from a child the child must be anesthetized, and everyone knows when he orders a general anesthetic that this procedure carries along with it a certain risk of death. As for the brain stem response I must dispute one of Hal's statements. We published last year on 81 patients ranging in age from 6 weeks premature to 15 years (Makatoff, B., Schulman-Galambos, C. and Galambos, R. Brain stem auditory responses in children. *Arch. Otolaryngol. 103:* 38-43, 1977); none was anesthetized and only five required sedation. This reflects my position that babies and children must be tested, if at all possible, without anesthetic or sedation. This rule is not difficult to follow; at the time the appointment is made the mother is told to bring the child in sleepy, at his nap time, with his favorite blanket and that sort of thing. The technicians are excellent at getting this point across and that is why in our clinic sedation is rarely used, and anesthetic never.

ISBN 0-12-514960-3

Now for the benefits. As this panel of experts has just shown, the brain stem response provides a comprehensive view of the auditory system from its origin in the cochlea up to the level of the inferior colliculus at least; the cochleogram, by contrast, gives information on the auditory nerve alone. Examination of a brain stem response apparently reveals what the cochleogram shows and in addition it can point out auditory disorders invisible to the cochleogram, namely, neurological lesions in the pathway ascending in the brain stem.

We have just heard that one can even estimate the audiogram by several techniques using the brain stem response. The procedure is quick, precise, informative, and it carries no risk; I would like to know, therefore, specifically what one can learn that will benefit the patient by doing an electrocochleogram in addition.

Davis: First of all, Bob, I stand corrected about the use of sedation. I did not have these very young babies in mind. We do not use sedation under 3 months of age. But for a period of quiet long enough for the audiometric determination of thresholds of four frequencies on each of the two ears, that calls for one hour of real relaxation; and such audiometry is our chief business with the older children.

Your question still stands, namely, what is the particular benefit of the electrocochleogram that is not obtained from brain stem. I think I can hear it coming: Cochlear microphonics, summating potentials, diagnosis of otologic pathology.

Galambos: But we just heard from Dr. Terkildsen that one can get cochlear microphonics by this technique.

Davis: Dr. Terkildsen, your name has been quoted here. Can we get cochlear microphonics with the brain stem technique?

Terkildsen: In normal young persons there is usually a small microphonic response at the vertex. It is much larger at the mastoid, but the interindividual variability is considerable.

This discussion about the need for sedation is really rather artificial. I agree with Dr. Galambos that infants below the age of ½ year readily fall asleep without sedation if they are handled properly.

Our main concern, however, is with the somewhat older children where the differential diagnostic possibilities are psychosis, mental retardation or multiple handicaps, with or without hearing impairment. In our hospital we are now at a point where objective hearing tests are mandatory in such patients. We can obtain a complete audiogram within one hour, but only if the child is asleep and here it is absolutely necessary to use sedation, short acting barbiturates or Valium.

It ought to be mentioned that children yield very large responses. When you go up in age groups the brain stem responses generally become more difficult to record. The beautiful responses seen in the literature are usually from young, pretty secretaries. When they get older their responses tend to diminish.

Davis: They just get hardheaded.

Terkildsen: Maybe. It is even more difficult to record from men. We have evidence that there is a gradual increase of J_5-latency in both sexes, 0.1 msec per decade. There also appears to be a sex difference so that the latency is 0.25 msec longer in men.

When we use this technique in neurological diagnostic work it is often a great advantage to use some kind of sedation. We prefer Valium given intravenously in the amount of 10 mg.

Galambos: Dr. Terkildsen and I have privately discussed the responses in old age. I did not bring it with me but I have a slide showing magnificent brain stem responses from a young woman on which is superimposed a virtually identical response from Baird Hastings, who is shortly going to celebrate his 83rd birthday. So, it is not invariably true that old people yield poorer responses than beautiful young women.

Terkildsen: There is certainly a considerable variability. My statement is based on statistics from a rather large population and your two subjects may be outside the 5 pct. confidence limits.

Thornton: Just one point about straightforward clinical application. I think I ought to mention this, seeing that it hasn't cropped up so far.

From the studies that have been carried out recently, using contralateral masking over a range of zero to 80 dB, the ipsilateral brain stem responses are not significantly altered. Of course this is useful in an audiological clinical context. It is clear, I think, from Arnold Starr's data, and it is confirmed with the way we have worked up a clinical approach to these recordings, that we would always record bilaterally. We would record using both monaural and binaural stimulation if necessary, for the most difficult cases, because those conditions allow you to sit down and really try to work out a diagnostic interpretation.

The surprising thing about these responses is that in neurological application they actually work. Our data, on patients who come to operation or post mortem, where we know the lesion site, has not thrown up any clear counterexample to the generating sites described by Buchwald and Huang.

With regard to multiple sclerosis patients, our work has shown latencies similar to those given by Arnold Starr. We studied a definite group, meeting Schumacher's criteria, where we are getting nearly 90% showing what are effectively subclinical lesions, or delays between wave 1 and wave 5.

What is perhaps more interesting, because for the definite group the neurologists already have a good diagnosis, are the results from a retrobulbar neuritis group. A 15-year follow-up recently published on patients presenting with optic neuritis who later developed M.S. came up with a figure of about 70%. The brain stem response data collected so far give a value of 65%. This seems a good diagnostic indication for this technique.

Davis: Dr. Gerken, do you have any nice afterthoughts?

Gerken: One point I didn't make has to do with the relation between psychophysical kinds of experiments and evoked potential measurements. In presenting a click and a masking noise, for example, the subject may hear the click but the potential will disappear, or vice versa. In the case of the masking noises that I was talking about, as one moves those bands of noise around on the frequency spectrum in the presence of the single-cycle clicks, the perceptual quality of the click changes. This could perhaps be explained in terms of the areas of the cochlea which are or are not being masked. The latencies of the responses that pop out on either side of that band of noise are also changed. These latency changes were apparent in my slides but were not emphasized (see Teas, Eldredge and Davis, 1962). In general the relationship between perception and evoked potentials is an area that has been largely neglected.

Terkildsen: According to our experience it is only rare that you need to apply contralateral masking in order to avoid cross hearing.

We have shielded headphones that are mounted in noise-protecting domes. With such an arrangement there is no cross-talk problem with stimulus intensities up to 105 dB p.e. SPL.

Davis: Dr. Starr, do you wish to respond with any rebuttals or further afterthoughts?

(Dr. Starr declines.)

I would like to ask one question of the panel myself before throwing it open to the audience: Have any of you encountered cases where you have been unable to record the brain stem response on Jewett 5 specifically but were convinced from behavioral evidence that the patient was hearing the signal?

Galambos: Let me try to answer that question in two ways. Some years ago, when I was new in this business, people would come to me and say, "We have tested a normal-hearing person and found he has no brain stem response". This used to worry me so much that I would visit their place and look, and invariably I discovered some deficiency in the machine being used or in the way the operator used it. I now tell such people, when they say such a thing, that I believe they ought not to advertise their finding because it is a demonstration that they are incompetent.

Next, I have been shown brain stem responses from two multiple sclerosis patients with normal audiograms in which only wave I was present. I interpret them as showing the disease has selectively inactivated the time-keeping portion of the auditory pathway with essential sparing of the rest of it. This is part of the reason why I pushed the anatomists so hard yesterday for evidence of a time-keeping sub-system in the outflow from the cochlear nucleus. These two cases are explained most simply by supposing that a brain stem pathway responsible for the brain stem response has been selectively attacked by the disease.

Thornton: The occasions when we have had a patient who had normal or near-normal audiogram, where we haven't seen a Jewett V response reflects the point made by Bob Galambos on timing. We have seen it in advanced multiple sclerosis cases where probably we are not getting an evoked response because we are not getting good synchronous activity. There is still a neural signal going through leading to normal detection, but I think Arnold Starr knows we have many more of these cases.

Starr: I think there is a paradox for those interested in "hearing" if you cannot record a wave V. The absence of wave V in someone who can "hear" implies a disorder of the central auditory pathway. One of the patients I showed with an acoustic neuroma had only a wave I and II and no hearing impairment as defined by his own impression as well as by audiometric testing. One interpretation is that the central lesion produced a loss of synchrony which affected the detection of wave V to a greater extent then "hearing". Alternatively, the brain stem potentials are generated only by a portion of the auditory system which is not essential for "hearing".

Davis: As I said at the beginning, our watchword is synchrony. You can lose responses either from a loss of anatomical units or blocking of conduction or from disruption of synchrony.

If you are not too thirsty, folks, we will accept some questions from the floor.

LaJoie: I have one big, long question which should open up some discussion, I hope. Is there any clinical value in evaluating auditory evoked responses either early or late in stroke patients particularly those with aphasia?

Starr: This is an important area to be studied. We did not discuss middle or long latency evoked potentials at all, which are the types of measures that are probably very relevant for cognitive processing as in aphasia. I do not have any data on the relationship of these longer latency potentials to the problem of aphasia.

Davis: I can't give any better answer than that myself. Are there other questions?

Carroll: Has anyone done any longitudinal studies working with multiple sclerosis patients where you have gotten some baseline measurements and then gone into monitoring progression, and so on?

Starr: We have tested our patients with multiple sclerosis repeatedly. In our experience an abnormality of evoked potentials persists after the patients recover symptomatically.

Galambos: Again, Stockard and Rossiter recently published a case with signs of multiple sclerosis in whom brain stem response latencies were all to long (Stockard, J.J. and Rossiter, V.S. Clinical and pathological correlates of brain stem auditory response abnormalities. *Neurology 24:* 316-325, 1977). Three weeks later, after treatment, her responses were nearly normal in latency. The patient also had recovery from her symptoms.

Thornton: We have quite a lot of serial studies on a few patients, not with ACTH treatment but with some other experimental treatment going on. We have good correlations between the latency decreasing during good periods and the latency getting a bit longer during bad periods, but invariably the patients are left with a deficit even though they may not have any clinical signs that are immediately observable.

Cohen: Dr. Starr, have you looked at rate functions, in these electrolytic studies, for clicks in these animals to see if waves are progressively displaced in latency or reduced in amplitude as a function of lesion location and/or extent of lesion.

Starr: Our rates are 25 per second. We have not studied higher rates of stimulus presentation.

Trahiotis: Dr. Gerken, with respect to auditory function, I have heard about a number of different stimuli: filtered clicks of one- or two-cycle sinewaves. For these stimuli the evoked potentials are looked at with respect to normal hearing. Will someone say something about temporal integration, or what do we mean by normal hearing? Does that really take into account only normal data from long-duration stimuli. Or do we mean the threshold a normal person would have with a particular pulse? How do these vary?

Gerken: That is a big one. I would rather speak to a related question, -- that of the critical stimulus elements in the generation of the evoked potential. When you use different stimuli the evoked potentials may or may not differ. Single cycle stimuli of different frequencies may yield discriminably different response waveforms. Other stimulus dimensions, however, do not seem to be critical. For example, duration; if you use 4 cycles instead of a single cycle, the potential doesn't change particularly. When using a single cycle stimulus it is clear that the evoked potential is a response to the onset of the stimulus.

When you are using a stimulus with a slow rise time, there is uncertainty as to what is the stimulus element (or elements) that is producing the response. Yes, we know that a slower rise time gives a narrower spectrum and presumably activates a more limited group of hair cells, but what is the exact stimulus? Is it the first measurable rarefaction cycle? Is it the second? Is there an interaction of some sort between the various cycles? These are all questions that can be approached experimentally. (See, for example, Kiang's discussion at this Symposium on the relation between single unit data and evoked potentials). As to how all this relates to normalcy of hearing, we will simply have to await the experimental results.

Galambos: Hecox et al., published on the effect of rise time, duration and interstimulus interval upon the brain stem evoked response (Hecox, K., Squires, N. and Galambos, R. Brainstem Auditory Evoked Responses in Man. I. Effect of stimulus rise-fall time and duration. *J. Acoust. Soc. Am. 60:* 1187-1192, 1976). The stimuli were noise bursts. The conclusion was that the onset is by far the most important variable.

Trahiotis: The question was misunderstood. I was not asking about the evoked response but the behavioral response. I am worrying about what is the normal audiogram. The behavioral response (threshold performance) can change tremendously as a function of the stimulus parameters. I was not asking about the electrical response.

Thornton: It is a problem we have been worried about. When one is trying to estimate threshold with evoked responses using clicks or short tone bursts, there is a possible calibration problem. Figure 1 (Thornton Discussion Fig.) shows the threshold by log duration for tone bursts for normal subjects. This shows the normal temporal integration function (curve A). If we ignore for the moment any errors or corrections in our evoked response threshold, we are going to measure an evoked response threshold with a short-duration stimulus, and we measure the value at E_1 for the normal population.

We then look at the standard long-duration audiometric tone threshold (S_1) and we work out a correction factor (X). This is the normal biological calibration procedure. What happens when we get results from patients? Let's consider the patient with an end-organ lesion. He has a hearing loss and he has a flat temporal integration function (curve B). We measure his evoked response threshold as E_2, add the correction factor X, and arrive at a value (T_2) that is actually better than his true audiometric threshold (S_2).

Actually, it may not be a real problem. With transtympanic ECoG we are using a response that comes between 1 and 4 msec latency. It is my understanding that although end-organ lesions can affect temporal function, the site where temporal integration actually occurs is very much higher in the system than the generation site of the N_1 response. So, I think that a biological calibration is viable. The problems involved do not have a clear-cut solution but it is this argument that underlies the rationale to calibrate short-duration signals in terms of dB peak equivalent hearing level.

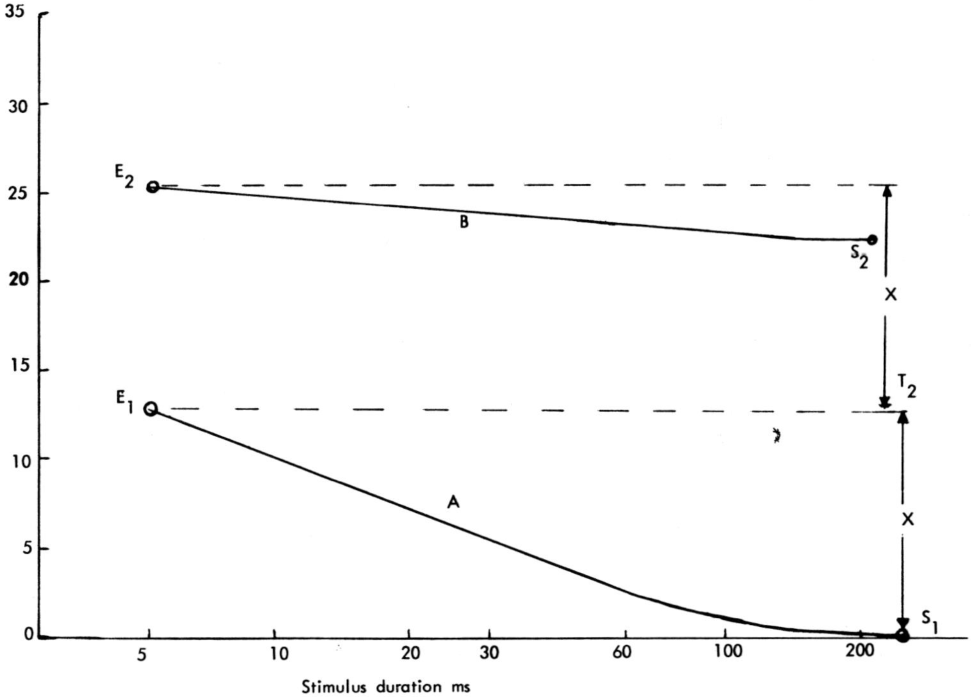

Thornton Discussion Fig. 1. See text.

Galambos: You are interested in the growth of loudness as noise burst duration increases from 2 msec to 200 msec?

Trahiotis: I am concerned that when the normal audiogram or hearing loss was defined it was not clear whether the same stimulus was used in all the conditions. If the stimuli were different across conditions the behavioral threshold would be different.

Davis: If we could only standardize our stimuli across labs it would help a lot.

Terkildsen: My two audiograms illustrate this point. In the first one our reference was the subjective threshold in normal listeners and we appear to be able to measure normal audiometric thresholds in the high frequencies.

These are old results and I believe it is wrong to use such a calibration procedure which yields a stimulus that is 20-25 dB more intense than the ISO-audiometric reference.

What we are up against is the temporal summation effect and, as Dr. Thornton rightly mentioned, this effect is greatly reduced in patients with a cochlear hearing impairment. If we had used the same kind of calibration in the patient with the ski-slope audiogram we would have overestimated the hearing.

These findings are in complete agreement with our knowledge about the physiology and the pathophysiology of hearing. What must be realized is that we cannot ascertain completely normal hearing by these methods. The response is determined within fractions of a msec without the benefit of temporal summation and the objective threshold in normal subjects will have to be at around 20-25 dB in ISO-audiometric norms or 30-35 dB in p.e. SPL.

CORTEX

Moderator: *Robert A. Butler*

THE AUDITORY CORTEX

Irving T. Diamond

Duke University

The purpose of this paper is to present recent evidence in support of the concept that the auditory cortex is a field consisting of a number of closely related subdivisions. The term "field" was first used in this sense by Rose (1949) and by Rose and Woolsey (1949), in an effort to revitalize the inquiry into the architectonic subdivisions of the cortex; this inquiry had become bogged down with questions such as, Is a single area absolutely uniform? The traditional view, as developed by Campbell (1905) for example, was that every architectonic subdivision was a functional unit, the borders of which corresponded to differences in connections. Thus, the visual sensory area of Campbell received projections from the lateral geniculate body and served visual sensory functions while the adjacent visual psychic area did *not* receive fibers from the lateral geniculate body and served in higher level visual functions such as visual memory, learning and perception of objects. The difficulties in the traditional view arose because not all cortical areas had sharp borders, because not all areas seemed to be uniform throughout and because the projection field of some thalamic nuclei, for example, the pulvinar nucleus, covered several architectonic subdivisions. Debates concerning how sharp a border must be proved to be increasingly unproductive and eventually led to a devastating criticism by Lashley and Clark (1946) in which the basic assumptions of the method of architectonic subdivision were questioned and even the reliability of the method was assailed.

Rose and Woolsey selected the auditory "field" in the cat to show why a functional unit was not uniform. They argued that the entire field consists of a number of closely related cytoarchitectonic subdivisions serving a common function; but each subdivision is functionally distinct to some degree. To support this idea they relied first on cytoarchitectonics and second on the results derived from the methods of retrograde degeneration and evoked potentials. For example, AI, AII and Ep alike were electrically responsive to auditory stimulation but AI and AII each had its own distinct tonotopic organization; further, AI, AII and Ep each received fibers from the auditory thalamus but only AI received essential projections from the principal part of the medial geniculate body. Later the auditory field was enlarged to include the insular and temporal areas so that today the auditory field of the cat includes an extensive region from the suprasylvian sulcus to the rhinal fissure (Diamond et al., 1958, Rose and Woolsey, 1958).

ISBN 0-12-514960-3

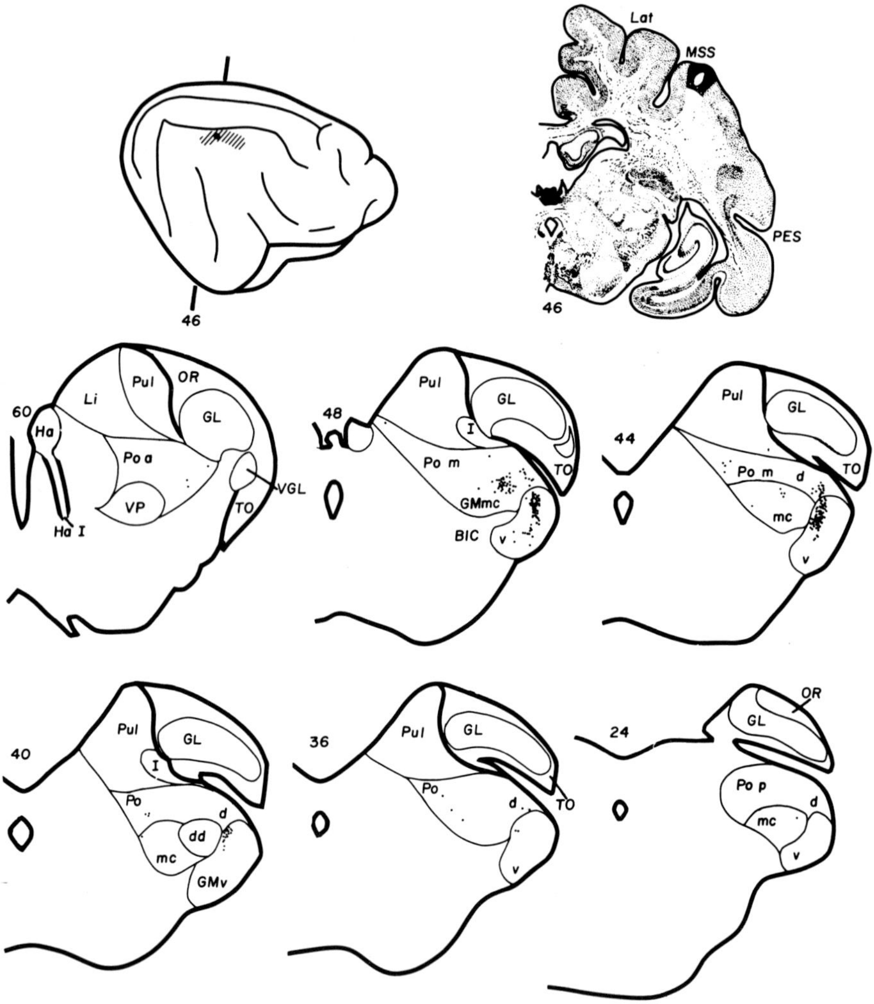

Fig. 1. To show the results of an injection of HRP into cortical AI in cat 893L. On the top of the figure the injection site is shown by a black dot while the diffusion of HRP is indicated by diagonal lines. To the right is a frontal section through the injection site. Here the needle track is shown in white surrounded by a black area to show the diffusion of HRP. Below are six sections through the thalamus and each labeled cell is indicated by a dot. The same format applies to the next four figures. The abbreviations in this and the subsequent figures are as follows: AES, anterior ectosylvian sulcus; BIC, brachium of the inferior colliculus; CM, centre median nucleus; dd, deep dorsal nucleus of the medial geniculate body; GL, dorsal lateral geniculate body; GMc, c, caudal division of the medial geniculate body; GMd, d, dorsal

RETROGRADE TRANSPORT STUDY OF THE AUDITORY CORTEX IN THE CAT

The method of retrograde transport of HRP supports this concept of a field unified by certain common connections and yet subdivided by differences between the various parts. For example, the evidence now to be presented will show that every subdivision of the auditory cortex in the cat receives fibers from the magnocellular division of the medial geniculate body (Winer et al., 1977). This is just the kind of evidence necessary to reveal the unity of the field. At the same time, no two subdivisions receive the same projections from the thalamus and indeed each cortical subdivision can be identified chiefly with one thalamic nucleus. The evidence will show that the ventral division of the medial geniculate body (which corresponds roughly with the anterior two-thirds of the principal division) projects only to cortical area AI and only in a highly topographic fashion (see Morest, 1964, for definition of ventral division).

Figure 1 shows the results of an injection of HRP into AI of cat 893L. The distribution of labeled cells is striking, with a densely populated band in the ventral division of the medial geniculate body and a diffusely distributed population of labeled cells in the magnocellular division of the medial geniculate body and in the posterior group. A lesser amount of HRP was injected into AI of the right hemisphere in cat 1136 (see Fig. 2). Correspondingly fewer cells were labeled in the thalamus. Still it is possible to recognize the essential pattern: a band of cells in the ventral division of the medial geniculate body and scattered cells widely distributed over several divisions, the magnocellular and dorsal divisions of the medial geniculate body and the anterior and medial parts of the posterior group.

Injections of each of the other cortical subdivisions also produced a distinctive pattern. In the case of the temporal cortex, the caudal division of the medial geniculate body had the greatest concentration of labeled cells (see Fig. 3 which illustrates the results of experiment 876L). After injecting the insular area, the medial division of the posterior group had the greatest concentration of labeled cells (see Fig. 4 which illustrates the results of experiment 910L). After injecting Ep the dorsal division of the medial geniculate body had the greatest concentration of labeled cells (see Fig. 5 illustrating experiment 920R). Distinctive patterns in the distribution of labeled cells were also produced by injections into AII and into the dorsal part of the posterior ectosylvian gyrus.

division of the medial geniculate body; GMmc, mc, magnocellular division of the medial geniculate body; GMv, v, ventral division of the medial geniculate body; Ha, habenula; Ha I, habenulo-interpenduncular tract; I, inferior subdivision of pulvinar nucleus; Lat, lateral gyrus; Li, lateral intermediate nucleus; MD, mediodorsal nucleus; MSS, middle suprasylvian sulcus; OR, optic radiation; PES, posterior ectosylvian sulcus; PO, posterior nuclear group of the thalamus; Po a, anterior sector of the posterior group; Po m, medial sector of the posterior group; Po p, posterior sector of the posterior group, PS, pseudosylvian sulcus; Pul, pulvinar nucleus; Rh, rhinal sulcus; TO, optic tract; VGL, ventral lateral geniculate body; VP, ventroposterior nucleus.

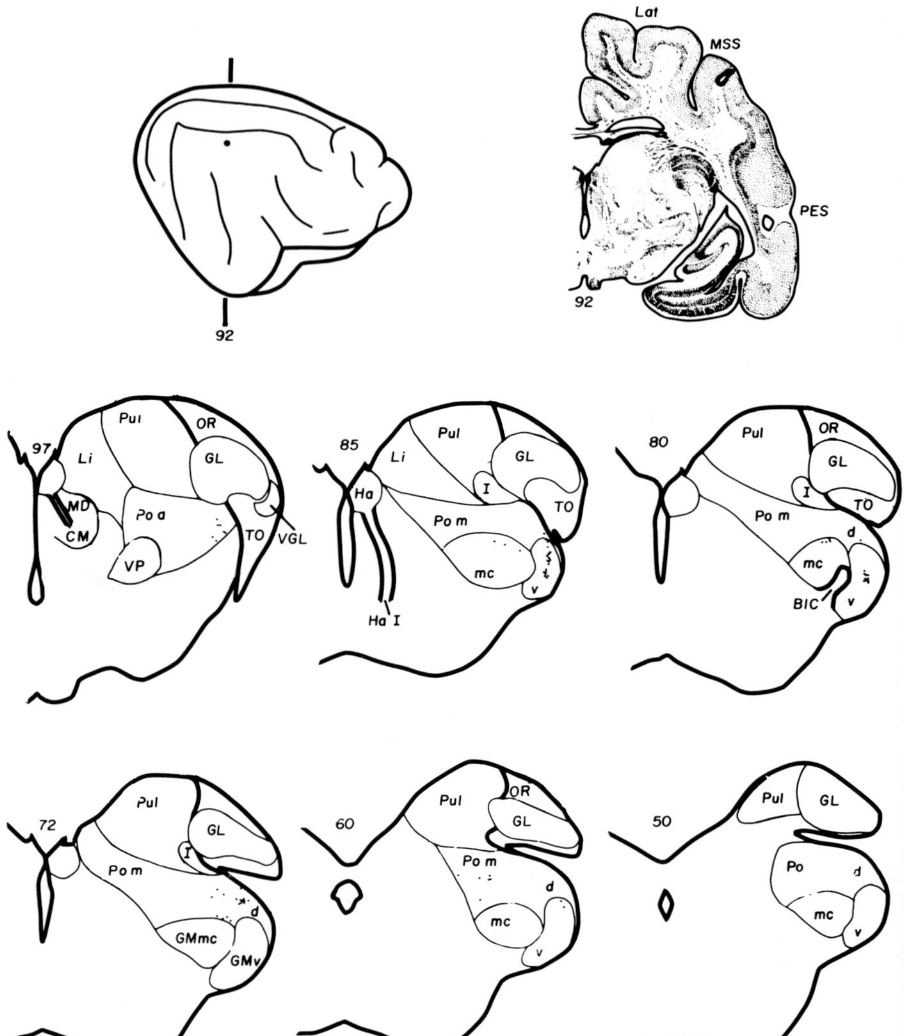

Fig. 2. To show the results of an injection of HRP into cortical area AI in cat 1136R.

Thus, every cortical subdivision appears to be the principal target of one thalamic subdivision but every thalamic subdivision, except for the ventral division which projects only to AI, projects to two or more cortical subdivisions; and in turn every cortical subdivision receives fibers from two or more thalamic subdivisions.

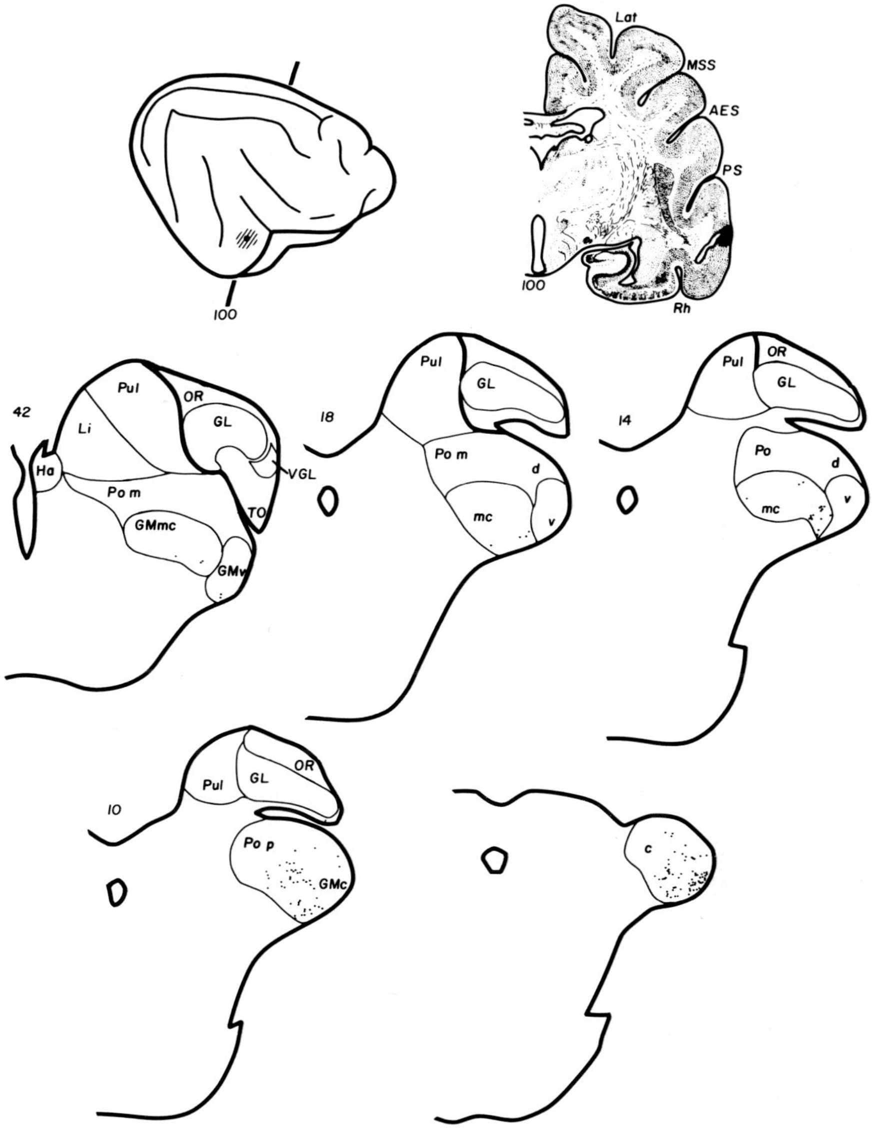

Fig. 3. To show the results of an injection of HRP into the temporal area of cat 876L.

Needless to add we have ruled out the possibility that these results can be attributed to the diffusion of HRP beyond the borders of a single cortical subdivision. In conclusion, there is an extensive overlap in the projections of thalamus to auditory cortex but this overlap is by no means haphazard and strictly follows orderly principles.

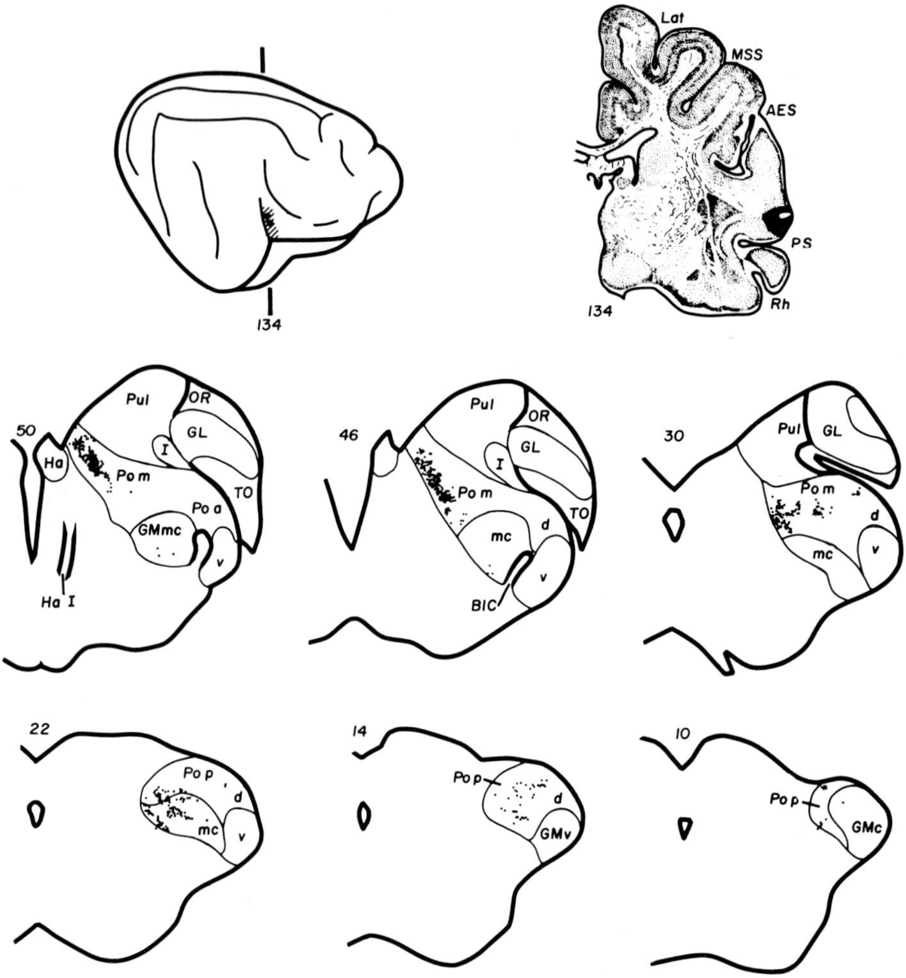

Fig. 4. To show an injection of HRP into the insular area of cat 910L.

IS THE AUDITORY CORTEX OF THE CAT CHARACTERISTIC OF MAMMALS? A COMPARISON OF CAT AND PRIMATE

The cat continues to be the favorite species of researchers who study the auditory pathways, but comparative studies especially of the visual system show that there are significant differences between the cat and other mammalian lines of descent (Diamond and Hall, 1969; Diamond, 1976). For example, the lateral

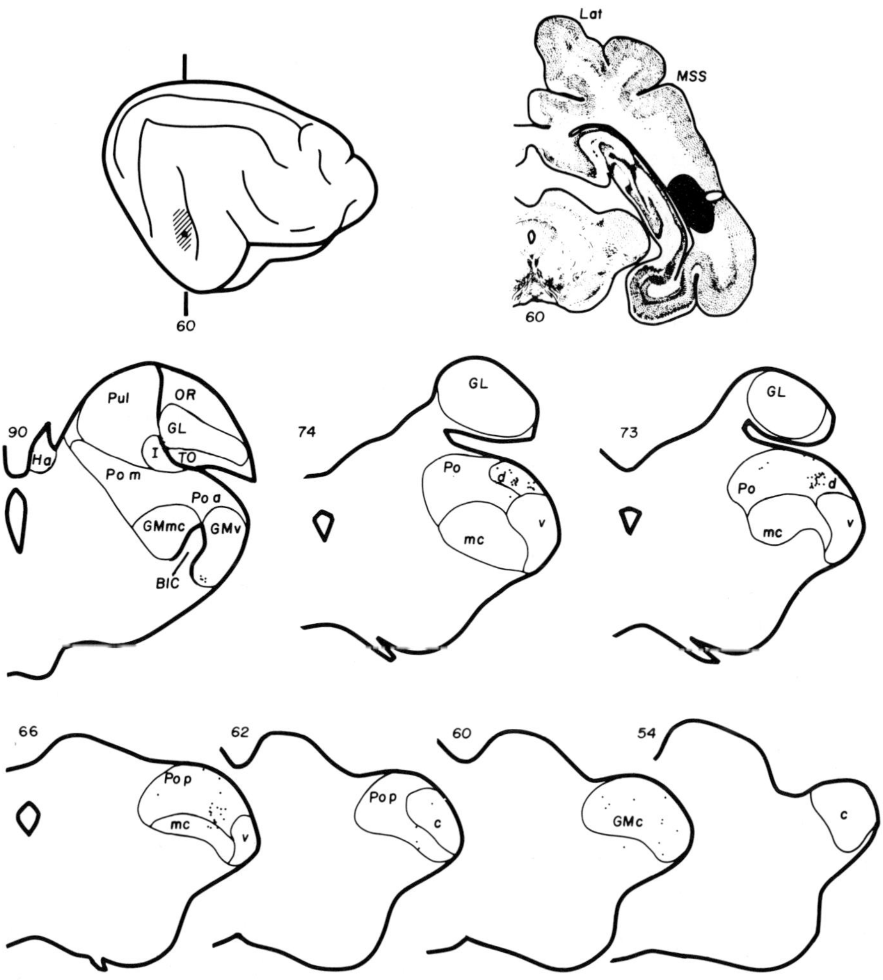

Fig. 5. To show an injection of HRP into cortical area Ep in cat 920R.

geniculate body of the cat projects to cortical areas outside of area 17, but there is no evidence of such an extrastriate target in primates or in tree shrews, a species we have been studying for a number of years. More significant for the present purpose, the cortical projections of the visual thalamus in the cat, which has a number of divisions including subdivisions of the lateral geniculate body itself, overlap extensively (Garey and Powell, 1967; Niimi and Sprague, 1970; Rosenquist et al., 1974). Perhaps the overlap in the projections to the auditory cortex of the cat reflects the nature of carnivores and is not characteristic of all mammals.

To answer this question we turned to the cortex of *Galago senegalensis*. We had been studying the visual cortex of the Galago intensively so it seemed natural to extend this study to the auditory system. This inquiry was first undertaken by Richard Ravizza, joined recently by David Fitzpatrick and Denis Raczkowski. First the auditory cortex was identified by cytoarchitectonic criteria. Since the cytoarchitectonic character of the visual cortex of cat differs significantly from both tree shrews and primates it was surprising to find that the auditory koniocortex in Galago fits almost exactly Rose's description of the first auditory area in the cat, AI. The chief characteristic of AI in the cat is that layers II, III and IV are fused and very densely populated with small cells. Presumably many of these cells are the so-called granular cells that constitute the principal cell type in layer IV of say area 17. Since layer V is very light and broad there is a striking contrast between the dark outer layers and the light inner layers. Precisely these features can be identified on the rostral pole of the temporal lobe of the bush baby *Galago senegalensis*. It seems fair to call this area AI even though the electrophysiological evidence which defines AI is missing. Further, area AI in the Galago like AI in the cat is surrounded by a belt which shares some of the cytoarchitectonic characteristics of the core notably the fusion of layers II, III and IV. In general, the difference between belt and core is that the density of cells in the superficial layers is less in the belt than in AI. One area of the belt is an exception and is distinct from the rest inasmuch as layer IV separates from layer III and layer V is darker as a result of a denser population of larger pyramids. This distinct area consists of a broad band that lies on the lateral surface of the temporal lobe and extends from one end of the sylvian fissure to the other. For the purpose of the present argument I will call this band "Ep" since it seems to resemble the posterior ectosylvian area of the cat.

The results now to be presented will show that this area has the same thalamic connections as "Ep" in the cat. In general the results of injecting the subdivisions of auditory cortex in the bush baby with HRP reveal a striking similarity between cats and this prosimian primate. Figure 6 diagrams the results of injecting a small amount of HRP into the first auditory subdivision or "AI" of Galago 1260. This and the following two figures are taken from Fitzpatrick et al. (1977). The figure shows a row of labeled cells in the ventral division of the medial geniculate body, in addition a few labeled cells can be identified in the magnocellular and dorsal divisions of the medial geniculate body. When the cortex below AI was injected as in Galago 1393, the labeled cells were concentrated in the caudal division of the medial geniculate body and the adjacent caudal part of the magnocellular division (see Fig. 7). A few labeled cells were also found in the dorsal division of the medial geniculate body. When the band called "Ep" was injected the labeled cells were found concentrated in the dorsal division with a scattering of cells in the magnocellular division and the posterior group (see Fig. 8).

Thus each cortical subdivision has one principal source for its afferent input from the thalamus but at the same time each division also receives projections from at least one other, secondary thalamic subdivision. Further, the magnocellular

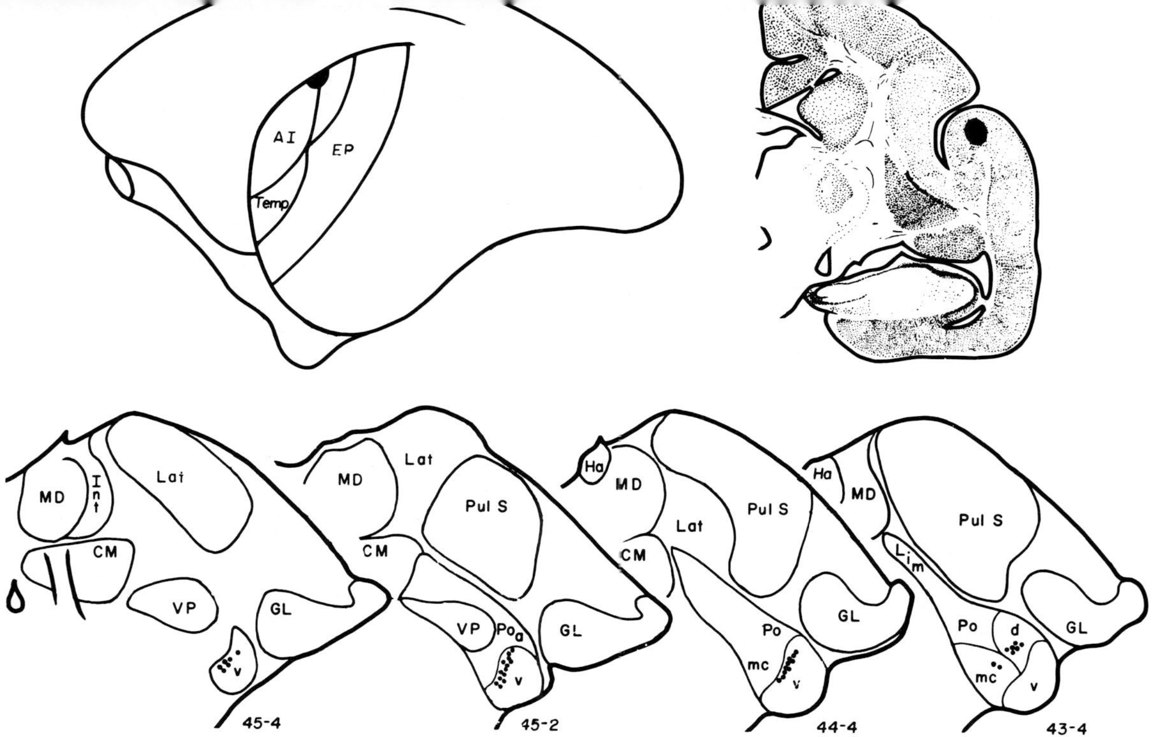

Fig. 6. To show the results of an injection of HRP into the cortical area AI in Galago 1260. The abbreviation in this and the subsequent two figures are as follows: AI, auditory area I; CM, centre median nucleus; Ep, posterior ectosylvian area; GL, dorsal lateral geniculate body; GM, medial geniculate body; GMc, c, caudal division of the medial geniculate body; GMd, d, dorsal division of the medial geniculate body; GMmc, mc, magnocellular division of the medial geniculate body; GMv, v, ventral division of the medial geniculate body; Ha, habenula; Im, medial part of the inferior subdivision of the pulvinar nucleus; Int, intralaminar nuclei; Lat, lateral nucleus; Lim, nucleus limitans; MD, mediodorsal nucleus; Po, posterior nuclear group of the thalamus; Po a, anterior sector of the posterior group; Pt, pretectum; Pul I, inferior division of the pulvinar nucleus; Pul S, superior division of the pulvinar nucleus; Sg, suprageniculate nucleus; Temp, temporal cortex; VP, ventroposterior nucleus.

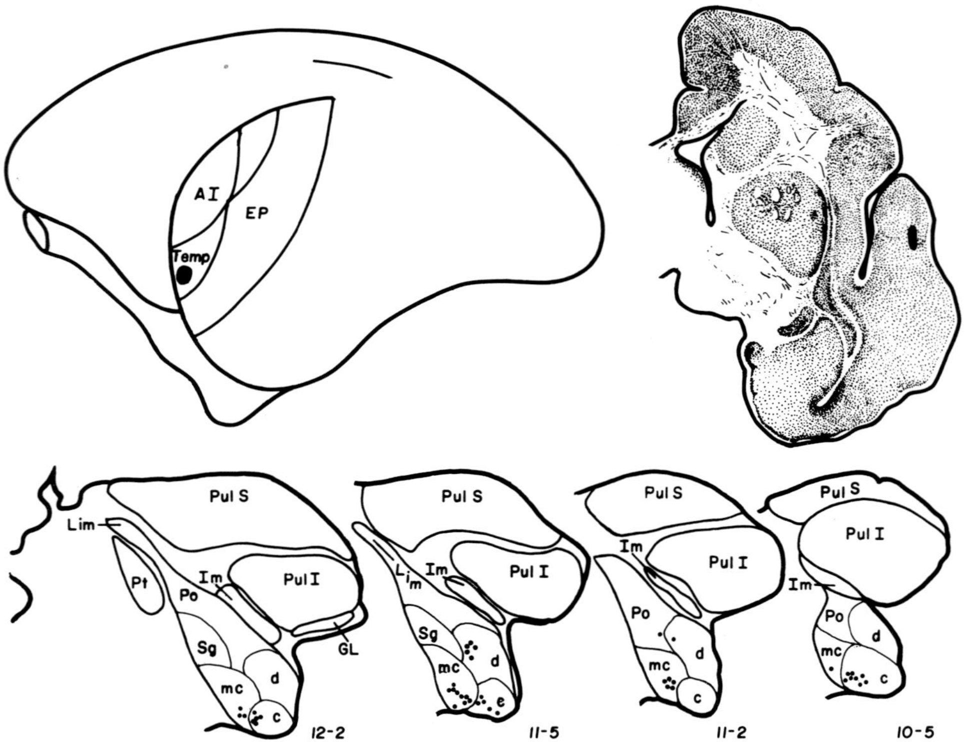

Fig. 7. To show the results of an injection of HRP into the temporal auditory cortex of Galago 1393.

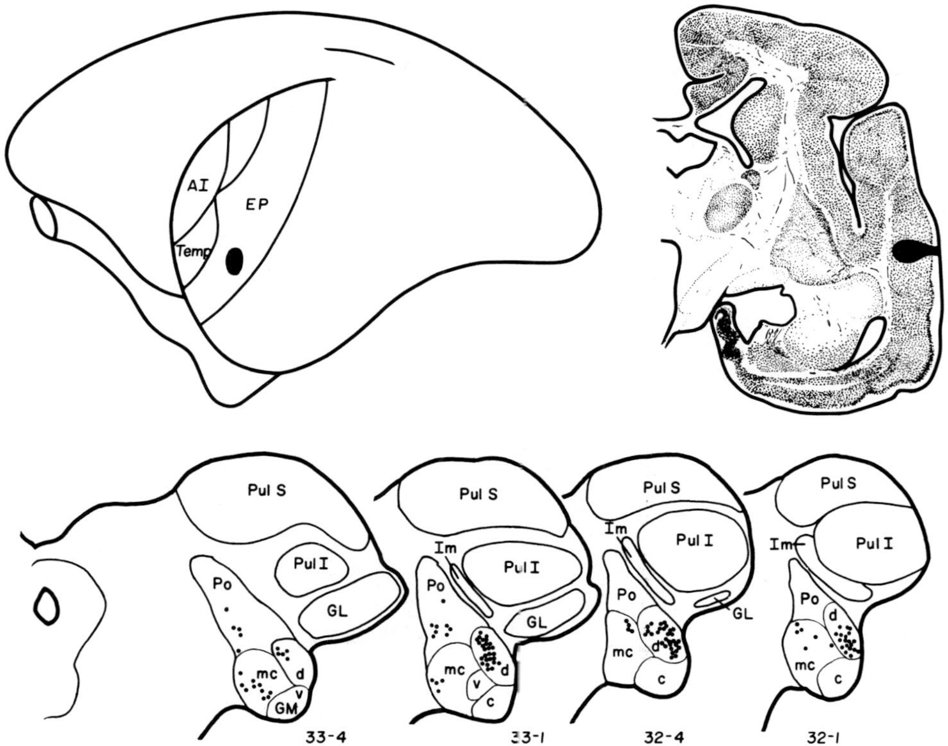

Fig. 8. To show the results of an injection of HRP into the cortical area Ep of Galago 1359.

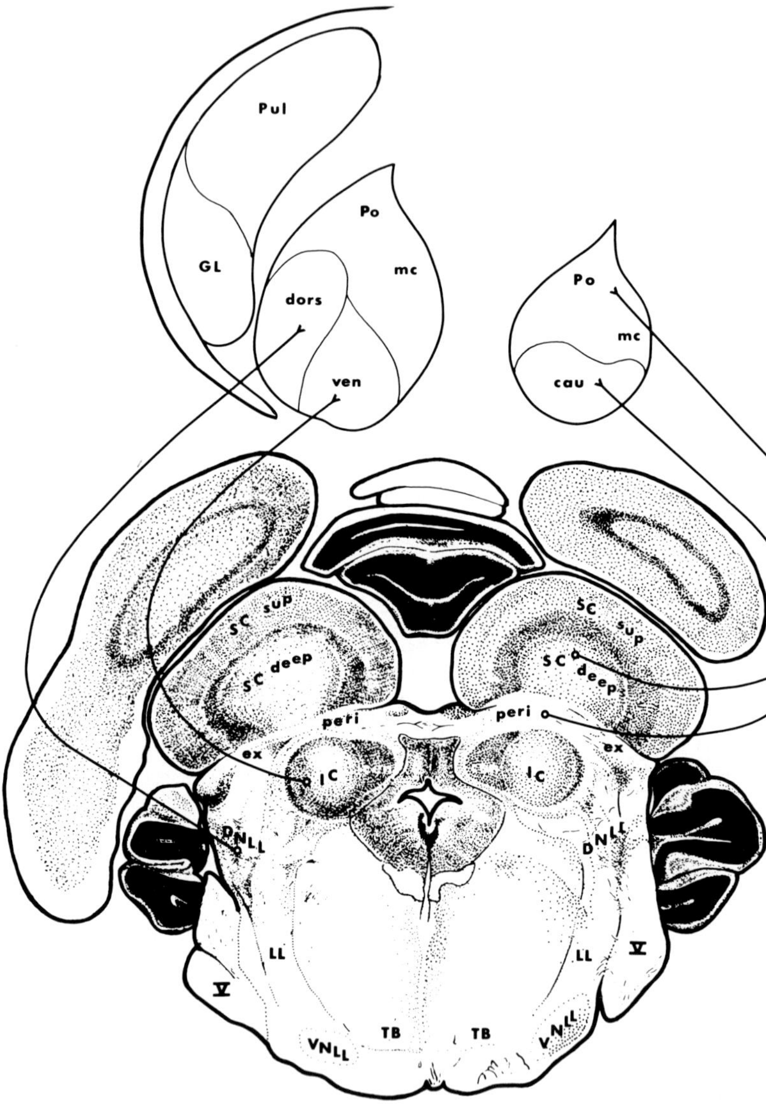

Fig. 9. Schematic drawing to diagram the pathways in *Tupaia glis,* from the midbrain to the thalamus. The figure shows four separate paths, 1) from the central nucleus of the inferior colliculus to the ventral division of the medial geniculate; 2) from the lateral tegmental area in the vicinity of the dorsal nucleus of the lateral lemniscus to the dorsal division of the medial geniculate body; 3) from the deep superior colliculus to the posterior nucleus; and 4) from the pericentral area of the inferior colliculus to the caudal division of the medial geniculate. Abbreviations for this figure are as follows: cau, caudal division of the medial geniculate body;

division of the medial geniculate seems to project to all cortical subdivisions; and finally the projections to the first auditory area are highly topographic. A single row of labeled cells is produced if the injection is small enough and the locus of this row moves from the lateral to medial border of the ventral division of the medial geniculate body as the locus of the injection in AI is varied.

As the same conclusions are derived from the experiments in the cat, it is fair to conclude that the same general principles hold for the organization of auditory cortex in all or most mammals.

ASCENDING AUDITORY PATHWAYS IN THE TREE SHREW, TUPAIA GLIS

These results confirm and justify the concept of a field as put forth by Rose (1949). But it can be argued that the functional significance of this organization remains obscure since the question of why there are subdivisions within the field, has simply been transferred from the cortex to the thalamus. In other words, it is fair to ask: "What is the functional significance of the thalamic subdivisions just described?" A starting point to the answer is that each one of these divisions has a different source for its auditory impulses, which is to say each subdivision may be a relay in a distinct pathway; and some of these pathways carry somatosensory as well as auditory impulses. To support this conclusion I will briefly review some results of experiments in the tree shrew, *Tupaia glis*. These results are taken from studies by Casseday et al., (1976) and by Oliver and Hall (1975), and are summarized by the diagram shown in Figure 9.

If a lesion is restricted to the central nucleus of the inferior colliculus and anterograde degeneration is traced forward to the thalamus, it is principally the ventral division of the medial geniculate body which contains axonal and terminal degeneration. To a lesser extent degeneration is located in the magnocellular division but the dorsal and caudal divisions of the medial geniculate body remain free of degeneration. The dorsal division on the other hand contains terminal degeneration while the ventral division is essentially free of degeneration following a lesion of the lateral lemniscus and surrounding tegmentum. Finally the caudal part of the medial geniculate body contains terminal degeneration whenever the lesion is in the pericentral areas of the inferior colliculus; add to these results the fact that the posterior group and the magnocellular division of the medial geniculate body contain terminal degeneration following lesions of the deep layers of the superior colliculus (Harting et al., 1973; Casagrande et al., 1972).

DNLL, dorsal nucleus of the lateral lemniscus; dors, dorsal division of the medial geniculate body; ex, external nucleus of the inferior colliculus; GL, lateral geniculate body; IC, central nucleus of the inferior colliculus; LL, lateral lemniscus; mc, magnocellular division of the medial geniculate body; peri, pericentral region of the inferior colliculus; Po, posterior nuclear group of the thalamus; Pul, pulvinar nucleus; SC deep, deep layers of the superior colliculus; SC sup, superficial layers of the superior colliculus; TB, trapezoid body; ven, ventral division of the medial geniculate body; VNLL, ventral nucleus of the lateral lemniscus; V, fifth cranial nerve.

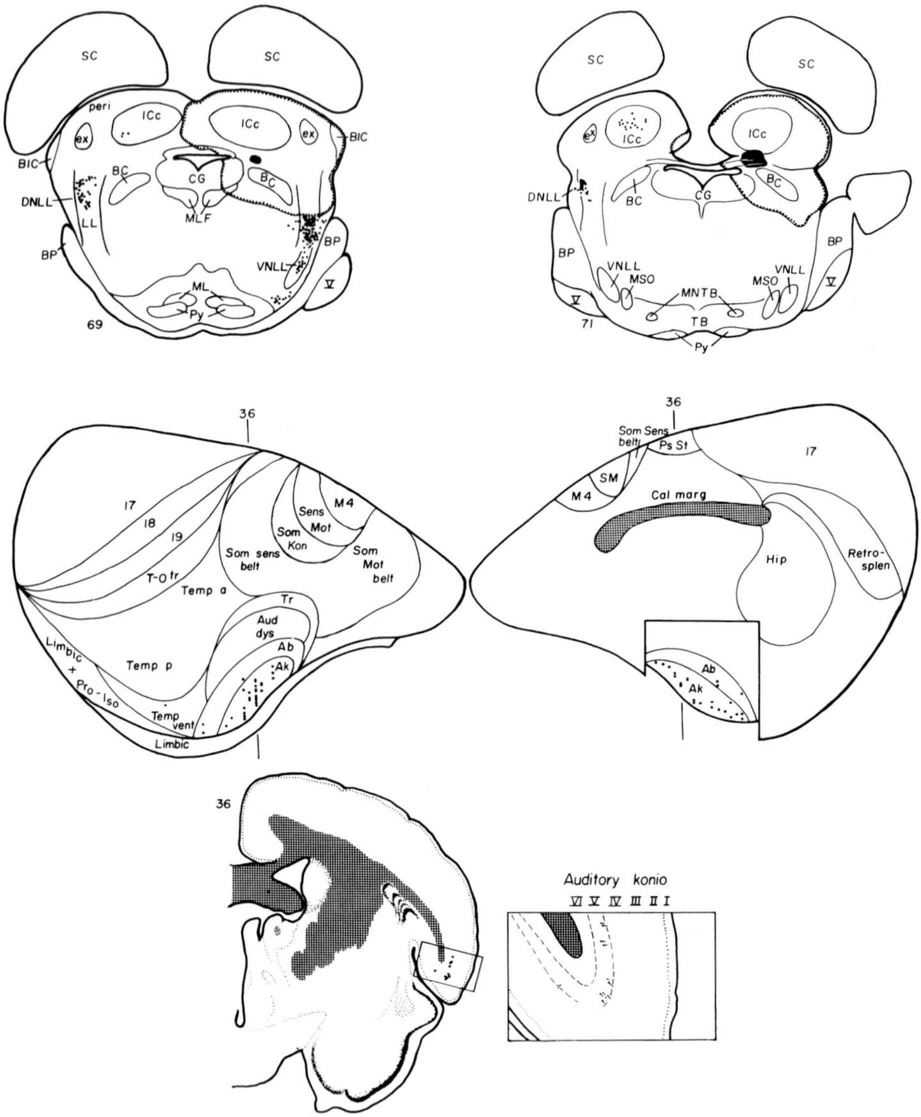

Fig. 10. To show the results of injecting HRP into the inferior colliculus of Tupaia 0206 and especially to show the cortical neurons which project to the injection site. The top of the figure shows two sections through the midbrain in which the injection site is depicted in black. It is clear that the HRP was injected chiefly below the central nucleus.

In the middle of the figure are two drawings, on the left a 45° view of the dorsal and lateral surface and on the right a 45° view of the dorsal and medial surface. Each dot represents a single labeled cell.

Finally below is a frontal section through the auditory koniocortex which reveals that all

It has not escaped our notice that some of these pathways are likely to be somatosensory as well as auditory. In any case the subdivisions of the auditory thalamus seem to depend on the existence of several parallel pathways by means of which impulses can ascend the brain stem to reach the thalamus.

In summary, the auditory field consists of a core, or AI, which is the target of the lemniscal path relaying in the central nucleus of the inferior colliculus and the ventral division of the medial geniculate body and a surrounding belt which is *not* the target of the lemniscal path. This belt consists of several subdivisions which seem to be related to the core functionally even though some of these probably receive somatic impulses as well as auditory.

FURTHER INTERCONNECTIONS WITHIN THE FIELD: CORTICO-CORTICAL CONNECTIONS AND DESCENDING PROJECTIONS

Two additional kinds of evidence support the view that the several subdivisions which make up the field are linked with each other, which is to say that there is further justification for the concept of a "field". First, the cortico-cortical projections within the auditory field are very intense while few fibers connect the auditory field with other cortical fields. For example, we have shown that AI projects to AII and that AII reciprocates by projecting back to AI; but AI does not, for example, project to the adjacent suprasylvian gyrus (Diamond et al., 1969).

The descending projections from the auditory field are as organized as the ascending projections and provide a new insight into the significance of the field. First, each cortical subdivision reciprocates its thalamic input by a descending projection. Thus, AI projects to the ventral division of the medial geniculate body, the temporal area projects to the caudal division of the medial geniculate body, etc. (see Diamond et al., 1969). In general these descending projections from cortex to

of the labeled cells are in the 5th layer.

The abbreviations in this and the following figure are as follows: AB, Aud b, auditory belt area; Ak, auditory koniocortex; Aud dys, auditory dysgranular area; BC, brachium conjunctivum; BIC, brachium of the inferior colliculus; BP, brachium pontis; Cal marg, callosal marginal area; CC, corpus callosum; CG, central grey; DNLL, dorsal nucleus of the lateral lemniscus; ex, external nucleus of the inferior colliculus; GP, griseum pontis; Hip, hippocampus; ICc, central nucleus of the inferior colliculus; Limbic, limbic cortical area; LL, lateral lemniscus; ML, medial lemniscus; MLF, medial longitudinal fasciculus; MNTB, medial nucleus of the trapezoid body; MSO, medial superior olive; M4, motor area 4; peri, pericentral zone of the inferior colliculus; Pg, parabigeminal nucleus; Pro Iso, proiso cortex; Ps st, pseudo striate area; Py, pyramidal tract; Retro splen, retrosplenial cortical area; SC, superior colliculus; SM, Sens mot, sensory motor area; Som Kon, somatic koniocortex; Som Mot belt, somatic motor belt; Som Sens belt, somatic sensory belt; TB, trapezoid body; Temp a, anterior Temporal area; Temp p, posterior Temporal area; Temp vent, ventral Temporal area; T-O trans, temporal occipital transition; VNLL, ventral nucleus of the lateral lemniscus; IV, trochlear nerve; V, trigeminal nerve; 17, cortical area 17; 18, cortical area 18; 19, cortical area 19.

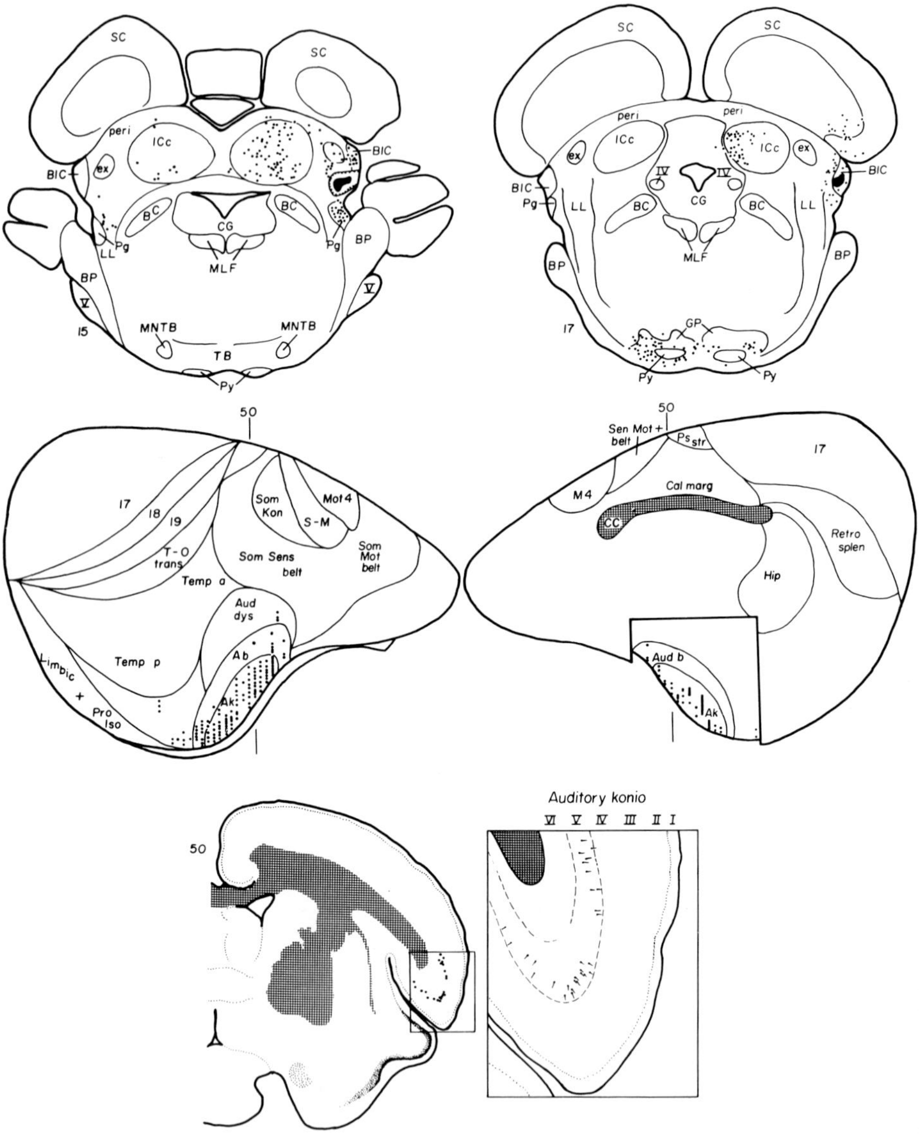

Fig. 11. To show the results of injecting HRP into the inferior colliculus of Tupaia 0168. The injection site as depicted at the top of the figure is at the lateral extremity of the inferior colliculus and lies outside both the central nucleus and the external nucleus. Again as in the previous experiment illiustrated in Figure 10, labeled cells in the cortex are almost restricted to the koniocortex or AI.

thalamus originate from neurons in layer VI. There are notable exceptions to this rule but the principle holds for the traditional relay nuclei of the thalamus. For example, layer VI of the striate cortex projects to the lateral geniculate body (Raczkowski and Diamond, 1978).

Neurons from layer V of the auditory cortex also send descending axons to the auditory centers of the brain stem. The organization of these projections is especially significant for the present argument, since the descending projections from a given cortical sector always appear to have targets in a parallel pathway and never in the same ascending pathway. To illustrate my meaning with a particular example, AI projects to the inferior colliculus but not to the central nucleus which is the tectal relay in the lemniscal-AI path.

This conclusion is derived from experiments by Jones et al. (1976) in which HRP was injected into various subdivisions of the tree shrew tectum. Figures 10 and 11 show the cells of layer V in auditory koniocortex which are labeled by HRP injections into the pericentral division of the inferior colliculus. If the central nucleus is injected with HRP no cortical cells are labeled. Thus the central nucleus of the inferior colliculus does not appear to be a target of descending projections from the cortex at least in tree shrew. If the deep layers of the superior colliculus are injected then cells of layer V of the auditory belt are labeled. The deep superior colliculus seems to be one of the few centers where impulses from the three chief neocortical modalities converge.

In summary, each cortical subdivision in the field is the primary target of one ascending path, -at least one thalamic nucleus. The overlap between projections from the various thalamic nuclei link the subdivisions of a field to each other. Different cortical subdivisions are also linked by descending projections. Thus area AI projects to tectal areas which in turn project to parts of the auditory belt.

IMPLICATIONS OF THE CONCEPT OF THE "AUDITORY FIELD"

The field as first defined by Rose was applied to adjacent cortical subdivisions closely related by cytoarchitectonic criteria. This concept put an end to the debate about the borders since only one feature need change to distinguish closely related subdivisions and even this single change need not be abrupt. More significantly, the cytoarchitectonic subdivisions defined by Rose could be correlated with the subdivisions defined by electrophysiology and thalamic connections.

I have tried to show that the various subdivisions within the auditory field of the cat probably are the targets of distinct parallel pathways. This conclusion must be qualified inasmuch as there is no simple one-to-one relationship between a thalamic subdivision and a cortical subdivision. Nevertheless, the key to understanding the significance of cortical subdivisions within a field appears to lie in the study of parallel ascending pathways within the same modality.

If we accept this starting point for the sake of the argument, a surprising extention or implication of the concept of the "field" emerges. Our comparative studies of the tree shrew and bush baby have demonstrated the presence of parallel

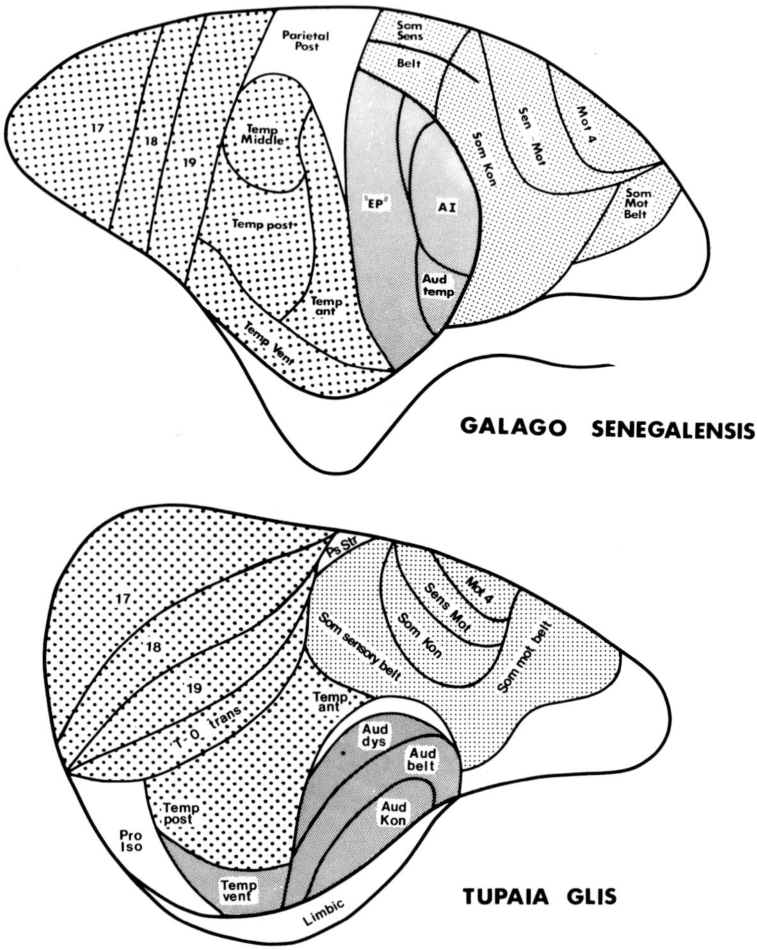

Fig. 12. To show the auditory, visual and somatic fields in *Galago senegalensis* (B) and in *Tupaia glis* (A).

B. Below is shown the homologous areas in the Galago. The visual field in Galago is subdivided into several parts including area 17 and a number of subdivisions in the occipital and temporal lobe. The somatic field is very much like that described below in the tree shrew. The auditory field has been discussed in the text.

A. In the tree shrew, the visual area consists of area 17 which is the target of the lateral geniculate, the extrastriate belt (areas 18, 19 and the transition zone), and the temporal area which is further divided into an anterior, posterior and ventral division. The entire region from the border of area 17 to the auditory cortex receives fibers from the pulvinar nucleus. The auditory field consists of several divisions, a core or konicortical area surrounded by a belt which in turn is subdivided into several regions. The two that are *visual* pathways with the result that the entire occipital lobe and most of the temporal lobe can be regarded as a single visual "field". To be sure the borders between subdivisions within the visual field are sharp, at least some of them are, so that the issues which beset the study of architectonics never would have arisen if the study of cortical architecture had been restricted to the striate cortex, for example. Nevertheless, I feel it is justified to argue that the same principles which characterize the auditory field can be applied to the visual field. First the cortico-cortical connections between subdivisions within the visual field are intense, while cortico-cortical connections between the visual and auditory fields or between the visual and somatosensory fields are relatively sparse.

Second, descending projections further reveal the close interrelationships between the various parts of the field. Thus, layer V of area 17 projects to the superficial layers of the superior colliculus and these project to the pulvinar nucleus, which in turn projects to the visual cortex of the temporal lobe; and layer V of the striate cortex projects directly to all subdivisions of the pulvinar nucleus at least in Galago (Raczkowski and Diamond, 1976; Raczkowski and Diamond, 1978).

Third, there are some thalamo-cortical projections which reveal the essential unity of the field. Just as the magnocellular division of the medial geniculate projects to whole auditory field, the pulvinar nucleus projects to the striate cortex as well as to the extrastriate visual belt and to the visual areas of the temporal lobe (Coleman et al., 1977; Raczkowski and Diamond, 1978). In summary, if a cortical field is defined as the target of two or more parallel pathways within a single modality having at least some common connections and having subdivisions closely interconnected by means of cortico-cortical, ascending and descending projections, then the result is the cortical maps of Tupaia and Galago shown in Figure 12A and 12B.

CORTICAL FIELDS AND CYTOARCHITECTONIC CRITERIA

It could be argued that in order to draw the three fields shown in Figures 12A and 12B the original meaning of the term field was so stretched as to eliminate cytoarchitectonic criteria as a basis for classifying. The prevailing view has been that cortical subdivisions fall into three classes: 1. primary sensory cortex; 2. motor cortex; and 3. association cortex. The classification proposed here assigns areas to the same class which have traditionally been regarded as poles apart, for example, the somatic sensory area and the motor area; and assigns areas to different classes

depicted here are called auditory belt which resembles the koniocortex inasmuch as areas II, III and IV are fused but layer V has larger pyramidal cells in the belt. In the adjacent region called the dysgranular auditory area the cells of layer V are even larger and darker and indeed layer V becomes darker than the superficial layer three layers. Finally the somatic field has several subdivisions, notably the primary motor area and the primary somatosensory area. A major point is that between these two areas is a zone called sensory motor which appears to be intermediate having a slight development of the 4th granular area.

have been regarded as in the same class, notably, the primary koniocortex. But the difference between the two views does not depend on the extent to which reliance is placed on cytoarchitecture but rather on the underlying view about the functional significance of the classification. There is as much ground for calling sensory and motor areas similar (layer V seems to be much alike throughout the somatic field) as there is for calling auditory and visual koniocortex alike. Indeed, the case for the differences between auditory and visual koniocortex is as strong as the case for similarities: thus the auditory koniocortex is characterized by a fusion of layers II, III and IV and visual koniocortex is characterized by a separation of layers II, III and IV. It makes no sense to argue that layer IV is more or less important for classification than layer V. The issue then turns on the underlying assumptions of function and the usefulness of the scheme to help understand functional organization. In my view all or most of the cortex is sensory inasmuch as it receives sensory

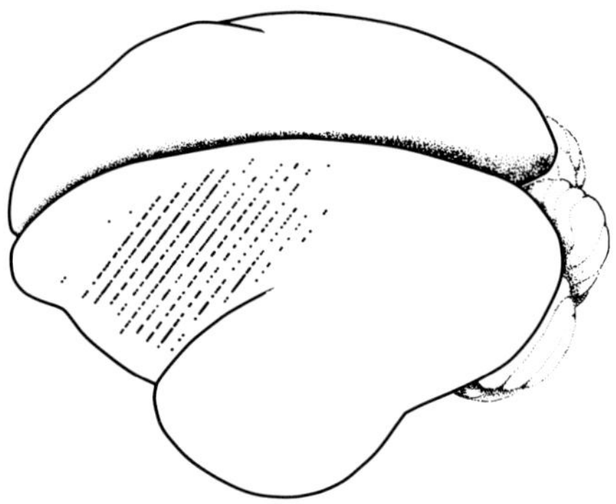

Fig. 13. To show the distribution of labeled cells in the cortex of Galago 1282 after an injection of HRP into the gracile and cuneate nuclei. The labeled cells in the cortex have been plotted and projected to the lateral surface in a series of sections through the whole brain. It is obvious that the area containing labeled cells corresponds exactly with the areas classified as the somatic field in figure 12A. This field includes the following areas, Motor 4, the sensory motor area, the somatic koniocortex and the belt around the sensory and motor areas. This figure was taken from experiments in progress by Glenn C. Thompson and Aldo Rustioni.

impulses from thalamic nuclei. In my experience there is no area of the cortex of Tupaia and Galago, certainly none shown in the maps of Figures 12A and 12B, which does not receive sensory input from the thalamus; and there is no nucleus of the thalamus which does not receive sensory impulses from brainstem centers or cortex. Even the pulvinar nucleus is sensory in so far as those subdivisions of the pulvinar not receiving tectal or pretectal fibers are recipients of fibers from layer V of area 17 (Raczkowski and Diamond, 1976). Further, all of the neocortex is motor in the sense that everywhere layer V is the source of fibers which descend to the tectum, pons, reticular formation, spinal cord, etc. Thus all of the somatic field projects to nuclei of the dorsal columns (see Figure 13).

In the traditional view, the function common to sensory areas was thought to be conscious experience of elementary sensory qualities such as pitch. There is little or no evidence for the assumption that auditory cortex is the basis for hearing pitch. The association areas were regarded as the site of converging impulses from the various sensory areas. There is little or no evidence, even anatomical evidence, of extensive cortical areas receiving converging fibers and little or no evidence that learning or association takes place by cortico-cortical paths from primary sensory areas to association areas. Finally, there is no evidence that the so-called motor cortex is the final common path of the cortex. Rather than being a compulsory relay in a pathway from sensory centers to motor centers, the motor cortex can be regarded as sensory cortex in the same sense as the traditional somato-sensory areas (3,2 or 1) since it receives thalamic fibers from the ventral group carrying "spinal cord information"; and the sensory cortex can be regarded as motor in the same sense as the traditional Motor area 4 since its layer V sends descending fibers to spinal cord.

Acknowledgements

I would like to thank Pamela Madren for her help in preparing this manuscript, Mrs. Nada Staddon and Mr. Leroy McMillan for their help in preparing the illustrations and the National Institute of Mental Health Grant MH04849 for their support.

REFERENCES

Campbell, A.W. *Histological studies on the localization of cerebral function.* Cambridge: Cambridge University Press, 1905.

Casagrande, V.A., Harting, J.K, Hall, W.C., Diamond, I.T. and Martin, G.F. Superior colliculus of the tree shrew: a structural and functional subdivision into superficial and deep layers. *Science 177:* 444-447, 1972.

Casseday, J.H., Diamond, I.T. and Harting, J.K. Auditory pathways to the cortex in *Tupaia glis. J. Comp. Neurol. 166:* 303-340, 1976.

Coleman, J., Diamond, I.T. and Winer, J.A. The visual cortex of the opossum: the retrograde transport of horseradish peroxidase to the lateral geniculate and lateral posterior nuclei. *Brain Res. 137:* 233-252, 1977.

Diamond, I.T. Organization of the visual cortex: comparative anatomical and behavioral studies. *Fed. Proc. 35:* 60-67, 1976.

Diamond, I.T., Chow, K.L. and Neff, W.D. Degeneration of caudal medial geniculate body following cortical lesions ventral to auditory area II in the cat. *J. Comp. Neurol. 109:* 349-362, 1958.

Diamond, I.T. and Hall, W.C. Evolution of neocortex. *Science 164:* 251-262, 1969.

Diamond, I.T., Jones, E.G. and Powell, T.P.S. The projection of the auditory cortex upon the diencephalon and brain stem in the cat. *Brain Res. 15:* 305-340, 1969.

Fitzpatrick, D., Raczkowski, D., Ravizza, R.J. and Diamond, I.T. Organization of the thalamocortical projections to the auditory cortex in *Galago senegalensis. Neurosci. Abst. 3:* 67, 1977.

Garey, L.J. and Powell, T.P.S. The projection of the lateral geniculate nucleus upon the cortex in the cat. *Proc. Roy. Soc. London 169:* 107-126, 1967.

Harting, J.K., Hall, W.C., Diamond, I.T. and Martin, G.F. Anterograde degeneration study of the superior colliculus in *Tupaia glis*: evidence for a subdivision between superficial and deep layers. *J. Comp. Neurol. 148:* 361-386, 1973.

Jones, D.R., Casseday, J.H. and Diamond, I.T. Further study of parallel auditory pathways in the tree shrew, *Tupaia glis. Anat. Rec. 184:* 438, 1976.

Lashley, K.S. and Clark, G. The cytoarchitecture of the cerebral cortex of *Ateles:* a critical examination of architectonic studies. *J. Comp. Neurol. 85:* 223-305, 1946.

Morest, D.K. The neuronal architecture of the medial geniculate body of the cat. *J. Anat. London 98:* 611-630, 1964.

Niimi, K. and Sprague, J.M. Thalamo-cortical organization of the visual system in the cat. *J. Comp. Neurol. 138:* 219-250, 1970.

Oliver, D.L. and Hall, W.C. Subdivisions of the medial geniculate body in the tree shrew *(Tupaia glis). Brain Res. 86:* 217-227, 1975.

Raczkowski, D. and Diamond, I.T. Projections from layers V and VI of the neocortex to the tectum and the thalamus of *Galago senegalensis. Neurosci Abst. 2:* 1086, 1976.

Raczkowski, D. and Diamond, I.T. Connections of the striate cortex of *Galago senegalensis. Brain Res.* In press, 1978.

Rose, J.E. The cellular structure of the auditory region of the cat. *J. Comp. Neurol. 91:* 409-440, 1949.

Rose, J.E. and Woolsey, C.N. The relations of thalamic connections, cellular structure and evocable electrical activity in the auditory region of the cat. *J. Comp. Neurol. 91:* 441-466, 1949.

Rose, J.E. and Woolsey, C.N. Cortical connections and functional organization of the thalamic auditory system of the cat. In: *Biological and Biochemical Bases of Behavior,* edited by H.F. Harlow and C.N. Woolsey. Madison: University of Wisconsin Press, 1958, p. 127-150.

Rosenquist, A.C., Edwards, S.B. and Palmer, L.A. An autoradiographic study of the projections of the dorsal lateral geniculate nucleus and posterior nucleus in the cat. *Brain Res. 80:* 71-93, 1974.

Thompson, C. and Rustioni, A. Descending projections of the somatic cortex in *Galago senegalensis.* Personnal communication.

Winer, J.A., Diamond, I.T. and Raczkowski, D. Subdivisions of the auditory cortex of the cat: the retrograde transport of horseradish peroxidase to the medial geniculate body and posterior thalamic nuclei. *J. Comp. Neurol. 176:* 387-418, 1977.

DISCUSSION

Galambos: Are you saying that there is uniformity with respect to the descending components even though the ascending inflows are surprisingly diverse? That the ascending is not so easy to understand while the descending connections are?

Diamond: I think that Bob is inviting me to comment on the relation between ascending and descending projections to the cortex. Ascending projections can be specific, such as the projection of the ventral division to AI or diffuse in the sense that the magnocellular division projects to all of the subdivisions of the auditory field. In the same way, descending projections are of two sorts, a number of cortical areas can converge on a single subcortical target as in the case of the projections from layer V or an extensive region of the cortex to the deep superior colliculus, or a single cortical subdivision such as AI can project to a given portion of the inferior colliculus. I am not saying the unity of the field can only be revealed by descending projections.

Galambos: But it is more clearly revealed by the descending than by the ascending?

Diamond: No. Look at the magnocellular division of the medial geniculate body. That is the diffuse auditory projection relay in the sense that it goes to all of the parts of the auditory cortex. Incidentally, you see how this organization can shed light on this whole controversy about the tonotopic organization. If GMmc projects to layer I in a diffuse way, and layer I is inactivated with anesthetic, then only the topographic organization of the ventral division, which is exquisite, will be recorded. If you leave the influence of GMmc intact then you are going to get a totally different picture.

Ritz: With your injections of HRP in the inferior colliculus, do you ever see uptake into the medial geniculate?

Diamond: No.

Rose: It is indeed a pleasure to see the evolution of the concept of an architectonic field. Personally, I think that what you have shown indicates strongly that there exists more than one valid cortical map as there exists more than one valid map of the United States. Depending on the criteria used one obtains different maps. Thus, eg., a map based on thalamo-cortical connections is likely to be different from that based say, on callosal connections, yet each is valid in its own right. You have shown very nicely the morphological significance of some of the connections. It is useful to realize that a cortical field can be often viewed as being composed of a number of segments each different slightly morphologically from its neighbors. Presumably, different sets of overlapping connections are responsible for the morphological gradients observed.

SOME RELATIONSHIPS OF BINAURAL RESPONSE PATTERNS OF SINGLE NEURONS TO CORTICAL COLUMNS AND INTERHEMISPHERIC CONNECTIONS OF AUDITORY AREA AI OF CAT CEREBRAL CORTEX

John F. Brugge and Thomas J. Imig

University of Wisconsin

INTRODUCTION

The primary auditory field (AI) in cat and monkey can be distinguished on cytoarchitectonic grounds from the auditory belt that surrounds it (Rose, 1949; Rose and Woolsey, 1949; Merzenich and Brugge, 1973; Pandya and Sanides, 1973; Imig et al., 1977). Many neurons within this area are tuned to a relatively narrow range of frequencies and together they form a complete topographic representation of the audible frequency spectrum that is coextensive with the cytoarchitectonic boundaries of AI (Goldstein et al., 1970; Merzenich and Brugge, 1973; Merzenich et al., 1975; Imig et al., 1977). Furthermore, the majority of neurons recorded within a radial cell column have very similar best frequencies (Hind et al., 1960; Abeles and Goldstein, 1970). In addition to being frequency selective, most of the neurons recorded in AI are also sensitive to binaural stimulation (Hall and Goldstein, 1968). Neurons responding at low stimulus frequencies, below about 4000 Hz, are sensitive to small disparities in time of arrival of the stimulus at the two ears (Brugge et al., 1969; Brugge and Merzenich, 1973; Benson and Teas, 1976). At higher stimulus frequencies cells of AI may be sensitive to changes in the sound pressure level of a binaural stimulus (Hall and Goldstein, 1968; Brugge et al., 1969; Brugge and Merzenich, 1973). Recently it has been shown that binaural neurons in the high frequency representation of AI form functional cell columns, some of which overlap the map of best frequency in an orderly way (Imig and Adrian, 1978). Further work has revealed that the pattern of some of the corticocortical connections made by AI relate not only to the frequency organization but to the distribution of binaural columns as well (Imig et al., 1977).

In this paper we discuss three aspects of binaural organization of AI in the cat. First we present data from single unit studies which show differential sensitivities among AI neurons to changes in binaural stimulus parameters. Second, we

ISBN 0-12-514960-3

show maps of functional cell columns formed by neurons with binaural properties. Finally, we present results from combined electrophysiological and anatomical experiments that show some relationships between the interhemispheric patterns of connections and the tonotopic and binaural organization of the primary auditory field.

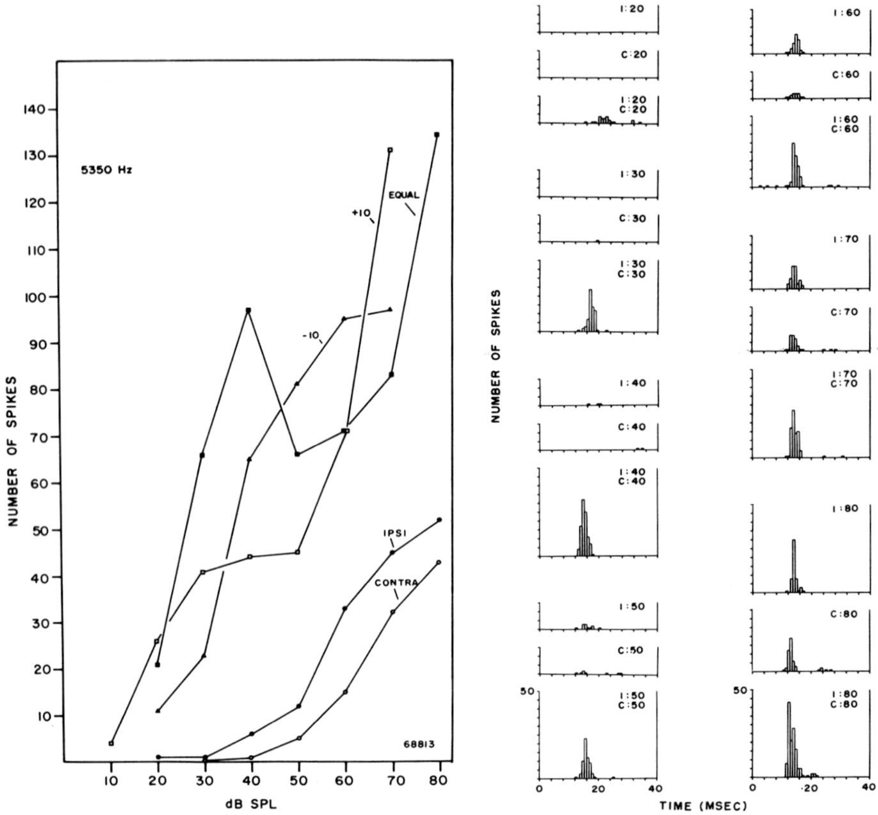

Fig. 1. Effect of raising stimulus intensity on monaural and binaural spike counts for a neuron in AI having a best frequency of 5350 Hz. Two monaural and three binaural curves are shown. One binaural curve was obtained when SPLs at the two ears, shown on the abscissa, were equal. The two others were obtained when the SPL at one ear was 10 dB greater or less than that at the opposite ear. Post-stimulus time histograms show response patterns to ipsilateral (I), contralateral (C) and binaural stimulation at the designated SPLs. Tone duration: 200 msec; repetition rate: 2/sec; 50 stimulus repetitions; sodium pentobarbital anesthesia; SPL re: 0.0002 dyne/cm².

NEURONS WITHIN AI SENSITIVE TO CHANGES IN BINAURAL INTENSITY

Based upon their responses to changes in intensity of a binaural stimulus, neurons in AI may be grouped into three categories. The first category includes those neurons which are excited by monotic stimulation of both the left and right ears and which, when the two ears are stimulated together, generate a significantly greater number of spikes than when either ear is stimulated alone. Figure 1 illustrates the response patterns from one such neuron. In this case monotic stimulation to either ear at best frequency results in spike-count functions which increase monotonically over a range of nearly 50 dB. Stimulation of the ipsilateral ear is

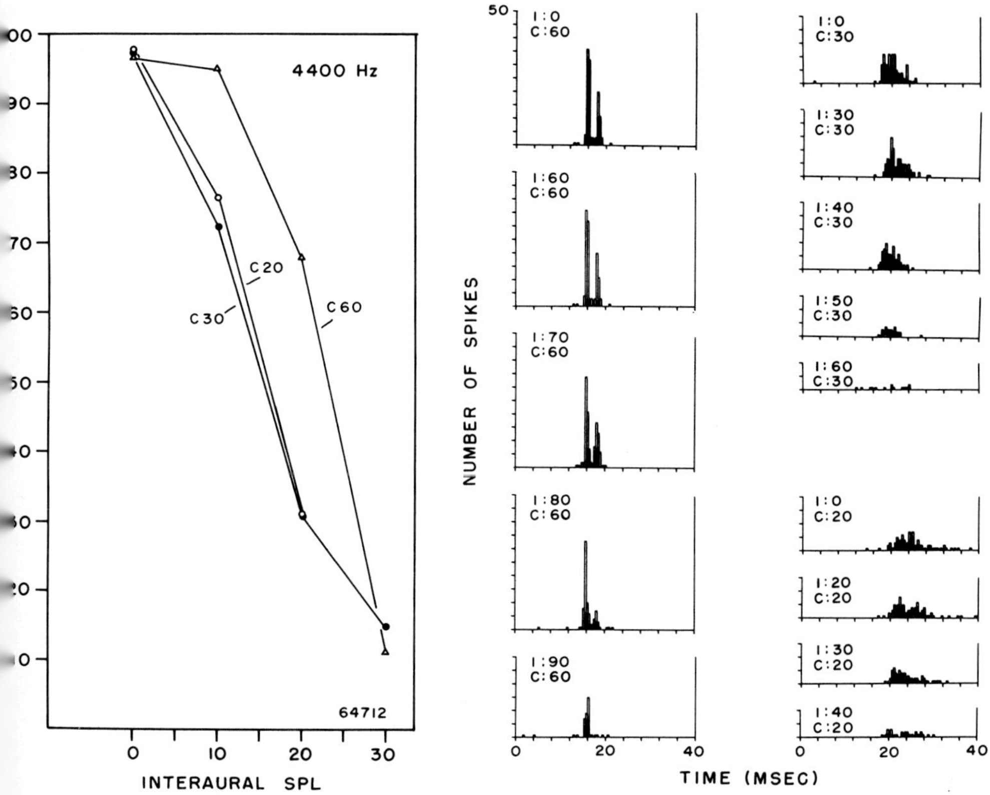

Fig. 2. Effect of raising SPL at the ipsilateral ear when the contralateral stimulus intensity was held constant at 20, 30 and 60 dB. Spike count is expressed as percentage of spikes evoked by monaural contralateral stimulation at each of the designated SPLs. Poststimulus time histograms show discharge patterns when the ipsilateral (I) and contralateral (C) ears were stimulated alone and when the stimuli were delivered simultaneously. Tone duration: 100 msec; repetition rate: 1/sec; 100 stimulus repetitions; best frequency: 4400 Hz; chloralose anesthesia.

more effective than contralateral ear stimulation at any given SPL. When both ears are stimulated simultaneously, either at the same SPL or under conditions where the interaural intensity difference is held at 10 dB the number of spikes evoked is substantially greater than the number evoked by monotic stimulation. For this neuron binaural stimulation results in an extended dynamic range since under these conditions threshold for activation of the cell is some 20 dB below that required by

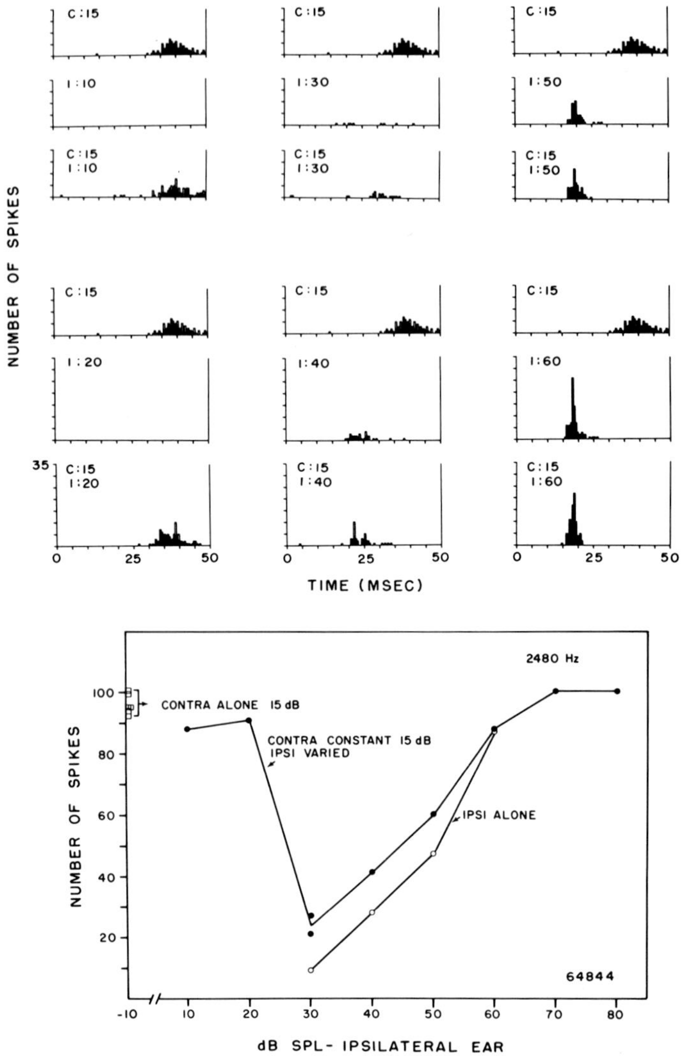

Fig. 3. Effect of raising SPL at the ipsilateral ear when the effective SPL at the contralateral ear is held constant at 15 dB. Poststimulus time histograms show firing patterns to monaural and binaural stimulation. Tone duration: 100 msec; repetition rate: 2/sec; 100 stimulus trials; best frequency: 2480 Hz; chloralose anesthesia.

stimulation of either ear alone. Compared to cells in the other classes, neurons in this category will be relatively sensitive to changes in sound pressure level anywhere in the sound field but will be relatively insensitive to the location of a sound source. Neurons with these properties constitute the majority of AI cortical neurons studied by Hall and Goldstein (1968).

The second category of binaural neurons in AI is comprised of cells which are sensitive to small changes in interaural sound pressure levels and hence may play roles in localization of the source of a sound in space. Because of some differences in the behavior of neurons within this category it is convenient to divide the class.

A first subcategory comprises cells which are excited by stimulation of only one ear, usually the contralateral one. Stimulation of the opposite ear alone shows no demonstrable effect upon the cell. However, a tone which appeared ineffective when delivered monaurally may show a powerful influence on the discharge of the cell when it is paired with a highly effective tone of the same frequency at the opposite ear. The cell illustrated in Figure 2 was driven only by contralateral ear stimulation. When a best frequency tone to the contralateral ear was paired at several SPLs with a tone of the same frequency at the ipsilateral ear the effect was a suppression of the discharge. Varying the interaural SPL over a range of about 30 dB reduced the number of spikes evoked by contralateral ear stimulation by nearly 90%. The binaural response approaches that obtained by stimulation of the ipsilateral ear alone at this SPL.

A second subcategory contains neurons which have some properties similar to those shown by the previously illustrated cell. The neuron in Figure 4 is excited maximally by contralateral ear stimulation over a wide range of SPLs between 15 and 70 dB. Stimulation of the ipsilateral ear alone, on the other hand, is seen to be effective in evoking spikes only at SPLs greater than 30 dB. In this experiment the contralateral ear is stimulated at 15 dB; the ipsilateral ear is stimulated simultaneously by tones of the same frequency at several different SPLs. The effect of raising the ipsilateral stimulus to 30 dB is to dramatically reduce the spike count to about 20% of its control level, a level which approaches that obtained by stimulation of the ipsilateral ear alone at that intensity. Further increases in ipsilateral intensity result in a steady increase in firing. Scrutiny of these data indicate that at low ipsilateral SPLs, below 20 dB, the joint response of the unit is identical to that obtained by stimulation of the contralateral ear alone. Raising the ipsilateral SPL to 30 dB results in a shift in the response pattern so that now the response approaches that of the ipsilateral ear alone, keeping in mind that the monotic ipsilateral response was but a few spikes. Indeed, further increases in ipsilateral SPL results in firing patterns which are nearly identical to those obtained by monotic ipsilateral stimulation.

A third major category includes those cells which are excited by monotic stimulation of both ears. In contrast to neurons previously described which also respond to monotic stimulation of the left and right ears, simultaneous binaural stimulation is no more or less effective in firing these cells than the more effective monotic stimulus. For the cell illustrated in Figure 4, monotonically increasing spike-count functions were obtained when the left and right ears were stimulated alone at SPLs between 10 and 50 dB. Stimulation of the contralateral ear evoked a greater number of spikes and shorter latent period to the first spike at any given SPL than did stimulation of the ipsilateral ear. At each binaural pairing over the unit's dynamic range the firing pattern was indistinguishable from that obtained by

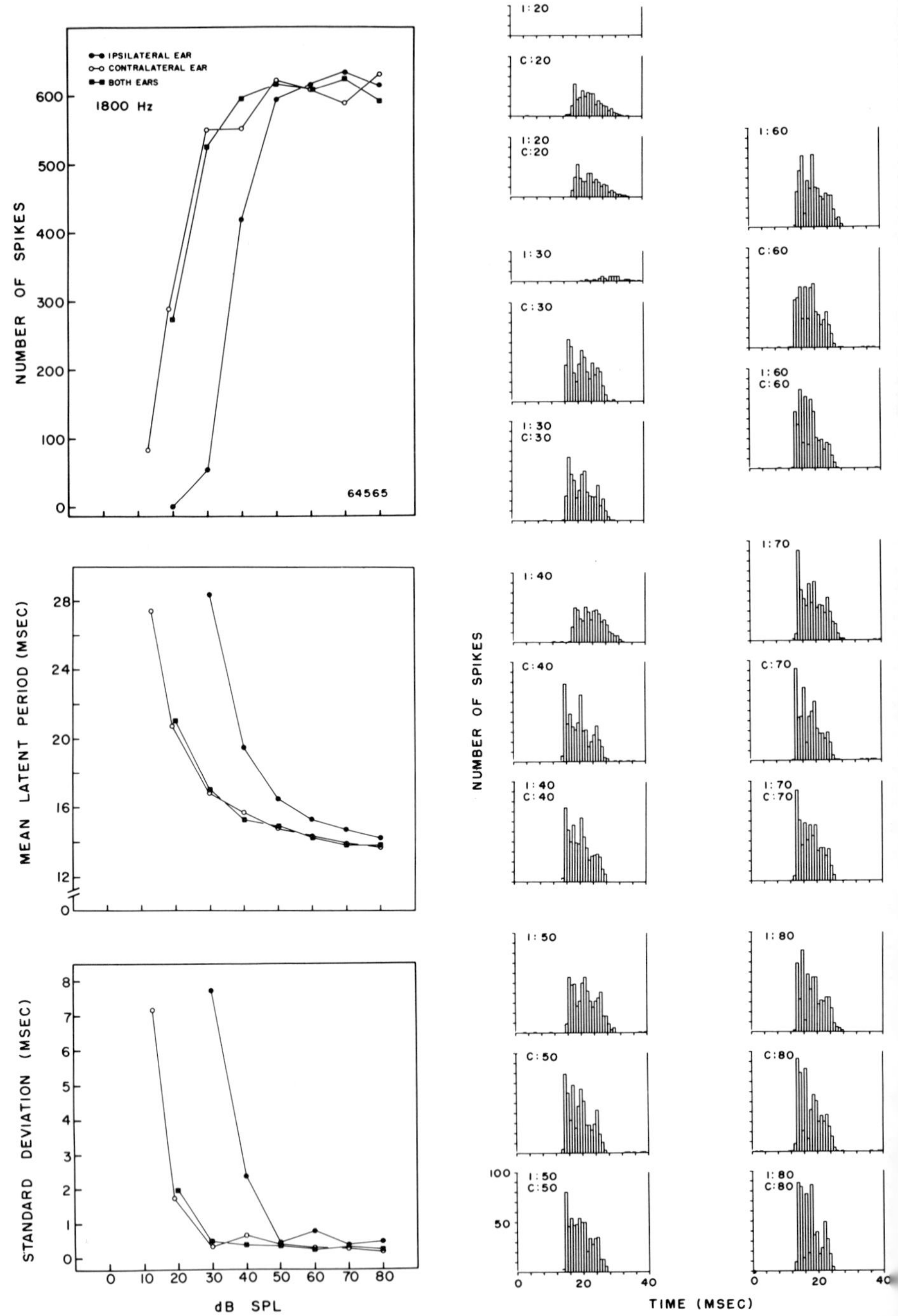

Fig. 4. Effect of raising SPL on monaural and binaural spike count and mean and standard deviation of first-spike latency. Poststimulus time histograms show firing patterns to monaural and binaural stimuli at each stimulus pairing. Tone duration 100 msec; repetition rate 1/sec; 100 stimulus trials; best frequency: 1800 Hz; chloralose anesthesia.

stimulation of the dominant (contralateral) ear alone. Stimulation of the ipsilateral ear, while very effective alone, made no demonstrable contribution to the joint response. At SPLs below about 60 dB the unit responded as though no ipsilateral stimulus was present; the information transmitted by this neuron over this intensity range related to the contralateral ear only. At saturation firing levels above 60 dB the joint response and the individual responses become almost indistinguishable. However, close examination of the first spike latency and response histograms shows that the contralateral ear continues to dominate the joint response up to about 80 dB.

We may summarize these findings by stating that in response to binaural stimulation, where only intensity changes are considered, three categories of cells are found within AI. The first comprises neurons which are relatively insensitive to interaural intensity but which are capable of detecting change in intensity anywhere in the sound field. This mechanism may provide for low sound thresholds and relatively wide dynamic ranges. The second category of cells contains those neurons which can detect the small intensity cues employed by a listener in localizing or lateralizing the source of a sound. These cells respond to a binaural stimulus in one of three modes. First, the firing pattern may be the same as that generated by stimulation of the contralateral ear alone. Second, the response may be identical to that obtained by monotic ipsilateral ear stimulation. And third, the response may resemble neither monotic response and hence reflects a powerful interaction of inputs from the two ears. Which mode prevails in the joint response depends upon the interaural intensity. The third cell category contains those neurons that are excited by stimulation of each ear but for which there appears to be little binaural interaction. The joint response is identical to that of the dominant ear.

ORGANIZATION OF BINAURAL NEURONS WITHIN AI

Neurons displaying similar binaural properties appear to aggregate within columns in AI (Imig and Adrian, 1977). Figure 5 shows the results of two experiments in which microelectrodes were inserted into AI in closely spaced penetrations and the binaural response properties of neurons and neuron clusters determined at regular short intervals. For each experiment the locations of the entrance of the penetrations are shown on a drawing of the lateral surface of the hemisphere. The path taken by each electrode is shown on a drawing of the tissue section within which the electrode tracks were located. Small electrolytic lesions were made at points along the penetration where changes in unit properties were detected. Neurons and neuron clusters were classified with respect to their monaural and binaural sensitivities at best frequency. The classification was based on the experimenter's judgement of the relative size of the neural response viewed on the oscilloscope screen and heard over the audiomonitor. While this procedure may overlook cells within a cluster which do not conform to the dominant cluster response it has the great advantage that the response properties of many closely spaced neurons can be sampled and mapped.

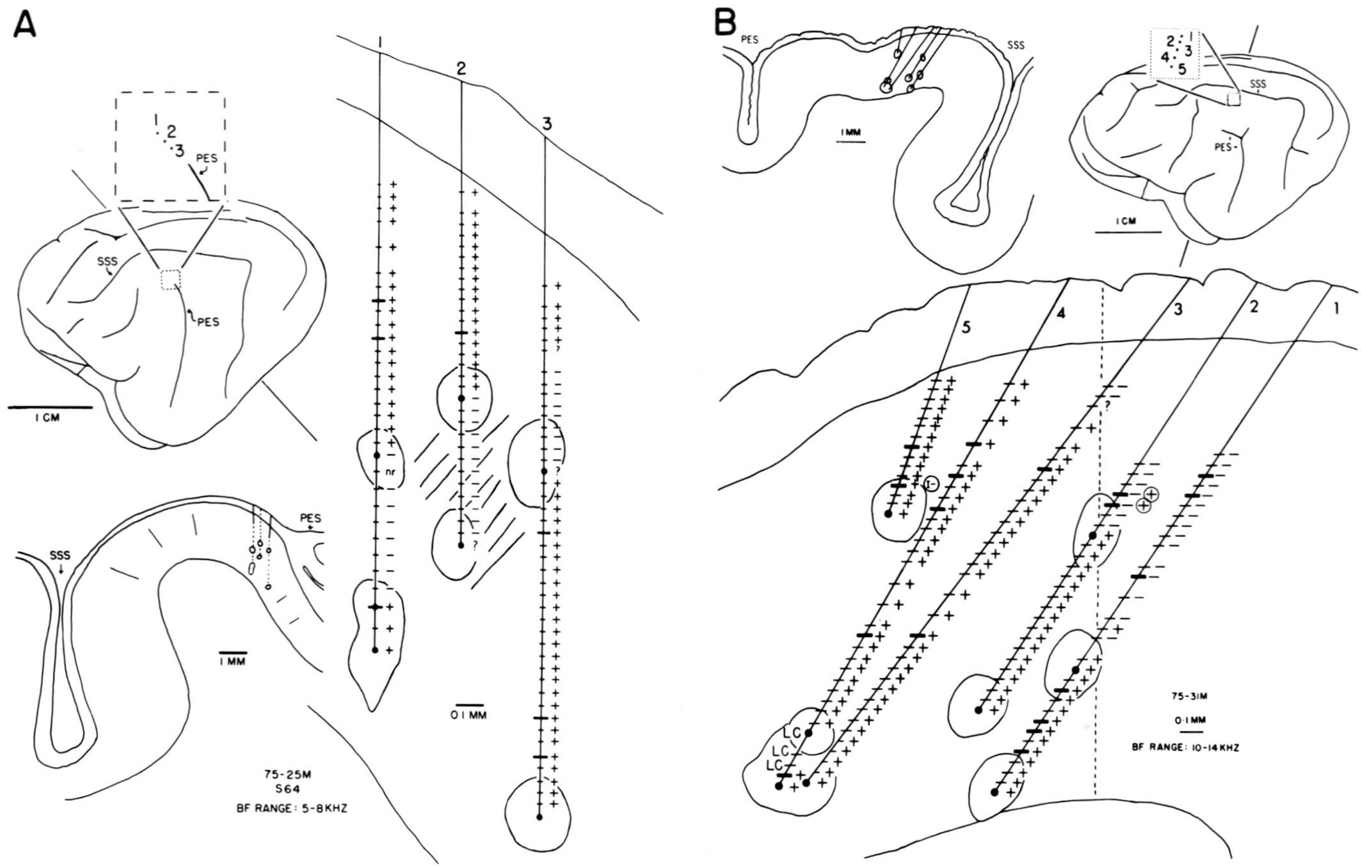
A
1
2
3
PES
SSS
PES
1 CM
SSS
PES
1 MM
nr
0.1 MM
75-25M
S64
BF RANGE: 5-8KHZ
B
PES
SSS
1 MM
2 1
3
4 5
SSS
PES
1 CM
1
2
3
4
5
LC
LC
LC
75-31M
0.1 MM
BF RANGE: 10-14KHZ

Fig. 5. Sequential distribution of binaural interactions of neurons or neuron clusters along closely spaced electrode penetrations into AI in two experiments. In both A and B are drawings of the lateral surfaces of the mapped hemispheres showing the location of each electrode penetration. Also shown are drawings of tissue sections with electrode tracks and lesions drawn in. In the enlarged drawings of each tissue section the type of binaural interaction recorded at sequential points is indicated. Heavy horizontal bars indicate isolated units, light bars unit clusters. Summation responses are indicated by (+) and suppression responses by (-); (n.r.) no response, (LC) latency change; SSS: suprasylvian sulcus; PES: posterior ectosylvian sulcus.

The great majority of neurons studied in these experiments were influenced by binaural stimulation. Some were excited only by stimulation of one ear, usually the contralateral one, while others were driven by monotic stimulation of each ear.

By far the most commonly encountered binaural interaction was one in which the response to binaural stimulation was judged to be greater in size than the response to stimulation of either ear alone at the same frequency and SPL. This interaction is referred to as *summation* and is no doubt the same interaction displayed by units in the category illustrated in Figure 1. Neurons in this class are indicated by a (+) in Figure 5.

Neurons which were excited less by binaural stimulation than by stimulation of the dominant ear alone at the same frequency and SPL were classified as showing *suppression*. Stimulation of the opposite ear alone at any SPL may be ineffective in driving some units; in other cases the cell is excited if the intensity at that ear is raised to relatively high levels. This class most probably includes the two subcategories of cells illustrated in Figures 2 and 3. Suppression responses are recorded as (-) in Figure 5. Most neurons and neuron clusters in these experiments were classified as summation or suppression. However, the response of a few neurons did not fit these categories. A few cells and cell clusters were excited by monaural stimulation of each ear; the binaural response could not be distinguished from that evoked by stimulation of the dominant ear alone. This type of response which is referred to as *occlusion*, may correspond to the response shown in Figure 4. There is also a small number of cells and cell clusters which responded only to stimulation of one ear and which failed to demonstrate binaural interactions.

In both experiments shown in Figure 5 the electrode tracks run obliquely with respect to radial cell columns through the cortical grey matter. Neurons displaying similar binaural interactions tend to occur at sequential points along each electrode penetration. At points along the penetration the sequence abruptly shifts to a sequence of units displaying a different binaural interaction. For example, in experiment 75-25M (Fig. 5A) the first 19 units and unit clusters encountered in penetration 1 showed summation responses. This was followed by a sequence of suppression responses which, in turn, abruptly changed to summation responses again near the end of the penetration. Slightly different, but nonetheless regular patterns of binaural responses were recorded in adjacent penetrations 2 and 3. Careful reconstruction of electrode penetrations and lesion sites in serial histological sections indicate that units displaying summation or suppression responses aggregate in regions which extend through layers III-VI of the cortical grey matter and hence which form cell columns. These regions which are dominated by neurons having the same binaural properties are referred to as *binaural columns.* In experiments illustrated in Figure 5A, penetrations 1 and 3 pass through a suppression column which is flanked on both sides by summation columns. In Figure 5B penetrations 1, 2 and 3 pass from a suppression column into a summation column.

Binaural columns may be quite extensive, often occupying several square millimeters of cortical surface area. Figure 6 illustrates two surface maps obtained by making many closely-spaced near-vertical penetrations into the cortex and deter-

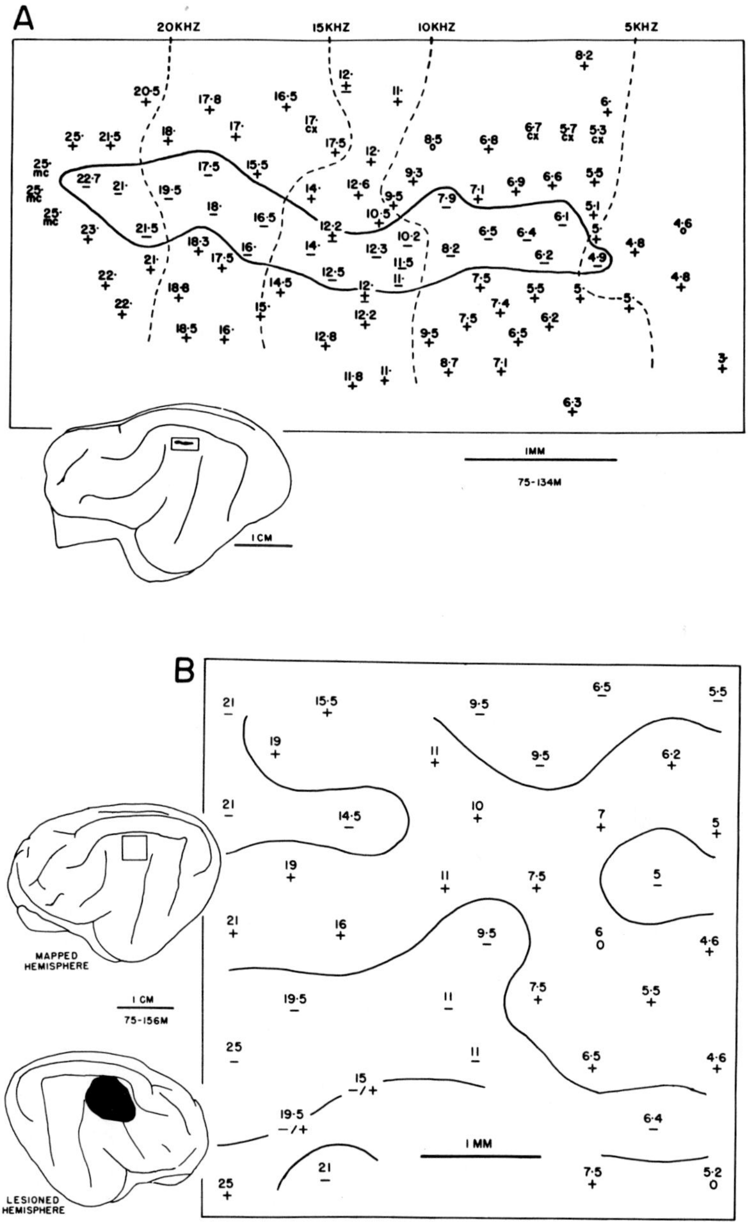

Fig. 6. Surface maps of portions of AI showing the topography of binaural columns. At each electrode penetration site, best frequency and binaural interaction is given. Binaural interactions of neurons or neuron clusters within each penetration: (+) summation; (-) suppression; (mc) monaural contralateral, (cx) mixed interactions; (±) summation at one depth within column, inhibition at another; (o) occlusion.

mining best frequency and binaural interactions at several cortical depths. Best frequency and binaural interactions of units or unit clusters within each penetration are shown on the map at the location of the penetration. In Figure 6A a small region of AI representing frequencies ranging from about 3 kHz to 25 kHz was mapped. Tonotopical organization of this region of AI is clearly seen. Dashed lines follow four isofrequency contours. In this experiment an entire suppression column was mapped. It extends along a narrow strip of cortex nearly orthogonal to the isofrequency lines. The column is about 0.5 mm wide and 4 mm long and spans more than two octaves of the frequency representation. Figure 5B shows another surface map of AI in an animal which sustained a large lesion of AI of the middle ectosylvian cortex of the opposite hemisphere a week before the map was obtained. Binaural columns are still in evidence in AI of this animal and no demonstrable differences between this map and those from normal animals could be attributed to the lesion. From detailed surface maps such as the one shown in Figure 5A it is estimated that suppression columns occupy about 28% of AI in the middle ectosylvian region while summation columns occupy about 66% of the same area. The remaining territory is taken up by units with mixed interaction, occlusion and monaural responses.

CALLOSAL INNERVATION PATTERN OF AI RELATED TO TONOTOPIC AND BINAURAL ORGANIZATION

Field AI has as one of its major targets the homotopic region in the opposite cerebral hemisphere (Diamond et al., 1968; Kawamura, 1973). Fibers connecting the two primary auditory fields travel within the splenium of the corpus callosum. We have been studying the projection patterns of AI callosal efferents by combining microelectrode mapping with tracing of the terminal distribution of fibers using autoradiographic and Fink-Heimer methods.

Figure 7 presents the results of one experiment where in the same animal electrophysiological mapping of best frequencies was combined with autoradiographic tracing of the pathway connecting the two primary fields. In this experiment a small sector of AI was mapped electrophysiologically as described in the previous section. Then an injection pipette was inserted into the cortex at the 5.5 kHz point on the map and 2.5μCi of 3-H proline dissolved in 0.025μl of saline was delivered under pressure. The region of AI on the opposite hemisphere which represented about the same range of best frequencies was mapped electrophysiologically. About 24 hours after the proline injection and after both hemispheres were mapped, the animal was perfused with saline and formol-saline. Serial histological sections through the mapped areas were subsequently processed autoradiographically to reveal the distribution of the label at the injection site and the distribution of the transported label at the target sites within the opposite hemisphere. The electrode penetrations were reconstructed from the same serial sections and combined frequency and autoradiographic maps were constructed. In the right hemisphere the label was heaviest in the immediate area of the injection site. With-

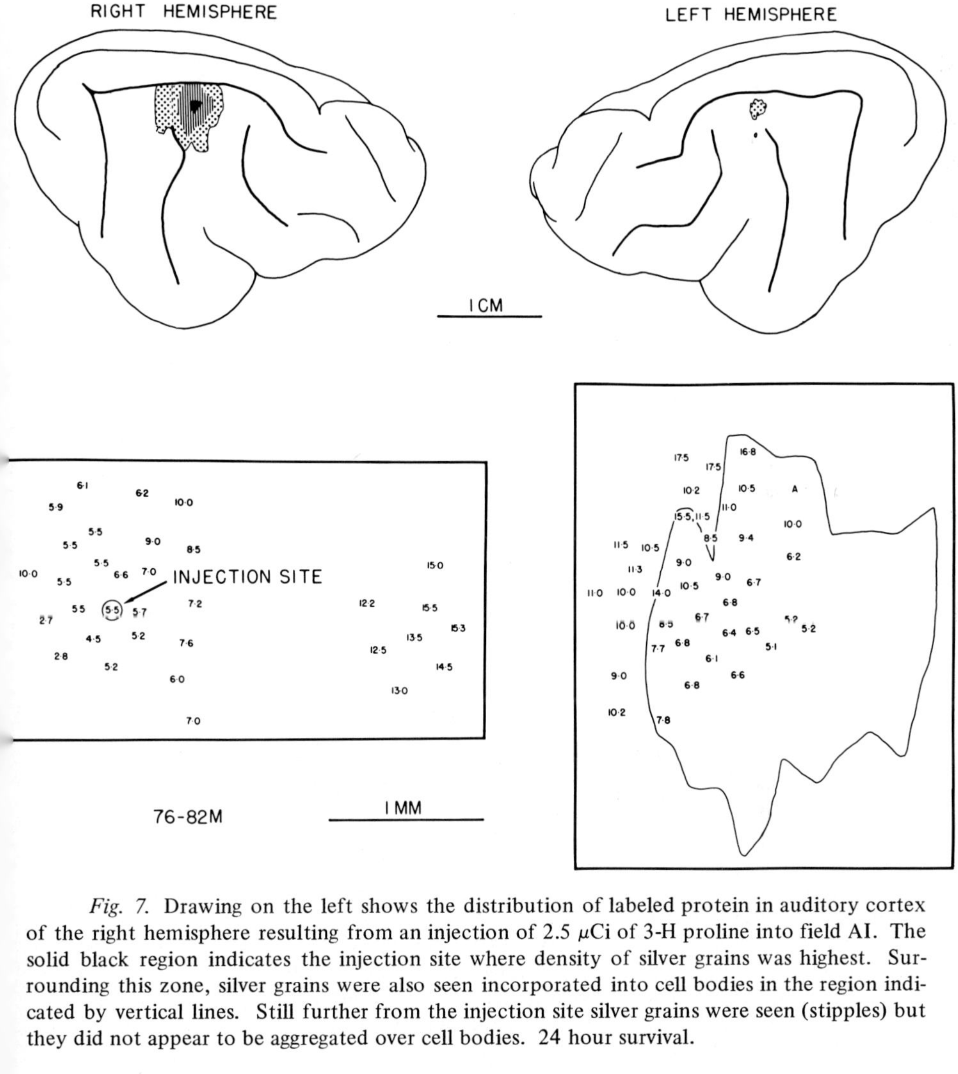

Fig. 7. Drawing on the left shows the distribution of labeled protein in auditory cortex of the right hemisphere resulting from an injection of 2.5 μCi of 3-H proline into field AI. The solid black region indicates the injection site where density of silver grains was highest. Surrounding this zone, silver grains were also seen incorporated into cell bodies in the region indicated by vertical lines. Still further from the injection site silver grains were seen (stipples) but they did not appear to be aggregated over cell bodies. 24 hour survival.

in the left hemisphere several patches of silver grains were seen, indicating terminal fields of neurons located within the right hemisphere near the injection site. One of the target sites was located within the region of AI mapped electrophysiologically. The target field within AI of the left hemisphere represents the same range of best frequencies as found in the region around the injection site, indicating that the regions of AI on the two hemispheres representing the same best frequencies are reciprocally connected.

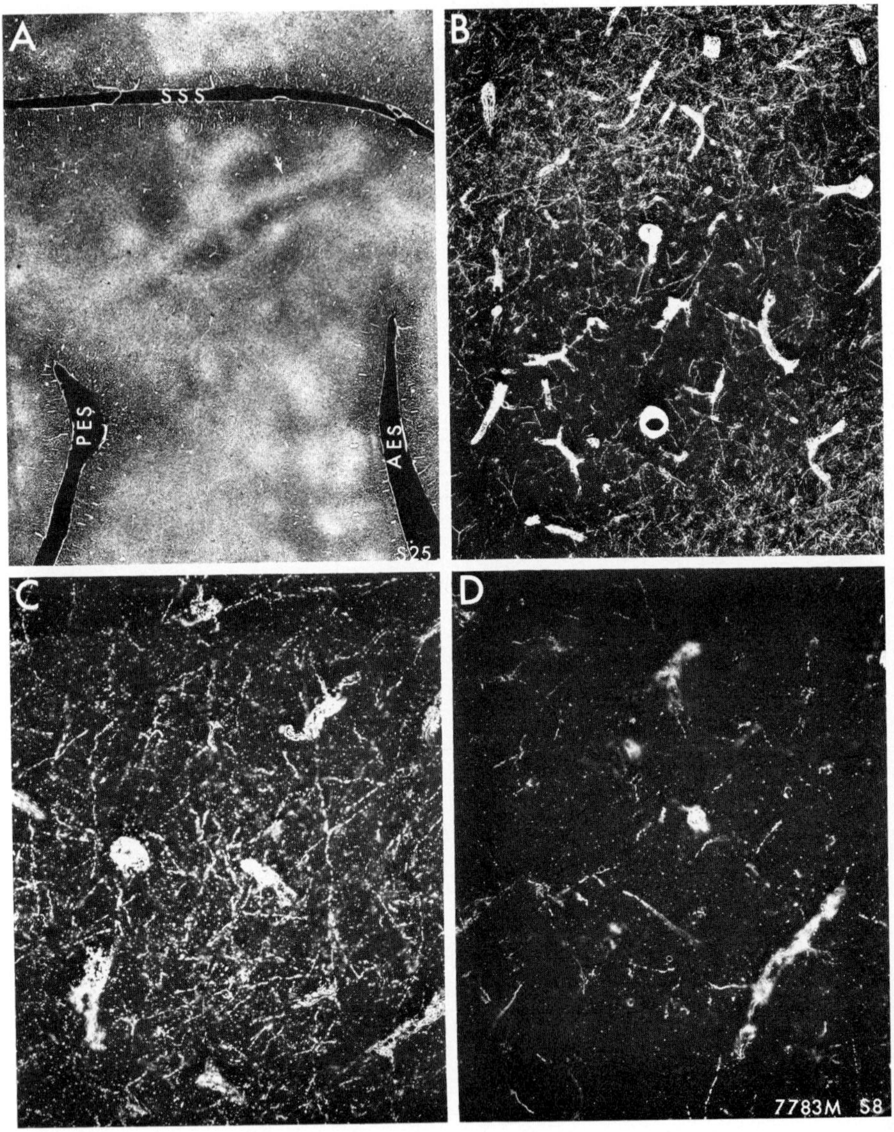

Fig. 8. A. Dark-field photomicrograph of Fink-Heimer stained tangential sectior through auditory cortex from an animal that was allowed to survive one week after the cauda portion of the corpus callosum was sectioned. Photomicrographs B–D are taken at highe power from the region around the arrow in A but from a tissue section more superficial than A Figures C and D are high power photomicrographs from the same section shown in B showin adjacent heavily and sparsely innervated regions of AI. SSS: suprasylvian sulcus; PES: posterio ectosylvian sulcus; AES: anterior ectosylvian sulcus.

Following a single injection of 3-H proline into AI, the density of labelling within the homotopic target site of the opposite hemisphere is not uniform. Rather, the label appears in patches with some areas of AI within the target zone receiving a heavier projection than others. The full pattern of callosal projection within AI of one hemisphere is shown in Figure 8. In this experiment the animal was allowed to survive one week after the caudal half of the corpus callosum was surgically sectioned. After transcardial perfusion with formol-saline, the relevant block of cortical tissue was removed, compressed lightly between glass slides in order to flatten the region beneath the suprasylvian sulcus and allowed to harden in formol-saline. Sections were taken parallel to the flattened surface and stained for degenerating fibers and terminals by the Fink-Heimer method. Figure 8A is a low-power dark-field photomicrograph of AI showing the resultant patterns of degeneration. In this figure degenerating axons and axon terminals appear white against the black background. Some of the patches of degeneration are elongated strips oriented in a direction along the axis of the low-to-high frequency gradient. Figures 8B and C are dark-field photomicrographs of the region marked by the arrow in 8A to show the relative density of the fiber and terminal degeneration within the target field.

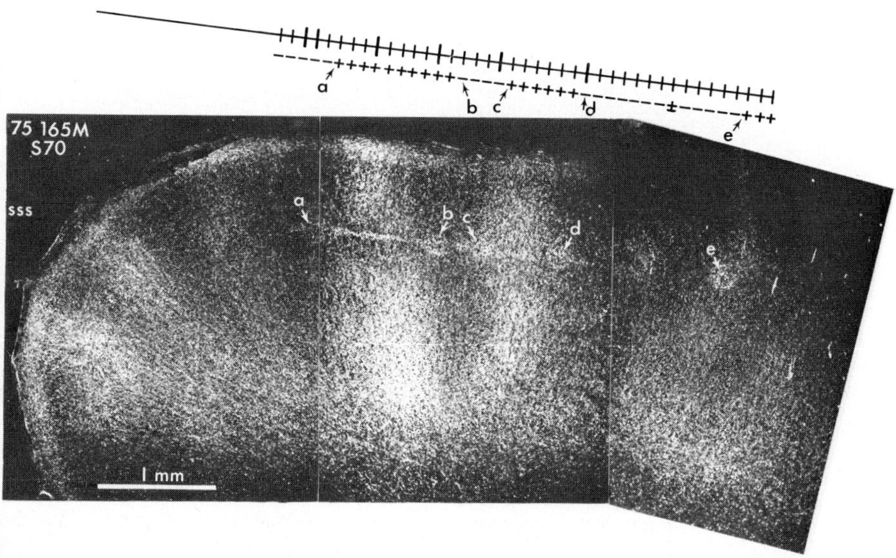

Fig. 9. Dark-field autoradiograph of a coronal section through AI showing the distribution of labeled protein resulting from multiple injections of 700 μCi of proline into the opposite AI 5 days earlier. Shown also is an electrode track with lesions (a–e) located along it. The sequence of binaural interactions recorded from single neurons and neuron clusters along this track as well as the lesion position are shown above the photomicrograph.

The non-uniform callosal projection pattern of middle ectosylvian AI cortex shown in Figure 8 bears a close resemblance to the pattern of binaural columns mapped electrophysiologically in this same region. Such a relationship is revealed directly in experiments which combine microelectrode mapping of binaural columns with autoradiographic tracing of the callosal pathway. The results of one such experiment are shown in Figure 9. In this experiment 700 μCi of 3-H proline was injected at multiple sites within AI using sterile surgical techniques. Five days later a dorso-ventral tangential electrode penetration was made into AI of the opposite hemisphere. As the electrode passed through middle cortical layers, binaural interactions of cells and cell clusters were determined at regular intervals and lesions placed where changes in binaural response properties appeared. Following the experiment the brain was processed for autoradiography. The electrode penetration was reconstructed in a single coronal section. Figure 9 is a dark-field photomicrograph of that section. Silver grains which appear white in this photomicrograph indicate the location within AI of afferent terminals and fibers whose cell bodies are in opposite AI. Silver grains are not distributed uniformly throughout the cortex. Rather, they appear as alternating light and dark bands. During electrophysiological mapping of this hemisphere the electrode passed through several binaural columns and lesions were placed to mark their borders. It is clear that summation columns are relatively heavily labeled whereas suppression columns are relatively devoid of silver grains. Reconstruction of serial autoradiographed sections from this brain reveals a surface pattern of silver grains which is similar to the pattern of degenerating terminals shown in Figure 8.

Acknowledgements

This work was supported by NSF Grant No. BNS76-19893 and NIH Grant No. 5 P01 NS12732.

REFERENCES

Abeles, M. and Goldstein, M.H.Jr. Functional architecture in cat primary cortex: columnar organization and organization according to depth. *J. Neurophysiol. 33:* 172-187, 1970.

Benson, D.A. and Teas, D.C. Single unit study of binaural interaction in the auditory cortex of the chinchilla. *Brain Res. 103:* 313-338, 1976.

Brugge, J.F., Dubrovsky, N.A., Aitkin, L.M. and Anderson, D.J. Sensitivity of single neurons in auditory cortex of cat to binaural tonal stimulation: effects of varying interaural time and intensity. *J. Neurophysiol. 32:* 1005-1024, 1969.

Brugge, J.F. and Merzenich, M.M. Responses of neurons in auditory cortex of the macaque monkey to monaural and binaural stimulation. *J. Neurophysiol. 36:* 1138-1158, 1973.

Diamond, I.T., Jones. E.G. and Powell, T.P.S. Interhemispheric fiber connections of the auditory cortex of the cat. *Brain Res. 11:* 177-193, 1968.

Goldstein, M.H.Jr., Abeles, M., Daly, R.L. and McIntosh, J. Functional architecture in cat primary auditory cortex: tonotopic organization. *J. Neurophysiol. 33:* 188-197, 1970.

Hall, J.L.II and Goldstein, M.H.Jr. Representation of binaural stimuli by single units in primary auditory cortex of unanesthetized cats. *J. Acoust. Soc. Am. 43:* 456-461, 1968.

Hind, J.E., Davies, P.W., Woolsey, C.N., Benjamin, R.M., Welker, W.I. and Thompson, R.F. Unit activity in the auditory cortex. In: *Neural Mechanisms of the Auditory and Vestibular Systems,* edited by G.L. Rasmussen and W.W. Windle. Springfield: Charles C Thomas, 1960.

Imig, T.J. and Adrián, H.O. Binaural columns in the primary field (AI) of cat auditory cortex. *Brain Res.* (In press).

Imig, T.J., Ruggero, M.A., Kitzes, L.M., Javel, E. and Brugge, J.F. Organization of auditory cortex in the owl monkey *(Aotus trivirgatus). J. Comp. Neurol. 171:* 111-128, 1977.

Imig, T.J., Reale, R. and Brugge, J.F. The origin and targets of primary field efferents related to tonotopic and binaural maps of cat auditory cortex. *Proc XXVII Intern. Cong. Physiol. Sci.,* 1977.

Kawamura, K. Corticocortical fiber connections of the cat cerebrum. I. The temporal region. *Brain Res. 51:* 1-21, 1973.

Merzenich, M.M. and Brugge, J.F. Representation of the cochlear partition on the superior temporal plane of the macaque monkey. *Brain Res. 50:* 275-296, 1973.

Merzenich, M.M., Knight, P.L. and Roth, G.L. Representation of cochlea within primary auditory cortex in the cat. *J. Neurophysiol. 38:* 231-249, 1975.

Pandya, D.N. and Sanides, F. Architectonic parcellation of the temporal operculum in rhesus monkey and its projection pattern. *Z. Anat. Entwicklungsgesch. 139:* 127-161, 1973.

Rose, J.E. The cellular structure of the auditory region of the cat. *J. Comp. Neurol. 91:* 409-440, 1949.

Rose, J.E. and Woolsey, C.N. The relations of thalamic connections, cellular structure and evocable electrical activity in the auditory region of the cat. *J. Comp. Neurol. 91:* 441-446, 1949.

DISCUSSION

McFadden: In recent years electrophysiologists working with the visual system have shown that areas believed to be classically visual are indeed more complicated. For example, there are apparently vestibular and auditory inputs into both superior colliculus and Area 17. My first question is: Do you know of anything like this with the auditory system? My second question is more specific: it concerns those cells which went through inhibition as a function of level to the ipsilateral ear and then an excitation. Might that simply be due to cross conduction?

Brugge: The answer to the first question is that within the auditory fields in the middle ectosylvian region there is no evidence I know of that there is any strong input from other modalities. There certainly is in other so-called association areas on the suprasylvian cortex.

The answer to the second question relates to a technical problem one might face. It is true that you can get cross conduction at high stimulus intensity. However, by looking closely at the time structure of the discharges we can usually eliminate the possibility that the binaural effect is the result of the cross conduction.

White: In one of your slides you showed a belt of suppressive units superimposed on a tonotopic map of the A1 region. Did you look for frequency selectivity in your suppression units? If so, what did you see?

Brugge: We do not measure the complete tuning curves of those cells. However, they are frequency selective.

THE SCALP DISTRIBUTION OF AUDITORY EVOKED POTENTIALS

William R. Goff

Yale University School of Medicine

It is well known that averaging the electroencephalogram (EEG) subsequent to, and synchronized with, the presentation of a repetitive auditory stimulus permits the recording of the Auditory Evoked Potential (AEP), a multiphasic series of electrical potentials beginning after the stimulus and lasting 400-500 msec. Figure 1 shows schematically the human AEP evoked by a click of approximately 70 dB and recorded from a normal awake adult not required to perform a specific task with regard to the stimulus. It has become common to refer to these potential peaks and troughs as components. Note that the X-axis representing time is on a log scale so that both the short latency, short duration brainstem evoked potentials (BEPs) and the slower, later components can be seen.

We follow the polarity-latency component nomenclature recommended by the Committee on Publication Criteria at the 1974 Brussels Symposium (Donchin et al., 1977). Thus P or N denotes positive or negative voltages and the number is the average latency of this component in normal adult subjects. Positive voltage is upward in our records. P2-P9 are subcortical components including BEPs. Components occurring between approximately 10 to 100 msec are frequently called middle latency components and the remaining components are referred to as long latency or late components.

Knowledge of the neural origins of evoked potential components is important if we are to exploit them maximally in the analysis of brain function for both clinical application and neuropsychological research. Since opportunities to record from the surface or depths of the human brain or to analyze systematically the effects of localized lesions are extremely limited, topographical analysis of scalp potentials is probably the best way available to gain information about evoked potential sources. The analysis is complicated, however. First, not all scalp recorded evoked potential components come from the brain. As first shown by Bickford et al. (1964), quite a few are generated in cranial musculature. These are termed myogenic components as distinguished from neurogenic brain potentials. To give an idea of the magnitude of the myogenic problem, those AEP components considered by us to be wholly or partly myogenic are circled or squared in Figure 1. Second, one rarely if ever records from the scalp evoked activity generated by one source, but rather records the resultant of contributions from multiple sources.

Despite this complexity, scalp topographies yield useful information about

ISBN 0-12-514960-3

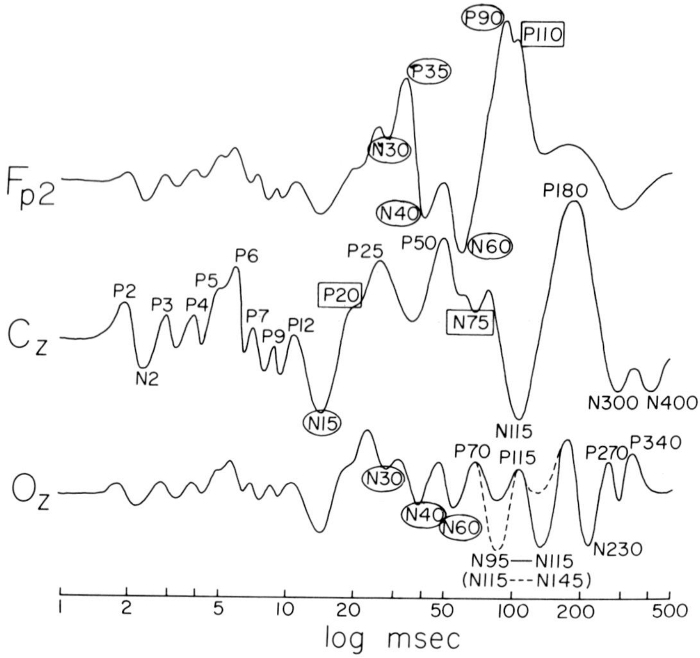

Fig. 1. Schematic representation of AEP evoked by binaural click of approximately 70 dB Sensation Level recorded from the 10-20 system electrodes indicated. For purposes of illustration, BEPs and the remaining components are not drawn to the same amplitude scale; BEPs are much smaller (typically .01-.03 μV) than later components (typically 2-20 μV). Three electrode locations are represented since not all components appear at all locations. Adopted from Goff et al. (1977a).

the anatomical sources of evoked potentials based both on theoretical results derived from field potential theory and on empirical comparisons between scalp and intracranially recorded evoked activity. I will review these results briefly; they are discussed in greater detail elsewhere (Goff et al., 1977a). First, in the absence of significant contamination from myogenic and other extracranial sources, evoked potentials recorded from the scalp provide a good representation of the morphology of intracranially recorded evoked activity. Second, the most important variables determining the relationship between intracranial and scalp-recorded potentials are the location, orientation, and spatial extent of the sources relative to the recording electrodes. For focal superficial sources, the degree of amplitude attenuation, often expressed as the "attenuation ratio" (AR, defined as the ratio of maximum cortical surface amplitude to maximum scalp amplitude), will be on the order of 10:1 to 100:1. In contrast, ARs for very deep sources like those of the BEPs approach 1:1. For both scalp and intracranially recorded potentials, spatial distributions of components are also strongly influenced by source location, orientation and spatial extent. For theoretical purposes EP sources are often modeled as current dipoles, and derivations from dipole theory are used to interpret empir-

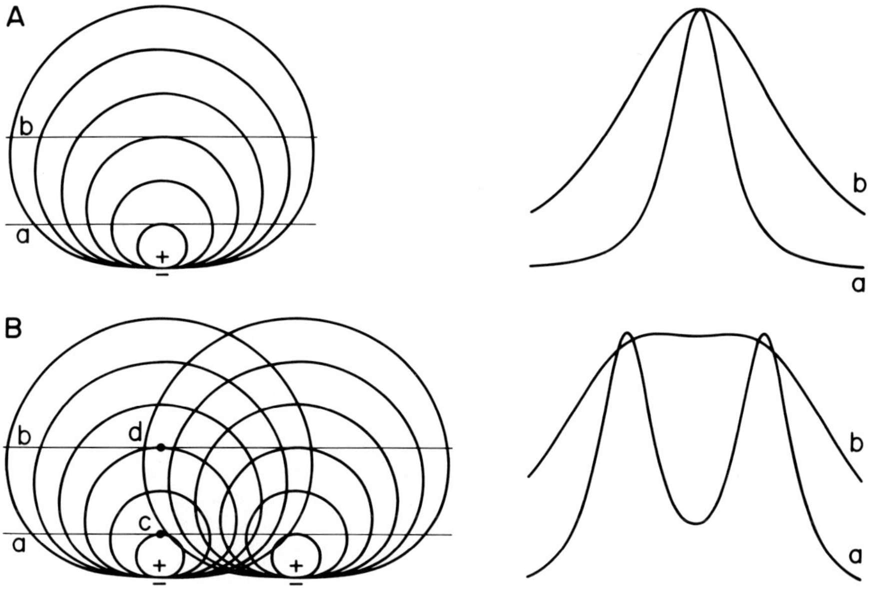

Fig. 2. Illustration of the effects of distance from dipole sources on spatial resolution and spatial averaging. A. The potential field generated by a single vertically oriented dipole source located in the plane of the figure is shown on the left. Amplitude distributions along horizontal lines a and b perpendicular to the dipole axis are shown on the right. B. Potential fields generated by two adjacent dipole sources identical to the one in A are shown on the left. Amplitude distributions along the same horizontal lines a and b are shown on the right. Points c and d lie along the vertical axis of the dipole on the left. Amplitudes are expressed as percent of maximum value in each distribution. Negative sides of the potential fields are not shown. From Goff et al. (1977a).

ical evoked potential data. This is illustrated in Figure 2. In this figure only the positive sides of dipole fields are shown; each field would have a negative side of identical shape pointed downward in the figure. Figure 2A presents the potential field generated by a single vertically oriented point dipole source located in the plane of the figure. The spatial distribution at two distances a and b from the source are shown on the right. Note that the distribution is broader at b, a greater distance from the source. Figure 2B illustrates spatial distributions derived from two point dipole sources each identical to that in Figure 2A. This example is particularly relevant to discussions of AEPs because an auditory stimulus generates activity bilaterally in many auditory structures. An electrode array relatively close to the sources (line a) will resolve two peaks as indicated on the right. However, an array located further from the sources (line b) will resolve only a single broad peak.

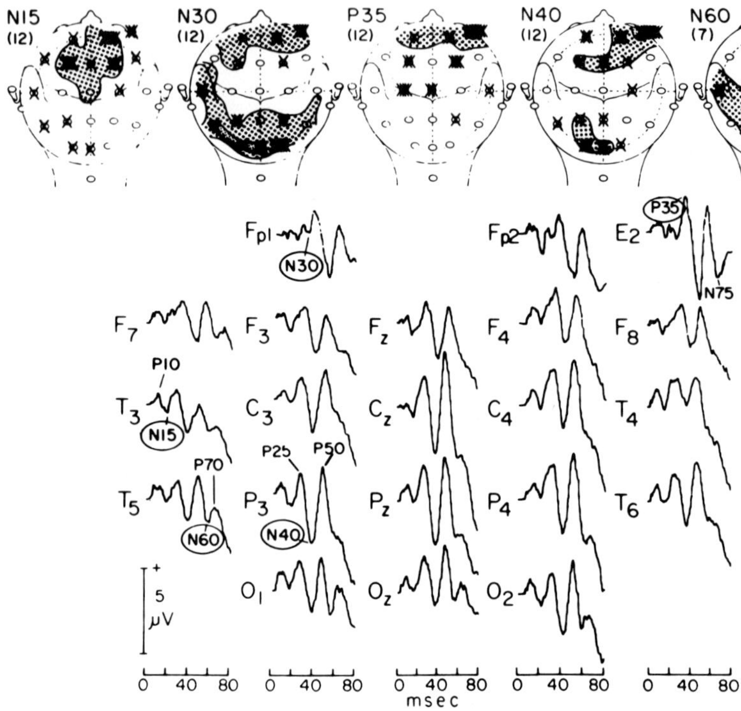

Fig. 3. Multiple latency AEP components recorded from a typical subject with topographies of those considered myogenic. Traces are the grand averages of eight replications of 64 responses each. In this and subsequent figures, numbers in parentheses indicate number of subjects upon whom topographies are based. Finely stippled areas are the estimated area where component was 75% or more of maximum; grossly stippled areas are estimated 50% or more of maximum. Crosses indicate locations in which the component was 90% or more of its maximum value in any subject. Positive voltage is upwards referenced to A2. From G.D. Goff et al. (1977).

We will see that a single broad, centrally focused peak is precisely the scalp topography found for several AEP components.

These empirical and theoretical relationships between scalp topographies and intracranial sources can be used to generate useful inferences about the neural origins of evoked potentials. These inferences must be made with great caution,

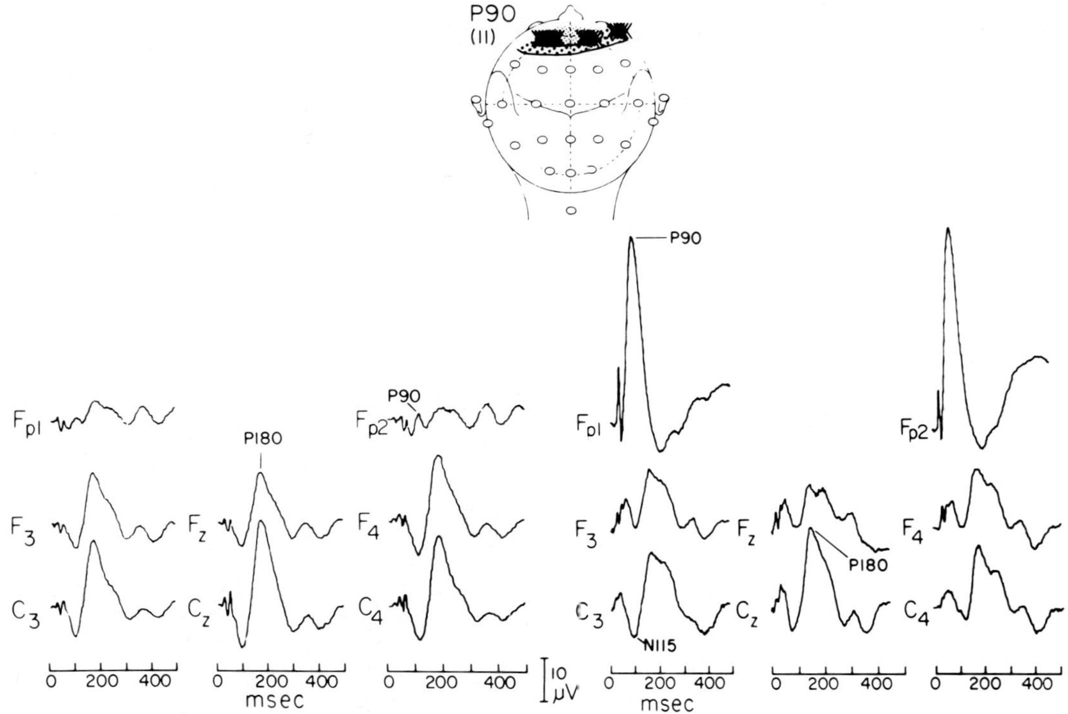

Fig. 4. P90 myogenic AEP component in an experienced (left) and inexperienced (right) subject in group topography for 11 subjects. Adapted from G.D. Goff et al. (1977).

however, since topographies can be misleading in the absence of supplementary information based on direct brain recording as we have shown in the somatosensory system (Goff et al., 1977b). Topographies can also be useful at the empirical level to identify probable myogenic components, estimate their degree of contamination of neurogenic components, and simply to know what components at what amplitude to expect at given electrode locations.

For these reasons we have examined the scalp topography of auditory, somatic, and visual evoked potentials, recording in twelve subjects from all electrodes in the 10-20 system plus additional electrodes (Allison et al., 1977; G.D. Goff et al., 1977). Auditory stimuli were clicks generated by 1.0 msec pulses from a Grass Model S4 stimulator modified in intensity by a Hewlett-Packard EO1350B attenuator and delivered by a Grason Stadler TDH 39 earphone to the right ear. Average click intensity was 85 to 87 dB SL. Recording was referential to A1. Because of the radically different recording parameters required to resolve BEPs, they were not examined in our study.

First let us consider myogenic components. Figure 3 shows for a typical subject the middle latency AEP components as recorded from the 10-20 electrode locations indicated. Those components we regard as wholly or partly myogenic are circled and their topographies are shown above. Details of component measurement and construction of isopotential maps are presented elsewhere (G.D. Goff et al., 1977). N15 is the negativity of what has been called the post-auricular response. The topography shown is accurate for an ear reference. However, in a supplementary study we checked topography using a noncephalic reference and the topography of N15 was limited to the ear mastoid region. Thus activity at the reference distorted the topography of N15 which emphasizes again the point made repeatedly by us and by others: The activity of a reference must be assessed for the components to be recorded. Otherwise there is a risk of distortion of the waveform, latency and topography of the response.

The topographies of N30, N40, and N60 suggest that we may be observing two different generating processes although two components could not be distinguished in terms of latency. N30 is regarded as wholly myogenic because of its highly peripheral distribution. N40 is the separation between P25 and P50 which on the basis of considerable other evidence are generally regarded as neurogenic. As we shall see shortly, the topography of P25 and P50 is predominantly in the central vertex area. N40 may appear largest where P25 and P50 are smallest, i.e., in the frontal and occipital areas. Nonetheless its distribution concentrated near the eye suggests a significant myogenic contribution. Similarly the amplitude of N60 may appear to be greatest where P50 is smallest; but again there appears to be a frontal musculature contribution.

It should be emphasized that on the basis of topography alone, the evidence for a muscular versus neural origin is equivocal for some components. In general, components which were largest only at peripheral electrodes overlying or close to muscles were regarded as myogenic, especially if they varied greatly in amplitude within or between subjects and tended to be larger in inexperienced subjects.

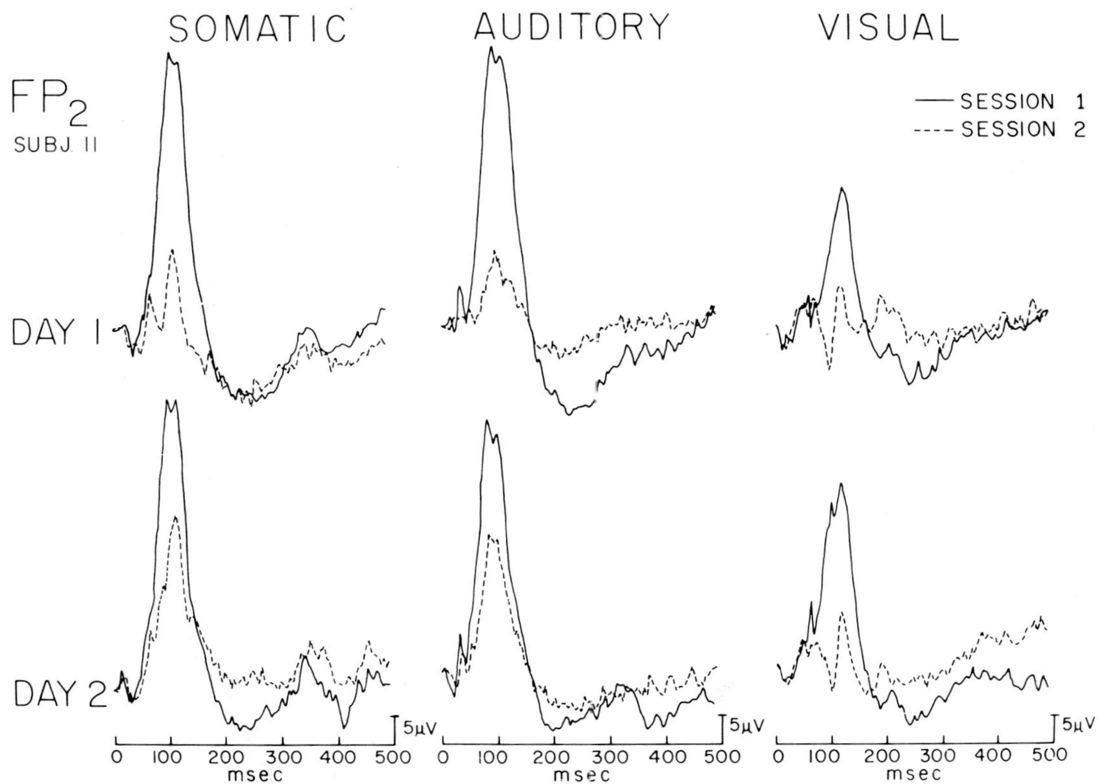

Fig. 5. Comparison in one subject of P90 myogenic AEP component with similar myogenic potentials evoked by somatic (median nerve shock) and visual (Maxwellian-view white light flash) stimuli. Each trace is the average of 64 responses.

Inexperienced subjects tend to be tense and myogenic potentials are known to be enhanced when the generating muscles are under tension (Bickford et al., 1964). We attempted to apply the muscle tension test but found that the resting waveform was so altered under muscle tension that the correspondence between components in the relaxed versus tense condition was unclear. Picton et al. (1974) and Streletz et al. (1977) have recorded AEPs as a function of muscle tension. Their designation of myogenic components is in general agreement with ours.

Some auditory evoked myogenic components can be very large even in the absence of overt muscle tension. Figure 4 illustrates this for a later component, P90. The left group of responses was recorded from a member of our laboratory who is very experienced in being a subject and therefore relaxed. Note the very small P90 at Fp_1 and Fp_2. The subject whose responses are shown on the right was a naive subject and presumably tense. Note the highly localized topography for the group of 11 subjects; so localized in fact that topographies of neighboring potentials for subjects with small P90 components were not markedly different from topographies based on subjects with large P90 components. For subjects with a large P90 component, some reflection of the component may be seen at frontal locations but it is not apparent at central locations.

The auditory P90 myogenic component has a somatic and visual counterpart as shown in Figure 5. Figure 5 also shows that P90 diminishes with experience within the same day's recording (Session 1 versus Session 2) and across days, presumably as the subject becomes more relaxed. This evoked myogenic component as well as some of the earlier ones apparently arise from orbicularis oculi muscles (Rushworth 1962; see Allison et al., 1977 for details). They are usually not associated with overt eyeblink. In some subjects a small reflex movement of the upper eyelid is detectable which does appear on the EEG monitor but is much smaller than the overt eyeblink. Perhaps the most important implication of the characteristics of all these frontal myogenic components is that we consider it imperative that a peripheral frontal electrode such as Fp_1 or Fp_2 be placed for all evoked potential recording (other than BEP) in all modalities so that possible distortion of neurogenic by myogenic components can be assessed.

Turning now to components which are entirely or predominantly neurogenic, middle latency components P25-N40-P50 are shown in Figure 6. These comprise the "W-shaped" waveform recorded by many investigators from the scalp and cortical surface. They are primarily neurogenic although they can be distorted by the temporally contiguous myogenic activity shown in Figure 3. P25 and P50 (like BEPs) are generally largest at the vertex.

A question of major importance to those of us who wish to utilize AEPs clinically is whether any of the early or middle latency AEP components represent the initial response of primary auditory cortex, or in other words the primary AEP. What is apparently the primary AEP recorded directly from auditory cortex in man has a latency of about 15 msec (Celesia 1976). Components are recorded in the same latency range from the scalp. We sought to determine if any of these components were indeed primary responses by recording from patients under barbiturate

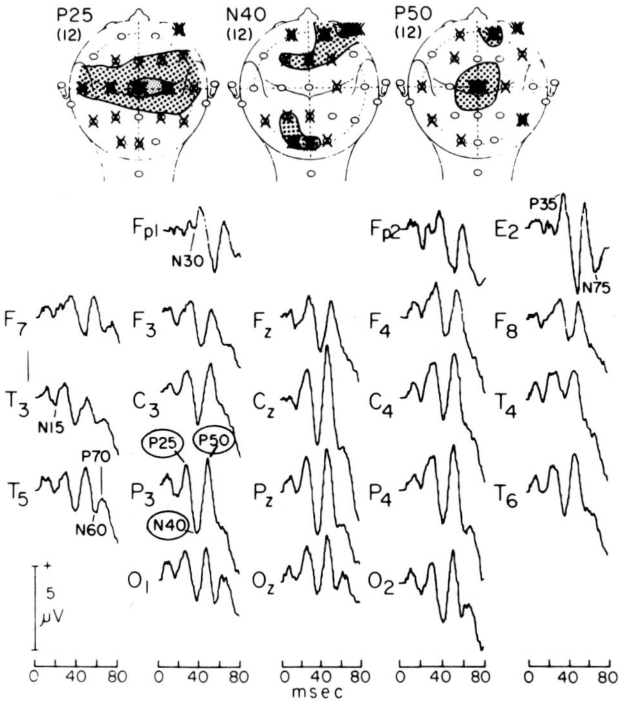

Fig. 6. Middle latency neurogenic (circled) AEP components from a typical subject, and group topographies. Records are grand averages of eight replications of 64 responses. Adapted from G.D. Goff et al. (1977).

anesthesia (Goff et al., 1977). The resistance of primary evoked potentials to barbiturates has been repeatedly demonstrated in animals including primates (see Goff et al., 1977a, for summary). We used this test many years ago to demonstrate that the early somatic evoked potential components N20-P30 represented the initial activity of primary somatic cortex (Abrahamian et al., 1963; Allison et al., 1963). For our auditory study, all patients were young males undergoing elective non-neurological surgery who volunteered for the study after discussion of the procedures and goals of the experiment. Prior to the day of surgery, control AEP recordings were made in the laboratory. In surgery, with the patient on the operating table but prior to the administration of anesthesia, additional AEPs were obtained as controls for the effects of premedications, typically diazepam and atropine sulphate. Then a total of 8.4 mg/kg thiopental was administered intravenous in three equal doses, the second two doses at 1 minute and 5 minutes after the first. Recording began after the second dose.

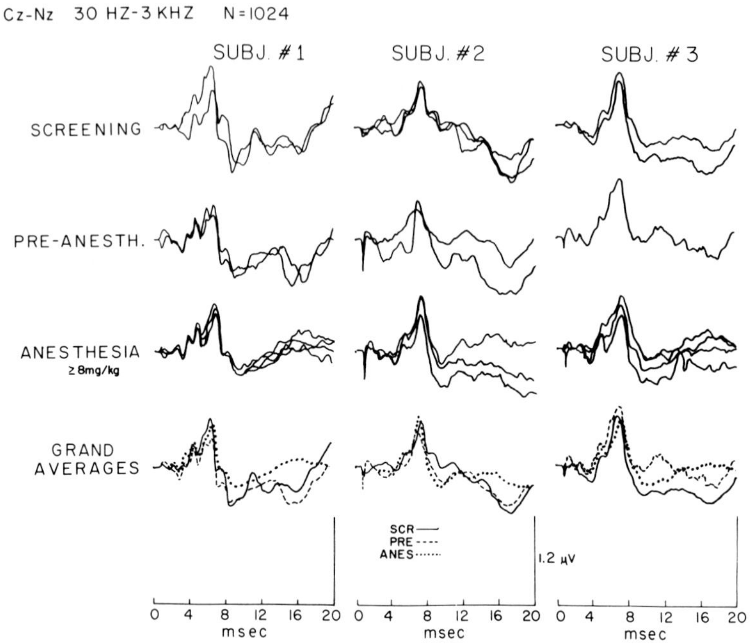

Fig. 7. Effects of barbiturate anesthesia on short latency AEPs in three subjects (columns). Except for grand averages, each record is the average of 1024 responses. Additional explanation in text. From Goff et al. (1977).

Figure 7 shows the effects of induction levels of barbiturate anesthesia on short latency AEPs. Three subjects are shown. "Screening" are the responses recorded in the laboratory; "pre-anesth." are the premedication controls taken in surgery; "anesthesia" is with the patient close to or at the induction level. Anesthesia had no effect on P2 through P6 as expected for responses of the synaptically secure, lemniscal afferent system. P7 and P9 were too small and inconsistent for quantification; our impression was that they were affected by anesthesia but not suppressed. This is consistent with the conclusion of Stockard and Rossiter (1977) that these components (their components VI and VII) reflect activity in medial geniculate and geniculo-cortical radiations respectively. P12, seen most clearly in the subject shown in the left column of Figure 7, is the only remaining neurogenic component occurring in the first 20 msec. It is suppressed by barbiturate anesthesia and therefore is not the primary cortical response. Subsequent neurogenic AEP components are too late for the primary cortical response and also are completely suppressed by barbiturate anesthesia (Goff et al., 1977).

Recent unpublished observations by Vaughan and colleagues (reported in Goff et al., 1977a) find early scalp components which are of maximum amplitude

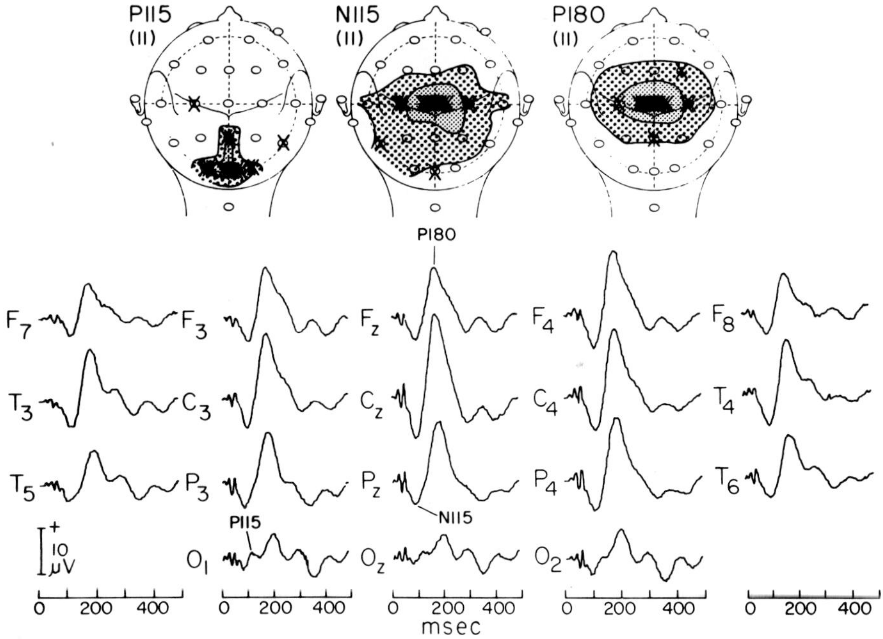

Fig. 8. Long latency AEP components from a typical subject and group topographies for components indicated. Each record is the grand average of eight replications of 64 responses. Adapted from G.D. Goff et al. (1977).

just superior to the estimated level of the Sylvian fissure and which invert in polarity below this level. Possibly these potentials may represent the primary auditory evoked potential but so far as I know they have not yet been subjected to the barbiturate test. In summary, then, with the averaging technique auditory activity can be recorded from subcortical nuclei including medial geniculate and from geniculo-cortical radiations. So far, however, we have not recorded activity which can be unequivocably identified as the primary cortical auditory evoked potential.

Now let us turn to long latency responses. The long latency components of maximal interest in the literature at present are the "T-complex" reported by Wolpaw and Penry (1975; 1977), the vertex potential, long used in evoked potential audiometry until recently supplanted in most cases by BEPs, and a series of still later potentials, sometimes called the late positive complex (LPC). Of the LPC, the so-called P300 wave has received considerable attention because of its responsiveness to psychological, especially cognitive, variables.

The T-complex is reported by Wolpaw and Penry to be a positivity at approximately 105 msec followed by a negativity at 150-160 msec which is localized bilaterally to the temporal area. Its latency is shorter contralateral than ipsilateral to the side of monaural stimulation. It tends to be obscured in scalp recordings by the temporally overlapping and larger amplitude vertex potential. According to Wolpaw and Penry, it is necessary to subtract the vertex potential from the combination of the two as recorded in the temporal area in order to resolve the T-complex.

Late components as we record them in a typical subject are shown in Figure 8. The vertex potential, N115-P180, dominates the record at most locations. As the topographies show, both components are maximal at the vertex; N115 is roughly bilaterally symmetrical and P180 is quite symmetrical. The only component we recorded which might correspond to the T-complex appeared as an interruption of the N115 component of the vertex potential. The topography of this component, which we call P115 (Fig. 8; 0_1) has an occipital rather than the expected temporal focus. This difference could be a result of the location of our reference electrode (Wolpaw and Penry used a balanced noncephalic reference), or the fact that we did not subtract out the vertex potential, or component P115 may have no relation to the T-complex. Neither did we observe a reliable negativity in the T-complex latency range, perhaps due to its being obscured by the positivity of the vertex potential.

In one patient, we have recorded directly from the lateral surface of the temporal lobe near the Sylvian fissure, a positive-negative sequence which corresponds well in latency and polarity with the T-complex. In Figure 9 AEP components at approximately P100-N200 are recorded from electrodes 6, 7, 11, and 13. This response is specific to the temporal lobe; a quite different response is recorded from immediately adjacent central cortex medial to the Sylvian fissure at electrodes 3, 5, and 4. The response is not resolved at the scalp location C_Z. The P100-N200 response is specific to auditory stimulation; somatosensory responses recorded from the same electrode locations shown at the right of the figure, are quite different. However, in other patients we have recorded from the cortical surface of the somatosensory area a somatic specific late response highly similar in polarity and latency to the auditory T-complex (Goff et al., 1977c). Thus it is possible that in both the auditory and the somatic system there is a modality specific late potential in the 100-200 msec range which is obscured in typical scalp recordings by the overpowering vertex potential. Wolpaw and Penry have suggested that the auditory response arises from the secondary auditory area.

Our topography for the vertex potential is in general agreement with the findings of others showing a maximum amplitude focus at the vertex and bilateral symmetry around it. The neural origins of vertex potentials and whether they are or are not modality specific is a subject of active controversy at present. Early reports suggested an origin in mesial cortex (Gastaut 1954; Hughes and Mazurowski 1964). Picton et al. (1974) reported a slightly more anterior distribution for the auditory vertex potential (see Fig. 11) and suggested that it arises largely from frontal association cortex. Both of these suggestions are compatible with the concept of a nonspecific origin. In contrast, Vaughan and Ritter (1970), on the basis of an observed polarity reversal in scalp recorded vertex potential components at the

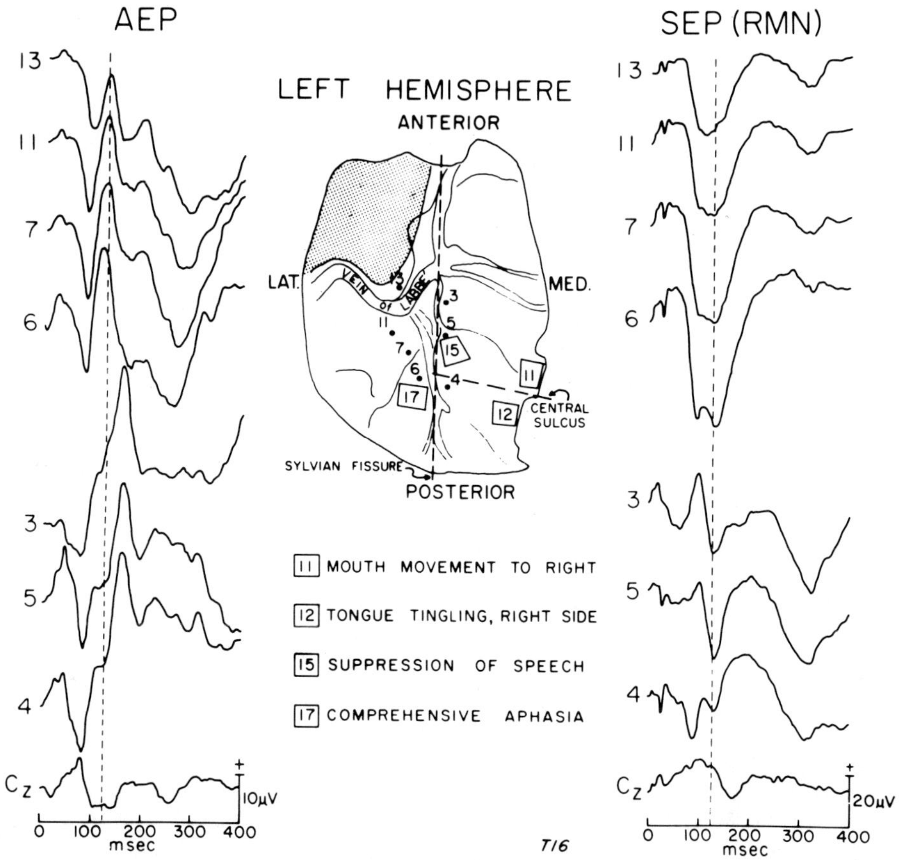

Fig. 9. Auditory and somatic evoked potentials from Peri-Sylvian cortical surface. AEPs were evoked by a 65 dB SL click delivered to the contralateral (right) ear. Somatic evoked potentials were evoked by shock to contralateral (right) median nerve at the wrist at 3 ma above thumb twitch threshold. Electrical stimulation of the cortex at locations indicated by box numbers produced the results listed and indicated the approximate location of the central sulcus. The records shown are the grand averages of three replications of 48 stimulations. All records are referential to linked ears. Stippled area indicates excision subsequent to recordings. From Goff et al. (1977a).

presumed level of the Sylvian fissure, proposed that they were generated in the auditory receiving area. There has been considerable controversy about the observations of Vaughan and Ritter and their interpretation of them (see Goff et al., 1977b, for review). The balance of the evidence seems to support the position of Vaughan and colleagues who believe that most, if not all, of AEP late components are generated in primary and secondary auditory cortex. Although our scalp topography of the vertex potential might seem to contradict the Vaughan position,

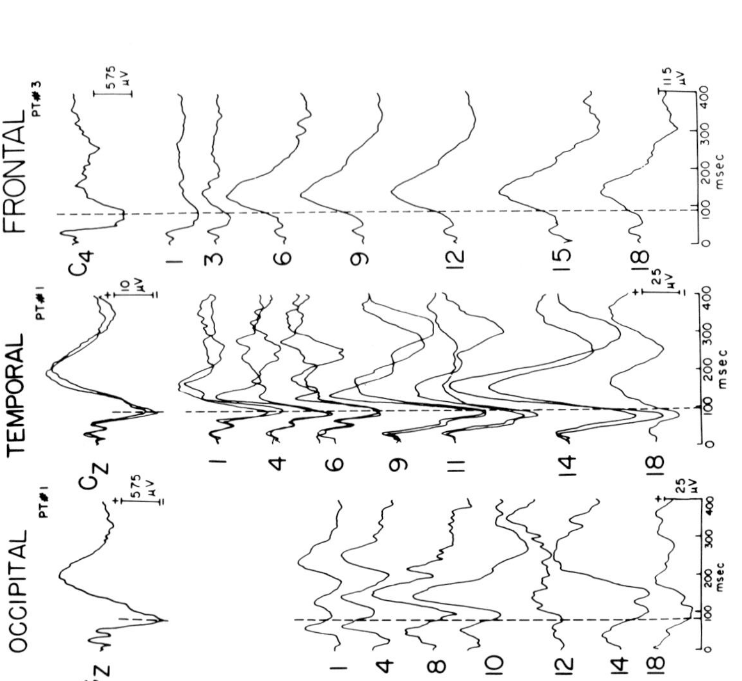

Fig. 10. AEPs from intracranial electrodes with 18 recording sites. Approximate electrode locations in the brain are indicated at the left. Cross bars on schematic electrodes indicate approximate location of each recording site from superficial (1) to deep (18). Occipital and temporal electrode AEPs are from the same patient; frontal AEPs are from a different patient. Each trace is the grand average of at least three replications to 64 responses each. Double traces on the temporal electrode are from different recording sessions. Adapted from Goff et al. (1977c).

the theoretical derivations shown in Figure 2B demonstrate that the potential field generated by two distinct dipole sources has a broad unimodal distribution when measured sufficiently far from the sources. Thus, the empirical scalp topographies currently available do not discriminate between the Vaughan position and other alternatives.

It might be expected that the issue would be resolved by intracranial recording. Unfortunately this has not proven to be the case for vertex potentials. We have had the opportunity to record from the depths of the brain in selected epileptic patients. The depth probes are placed stereotactically for the clinical purpose of localizing epileptogenic tissue for possible neurosurgical excision. Evoked potential recording proceeds concurrently with clinical monitoring. Details of procedure are given elsewhere (Goff et al., 1977c). Briefly, the depth probes are implanted bilaterally in frontal, central, and occipital areas. The frontal electrodes sample activity from mesial frontal and orbital cortex; the tips of the central and occipital probes terminate in the anterior pole of the temporal lobe. Each probe has 18 recording sites. Figure 10 is a composite of intracranial records presented in detail elsewhere (Goff et al., 1977c). Because it is a composite, electrode locations shown on the schematic brain are typical but not precise for the patients shown. Also the occipital and temporal probe records are from the same patient, but the frontal records are from a different patient. Central scalp locations are shown for comparison to depth probes. The general finding is that evoked potentials apparently corresponding to auditory vertex potentials are seen diffusely and with bilateral symmetry throughout the depth of the brain. There seems to be a maximum amplitude focus in the mid central region (temporal probe location 14; occipital probe locations 8 and 10) which would support the theory of a modality specific response originating in auditory cortex. However a virtually identical waveform and maximum amplitude focus is observed to somatic stimulation suggesting the possibility of a nonspecific origin in central subcortical structures. Future research, including primate models, will be required to establish the neural origins of vertex potentials. Unfortunately, it has not yet been demonstrated that primates have vertex potentials.

Evoked potential components up to and including the vertex potential are sometimes referred to as exogenous potentials because they are considered to be principally determined by the evoking stimulus parameters and to reflect "obligatory" neural events. When some aspect of the stimulus unexpectedly changes, or it carries information relevant to the performance of the task, marked changes appear in the LPC. The P300 wave, sometimes called the P_3 wave, has received the most attention. The 300 msec is an average latency; actual latencies range from 250 to over 450 msec. P300 is often termed an endogenous potential and is said to be emitted rather than evoked under conditions generally subsumed by the concept of orienting, or cognitive stimulus evaluation. Specific examples of conditions which caused the P300 to be emitted are when information is embodied in the stimulus which resolves the subject's prior uncertainty, when target stimuli are recognized, when stimuli command a prompt motor reaction, when there is a sudden change in the stimulus, or when there is an omission of a repetitive stimulus.

Hillyard et al. (1976) have obtained perhaps the most comprehensive topographies for auditory P300 waves. They did 16-channel mapping for P300 during five different decision tasks. Figure 11, taken from their article, compares the distribution of the positivity of the vertex potential (their P2; our P180) to P300 for a task involving detection of a randomly presented tone pip at threshold intensity, and for an omitted stimulus. The two P300's are virtually identical in topography and are more widespread laterally and posteriorly than P2. Topo-

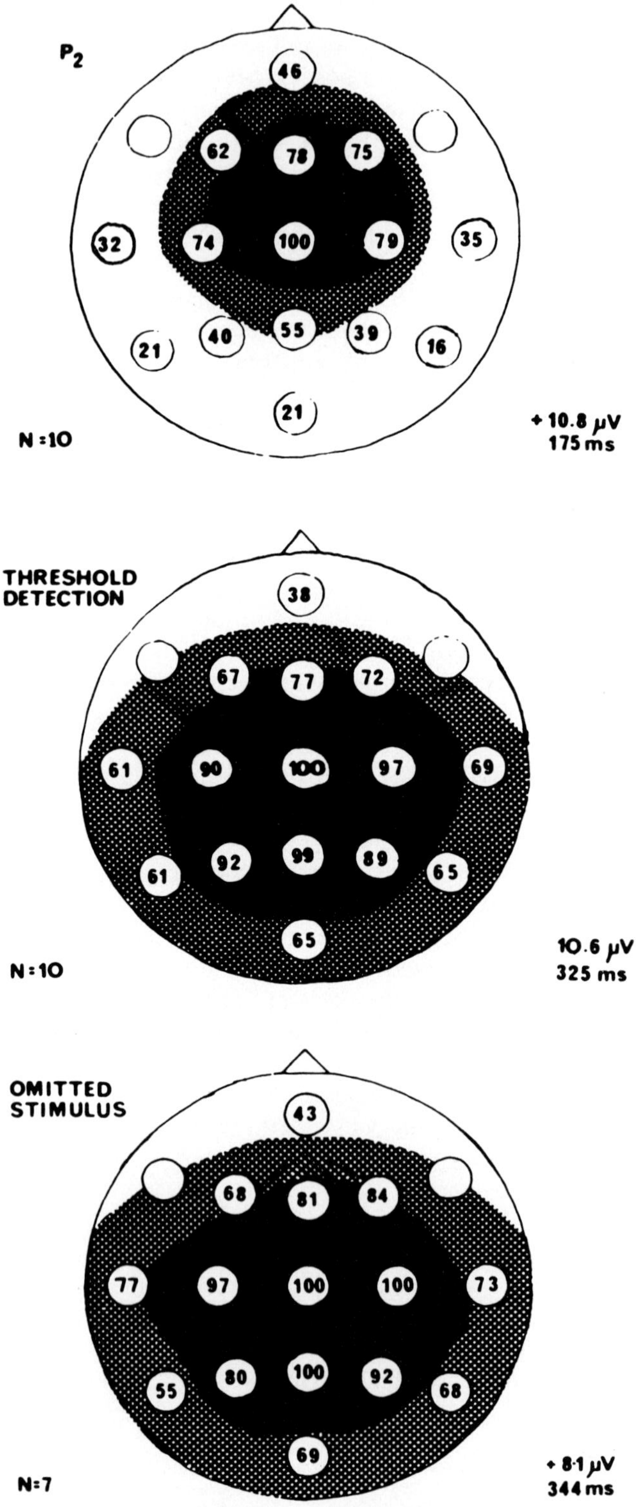
P2
46
62
78
75
32
74
100
79
35
21
40
55
39
16
21
N =10
+ 10.8 μV
175 ms
THRESHOLD
DETECTION
38
67
77
72
61
90
100
97
69
61
92
99
89
65
65
N=10
10.6 μV
325 ms
OMITTED
STIMULUS
43
68
81
84
77
97
100
100
73
55
80
100
92
68
69
N=7
+ 8·1 μV
344 ms

graphies for the three other tasks were similar. While similarity of latency and topography suggests common neural origins for the P300 and other late components, most recently evidence has begun to emerge suggesting that different components react differentially to different stimulus paradigms and that a given component has different topographies according to the modality of the eliciting stimulus (Simson et al., 1976, 1977). This literature has been reviewed elsewhere (Goff et al., 1977a).

SUMMARY

Auditory evoked potentials recorded from the scalp begin almost immediately after stimulus presentation and last at least 450 msec in a normal awake adult. No early components have as yet been unequivocably shown to represent the primary response of the auditory receiving area. Recordings of early and middle latency components are subject to distortion by the occurrence of concurrent evoked myogenic potentials. Topographical analysis shows the myogenic components to be largest at peripheral scalp areas overlying or adjacent to cranial muscles. They are most prominent in the frontal region apparently arising from periocular and forehead musculature. Evoked potentials regarded as wholly or predominantly neurogenic appear maximally in the vertex and posterior parietal regions and are mostly bilaterally symmetrical regardless of whether the stimulus is monaural or binaural.

Those components occurring subsequent to approximately 100 msec are termed late components. An auditory late component (the T-complex) occurring in the 100-200 msec range has been reported to be resolved in scalp recordings by special procedures and a similar response has been recorded from temporal cortex in one patient. It has been suggested that this complex arises from the secondary auditory cortex. With typical recording methods this complex tends to be obscured by the larger vertex potential which occurs in the same latency range. The vertex potential (N115-P180), like earlier neurogenic components, is symmetrically distributed about a vertex maximum. Its origins are controversial; some have suggested that it is a modality specific response arising from the auditory receiving area, while other evidence suggests a modality non-specific origin in mid-central subcortical structures. Components succeeding the vertex potential appear to be determined less by the physical stimulus parameters than by the psychological significance of the stimulus. These potentials are sometimes said to be emitted rather than evoked. In scalp topography, they also tend to be symmetrically distributed around vertex maximum but their topography can vary with the task and modality of stimulation.

Fig. 11. Topography of the positive component (P2) of the auditory vertex potential evoked by a 50 dB tone pip, and P300 topographies to correctly detected threshold stimuli and omitted stimuli. Each map is a grand average of the percentage of maximum from N individual subjects. Black zone depicts regions of over 75% relative amplitude and hatched zone between 50 and 75%. From Hillyard et al. (1976).

Acknowledgements

Supported by the Medical Research Service of the Veterans Administration and by USPHS NIMH Grant MH-05286. I acknowledge gratefully the constructive crticisms and helpful suggestions of my colleagues, Drs. T. Allison and C.C. Wood.

REFERENCES

Abrahamian, H.A., Allison, T., Goff, W.R. and Rosner, B.S. Effects of thiopental on human cerebral evoked responses. *Anesthesiology 24:* 650-657, 1963.

Allison, T., Goff, W.R., Abrahamian, H.A. and Rosner, B.S. The effects of barbiturate anesthesia upon human somatosensory evoked responses. *Electroencephalogr. Clin. Neurophysiol.* Suppl. *24:* 68-75, 1963.

Allison, T., Matsumiya, Y., Goff, G.D. and Goff, W.R. The scalp topography of human visual evoked potentials. *Electroencephalogr. Clin. Neurophysiol. 42:* 185-197, 1977.

Bickford, R.G., Jacobson, J.L. and Cody, D.T.R. Nature of average evoked potentials to sound and other stimuli in man. *Ann. N.Y. Acad. Sci. 112:* 204-223, 1964.

Celesia, G.G. Organization of auditory cortical areas in man. *Brain 99:* 403-414, 1976.

Donchin, E., Callaway, E., Cooper, R., Desmedt, J.E., Goff, W.R., Hillyard, S.A. and Sutton, S. Publication criteria for studies of evoked potentials (EP) in man. Report of a Committee. In: *Attention, Voluntary Contraction and Event-Related Cerebral Potentials,* edited by J.E. Desmedt. *Prog. Clin. Neurophysiol. 1:* 1-11, 1977.

Gastaut, H. The brain stem and cerebral electrogenesis in relation to consciousness, *Brain Mechanisms and Consciousness,* edited by J.F. Delafresnaye. Springfield: Charles C Thomas, 1954, p. 249-283.

Goff, G.D., Matsumiya, Y., Allison, T. and Goff, W.R. The scalp topography of human somatosensory and auditory evoked potentials. *Electroencephalogr. Clin. Neurophysiol. 42:* 57-76, 1977.

Goff, W.R., Allison, T., Lyons, W., Fisher, T.C. and Conte, R. Origins of short latency auditory evoked potentials in man. In: *Auditory Evoked Potentials in Man. Psychopharmacology Correlates of EPs,* edited by J.E. Desmedt. *Prog. Clin. Neurophysiol. 2:* 30-44, 1977.

Goff, W.R., Allison, T. and Vaughan, H.G.Jr. The functional neuroanatomy of event related potentials. In: *Event Related Brain Potentials in Man,* edited by E. Callaway and S.H. Koslow. New York: Academic Press. In press, 1977a.

Goff, W.R., Allison, T., Williamson, P.D. and VanGilder, J.C. Scalp topography in the localization of intracranial evoked potential sources. In: *Multidisciplinary Perspectives in Event-Related Brain Potential Research,* edited by D. Otto. U.S. Government Printing Office. In press, 1977b.

Goff, W.R., Williamson, P.D., VanGilder, J.C., Allison, T. and Fisher, T.C. Neural origins of long latency evoked potentials recorded from the depth and cortical surface of the brain in man. In: *Somatosensory Evoked Potentials and their Clinical Uses,* edited by J.E. Desmedt. *Prog. Clin. Neurophysiol. Vol. 7.* In press, 1977c.

Hillyard, S.A., Courchesne, E., Krausz, H.I. and Picton, T.W. Scalp topography of the P_3 wave in different auditory decision tasks. In: *The Responsive Brain,* edited by W.C. McCallum and J.R. Knott. Bristol: Wright, 1976, p. 81-87.

Hughes, J.R. and Mazurowski, J.A. Studies on the supracallosal mesial cortex of unanesthetized, conscious mammals. II. Monkey. D. Vertex sharp waves and epileptiform activity. *Electroencephalogr. Clin. Neurophysiol. 16:* 561-574, 1964.

Picton, T.W., Hillyard, S.A., Krausz, H.I. and Galambos, R. Human auditory evoked potentials. I. Evaluation of components. *Electroencephalogr. Clin. Neurophysiol. 36:* 179-190, 1974.

Rushworth, G. Observations on blink reflexes. *J. Neurol. Neurosurg. Psychiat. 25:* 93-108, 1962.

Simson, R., Vaughan, H.G.Jr. and Ritter, W. The scalp topography of potentials associated with missing visual or auditory stimuli. *Electroencephalogr. Clin. Neurophysiol. 40:* 33-42, 1976.

Simson, R., Vaughan, H.G.Jr. and Ritter, W. The scalp topography of potentials in auditory and visual discrimination tasks. *Electroencephalogr. Clin. Neurophysiol. 42:* 528-535, 1977.

Simson, R.C., Vaughan, H.G.Jr. and Ritter, W. The scalp topography of potentials in auditory and visual go-no-go tasks. *Electroencephalogr. Clin. Neurophysiol.* In press, 1977.

Stockard, J.J. and Rossiter, V.S. Clinical and pathological correlates of brain stem auditory response abnormalities. *Neurology 27:* 316-325, 1977.

Streletz, L.J., Katz, L., Hohenberger, M. and Cracco, R.Q. Scalp recorded auditory evoked potentials and sonomotor responses: an evaluation of components and recording techniques. *Electroencephalogr. Clin. Neurophysiol. 43:* 192-206, 1977.

Vaughan, H.G.Jr. and Ritter, W. The sources of auditory evoked response recorded from the human scalp. *Electroencephalogr. Clin. Neurophysiol. 28:* 360-367, 1970.

Wolpaw, J.R. and Penry, J.K. A temporal component of the auditory evoked response. *Electroencephalogr. Clin. Neurophysiol. 39:* 609-620, 1975.

Wolpaw, J.R. and Penry, J.K. Hemispheric differences in the monaural and binaural auditory evoked responses. *Electroencephalogr. Clin. Neurophysiol. 42:* 728-729, 1977.

DISCUSSION

Gerken: Did you identify a possible medial geniculate potential in terms of waveform number and location on the scalp?

Goff: We and others record brain stem components VI and VII. We have not identified their origin but Stockard and Rossiter (Stockard, J.J. and Rossiter, V.S. Clinical and pathologic correlates of brain stem auditory response abnormalities. *Neurology 27:* 316-325, 1977), on the basis of correlations between response abnormalities and postmortem or radiologically localized brain stem lesions, have suggested that component VI arises from medial geniculate and VII arises from thalamus or auditory radiations.

Galambos: I like the offhand way in which you toss off the statement you have 109--!

Goff: 108 recording sites.

Galambos: That is really remarkable; it has been a long time since anybody has had such a large population of these patients and I hope you will get excellent information from them.

You made a provocative remark. You said that the P300 is of no value in the clinical situation.

Goff: I didn't make that value judgment. I said so far it hasn't been demonstrated to be of clinical value.

Galambos: Not even in your place?

Goff: No, not yet.

Galambos: Have you tried?

Goff: No, we had not, which is why I did not say it was of no value but rather that it had not been demonstrated to be of value. With regard to the intracranial recordings, we have reported preliminary results (Goff, W.R., Williamson, P. D., VanGilder, J.C., Allison, T. and Fisher, T.C. Neural origins of long latency evoked potentials recorded from the depth and cortical surface of the brain in man. In: *Somatosensory Evoked Potentials and their Clinical Uses,* edited by J.E. Desmedt. *Prog. Clin. Neurophysiol. Vol. 7.* Basal: Karger. In press). The probes are placed for clinical monitoring to attempt to localize an epileptic focus for possible neurosurgical exision. We are able to record concurrently with the clinical monitoring. Up to six probes are implanted. Each probe has 18 recording sites so we can make an extensive survey of evoked activity.

Terkildsen: Did I hear you say that the activity in the time period from 20 to 50 msec after stimulus onset would be completely eliminated by barbiturate anesthesia?

Goff: It is our finding that the only components remaining after barbiturate anesthesia induction are the brain stem potentials. All subsequent activity is absent or markedly suppressed by sodium thiopental (Goff, W.R., Allison, T., Lyons, W., Fisher, T.C. and Conte, R. Origins of short latency auditory evoked potentials in man. In: *Auditory Evoked Potentials in Man. Psychopharmacology Correlates of EPs,* edited by J.E. Desmedt. *Prog. Clin. Neurophysiol. Vol. 2.* Basel: Karger. 1977, p. 30-44).

Nodar: When you said peak P7 probably originated at the level of the medial geniculate body, was that to an ipsilateral or contralateral stimulus?

Goff: I referred to the work of Stockard and Rossiter (1977) and I do not recall that information.

PROBLEMS AND METHODS IN PEDOAUDIOLOGICAL ERA

Jesper Barfod and Gerhard Salomon

Gentofte University Hospital

INTRODUCTION

Based upon the pioneering work of Davis (1939), Mituyosi (1954), Geisler et al. (1958) and others, ERA was introduced in the late 60's as a clinical audiometric tool applicable to the very young and the difficult-to-test neurologically or mentally disabled child. In the early 70's it was realized that the vertex response with latencies from 50-400 msec was only of limited value (Cohen et al., 1971; Rose et al., 1971) and research centers seemed to focus their attention on a variety of reasons for the failures in ERA.

This paper will attempt to analyze the problems involved in paedoaudiological vertex ERA (part I) and will try to evaluate different techniques applied in order to make vertex ERA a reliable clinical tool (part II).

Besides mentioning the generally known procedures applied to overcome some of the problems, we will specifically be concerned with the recent developments from our own laboratory and will report the first systematic results obtained with adaptive signal processing of vertex ERA in small children.

PART I

ERA from the vertex makes use of the principle that the average of a series of synchronized post-stimulus EEG epochs, presumably containing a time-locked sound-evoked response with a constant shape, will display the response patterns with a reasonable visual detectability. Whereas a hearing threshold response under certain lax restrictions can easily be visually detected after about 100 repetitive sound stimulations in adults, the discouraging results in small children are generally agreed to be due to four main reasons:

I. A very low signal-to-noise ratio
II. Difficulty in visual recognition of the response
III. Presence of frequent and intensive artifacts
IV. Great variability of response shape and latency

ISBN 0-12-514960-3

In children the signal-to-noise ratio (S/N) is small compared to adults. The amplitude of the evoked response appears to be in the same range in all age groups, varying from a few to 20μV. However, the background activity in children may be 4 times higher than for adults, where it is in the range 20-100μV. The S/N ratio decreases with decreasing stimulus intensity and the resulting impaired recognition of responses introduces a risk of considerable errors in threshold determination in children.

The criteria for the visual detection of responses are based on a subjective and very imprecise notion of what type of pattern can be expected. In contrast to the vertex response in adults, which shows a reasonable resemblance between subjects, the young children have "immature" and unpredictable response patterns (Salomon, 1975; Lentz and McCandless, 1971). This pattern shows an individual "maturation" and reaches more predictable configurations towards 4 years of age. In the brain-damaged child and in psychotic patients (Salomon, 1970) unusual patterns may likewise be observed. Hence, visual observers must be open-minded to any type of response pattern which appears reproducible. This variability is a potential source of false-positive recognitions (Schimmel et al., 1974; Salomon, et al., 1973).

Vertex ERA especially in children is troubled by a very pronounced artifact problem. The artifacts may originate from such technical sources as movement of the electrodes or wires; they may be of local biological origin, like transient EEG signals in epilepsy, or large DC potential shifts in connection with changes in brain activity or perception. Artifacts may also be produced by biological generators outside the brain (EMG, retinal potential, etc.).

Averaging will permit recognition of the evoked response by reducing the noise background, ideally in proportion to the square root of the number of epochs averaged. In the clinical situation measuring periods of more than five minutes on children are generally unfeasible. This permits about 100 epochs to be recorded and averaged which means that only a rather uniform noise will be sufficiently reduced. Any sudden large (10-100 fold) noise deflection will not be effectively removed by averaging, and the remnant may erroneously be interpreted as a response.

The "vigilance" problem results in fluctuation of the response pattern from second to second with changing activity of the brain caused by changes in attention. This change of pattern also produces latency fluctuations (Spreng, 1970). The variations result in an average response which originates from an ensemble of different response shapes (Salomon, 1975). This condition violates the ideal presumptions for averaging and obscures the shape of the pattern to be identified. Furthermore, possible secondary potentials like the perstimulatory negative DC shift, expectancy wave, and the P300 activity related to perception mechanisms may vary violently and uncontrollably.

Countermeasures

The four groups of methodological problems have been attacked principally by changing the biological procedure in the test, or by introducing technical and statistical remedies. Table I displays a number of adequate procedures. In the following, these countermeasures will be evaluated with reference to paedoaudiology, where restlessness of the child is a serious clinical problem and where ERA may be the only way to establish a sufficient audiological evaluation.

	PROBLEM	COUNTERMEASURES A. BIOLOGICAL	COUNTERMEASURES B. TECHNICAL
I	Low signal-to-noise ratio	1) Increased stimulus interval 2) Direction of attention, conditioning (CNV)	1) Filtering 2) Increased number of stimuli
II	Recognition of response	Experience in visual detection	Enhanced visual or automatic detection using 1) Multichannel recordings 2) Signal processing 3) Statistical analysis
III	Artifacts	Behavioral control	1) Needle electrodes 2) High CMRR, shielded room, short leads etc. 3) Artifact rejection
IV	Response fluctuation	Vigilance control	1) Clustering methods 2) Adaptive filtering

I. Signal-to-noise Ratio

Various biological conditions influence the signal-to-noise ratio in single EEG epochs. The trade-off between stimulus repetition rates and response amplitude indicates an optimum in adults for stimulus intervals of 1-2 seconds (Davis et al., 1966). Sparse experiments in children (Saloman, 1975) do not dispute this range. The impressive results of training and conditioning which produce directly (ie. without averaging) visible expectancy DC shifts (Brix, 1977) are obviously inapplicable in very small children. Consequently, only adjustment of stimulus rate seems to be an applicable biological procedure for improvement of signal-to-noise ratio.

On the technical side, the fact that signal and noise seem to have similar frequency characteristics reduces the possibilities for improving signal-to-noise ratio dramatically by filtering.

II. Response Recognition

The ability to judge subjectively will in general improve with experience provided the necessary feedback is present, but the result can be rather unsatisfactory, even with many years of experience.

Feedback obtained through experience does not generally improve detection ability, but will rather influence the relationship between false-positive and false-negative decisions characterizing the decision maker (Schimmel et al., 1974; Salomon, 1976). While a naive judge will try to maintain an equal number of false-positive and false-negative detections, assuming that errors are equally serious, a trained clinician will try to reduce the number of false-positive judgments (Suzuki et al., 1976).

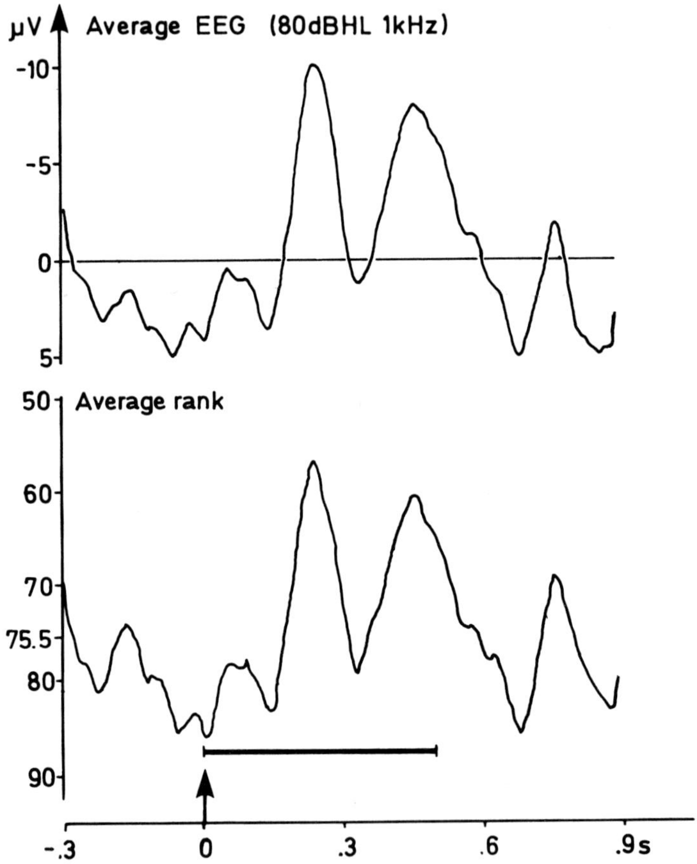

Fig. 1. Top: Average of sample values of 91 EEG epochs. Bottom: Average of rank of sample values of the same data as above. Ranking is performed for each EEG epoch (150 sample values).

On the technical side, subjective judgment can be improved by a multichannel recording system (Burian and Gestring, 1971) and subsequent application of visual (or mathematical) correlation techniques.

Another approach aiding visual judgment is preprocessing of single or averaged sweeps, eventually followed by a statistical evaluation of the averaged response.

Linear filtering has already been mentioned and seems to have only little effect. However, nonlinear filtering using ranking procedures has proved rather successful and will be treated in more detail. One of the problems in applying statistically-based methods for detection of responses in average EEGs is the large difference in the statistical properties of the data from sweep to sweep. Another problem is the presence of large DC shifts or large spikes, which, despite the application of averaging, may penetrate and influence the shape of the averaged sweep. In statistical terms the problem is that the distribution of signal values that are averaged is irregular. A method to overcome this problem in vertex ERA is proposed by Salomon (1974), using ranking statistics (Friedmann, 1937). Within each sweep all sample values are ranked according to their amplitudes; averaging now takes place on the ranks instead of on the measured values. The presence of a response will be reflected by deflections from the average rank values as for conventional average EEGs. Figure 1 shows both average EEG and average ranked EEG based on 91 epochs. The resemblance between the two displays is remarkable and indicates that only little information is lost when using the ranking procedure in connection with averaging. The ranking procedure effectively prevents a spike in a sweep from severely penetrating to the averaged sweep. Furthermore, it has a positive effect on DC fluctuations and, provided that no response signal is present and the background activity is random (and uncorrelated to the stimulus), the distribution of the sample values will be rectangular with mean $(n+1)/2$ and variance $n(n+1)/12$, where n is the number of sampling points being ranked in each recorded epoch. Averaging a number N of ranked sweeps will yield rank averages which, for $N>10$, with a good approximation is normally distributed with mean

$$\mu = (n+1)/2$$

and variance

$$\sigma^2 = n(n+1)/12N$$

Since the ranking procedure is nonlinear, the results of averaging will, in an irreversible manner, be dependent on any linear filtering of the signals before ranking.

The method proposed by Salomon (1974) comprises examination of the EEG after high-pass filtering (differentiation) and selection of sample points with increased density in regions where responses are to be expected. The average ranks for these sample points are normalized with respect to mean and variance from (1), squared and summed, and using a chi-square test the probability of a response being present is evaluated.

The method is advantageous because it is independent of the shape of the response, it is able to take advantage of response DC shifts, and it yields a single decision variable characterizing the total measurement. The method, however, is disadvantageous in that it is relatively dependent on a knowledge of where the response is present, in order to permit an effective selection of data points, and that it does not reveal any information on the latency of the response since it is based on distributed samples. Moreover, since the EEG is of relatively low bandwidth, conventionally used sample intervals (5-20 msec) will produce data values which are not uncorrelated. This again will influence the statistical foundation of the chi-square test, possibly leading to a larger number of false positives than the test significance-level indicates.

Another method also using the advantageous statistical properties of average ranks evaluates the probability of committing a false-positive judgment in relation to the size of the largest negative peak in the average rank epoch within a predetermined observation window. The negative deflection (vertex negative) is chosen, since it is a common experience that it is the most pronounced. Hence, one-sided statistical evaluation may be applied. Normalizing all data points in the averaged ranked sweep using the mean and variance from (1) yields data which are approximately normally distributed with zero mean and unit variance, provided no response is present. The distribution of the largest deflection to one side among a number of independent values with Normal distribution may easily be computed

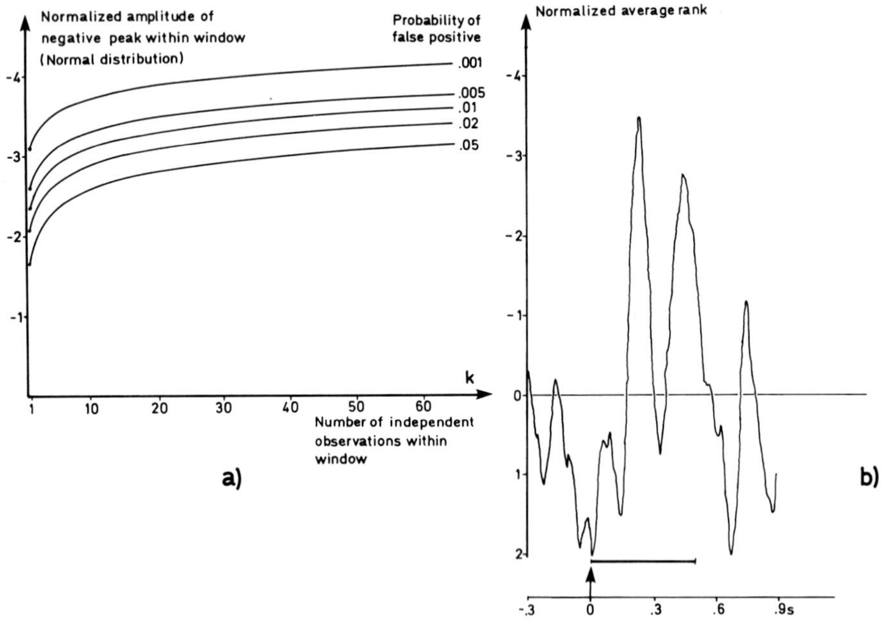

Fig. 2.a. Relationship between probability of false-positive detection and the normalized amplitude of the largest peak observed within a window of size k. Based on normal distribution and the assumption that observations within the window are independent.

b. Average ranks from Figure 1, normalized according to the known mean (75.5) and variance (20.7) (formula (1) N = 91, n = 150).

(see Appendix II). Presuming that no response is present, Figure 2a shows the correspondance between the normalized size of the largest deflection, the number k of observations within the window and the associated probability of obtaining a (negative) deflection equal to or larger than indicated. Figure 2b shows the normalized average ranked epoch from Figure 1. The assumption that all data points within the predetermined window are independent will ensure a safe base for judgment, since the correlation between data points presumably present will actually be equivalent in a smaller degree of freedom (ie. a smaller k). Some attempts have been made to estimate an equivalent degree of freedom based on the property of the EEG signal; Thornton (1977) concluded that data points more than approximately 40-50 msec apart may be regarded as being independent. However, the consequences of compensating for correlated data through a reduction of the degree of freedom are so far largely unexplored. Extreme caution should therefore be exercised when using these approaches in order to avoid overinterpretation of the data.

The delineation of Figure 2b is also useful in another aspect, since it indicates the relative significance of different signal components for the shape of the response.

III. Artifacts

The artifact problem has been approached largely by sedating the patient. Sedation should, however, be avoided, since it causes large variability of both response pattern and background activity (Salomon et al., 1973; Suzuki et al., (1976). Verbal instruction to small children to stay relaxed is, of course, inapplicable. However, it is possible to keep the child relatively calm by cooperation from parents or a nurse, or by repeating the test until familiarity with the test situation is achieved.

On the technical side, we have found that needle electrodes placed after local anesthesia are very stable and movement artifacts originating in capacitive couplings to and between the leads can be avoided by proper fixation of the leads and by having a differential amplifier with high common mode rejection. Most important, however, is the introduction of an effective artifact rejection system similar to the adaptive system proposed by Skogstad Nielsen et al. (1971) and/or the application of ranking methods which can minimize the influence of artifacts.

IV. Response Variability

The most important condition for a successful application of averaging in order to improve signal-to-noise ratio and permit detection of a response is constancy of latency and shape of the evoked response. This condition is only met with approximation in adults, but instruction and control of both physical and mental behavior may secure reasonable constancy. In children, instructions to count the stimuli, to read, or otherwise ignore stimuli are unfeasible and the only useful action seems to be nursing and entertainment to minimize vigilance.

The technical consequence of varying shape and latency of the response is, as mentioned, an eroded, degenerate, and unpredictable average response. In our previous work (Salomon and Barfod, 1977), we showed that average evoked responses based on cluster analysis, which groups sweeps with comparable background activity, showed improved distinction of the responses within a cluster. This seems to indicate a correspondance between the response shape and the EEG background activity. In consequence, we considered the concept of adaptive filtering which aims at establishing time series which are more suitable for averaging than the observed EEG epochs. The aim of adaptive filtering is hence to establish filtered sweeps in which the response is of a more fixed latency and a more constant shape than in the original sweeps. However, the only basis for estimating the filter is the background activity since, as mentioned, the signal-to-noise ratio is very low, especially in children. A multitude of filter models could satisfy the condition of conforming the properties of the background noise to constitute a homogeneous ensemble. These approaches, however, will have different influence on the phase properties and thereby change the shape of a possible response in different ways. The model, which has been extensively investigated by us, is an all-pole filter model of adaptively varying order from 2 to 9 in which the parameters are determined by autoregression analysis on the single observed (demeaned and detrended) EEG epochs (Salomon and Barfod, 1977). Applying this model to the data is equivalent to assuming that the EEG and the evoked response are generated from a white noise source and an invariant impulse source, respectively, then adding and subsequently filtering through a common, but time-varying, all-pole filter generating the observed EEG at its output. Hence, to obtain the input to this filter, presumably suitable for averaging, the individual EEG epochs must be inversely filtered through an all-pole filter individually estimated for every recorded epoch. Averaging the derived input sequences thus obtained showed the presence of a transient-like distinct shape representing the evoked response. Furthermore, investigations on adults with induced alpha and beta rhythm, respectively, showed that the pulse shape in the averaged derived input is roughly independent of the type of background activity, whereas it may differ to some extent between individuals (Salomon and Barfod, 1977).

Evaluation of visual and automatic detection procedures based on average derived input epochs in comparison with the methods mentioned previously will be reported for 10 normally hearing children in the range ½ to 3½ years.

Evaluation of Detection Methods

In order confidently to apply a decision variable in the detection of the presence or absence of a response, it is necessary to know some principal statistical properties of this variable. Due to the possible severe consequences, the main clinical concern is a knowledge of the probability of false-positives.

A possibly difficult and inaccurate estimate of the degree of freedom and/or imperfect knowledge of the distribution of the decision variable may have severe effect on the performance of the statistical test applied. In visual determination the evaluation mechanisms and the strategy for making the decision are largely unknown. Consequently the important clinical parameter, -the probability of false-positives, cannot be evaluated on theoretical grounds. A solution to this problem requires evaluation methods independent of a specific knowledge of the statistical properties.

An efficient evaluation procedure based on empirical means is as follows. A signal processor and detector, usually termed receiver, can be described by the block diagram shown in Figure 3 and may be symbolized by the diagram of Figure 1. Here the two possible stimulus conditions, signal present (S) or no signal present ($\bar{S}$) is the input, and the two possible outcomes, a positive detection (D) and a negative detection ($\bar{D}$), are shown. The various combinations of these conditions are indicated inside the block and the erroneous conditions are symbolized with their

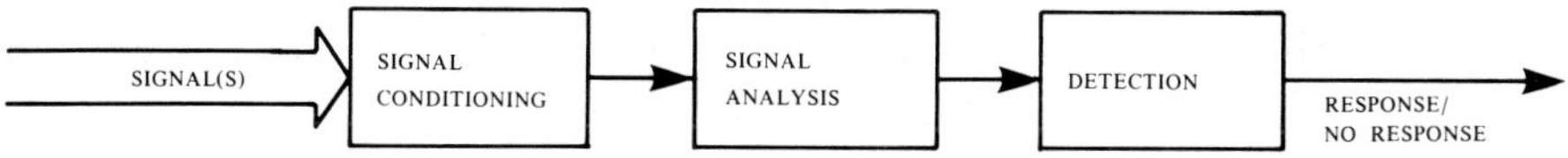

Fig. 3. Principal block diagram of an ERA receiver.

error type. Hence, detecting the signal when no signal was present is a type II error according to common nomenclature. For most types of receivers, the ratio between the two types of errors (false-positives and false-negatives) may be changed by changing the value of a single variable, often termed the criterion.

In order to evaluate a receiver, it is necessary to know the truth, ie. when signal was actually present or absent at the input of the receiver. To consider this problem in connection with ERA, it is necessary to decide whether hearing ability is associated with perception, comprehension and elicitation of an evoked response or rather the presence of the potential to perceive. Choosing the latter definition when evaluating enables us to define the truth as the presence of sound levels above normal threshold in the ears of a child who is unsuspected of audiological deficiencies and who from any other viewpoint is judged normal. The effect of this assumption on the evaluation method is discussed in Appendix I.

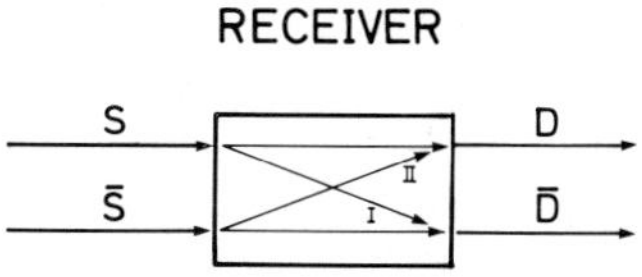

Fig. 4. Functional diagram of receiver. (See text.)

Provided information on the input condition is accessible, the performance of any receiver which conforms to the scheme of Figure 4 may be evaluated using the receiver operation characteristics (ROC) which maps the proportion of true-positive detections and corresponding properties of type II error for all possible criterion values (Fig. 5) (see Appendix I). Since the two variables generating the ROC are cumulative values, the ROC will be non-decreasing. In Figure 5, points corresponding to three values of the criterion are indicated.

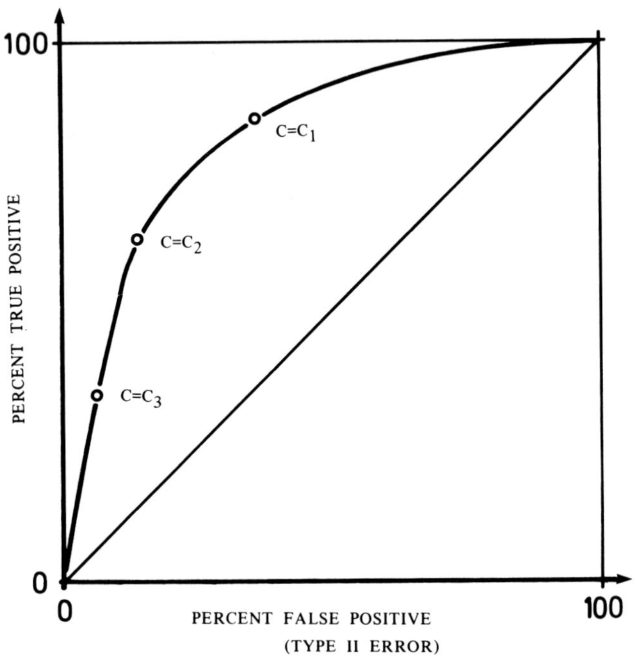

Fig. 5. Example of receiver operating characteristic. Points corresponding to three different values of the criterion are indicated.

A receiver which is incapable of distinguishing the presence of signal plus noise from noise alone at the input to the receiver will generate an ROC curve corresponding to the straight oblique (identity) line indicated in Figure 5. On this line the probability of positive detections (true-positives) is equal to the probability of false-positives, corresponding to guessing. Contrarily, a receiver which is very effective in discriminating presence of signal from no signal will have an ROC approaching the upper left corner of the figure. The ROC uniquely determines the performance of a receiver for all criterion values and readily gives information on the expected probability of false-positive detections.

Hence, to evaluate a receiver a large number of decision variables should be produced. Preferably half of the decision variables should be produced with stimulus and the other half without. The proportions of true-positive and false-positive detections in the observed data may then be evaluated for each of a number of selected criterion values. Plotting these data will generate an experimental ROC.

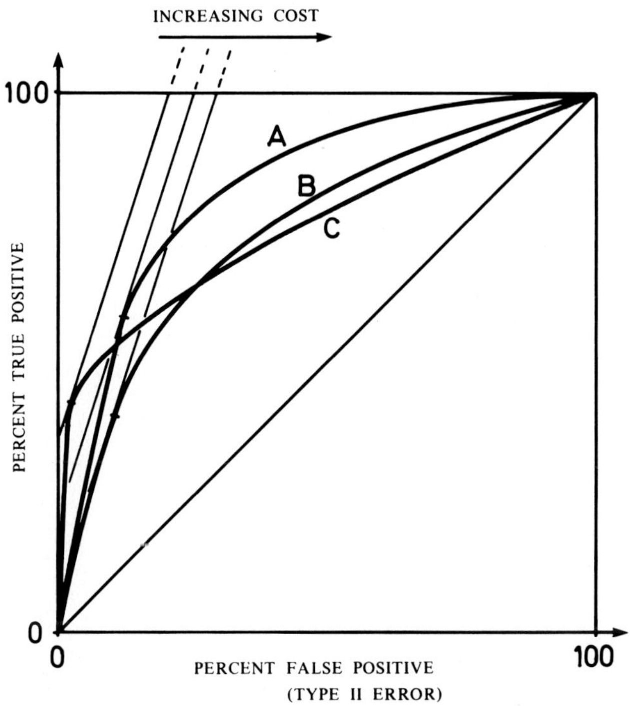

Fig. 6. Comparison between receiver operating characteristics for three hypothetical receivers A, B, and C. Optimum equal cost lines and optimum working points of the characteristics are indicated.

The properties of any receiver may now be compared to the properties of another receiver by comparing their ROC. Figure 6 illustrates examples of idealized ROCs. Several strategies exist for the comparison between ROCs. One is the Neyman-Pearson criterion, which, for a chosen probability of false-positive detections, eg. 5%, selects the receiver with the highest probability of true-positive detection. Another is the Bayesian strategy in which the excessive costs of erroneous decisions are evaluated. Lines of equal cost will have slopes determined by the ratio between the excessive cost of a type II error and the excessive cost of a type I error (see Appendix I). Figure 6 shows a field of equal-cost lines. The optimum criterion value to be chosen for any given ROC is the one which corresponds to a point for which the associated equal-cost line has the smallest cost. This equal-cost line will be a tangent to the ROC. Thus, the receiver to be preferred in the comparison of two receivers is the one associated with lowest cost for the optimum criterion. Hence, for the situation depicted in Figure 6, the receiver which has generated ROC 'C' should be preferred.

PART II

In our previous studies the clinical ERA results obtained in children below 4 years of age have been reported. The following attempts to minimize three of the four principal problems in vertex ERA in children were implemented:

I. In an attempt to enhance signal-to-noise ratio, the EEG was recorded with a 13 Hz low pass filter and a time constant varying from 3-10 sec, trying also to record the possible perstimulatory DC shift in response to 500 msec tone bursts. The stimulus interval was 2 sec.

II. To improve visual detection a multichannel write-out system was applied. Furthermore, response detection was aided by rank statistics (Salomon et al., 1973).

III. To reduce artifacts, an adaptive rejection system was used (Skogstad Nielsen et al., 1971). The use of drugs was avoided.

Using these countermeasures, and based on later subjective audiometry, less than 10% of the audiometric results were clinical errors (more than 30 dB difference), 85% of the determinations were within 20 dB and 65% within 10 dB (Salomon, 1975; 1976).

To evaluate the new development for a technical solution to the problem of response variability (IV), we have performed ERA using adaptive filtering and previously applied methods in a group of presumably normally-hearing children. In this study the artifact rejection system was excluded to avoid interaction in the comparison between the different response indicators. The evaluation was performed by visual inspection as well as by non-optimized automatic evaluation. Visual evaluation was included for two reasons: 1. visual evaluation of curves gives a good a priori impression of the pattern of a response, which in turn will help to choose the proper method for automatic evaluation; and 2. visual inspection of EEG audiometry is still the prevailing method.

Material

Five normal children between 6 months and 1 year and 5 normal children between 1½ and 3½ years were tested. Without any sedation, recordings were made between vertex and the mastoid with chlorided silver needles through an amplification system with a time constant of 10 seconds and an upper limiting frequency of 22 Hz (6 dB/octave). Fifty tone pips of 1000 Hz with a duration of 500 msec were delivered every 5 seconds. For each stimulus, two EEG epochs with a duration of 2400 msec were sampled, one starting 300 msec before the stimulus, and as a control, one interval containing only background noise starting 2200 msec after the stimulus. The sampling frequency was 62.5 Hz. The stimulus intensities delivered were aimed at 25, 55, and 85 dB SL using estimated corrections up to 10 dB based on otoscopic findings and measurement of middle ear pressure. In some children it was only possible to perform part of the test program due to restlessness.

Each EEG epoch was treated in the following way (Salomon and Barfod, 1977): After demeaning and detrending the EEG epoch the coefficient of an autoregressive series was determined for each post-stimulus epoch. The minimum number of coefficients (2-9) necessary for an adequate description of the epoch was determined adaptively for each epoch. By inverse filtering of each EEG epoch through the all-pole filter corresponding to the autoregressive series, input time series were derived for each EEG epoch.

Average EEGs and averaged derived inputs were produced for both observation and control epochs for each of the three stimulation intensities. A 15 Hz low-pass filtered version of the averaged derived input was also produced. Figure 7 shows examples of these curves from a child; to the left, the average EEG; in the middle column, the averaged derived input; and in the right column the 15 Hz low pass filtered version of the averaged derived input. Note how the derived input background is much more uniform than the EEG background.

Evaluation Methods

Double-blind visual evaluation was performed by two trained audiologists and two audio-engineers. The instruction for evaluation was that the responses could be expected in the interval between 80 and 400 msec post-stimulus. Each curve had to be classified "+" or "-" by forced choice, whereby 5 levels of detection were obtained: 4 +s, 3 +s, 2 +s, 1 +s, and 0 +s.

The objective evaluation was based on rank statistics as described earlier (Salomon, 1973) (model 1, based on ranking of dV/dt and using selected sample points in the interval -140 msec to +1300 msec relative to the stimulus onset). For derived input and derived input 15 Hz low-pass filtered, a simple preliminary decision variable was used. This was the ratio between the RMS value in the time interval between 84 and 404 msec, presumably containing both signal and noise, and the RMS value in the interval from 516 to 1620 msec post-stimulus only containing noise. Portions at the beginning and end of the derived epoch were avoided, since they may contain artifacts from the inverse filtering procedure applied.

Results

The ROC curve for visual scoring of the averaged EEG at 85 and 55 dB is shown in Figure 8. This scoring is very inefficient: with 5% false-positive recognitions only 12% correct recognitions have been made at 55 dB and 42% at 85 dB. The characteristic at 25 dB is not drawn, because it does not deviate significantly from the oblique line. Although some improvement could be expected by increasing the number of post-stimulus epochs and possibly by introducing artifact rejection, the performance outline may well be representative of the ERA performance in many clinics.

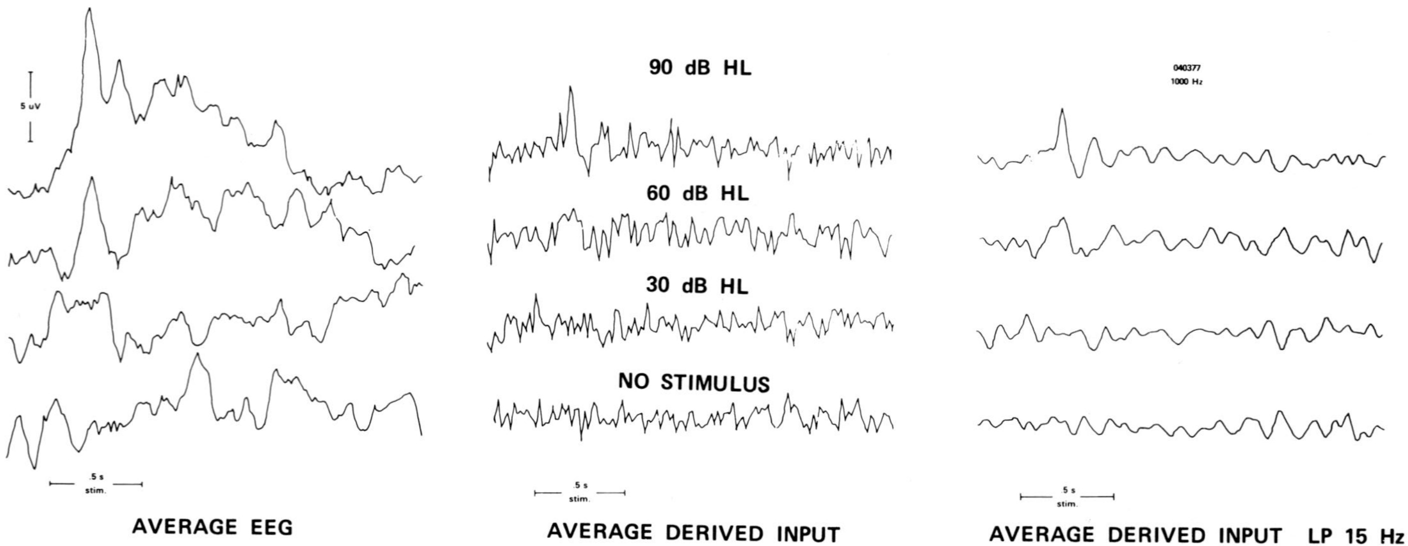

Fig. 7. Example of adaptive filtering of EEG for four stimulus conditions. Left: Averages without processing; center: average of derived input after adaptive inverse filtering; right: average derived input low-pass filtered with 15Hz cut-off frequency. Averages are based on 50 epochs.

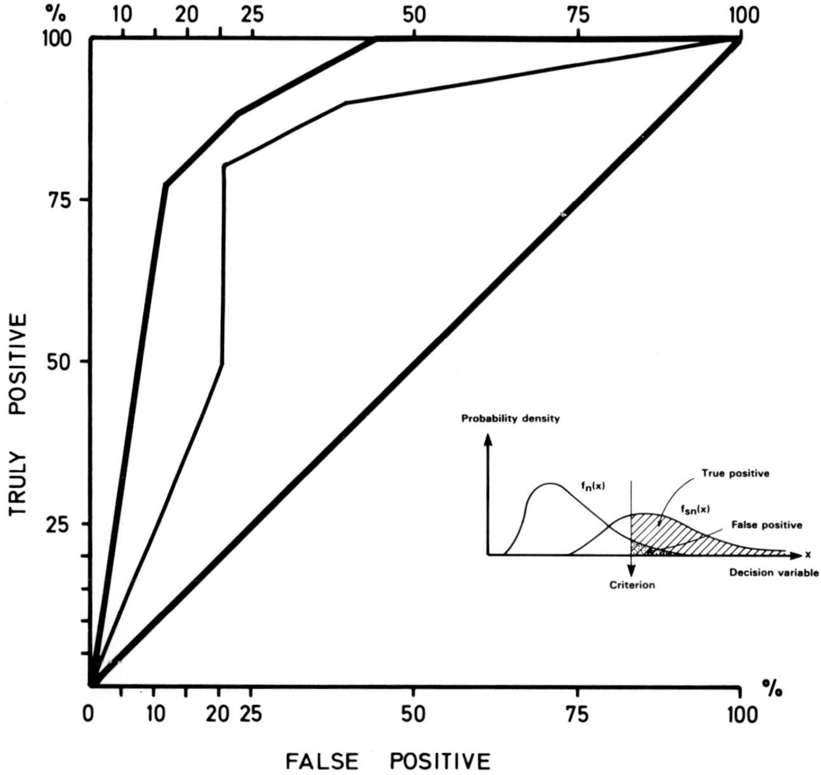

Fig. 8. ROC for detection of sound evoked vertex response based on visual recognition and averaged EEG epochs. Heavy line: 85dB SL, light line: 55dB SL.

The visual scoring of the derived input shown in Figure 9 compares favorably with the EEG scoring. With a 5% false-positive score rate a 70% correct positive recognition is made, both at 55 and 85 dB. The characteristic at 25 dB is not shown, because it does not deviate significantly from the oblique line. The extremely good performance at 85 dB is not reflected in the objective scoring of the derived input with our present method (see later).

From the type of recording shown in Figure 7 we expected an improvement in visual scoring by low-pass filtering compared to the unfiltered version of the derived input. As shown in Figure 10, the 55 dB curve does, in fact, show a slight improvement, but only for unacceptably high rates of false-positive scores (such as 20%). The characteristic at 85 dB deteriorates very much compared with the unfiltered version, probably because the low-pass filtering is preventing visual recognition of the sharp peak in the response.

The performance at 25 dB could raise the suspicion that no response was present at all. Consequently, we produced an ROC by combining all visual scores. This compounded ROC is shown in Figure 11 and demonstrates that the 25 dB stimulus does, in fact, produce a response; our future goal must be to detect this response with a limited number of stimuli.

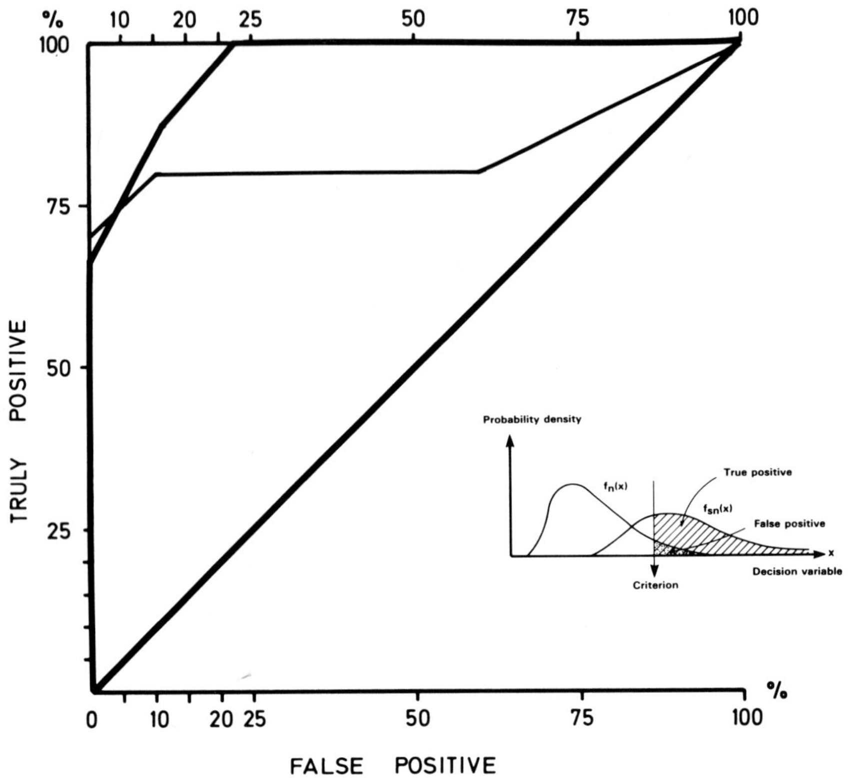

Fig. 9. ROC for detection of sound-evoked vertex response based on visual scoring of averaged derived input. Heavy line: 85dB SL, light line: 55dB SL.

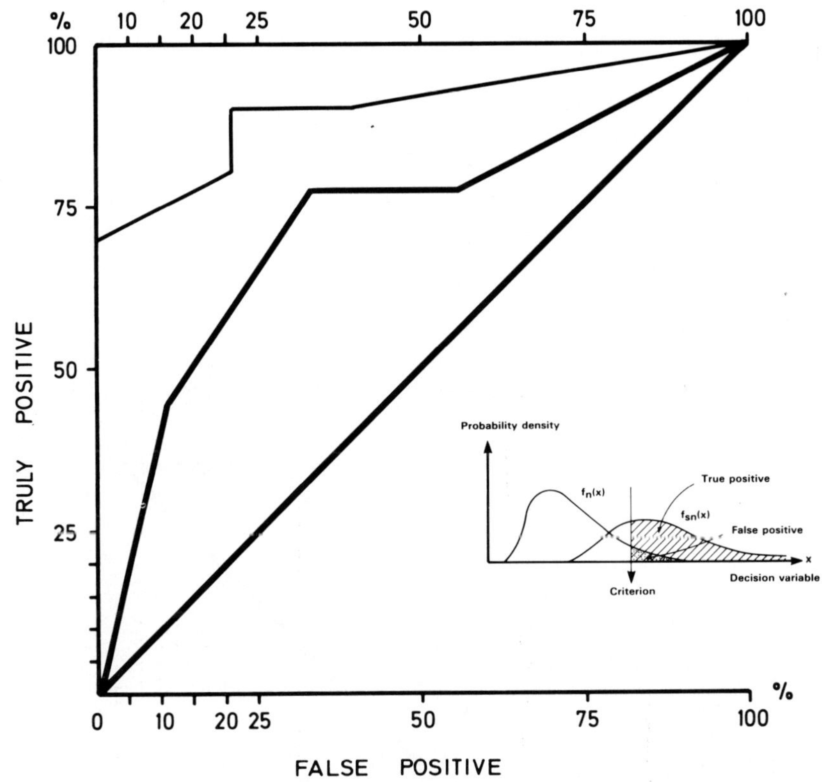

Fig. 10. ROC for detection of sound-evoked vertex response based on visual scoring of averaged derived input, low pass filtered at 15Hz. Heavy line: 85dB SL, light line: 55dB SL.

To evaluate the efficiency of using rank statistics, this procedure is compared to visual judgment. In Figure 12 the ROC of visual identification of the EEG response is superimposed on the ROC of response recognition based on rank statistics. At a criterion value producing 5% false-positive scores, an increase from about 30% to 90% is seen at 85 dB in the percentage of correct scores, and an increase from 12% to 25% at 55 dB. Thus, our earlier findings (Salomon, 1975, 1976) that rank statistics serve as an efficient tool in the clinic and that automatic procedures must be preferred to visual scoring are substantiated. Note how close the rank statistic curve comes to the ROC of a perfect receiver at 85 dB.

To compare determinations based on rank statistics of EEG with automatic scoring of derived input 15 Hz low-pass filtered, the ROC curves for the two procedures were superimposed. Figure 13 shows these superimposed curves at 85 dB. The ROC for derived input without low-pass filtering are approximately equal to the curve for the filtered version. The ROC curve for objective scoring of derived input does not perform very impressively in contrast to the ROC curve for visual scoring of derived input (Fig. 9), which performs very much like the rank statistic curve outlined here. This indicates that the automatic scoring of derived input

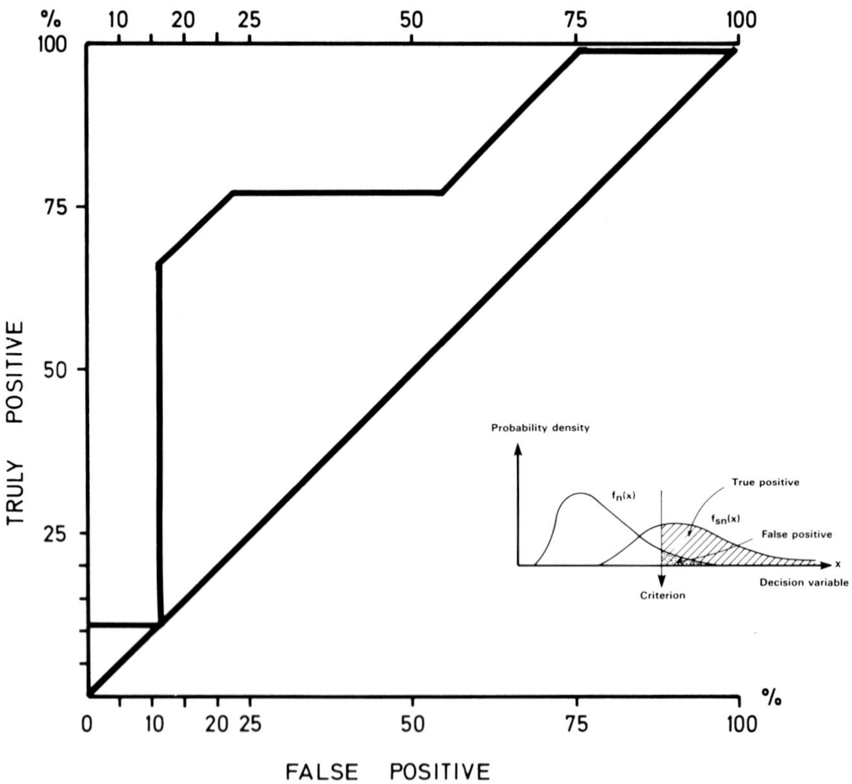

Fig. 11. ROC for detection of sound-evoked vertex response from 25dB SL using visual scores from both averaged EEGs, averaged derived input, and averaged low pass filtered derived input.

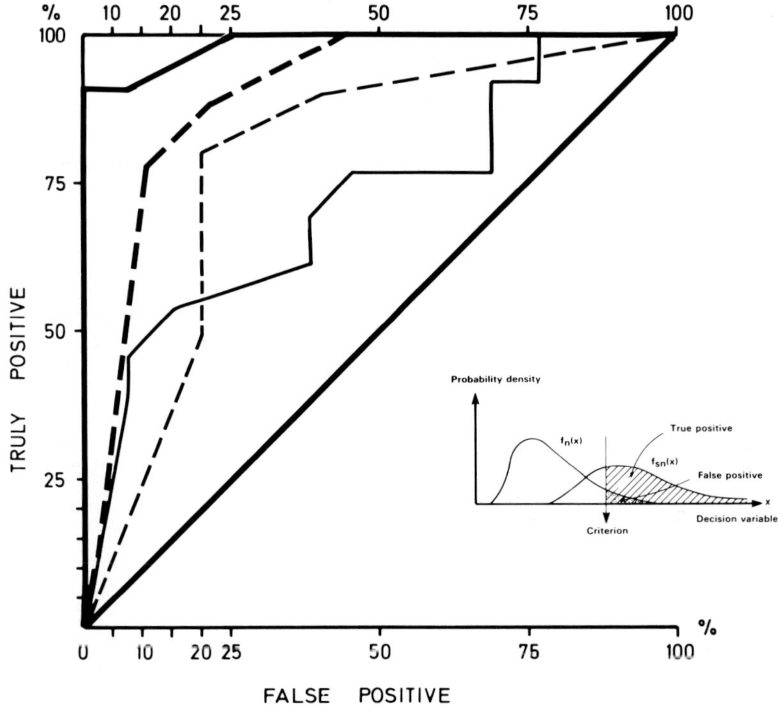

Fig. 12. ROC for detection of sound-evoked vertex response. Comparison between visual recognition in average EEG epochs (broken lines) and detection based on rank statistics (solid lines). Heavy lines: 85dB SL, light lines: 55dB SL.

using the present decision variable is inferior at 85 dB in its ability to identify the response. The lack of identification of the sound-evoked signal may be caused by the fact that the RMS value after the response at this intensity still contains stimulus-evoked activity. At the same time impressive performance using visual scores could be more dependent on changes of pattern than on changes in amplitude. An improved automatic scoring should give the same good results as the visual scores of derived input and should be expected to show at least the same performance at high intensities as rank statistics based on EEG. The superimposed ROC curves for determinations based on rank statistics and on derived input at 55 dB (Fig. 14) show that the automatic scoring of derived input is highly superior to rank statistics and nearly identical to the visual scoring of the same data (Fig. 9). At 5% rate of false-positive scores, approximately 80% correct positive scores are obtained. Consequently the use of automatic scoring on derived input is superior to rank statistics at lower intensities, i.e. smaller response amplitudes, which is most important for audiometric application.

Discussion

The detectability of a sound-evoked late vertex response in the clinical situation can be enhanced by a series of procedures, most of which are dependent on access to statistical methods involving the original data from each post-stimulus epoch. Access to single epochs is also a prerequisite for efficient adaptive artifact rejection. This seems to argue strongly against simple hard-wired averagers for vertex audiometry.

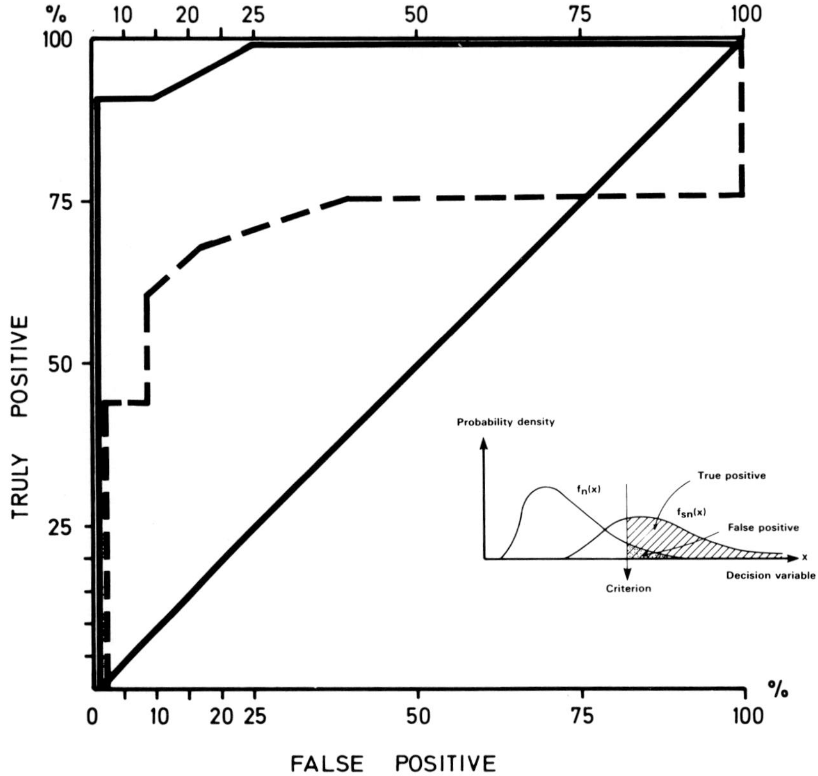

Fig. 13. ROC for detection of sound-evoked vertex response. Comparison between detection based on rank statistics (solid line) and detection based on ratio between energy in different parts of 15 Hz low pass filtered derived input. 85dB SL, 1 kHz.

The effect on the detectability of substituting the original EEG with a derived input must be evaluated by taking the following considerations into account: normally, a clinical trial will be based on approximately 100 stimuli and not on 50, as in the tests reported. The procedure will include artifact rejection and, most important, the children with cochlear hearing loss will normally show recruitment. Thus medium sensations of loudness and medium response amplitudes will be obtained at only 10-20 dB above threshold. A clinical follow-up on the use of the

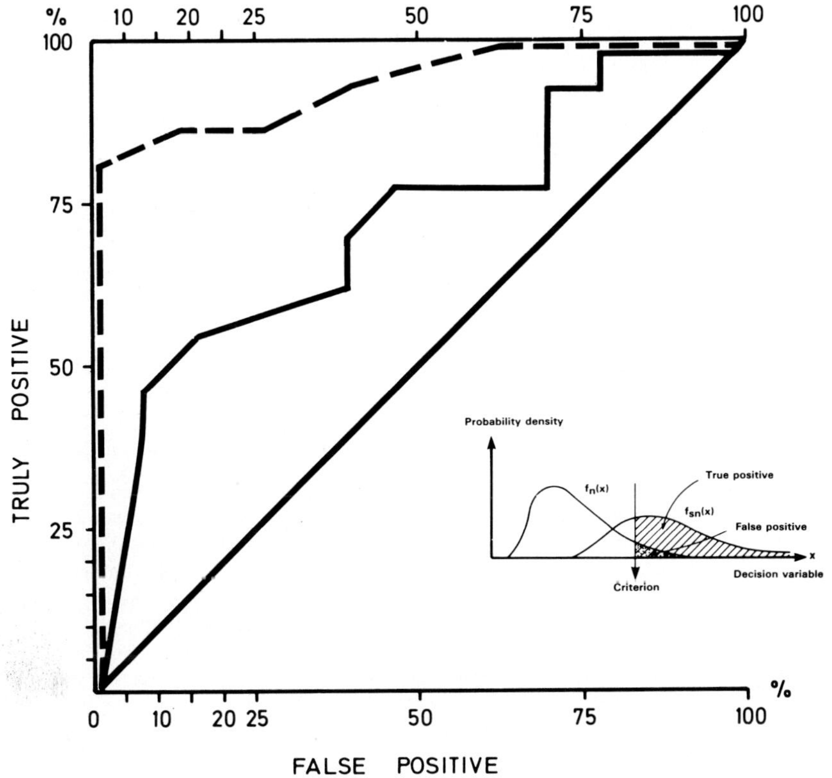

Fig. 14. ROC for detection of sound-evoked vertex response. Comparison between detection based on rank statistics (solid line) and detection based on ratio between energy in different parts of 15 Hz low pass filtered derived input. 55dB SL, 1 kHz.

adaptive filtering procedure proposed could thus be expected to improve the clinical results compared with earlier follow-up studies (Salomon, 1976).

For vertex ERA to be an effective supplement to other electrophysiological methods (ECoG & BSER) and not merely an unreliable competitor, it is necessary that the results from vertex ERA confidently reflect real malfunctions. To achieve this, it is necessary to apply advanced methodology and statistical evaluation procedures such as are outlined here.

The results obtained using the technical improvements mentioned are encouraging. Further investigations covering the applicability of the concept of adaptive inverse filtering in other conditions and further improvements of automatic detection procedures are necessary and in progress.

APPENDIX I

Receiver Operating Characteristic

Most receivers would be adequately described as consisting of a signal processing part producing a decision variable and a detector making the decisions according to some criterion (Fig. A1). The detector is most often of a type which compares the decision variable to the criterion and indicates a detection when the decision variable exceeds the criterion. If the statistical destribution of the decision variable is known in cases when only noise is present and

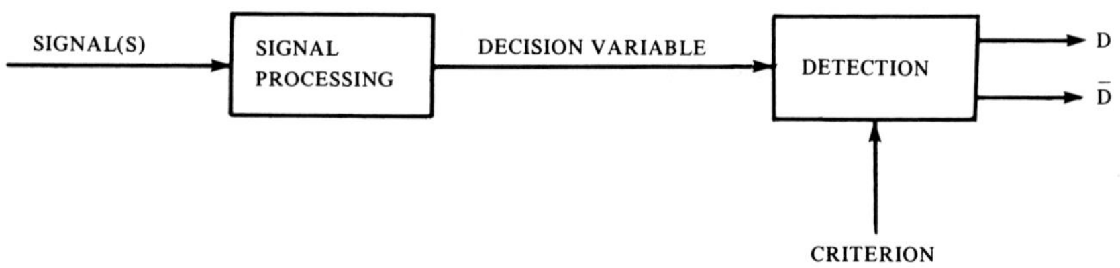

Fig. A1. Block diagram of receiver.

in cases when both signal and noise are present, the situation may be as in Figure A2. If the decision variable on any occasion exceeds the criterion indicated, the detector would announce a positive detection. The probability of erroneous detections are indicated by the shaded areas of Figure A2. False-negative (1-P (true positive)) decisions are also named type I errors, while false-positives are named type II errors. Changing the criterion will change the performance of the receiver by changing the proportion of true positives and trading the frequency of one type of error for the other. Establishing the relationship between the probability of false-positive detections (type II errors) and the probability of true positive detections for all possible criterion values will generate a receiver operating characteristic (ROC) which is illustrated in Figure 5. (See Lusted, 1968, for a comprehensive treatment with many practical examples related to medical science).

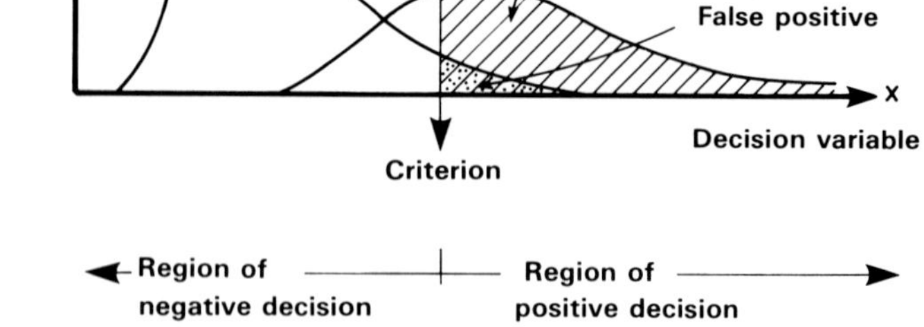

Fig. A2. Hypothetical distributions of the decision variables x, when only noise is present ($f_n(x)$) and when both signal and noise are present ($f_{sn}(x)$). Areas equal to the probability of true positive detection and false-positive detections for the shown criterion are indicated.

Determination of Bayes Criterion

The Bayes approach for decision making is based on an evaluation of the costs involved. Denoting the excessive costs for erroneous decisions C_I and C_{II} respectively, permits the evaluation of the entire cost C:

$$C = C_{II}p_{II} + C_I p_I$$

where p_I is the probability of type I error and p_{II} is the probability of type II errors.

This formula is equivalent to:

$$p_D = (1-p_I) = C_{II}p_{II}/C_I + 1 - C/C_I \tag{1}$$

where p_D denotes the probability of true positive detections (ordinate on the ROC).

Keeping C constant, (1) will produce a straight line in the ROC space with slope C_{II}/C_I. Hence, lines of slope C_{II}/C_I are lines of equal cost (Fig. 6).

An interesting consequence of this evaluation is that if an ROC at no point has a slope equal to or exceeding C_{II}/C_I, it would be desirable not to perform the investigation at all, but to assume that no positive response is present in all cases. The implication is that although a receiver performs significantly better than guessing, it should be avoided, not because of the cost of applying the receiver, but because of the relationship between costs of erroneous decisions. This again means that if the cost relationship is changed, a previously discarded receiver may prove to be a good choice.

Effect of Uncontrolled Response Suppression in the System Under Test

The evaluation performed is based on the assumption that a signal (evoked response) is present to the receiver when an acoustic signal having a level above normal threshold is presented to a normal subject's ear. A model of the system taking into account that this may not be true is given in Figure A3. Here the gate switches off the signal transmission with proba-

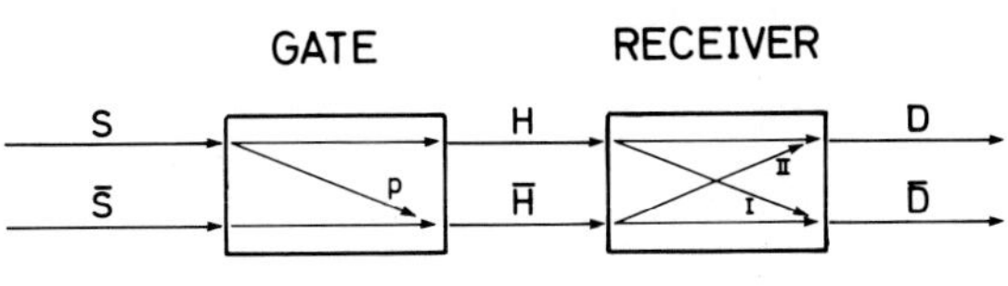

Fig. A3. Diagram of receiver system including signal suppression gate operating with unknown probability p.

bility p and the input to the receiver is now whether the condition H or H̄ is present. Assuming that the ROC for the receiver only is given (primed symbols) the ROC for the entire system including the gate may be computed:

$$p'_D = p'_D (1-p) + pp'_{II} = p'_D - p\,(p'_D - p'_{II})$$

$$p_{II} = p'_{II}$$

Hence, the ROC of the receiver including the gate will approach the 'guessing' line for $p \rightarrow 1$ and will be inferior to the ROC of the real receiver at all points, provided $p'_D > p'_2$ which is the case for operational receivers.

APPENDIX II

Distribution of Extreme Values

Let $x_1, x_2, x_3 \ldots\ldots x_n$ be equally and independently distributed with distribution function F(x).

The probability that the largest x_i among n is greater than C is complementary to that no x_i exceeds C. The probability of $x_i < C$ is F(C). The probability that all x_i (i = 1,n) does not exceed C is $F(C)^n$. Hence, the probability that the largest x_i exceeds C is $1 - F(C)^n$. Correspondingly, the probability that the smallest x_i is below C is $1 - (1\text{-}F(C))^n$.

REFERENCES

Brix, R. The significance "CNV-audiometry" and their relationship to the "late evoked potentials". Paper presented at the Vth Biennal International Symposium of the International Electric Response Audiometry Study Group, Jerusalem, 1977.

Burian, K. and Gestring, G.F. Discrepancies between subjective and objective acoustic thresholds. *Arch. Ohr.-Nas-Keilk. 198:* 73-82, 1971.

Cohen, M.M., Rapin, I., Lyttle, M. and Schimmel, H. Auditory evoked response. *Arch. Otolaryngol. 94:* 214-219, 1971.

Davis, P.A. Effect of acoustic stimuli on the waken human brain. *J. Neurophysiol. 2:* 494-499, 1939.

Davis, H., Mast, T. and Yoshie, N. The slow response of the humane cortex to auditory stimuli: recovery process. *Electroencephalogr. Clin. Neurophysiol. 21:* 105-113, 1966.

Friedmann, M. The use of ranks to avoid the assumption of normality implicit in the analysis of variance. *J. Am. Stat. Ass. 32:* 675, 1937.

Geisler, C.D., Frishkopf, L.S. and Rosenblith, W.A. Extra cranial response to acoustic clicks in man. *Science 128:* 1210-1211, 1958.

Lentz, W.E. and McCandless, G.A. Averaged electroencephalic audiometry in infants. *J. Speech Hear. Dis. 36:* 19-28, 1971.

Lusted, L.B. *Introduction to medical decision making.* Springfield; Charles C Thomas, 1968.

Mituyosi, A. Electrical responses of the human brain to acoustic stimulus. *Tohoku J. Exp. Med. 60:* 47-58, 1954.

Rose, D.E., Keating, L.W., Hedgecock, L.D., Selreurs, K.K. and Miller, K.E. Aspects of Acoustically evoked responses. *Arch. Otolaryngol. 94:* 347-350, 1971.

Salomon, G. Clinical "electrical response audiometry" on a general-purpose computer (IBM 1800). *Acta Otolaryngol.* Suppl. *263:* 238-241, 1970.

Salomon, G., Beck, O. and Elberling, C. The role of sedation in ERA from the vertex. *Audiology 12:* 150-166, 1973.

Salomon, G. Electric response audiometry (ERA) based on rank correlation. *Audiology 13:* 181-194, 1974.

Salomon, G. Automatic evaluation of human auditory evoked potentials from the vertex. *Symp. Zool. Soc. London 37:* 205-236, 1975.

Salomon, G. The electric response audiometry (ERA) from the vertex in paedoaudiology. Technical basis, clinical results and new developments. *J. Audiol. Tech. 15:* 2-27, 1976.

Salomon, G. and Barfod, J. A new concept of vertex ERA and EEG analysis applying inverse filtering. *Acta Otolaryngol. 83:* 200-210, 1977.

Schimmel, H., Rapin, I. and Cohen, M.M. Improving evoked response audiometry with special reference to the use of machine scoring. *Audiology 13:* 33-65, 1974.

Skogstad Nielsen, S., Salomon, G. and Elberling, C. Evoked response audiometry from the vertex using an IBM 1800 time-sharing system in clinical use. *Comp. Prog. Biomed. 2:* 24-35, 1971.

Spreng, M. Detection of influence of latency variability upon the averaged evoked responses. *Int. Audiol. 9:* 304-308, 1970.

Suzuki, T., Yamamoto, K., Taguchi, K. and Sakabe, N. Reliability and validity of late vertex-evoked response audiometry. *Audiology 15:* 357-369, 1976.

Thornton, A.R.D. Averaged evoked brain stem responses and their analysis for diagnostic application. Proceedings of Symposium in Application of Time Series Analysis. Southampton University, 1977.

DISCUSSION

Galambos: Can you give an estimate of what we must add to our computers to accomplish this analysis of yours?

Salomon: You will have to add a 16k unit, but you could get it fix-wired, so in money it would not be more than maybe $5,000 or something like that. But then you can use it for a lot of other types of statistics in your clinic at the same time.

Black: I am curious to know what the spectral coherence values of the outputs were from the noise stimuli.

Salomon: I didn't get what you asked.

Black: I was curious to know what the spectral coherence values were for the outputs when you used the white noise inputs.

Salomon: We derived the white noise and checked that it was a white noise by autocorrelation.

Black: I am asking whether part of the insensitivity of the technique may be due to the fact that you can't differentiate CNS noise from the signal, and whether the coherence values would estimate how much of the recorded evoked potential is correlated with your signal and how much of the signal is due to "background" noise. The sensitivity of the method may be related to how much uncontrolled input exists from other sources. How much limitation is there in the technique, because the EEG is such an indirect method relating the input to response?

Salomon: What you are really asking is, is it possible to estimate such a filter?

Black: That is correct.

Salomon: The answer is yes, but the autoregressive estimate gets very complicated with some EEG waveforms, and you have to use more and more coefficients in your autoregression to get the noise. Sometimes you will not be able to get it at all. We adapt the number of coefficients all the time to control that we really get white noise on the input side.

Black: If I understood you correctly, you did average the response.

Salomon: The average response?

Black: Period average the responses. How many periods do you have to average as a general rule, would you say?

Salomon: We derive the input from each post-stimulus epoch at the time.

Black: You did the derivation before you did the averaging?

Salomon: Oh yes, certainly.

EVOKED POTENTIAL AUDIOMETRY IN NEUROLOGICALLY IMPAIRED CHILDREN

Manuel M. Cohen and Isabelle Rapin

Albert Einstein College of Medicine

INTRODUCTION

The power of auditory evoked potentials (AEP) for audiometry in children too young or too impaired neurologically to cooperate for valid behavioral testing was recognized as soon as the technique became available. A decade ago, Rapin and Graziani (1967) described their findings in 21 infants under 3 years of age with brain pathology in whom they recorded late cortical AEPs. Rapin et al. (1970) later extended these observations to 30 brain damaged infants under one year of age. Fifty-one children with congenital rubella, 26 of whom were moderately to severely impaired neurologically, were also studied (Rapin et al., 1969). Our conclusion from these studies was that assessment of auditory function by late cortical evoked potentials in severely retarded infants and children was likely to yield a lower threshold than behavioral testing because low intensity stimuli do not elicit explicit behavioral responses reliably in these children. We noted that severely abnormal EEGs might interfere with threshold detection by late AEPs and that, as one might expect, no AEPs were recordable in children with isoelectric EEGs. We found asymmetric AEPs with lower voltage and higher threshold on the side of greater brain damage in one infant (Rapin and Graziani 1967) and Peronnet et al. (1974) reported AEPs of lower amplitude over the left hemisphere in aphasic patients. Unreliability in the assessment of auditory threshold with late AEPs when the EEG is very abnormal was also evident in a study by Hogan (1971) who studied 15 institutionalized adults with mental retardation and cerebral palsy: two of the 15, both of whom had high voltage abnormal EEGs, did not have detectable AEPs at 50 dB HL, unlike all but one of the others and all 15 controls. The question of whether late AEPs are masked by the abnormal EEG or whether the brain is so abnormal as to preclude their generation in a given patient is unanswered and must await the elucidation of the generators for late AEPs.

Brain damage does not necessarily decrease the amplitude of AEPs. Bigum et al. (1970) and Barnet et al. (1971) noted that the amplitude of visual, somatosensory and auditory evoked potentials was higher in children with trisomy 21 (Down's syndrome) than in normal children because of failure to habituate on

ISBN 0-12-514960-3

repeated stimulus presentation. Ornitz et al. (1968) found that in autistic children the amplitude of the N_2 wave of the late auditory cortical evoked response was greater than in normals during rapid eye movement sleep and, specifically, during the bursts of eye movements. These three studies did not address themselves to the question of threshold detection by late AEPs.

As one would expect, some children with brain damage, particularly those with rubella, kernicterus, and the sequellae of purulent meningitis, are likely to sustain damage both to the brain and to the cochlea. When an elevated threshold for late AEPs is found in these patients it is impossible to be sure of the site of pathology within the auditory pathway unless other measures are available. Advances in the past decade now enable us to resolve this dilemma.

Electrocochleography (Ruben et al., 1976) consists in recording the cochlear microphonic (receptor potential) and action potential of the acoustic nerve, but in most laboratories is carried out after insertion of a transtympanic electrode under general anesthesia in young children. Early AEPs are considered to reflect activation of the various subcortical auditory relay nuclei (Jewett and Williston, 1971), based on information from animal experiments and from patients with documented focal lesions in the brain stem (Starr and Achor, 1975; Sohmer et al., 1974; Stockard and Rossiter, 1977). It may be possible to pinpoint the site of pathology in cases where both cochlear and brain stem potentials can be recorded from surface electrodes (Tanahashi et al., 1976; Feinmesser and Sohmer, 1976). Onishi and Manabe (1976) reported a strong correlation between their patients' pure tone behavioral audiograms and acoustic thresholds based on cochleography and early AEPs for a one cycle 4000 Hz stimulus. Both the acoustic nerve action potential and brain stem response predominantly reflect activity at the basal end of the cochlea.

The relative ease of recording early AEPs (in contrast to late AEPs, they are resistant to sedation and anesthetics and do not vary with the phase of sleep) has led them to supplant late AEPs for audiometry in many laboratories, especially in young children with hearing impairment and brain damage (Onishi and Manabe, 1976; Mokotoff et al., 1977). They are easily recorded in newborns and prematures (Hecox and Galambos, 1974; Schulman-Galambos and Galambos, 1975). The latency of wave V decreases with maturation (Salamy et al., 1976) reflecting increasing conduction velocity with age. Sohmer et al. (1974) described several brain damaged children in whom the electrocochleogram was normal and/or in whom one or more of the later waves of the early AEP were detected even though the children appeared hearing impaired. While that study did not provide information about late AEPs, Galambos and Hecox (1977) reported a patient with a diffuse metabolic disease of the brain in whom absent late AEPs with preserved early AEPs was correlated with lack of behavioral response to sound.

The present study compares auditory thresholds based on behavioral tests with those indicated by early and late AEP recordings in a group of children with a variety of neurologic impairments, in order to examine the usefulness of these two approaches to electrophysiologic audiometry in the clinical assessment of multiply handicapped children.

METHODS

Children considered for inclusion in this study had a suspected hearing loss or delayed language development and had been referred for testing with AEP because reliable behavioral audiometry could not be obtained because of their young age or of associated deficits. The clinical records of all children tested in the AEP laboratory between 1975 and 1977 were reviewed. Charts of children whose only deficit was a hearing loss were discarded; all others were retained. The children's lack of responsiveness to sound and/or delayed or absent language development was associated with a variety of handicaps such as mental retardation, motor deficits, hyperkinetic behavior, autistic behavior and blindness. Data pertaining to medical diagnosis, findings on neurologic examination, EEG and special investigations, and assessment of behavior and intellectual function were abstracted, as were the results of behavioral and impedance audiometry. All but a few had been investigated in hospitals associated with the Albert Einstein College of Medicine. A minority of the children had been examined clinically by one or both of the authors. No child had to be discarded from the study for lack of clinical information, although clinical data were not necessarily complete for every child.

AEP testing was carried out in a sound proof room, usually with the child asleep and watched by his mother. Most were sedated with chloral hydrate, promethazine (Phenergan) and/or chlorpromazine (Thorazine). Gold cup electrodes were attached to the scalp at C_Z, T_4, T_3 according to the international 10-20 EEG electrode placement system, using linked mastoid or earlobe electrodes as reference. For those children in whom visual evoked potentials (VEP) were recorded, electrodes were placed at 0_2 and 0_1. Interelectrode resistance was kept below 10K ohms.

For recording early AEPs stimuli were 2000 to 4000 clicks (0.125 msec square waves) or tone pips (rise and decay of 1.5 msec, plateau 1 msec) at 2000 and and/or 4000 Hz delivered at a rate of 10 or 27 per second to each of the ears through TDH-39 earphones. For recording late AEPs stimuli were 64 tones with frequencies of 500 and 2000 Hz (20 msec rise and decay, 400 msec plateau) delivered approximately once every 2.2 seconds through an overhead speaker. Tone pip and click intensity levels were expressed in dB relative to subjective threshold of 5 normal-hearing adult listeners with pure tone thresholds between 0 and 5 dB HL (ANSI 1969) for frequencies between 250 and 8000 Hz. Intensities of the pure tones were expressed in dB HL (ANSI 1969). For early potentials the first intensity tested was 60 dB. If a response was detected, stimulus intensity was lowered to 30 dB and threshold estimated in 10 dB steps. If no response was detected at 60 dB, intensity was raised to 100 dB. If a response was present, intensity was then lowered and threshold estimated in 10 dB steps. Each intensity level was presented 3 times on the average. For late potentials intensities tested included 30, 50, 70, 80 and 100 dB HL. Stimuli at one intensity level were delivered in a block, with intensity varied quasi-randomly between blocks. Each intensity was presented 4 times on the average. Visual evoked potentials were obtained with monocular flash stimulation using a Grass PS-2 photo stimulator set at intensity 16, placed at approximately 2 feet from the child's face, and delivered 100 times in the presence of sufficient white noise masking to render its click inaudible. For all stimulus conditions, control runs without a stimulus were also recorded. To provide an estimate of the background EEG during the sampling epoch, a (±) reference channel (Schimmel, 1967) was used in which EEG samples were alternately added and subtracted, thereby cancelling time-locked components.

For early AEPs the EEG was amplified 400,000 times and a pass band of 90 to 3000 Hz was recorded. For late AEPs amplification was 10,000 times and the pass band 1 to 100 Hz. The EEG was fed into a CAT 1000 averager, monitored on an oscilloscope and recorded on paper in order to detect movement and muscle artifacts so that contaminated records could be discarded. AEP records were scored visually without knowledge of the stimulus conditions or identity of the child. A stimulus condition was scored as suprathreshold if at least two out of four records were scored as positive. The records without stimuli were used to evaluate the probability of false positive scores in each patient when threshold detection was uncertain.

All behavioral audiograms were obtained by two audiologists in a sound treated booth. For the few children who were conditionable, play audiometry or conditioned orienting response (COR) audiometry was utilized. Even in these children, threshold estimate was not totally reliable, although it ruled out a severe or profound hearing loss. For the majority of children in whom retardation, blindness or brain damage did not permit the use of conditioning techniques, testing was limited to behavioral observation of unconditioned responses to sound. Most patients had 2 or more behavioral tests. Most children were also tested with impedance audiometry.

Comparisons were made between AEP threshold estimates and the most reliable behavioral threshold estimate obtained at about the date of the AEP test. Hearing threshold estimated by early AEPs was assumed to lie 10 dB below the lowest intensity that evoked a brain stem potential. Hearing threshold by late AEPs was assumed to lie 20 dB below the lowest intensity that evoked a late cortical potential (Rapin et al., 1970; Mendel et al., 1975). The categories used for the degree of hearing loss were derived from those of Katz (1972), and included normal-mild (0-40 dB), moderate (41-70), severe (71-90) and profound (> 90 dB). When late AEPs were detected at one intensity level and inconsistently at the next lower level, hearing threshold by AEP was assumed to lie somewhere between the two levels tested, e.g. between moderate and severe levels. For the purposes of constructing graphs comparing behavioral and AEP threshold estimates, the category of loss chosen was always the less severe of the two categories between which threshold was assumed to fall.

Comparisons between behavioral and electrophysiologic estimates of hearing are displayed in Figures 1, 2, 4-7. In all figures, behavioral estimates of hearing threshold are displayed on the abscissa, and AEP estimates of hearing threshold on the ordinate. Open symbols refer to late cortical potentials, closed symbols to early brain stem potentials. Each symbol represents an individual child. When a closed

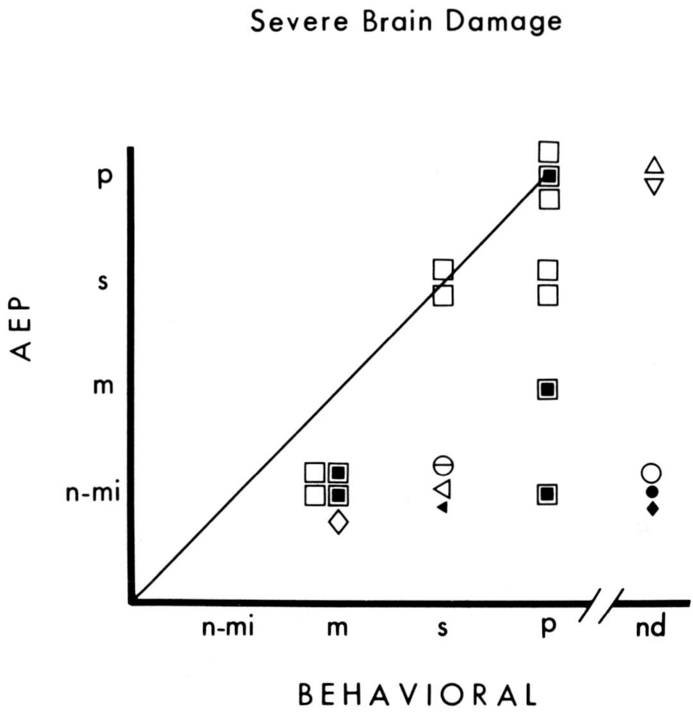

Fig. 1. Correlation of hearing thresholds obtained by AEP techniques with those obtained by behavioral audiometry in a group of 19 severely brain damaged and retarded children (median age 25 months). The letters located on the ordinate and abscissa of this and all succeeding figures indicate the severity of hearing loss as follows: n-mi (normal–mild), m (moderate), s (severe), p (profound). On the abscissa nd represents those cases where no data were available by behavioral audiometry at the specific frequency used for the AEP, or cases where a particular child was untestable by behavioral methods. Each open symbol represents the late AEP threshold estimate of a different child while closed symbols represent their early AEP threshold estimates. When early and late AEP threshold estimates were obtained for the same frequency (e.g. 2k Hz) and were in agreement, they appear as closed within open symbols. However, when a child's closed and open symbols do not coincide, this indicates that early and late AEPs were obtained for different stimulus frequencies.

symbol is depicted within an open symbol, threshold for early and late potentials for the same frequency for that child coincide. When early and late potentials for a child appear one above the other at the same or different intensity levels, they were obtained at different frequencies (usually the late potentials at 500 Hz, the early at 2000 and/or 4000 Hz). Behavioral levels always refer to threshold for the frequency at which the AEP threshold was obtained. For the sake of clarity, the data for only one frequency (usually 2000 Hz) per child were included in the figures, except in those cases where behavioral, early and late potentials were not available for the same frequency. For all figures, symbols falling on the diagonal indicate agreement between behavioral and electrophysiologic thresholds of hearing. Symbols falling below the diagonal indicate that electrophysiologic were lower than behavioral thresholds; symbols above the diagonal indicate that behavioral were below electrophysiologic estimates. In the absence of independent methods for assessing auditory threshold, it is not possible to determine whether a higher estimate of threshold by one method represents a lack of sensitivity of that method (type I error), or whether the lower threshold by the other method is erroneous and reflects a false-positive result (type II error for the method with lower threshold).

RESULTS

As one would expect from a sample of patients referred to a clinical facility for testing, the population was heterogeneous with respect to clinical diagnosis, severity and variety of handicaps. For the purposes of this study, the children were separated into several clinical subgroups in order to evaluate the results of evoked response audiometry (ERA) as a function of neurologic status.

Severely Brain Damaged Children

The largest sample was made up of 38 children with gross brain damage. Excluded from this group were children in whom a communication disorder was the presenting sign of cerebral dysfunction. Clinical characteristics of this sample of 38 children are presented in Table 1.

Comparison between behavioral data, early and late AEP in this severely brain damaged group are displayed in Figures 1, 2, and 4. Figure 1 compares behavioral and AEP threshold estimates in 19 children with severe brain damage and severe or profound mental retardation whose EEG was not hypsarhythmic. In 11 of the 19 children, electrophysiologic thresholds were lower than behavioral thresholds. In the 7 children in whom both early and late potentials were available, estimates by these two methods agreed. The generally higher behavioral than electrophysiologic thresholds reflect severely retarded children's lack of behavioral responsiveness to sound. It would be unwise to conclude, however, that profoundly neurologically impaired children may not have peripheral hearing losses: one child with a chromosome 18 deletion syndrome, who appeared profoundly deaf behaviorally, was shown by both early and late AEPs to have a moderate hearing loss which was probably conductive, judging from the results of impedance testing. Another child who sustained a severe neonatal insult and showed essentially no behavioral development but had visual evoked responses was profoundly deaf according to early and late AEPs as well as by behavioral assessment; in her case, it is impossible to judge whether the lack of early (and late) AEPs reflected cochlear damage or severe brain stem pathology. Recording of the cochlear microphonic and N_1 wave would be required in order to make this distinction.

The effect of a very abnormal EEG on late components of the AEP is dramatically illustrated by our findings in 6 children whose EEG was hypsarhythmic (Fig. 2). Hypsarhythmia refers to an EEG pattern seen only in infants and very young children in whom virtually the entire record consists of high voltage spikes and slow waves and is usually accompanied by myoclonic jerks called infantile spasms.

Table I

Clinical Characteristics of 38 Children with Gross Brain Pathology

(N = 38)

Age	range 5 - 127 months	
	median 34 months	
Diagnosis	congenital anomalies	8
	hydrocephalus	2
	genetic metabolic disease	5
	acquired static encephalopathy	21
	intrauterine infection	2
Mental retardation	moderate to severe	9
	severe to profound	29
Blindness		15
EEG	hypsarythmic	6
	other abnormality	15
	normal	4
	no data	13

Hypsarhythmia is not diagnostic of any one disease process but reflects profound alteration of cortical activity. It is usually indicative of diffuse irreversible brain damage resulting in severe or profound mental retardation, except in the few children where it can be successfully treated and the EEG pattern reversed by appropriate drug therapy. Note the dramatic dissociation illustrated in Figure 2 between early and late potentials in four of the five children in whom both were available, hearing estimates by late potentials suggested severe or profound hearing losses while early potentials indicated normal or near normal peripheral sensitivity. From a clinical standpoint, the lack of late components accurately reflects lack of behavioral responsiveness to sound despite normal thresholds for brain stem potentials. It is clear from the early potentials that amplification would have little to offer therapeutically. Note, however, that one child with hypsarhythmia appears profoundly deaf according to both early and late potentials as well as by behavioral

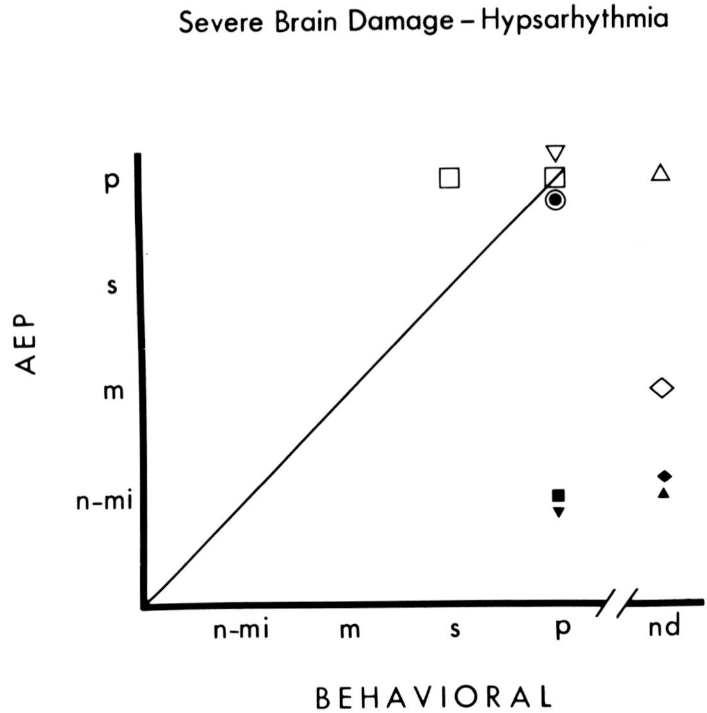

Fig. 2. Correlation of hearing thresholds estimated by AEP techniques with thresholds obtained by behavioral audiometry in a group of 6 severely brain damaged and retarded infants (median age 13.5 months) whose EEG was hypsarhythmic. Note the dramatic difference between early and late AEP threshold estimates in 4 of 5 children.

criteria. The same comment applies to him as to the other profoundly deaf child depicted in Figure 1 and discussed earlier.

We examined test results in 11 children represented in Figure 1 whose EEGs were abnormal without being hypsarhythmic. In 3 of these children, early and late AEPs yielded similar threshold estimates. In the remaining 8 children, tested more than a year ago, only late cortical responses were available. In one child the late AEPs suggested a normal threshold, in 3 a severe loss, and in 4 a profound loss. It is impossible to say whether, had early potentials been available in the 7 children with abnormal EEGs whose late potentials suggested severely impaired hearing, lower threshold estimates would have been obtained by brain stem potentials. The data in these 11 children with abnormal EEGs and in the 6 with hypsarhythmia indicate that whenever a child has a very abnormal EEG, it is essential to record both early and late potentials, early potentials to reflect the state of the cochlea and brain stem relay nuclei, and late potentials the ability of cortical neurons to respond to sound.

To further evaluate the relationship between cortical evoked potentials and

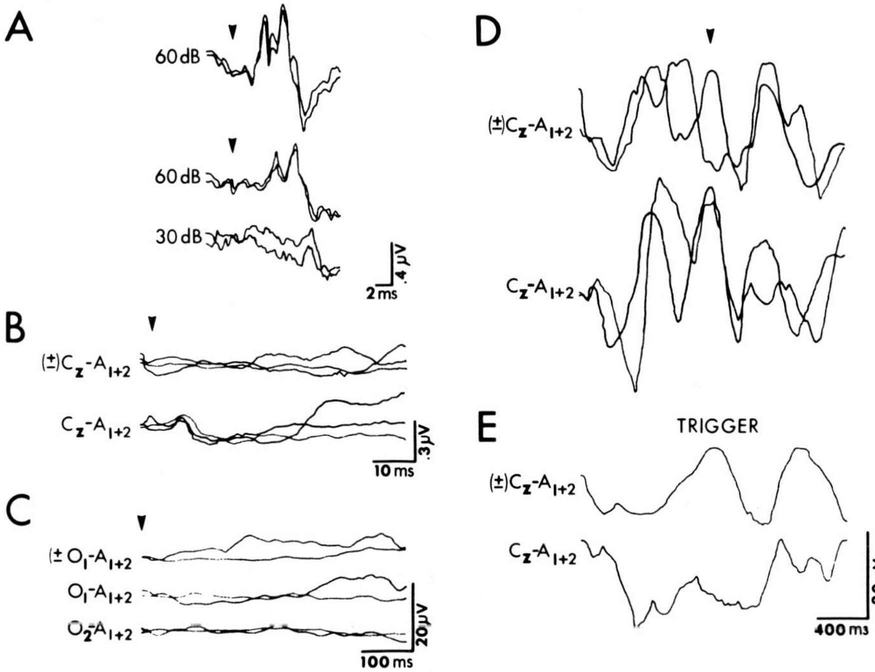

Fig. 3. Auditory and visual evoked potentials in a 7 month old infant with a hypsarhythmic EEG and profound behavioral retardation. Upward deflection reflects positivity at the active electrode. Stimulus delivered at the time indicated by the arrowhead.

A. Early AEPs recorded from C_z - A_2 at 10 stimuli/sec., N=3000, one replication; top trace: clicks; middle and bottom traces: 2k Hz tone pips.

B. Middle latency AEPs, recorded from C_z referred to linked ears, to 60 dB clicks at 10/sec., N=1500, two replications, bandpass 10-300 Hz. No middle latency potential is detected, but note the presence of a positive deflection with short latency in the bottom but not the (±) traces. This deflection probably represents an early AEP after low pass band filtering.

C. VEPs recorded to 100 monocular flashes presented at 2/sec., N=100, one replication. No response detected.

D. Late AEPs to 60 dB clicks presented at 1/2.2 sec., N=64, one replication. Note similarity of wave form between top (±) and bottom traces. This similarity denotes absence of late AEP components. The high voltage background in traces D and E reflects the high voltage abnormal EEG.

E. Trigger run; no stimulus.

abnormal EEGs, we also examined the records of 10 children with severe brain damage and abnormal EEG who did not have pathology of the eye and in whom visual evoked response records were available. In one child, both visual and late auditory evoked responses were well preserved. In 6 children, 3 of them with hypsarhythmic EEGs, neither visual nor auditory evoked responses were obtained. In 2 of these children, one of whom is illustrated in Figure 3, brain stem potentials

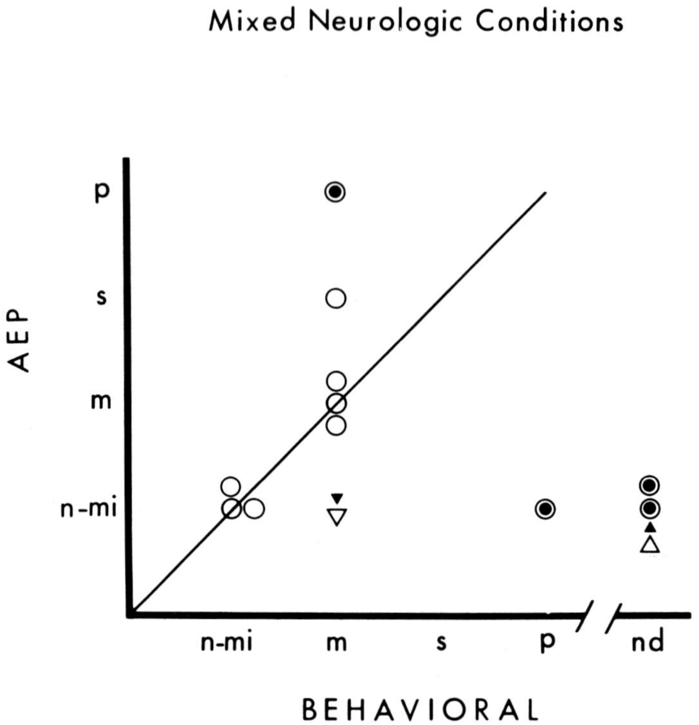

Fig. 4. Correlation of hearing thresholds estimated by AEP techniques with thresholds obtained by behavioral audiometry in a group of 13 children with a variety of neurologic conditions (median age 44 months).

were obtained at normal thresholds, ruling out a peripheral hearing loss as an explanation for lack of late auditory evoked responses. In these 6 children, functional if not organic cortical blindness and deafness may be inferred. Two children who appeared to have a profound hearing loss by late evoked responses had normal visual evoked responses; brain stem responses would have helped in these cases to clarify the differential diagnosis between a peripheral hearing loss and damage to cortical or subcortical auditory pathways. The 10th child had absent visual evoked responses and normal auditory evoked responses; he was a child with adrenoleukodystrophy, cortical blindness and verbal auditory agnosia who could not decode acoustic speech but whose behavioral sensitivity to pure tones was normal.

The data were examined to see whether asymmetries would be detected in 4 children, 3 of them belonging to the sample of children with primary language disorders to be discussed later, known to have asymmetric brain damage on the basis of their neurologic examination, seizure pattern, or EEG. Amplitude (in mm) of all detectable late AEPs at T_3 and T_4 electrodes were summed. In 3 of the 4 children, amplitude was slightly lower on the left, affected, side, but in one the difference was in the opposite direction. In only one child, in whom x-ray studies revealed a subtemporal extracerebral cyst, was the amplitude difference large enough to appear reliable.

Figure 4 compares the results of testing in a group of 13 children with miscellaneous neurologic conditions whose brain damage was less severe than in the children depicted in Figure 1 and 2. In contrast to more severely affected children, four children in the sample were normally responsive to sound behaviorally. In 3 others, late cortical potentials and behavioral audiometry both suggested moderate hearing losses. In the 2 children depicted by the symbols above the diagonal, behavioral estimates were lower than electrophysiologic estimates and, in at least one child, probably underestimated the severity of the hearing loss. This child, in whom both early and late potentials indicated a profound hearing loss, suffered from congenital cytomegalovirus infection, an agent known to affect the cochlea as well as the brain. In the 5 children depicted below the diagonal, behavioral thresholds overestimated the severity of the hearing impairment as in the other children with severe neurologic damage discussed earlier.

Children with Communication Disorders

There were 26 children whose main deficit was a communication disorder. Their clinical characteristics are summarized in Table 2. Among them were 11 children in whom a sensorineural hearing loss was associated with blindness (1 child), hyperkinetic behavior (3 children), retardation of moderate-to-severe degree (6 children) or severe-to-profound degree (2 children), motor deficits (6 children), congenital anomalies (1 child), and other handicaps. Autistic behavior without gross motor handicap was the most striking feature in 7 nonverbal children, one of whom was also blind. There were 8 children who had a language disorder without autistic behavior. Four of these children were viewed as suffering from verbal auditory agnosia, a syndrome in which temporal lobe dysfunction impairs phonologic decoding of acoustic language (Rapin et al., 1977); in the boy with adrenoleukodystrophy mentioned earlier, a CT scan indicated that demyelination had reached the temporal lobes at the time of testing, while in 3 children the EEG showed paroxysmal activity affecting the left or both temporo-parietal regions. Two other children with severe receptive deficits for acoustic language did not have EEG abnormalities although one had occasional brief staring spells. In contrast to the first group with severe brain damage (Table 1) where the sexes were equally represented, boys outnumbered girls 11 to 4 among children with autistic behavior and primary language disorders.

Figure 5 compares the results of ERA with behavioral audiometry in the 8 children with primary language disability. Note that all but one were found to have normal or near normal hearing by both methods (2 children with classic verbal auditory agnosia were thought to have mild hearing losses by pure tone behavioral audiometry. Inability to respond to pure tones at normal threshold levels has been

Table II

Clinical Characteristics of Children with Communicative Disorders

(N = 26)

Age	range 6-137 months median 61.5 months	
Diagnosis	sensorineural hearing loss with brain damage or other handicap	11
	primary language disability	15
	with autistic behavior	9
Mental retardation	none or mild	14
	moderate to severe	6
	severe to profound	6
Blindness		3
EEG	abnormal	6
	normal	10
	no data	10

found in other children with this syndrome but does not represent a true loss of auditory sensitivity (Rapin et al., 1977).) One child was thought to have a severe hearing loss behaviorally but was normal by both early and late evoked potentials.

Figure 6 shows the results in the 7 children with severely autistic behavior. Late potentials suggested moderate hearing losses in 3 children who, unfortunately, were tested before the time when we were able to record early potentials. All 3 had seizures and/or abnormal EEGs, so we cannot determine whether the late potential estimates were accurate or under-estimated peripheral hearing sensitivity. Hearing sensitivity was normal in the other 4 children.

Figure 7 depicts the results of testing in 11 children with hearing losses complicated by other handicaps. Early and late potentials agreed in all cases where both were available, with the exception of one child who may have had a high tone loss and therefore better hearing at 500 Hz (late potentials) than at 2000 Hz (early potentials). In one child with motor deficits and mental retardation as well as impaired hearing, early and late potentials suggested that behavioral audiometry may have underestimated the severity of the hearing loss. Unfortunately, he was one of the children in whom impedance testing was not carried out.

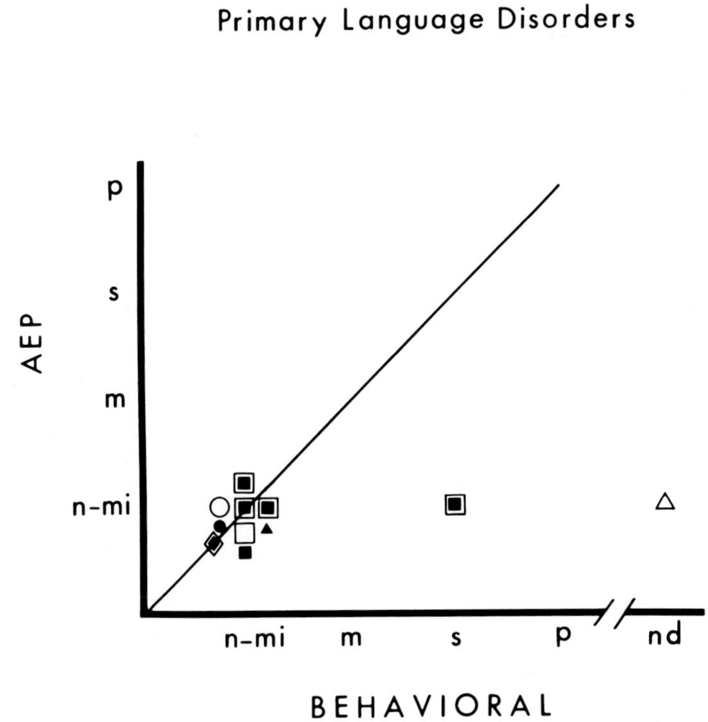

Fig. 5. Correlation of hearing thresholds estimated by AEP techniques with thresholds obtained by behavioral audiometry in a group of 8 children (median age 65 months) with primary language disorders.

DISCUSSION

This study confirms, in an entirely new sample of children with serious brain pathology, that auditory evoked potentials (AEPs) provide a clinically useful and, in severely handicapped children, the only available means for measuring auditory sensitivity. It also confirms that in many children the electrophysiologic threshold is lower than the behavioral one, reflecting the fact that retarded children fail to produce explicit behavioral responses to sensory stimuli at low intensities.

There are many conditions, like intrauterine rubella and cytomegalovirus infections, neonatal hyperbilirubinemia, and purulent meningitis that are capable of damaging the cochlea, the brain, or both. It is crucial in the adequate habilitation of such children to be able to decide whether peripheral deafness or brain damage accounts for lack of language development and poor response to sound. The introduction of early AEPs has added a new dimension to the assessment of these and other neurologically handicapped patients. When threshold for late AEPs was elevated, it used to be impossible to say whether the child was peripherally hearing impaired or whether the cortical evoked potential was masked by high voltage EEG abnormalities or blocked by cortical or subcortical pathology. Availability of impedance audiometry and early potentials now makes it possible to resolve this problem, as was illustrated by several children in this study and in others in the literature (e.g. Galambos and Hecox, 1977). Lack of late responses with preserved early ones is the hallmark of dysfunction in the central acoustic pathway.

Interference by an abnormal EEG with the recording of late AEPs and visual evoked potentials was most strikingly demonstrated by the children who had hypsa-

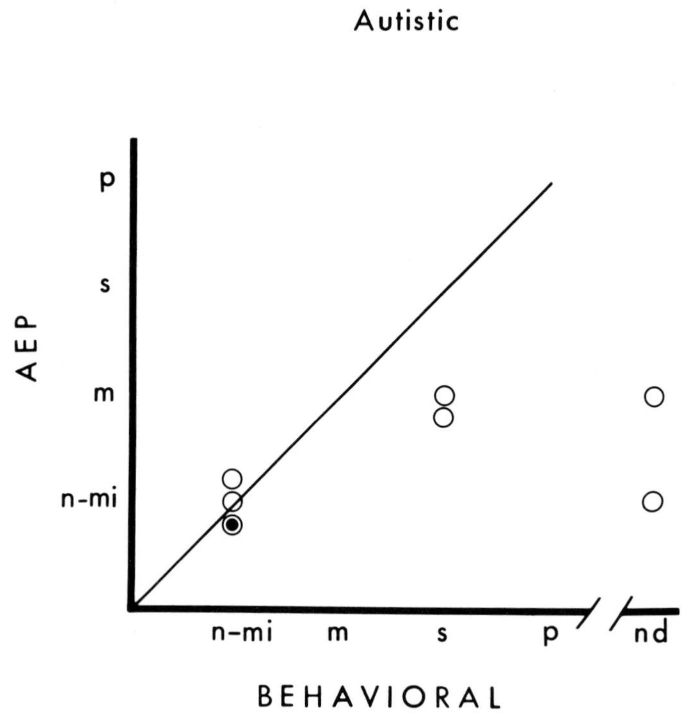

Fig. 6. Correlation of hearing thresholds estimated by AEP techniques with thresholds obtained by behavioral audiometry in a group of 7 children (median age 53 months) with autistic behavior and profound disorders of communication.

rhythmic EEGs. (Our earlier studies had shown that an absent EEG, presumably reflecting an absent or functionally dead cortex, also precludes the recording of late AEPs (Rapin and Graziani, 1967; Rapin and Ruben, 1970)). As pointed out earlier, it is not clear in the individual child whether the abnormal EEG interferes with the recording of late AEPs because it masks the AEP or, more likely, because it reflects a cortex whose function is so abnormal that it cannot generate an evoked response.

When brain stem potentials yield a normal acoustic threshold in these children, one can confidently rule out cochlear pathology as an explanation for lack of behavioral response to sound. But when there are neither early nor late AEPs, as was the case in 3 of our most severely damaged patients, recording of the cochlear microphonic and auditory nerve action potential would be required in order to distinguish a peripheral hearing loss from pathology affecting the brain stem as well as the cerebral hemispheres. Wave N_1 of the brainstem response, if present, would suggest a functioning cochlea, at least for high frequencies, since it is thought to represent the action potential of the acoustic nerve in response to the activation of the hair cells in the basal end of the cochlea.

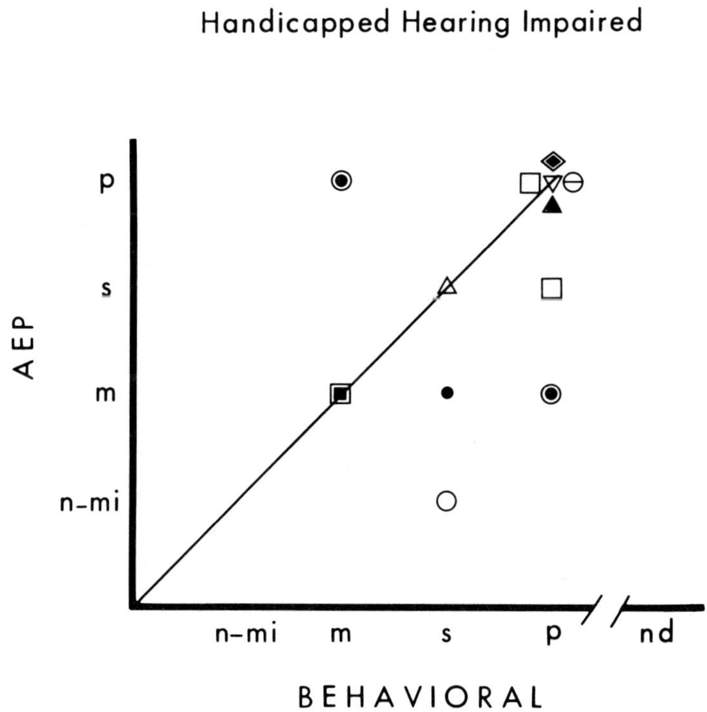

Fig. 7. Correlation of hearing thresholds estimated by AEP techniques with thresholds obtained by behavioral audiometry in a group of 11 children (median age 49 months) with sensorineural hearing loss and other handicaps.

This study included no child with severe pathology lateralized to a single hemisphere, with the exception of one child with a large cyst under the left temporal lobe. Our previous experience (Rapin and Graziani, 1967) and that of Peronnet et al., (1974) indicates that unilateral brain lesions may result in ipsilateral cortical responses with decreased amplitude and a higher threshold than on the normal side. In older patients who cannot cooperate with sophisticated receptive tests for speech, this evoked response asymmetry can be correlated with impaired processing of acoustic language and can be taken to reflect dysfunction at the higher levels of the auditory channel (Peronnet et al., 1974). Provided proper technical precautions have been taken, the finding of asymmetric late AEPs in a young child can thus be looked upon as significant and possibly reflecting lateralized cortical or subcortical dysfunction affecting audition. This potentially valuable information is lost if only vertex electrodes are used.

Another group of children in whom the AEP has provided useful data are those whose communication disorder, whether or not it is associated with autistic features, precludes reliable standard pure tone audiometry. Even when behavioral observation indicates that the children are not deaf, it is very important to be certain that they are not hard of hearing and especially to rule out a high tone loss. Too many children with poor language and atypical behavior who have been called developmentally language impaired turn out later to be hearing impaired with secondary psychiatric symptoms. We believe that all these children should be tested with both early and late AEPs in order to have information about as many levels of the acoustic pathway as possible.

Should one be content to record only early AEPs? Their lack of change with sleep or sedation is a great advantage when testing uncooperative children. Sedated sleep monitored by a parent has been entirely satisfactory and safe in our hands. There is no doubt that in otherwise-normal children suspected of a hearing loss in whom the goal is to decide whether amplification is needed, brainstem responses may provide adequate data for clinical use. Their usefulness will be enhanced if techniques such as high pass masking and the recording of frequency following responses extend the information they provide to the low frequency end of the spectrum (Davis and Hirsh, 1976). Since late cortical potentials to low frequency tones have a higher amplitude than those to high frequencies (Rapin et al., 1966), they can be used to supplement the sensitive information about high frequencies provided by early AEPs.

The greatest drawback of early AEPs is that they do not provide information about the cortical end of the acoustic pathway which is, after all, the portion concerned with complex auditory and linguistic processing. At this time, while we no longer rely solely on late potentials for assessing peripheral auditory sensitivity because of the difficulty with visual scoring of records, fluctuating threshold with phases of sleep (Osterhammel et al., 1973; Rapin et al., 1972), and greater time required for testing, we do use them to confirm and extend the results of early AEP testing. Even though we pointed out that a grossly abnormal EEG or severe brain pathology interferes with the detection of late AEPs and that, alone, they might be misleading in terms of assessing peripheral hearing sensitivity, lack of late AEPs in the presence of early AEPs is useful and correct information concerning the functional state of the higher levels of the acoustic pathway and the child's ability to process acoustic information. We feel this information should not be dispensed with.

Our conclusion is that, faced with a child with a complex clinical problem affecting his auditory communication channel, one needs to secure all the information one can. We choose to record early and late AEPs and to place electrodes over each of the hemispheres as well as at the vertex. We believe that we are at the threshold of a much more sophisticated era in evoked response audiometry. In the future one will not be content just to measure the sensitivity of the cochlea in order to prescribe an appropriate hearing aid or rule out a peripheral hearing loss, one will look for meaningful distortions in wave forms to detect pathology at various levels of the auditory system. Perception will be tested using discrimination and vigilance paradigms. One can forsee that much more complex acoustic and linguistic stimuli will be used routinely in order adequately to challenge the sophistication of the acoustic system. With the problem of automatic detection of AEPs largely solved (Salomon, 1975; Schimmel et al., 1975), mapping of threshold to pure tones and simple stimuli will require less time. One will then be able to ask more interesting and, ultimately, more meaningful questions concerning the capabilities of the brain damaged patient's entire auditory system, not just about his most peripheral receptor.

SUMMARY

Sixty-four children aged 5 months to 11½ years (median 44 months) were selected among all children referred for evoked response audiometry because their hearing could not be assessed reliably by behavioral audiometry. They were selected on the basis of the presence of additional handicaps besides suspected hearing loss or language deficit, such as severe brain lesions, mental retardation, hyperkinetic or autistic behavior, seisures, and blindness. Late (cortical) auditory evoked potentials (AEPs) and, more recently, early (brain stem) AEPs were recorded, usually during sleep. Threshold detection by behavioral audiometry and by early and late AEPs was compared.

Early and late AEP thresholds usually agree, except in some children with very abnormal EEGs (hypsarhythmia) where early potentials indicated normal auditory sensitivity and late AEPs to even high intensity tones were absent, indicating dysfunction in the upper levels of the auditory pathway. In severely brain damaged children, AEP thresholds tended to be lower than behavioral ones, reflecting such children's lack of responsiveness to low intensity sensory stimulation. In a few children with severe brain damage and abnormal EEGs in whom both early and late AEPs were absent, it was uncertain whether the site of pathology was in the cochlea or the brain stem. A number of other children were clearly both brain damaged and hearing impaired.

Early and late AEPs are viewed as complementary methods. While early AEPs alone may be sufficient in order to prescribe amplification for children with uncomplicated hearing losses, in those with complex communication disorders late AEPs supplement information about subcortical relays with essential data about the functioning of the cortical portion of the acoustic channel.

Acknowledgement

This work supported in part by grants NS 3356 and 2 TI NS 5325 from the National Institute of Neurological and Communicative Disorders and Stroke, and grant GRSG 613-4799 from the Department of Health Education and Welfare.

The authors gratefully acknowledge Ms. A. Brattson for her assistance during the course of data collection and analysis.

REFERENCES

Barnet, A.B, Ohlrich, E.S. and Shanks, B.L. EEG evoked responses to repetitive auditory stimulation in normal and Down's syndrome infants. *Dev. Med. Child Neurol. 13:* 321-329, 1971.

Bigum, H.B., Dustman, R.E. and Beck, E.C. Visual and somato-sensory evoked responses from mongoloid and normal children. *Electroencephalogr. Clin. Neurophysiol. 28:* 576-585, 1970.

Davis, H. and Hirsh, S.K. The audiometric utility of brain stem responses to low-frequency sounds. *Audiology 15:* 181-195, 1976.

Feinmesser, M. and Sohmer, H. Contribution of cochlear, brain stem and cortical responses to differential diagnosis and lesion localization in hearing loss. In: *Hearing and Davis: Essays honoring Hallowell Davis,* edited by S.K. Hirsh, D.H. Eldredge, I.J. Hirsh and S.R. Silverman. St. Louis: Washington University Press, 1976, p. 393-402.

Galambos, R. and Hecox, K. Clinical application of the brain stem auditory evoked potentials. In: *Auditory Evoked Potentials in Man Psychopharmacology Correlates of Evoked Potentials,* edited by J.E. Desmedt. Basel: S. Karger, 1977, p. 1-19.

Hecox, K. and Galambos, R. Brain stem auditory evoked responses in human infants and adults. *Arch. Otolaryngol. 99:* 30-33, 1974.

Hogan, D.D. Cortical response of retardates for AER audiometry. *Am. J. Ment. Defic. 75:* 474-477, 1971.

Jewett, D.L. and Williston, J.S. Auditory evoked far-fields averaged from the scalp of humans. *Brain 94:* 681-696, 1971.

Mendel, M.I., Hosick, E.C., Windman, T.R., Davis, H., Hirsh, S.K. and Dinges, D.F. Audiometric comparison of the middle and late components of the adult auditory evoked potentials awake and asleep. *Electroencephologr. Clin. Neurophysiol. 38:* 27-33, 1975.

Mokotoff, B., Schulman-Galambos, C. and Galambos, R. Brain stem auditory evoked responses in children. *Arch. Otolaryngol. 103:* 38-43, 1977.

Onishi, S. and Manabe, T. A comparison of the ERA fast responses with pure tone audiograms and their clinical use. In: *Hearing and Davis: Essays Honoring Hallowell Davis,* edited by S.K. Hirsh, D.H. Eldredge, I.J. Hirsh, and S.R. Silverman. St. Louis: Washington University Press, 1976, p. 435-443.

Ornitz, E.M., Ritvo, E.R., Panman, L.M., Lee, Y.H., Carr, E.M. and Walter, R.D. The auditory evoked response in normal and autistic children during sleep. *Electroencephalogr. Clin. Neurophysiol. 25:* 221-230, 1968.

Osterhammel, P.A., Davis, H., Wier, C.C. and Hirsh, S.K. Auditory evoked vertex potentials in sleep. *Audiology 12:* 116-128, 1973.

Peronnet, F., Michel, F., Echallier, J.F. and Girod, J. Coronal topography of human auditory evoked responses. *Electroencephalogr. Clin. Neurophysiol. 37:* 225-230, 1974.

Rapin, I., Schimmel, H., Tourk, L.M., Krasnegor, N.A. and Pollack, C. Evoked responses to clicks and tones of varying intensity in waking adults. *Electroencephalogr. Clin. Neurophysiol. 21:* 335-344, 1966.

Rapin, I. and Graziani, L.J. Auditory-evoked responses in normal, brain damaged, and deaf infants. *Neurology 17:* 881-894, 1967.

Rapin, I., Graziani, L.J. and Lyttle, M. Summated auditory evoked responses for audiometry: experience in 51 children with congenital rubella. *Int. Audiol. 8:* 371-376, 1969.

Rapin, I., Ruben, R.J. and Lyttle, M. Diagnosis of hearing loss in infants using auditory evoked responses. *Laryngoscope 80:* 717-722, 1970.

Rapin, I., Schimmel, H. and Cohen, M.M. Reliability in detecting the auditory evoked response (AER) for audiometry in sleeping subjects. *Electroencephalogr. Clin. Neurophysiol. 32:* 734-738, 1972.

Rapin, I., Mattis, S., Rowan, A.J. and Golden, G.G. Verbal auditory agnosia in children. *Dev. Med. Child Neurol. 19:* 192-207, 1977.

Ruben, R.J., Elberling, C. and Salomon, G. *Electrocochleography.* Baltimore: University Park Press, 1976.

Salamy, A., McKean, C. and Buda, F. Maturational changes in auditory transmission as reflected in human brain stem potentials. *Brain Res. 96:* 361-366, 1976.

Salomon, G. Automatic evaluation of human auditory evoked potentials from the vertex. *Symp. Zool. Soc. Lond. 37:* 205-236, 1975.

Schimmel, H. The (±) reference: accuracy of estimated mean components in average response studies. *Science 157:* 92-94, 1967.

Schimmel, H., Rapin, I. and Cohen, M.M. Improving evoked response audiometry. Results of normative studies for machine scoring. *Audiology 14:* 466-479, 1975.

Schulman-Galambos, C. and Galambos, R. Brain stem auditory evoked responses in premature infants. *J. Speech Hear. Res. 18:* 456-465, 1975.

Sohmer, H., Feinmesser, M. and Szabo, G. Sources of electrocochleographic responses as studied in patients with brain damage. *Electroencephalogr. Clin. Neurophysiol. 37:* 663-669, 1974.

Starr, A. and Achor, L.J. Auditory brain stem responses in neurological disease. *Arch. Neurol. 32:* 761-768, 1975.

Stockard, J.J. and Rossiter, V.S. Clinical and pathologic correlates of brain stem auditory response abnormalities. *Neurology 27:* 316-325, 1977.

Tanahashi, T., Matsumura, K., Niwa, H. and Iwata, H. Cochlear microphonics and eighth nerve action potentials: clinical and experimental studies. In: *Electrocochleography,* edited by R.J. Ruben, C. Elberling and G. Salomon. Baltimore: University Park Press, 1976, p. 479-499.

DISCUSSION

Starr: This is a very nice demonstration of the wide use of evoked responses for assessing neurological problems. Do you have any information on changes in the scalp distribution of the middle or late potentials in these young children with neurological problems?

Rapin: I didn't have time to go into this in my oral presentation. We did look for possible asymmetries in children in whom we thought there might be some asymmetric distribution of brain damage. We had no children in the present study with a severe lateralized brain lesion, except for one child who had a subtemporal arachnoidal cyst. In that child there was about a 25 per cent difference in the amplitude of the evoked response recorded over the right and left hemispheres.

We routinely use not only vertex but right and left electrodes. We had noted asymmetries in one of our earlier studies (*Neurology, 17,* 881, 1967), in which we had shown that not only is the response smaller on the side overlying the abnormal cortex, but threshold for the appearance of a detectable response may be higher. I think this type of information may be quite useful.

Deuel: Aside from the group of children whose problem you labeled "auditory agnosia" (and such children mostly have markedly abnormal EEGs, so you would expect to have some technical difficulties) have you used this method on children who have more severe language disorders?

Rapin: Yes. In the first group of children with language disorders we showed, about half were children you would label as having a verbal auditory agnosia. Only two of these had very severely abnormal EEGs at the time the test was done; the others did not. They just had staring spells. Most in this small sample of eight children had normal hearing sensitivity by electrophysiologic means, and none had a grossly detectable asymmetry between right and left hemispheres.

Deuel: Have you done cortical evoked potentials on any children who have severe language delay, but no other handicap that you have been able to find?

Rapin: Yes, but I don't recall that there were any in this group. I would reiterate the same statement, that the electrophysiologic method permits you to exclude a peripheral hearing loss. In general late potentials have not been very useful for finding an interhemispheric asymmetry in these children.

Butler: A great deal of interest has been directed toward the neural source of the auditory evoked potentials. Experimental approaches to this problem have ranged from the simple, non-invasive procedure of manipulating electrode placement on the scalp, to the recording from implanted electrodes in man and the systematic ablation of auditory neural structures in animals. There are other approaches; for example, one can draw inferences about the generators of the various components of the auditory evoked potentials simply on the basis of their morphology. I have asked Dr. Kiang to provide us with some sort of framework that could serve to organize our thinking along this line. Perhaps, Nelson, you might take about five minutes or so to discuss this question?

Kiang: There are at least three major factors in determining the shapes and sizes of gross responses. These are: 1. The shape and size of the contribution from each element, the so-called "unit potential"; 2. The synchrony or time relation of the units potentials; and 3. The spatial orientation of the elements. Each of these factors can be influenced by many considerations. For example, the unit potential as seen by the gross electrode would be influenced not only by the nature of the potential developed at the active region but also by the current paths. Moise Goldstein and I once wrote a paper in which we noted that the shape of the unit potential interacts with synchrony in such a way that a small degree of desynchronization will affect gross potentials with sharp waveform more than those with broader waveforms. For instance, the N_1 potential from the auditory nerve has a waveform nearly as sharp as an action potential from myelinated fibers of the appropriate size. A small decrease in synchrony that eliminates N_1 will leave slower potentials such as evoked cortical responses relatively intact. The third factor of spatial orientation of the active elements is extremely important. If the elements are randomly oriented, perfectly synchronized, the resultant will be no recordable gross response.

For evoked brain potentials we need information on all these three factors before we can satisfactorily establish the sources. If one records activity from single units in the brain you see at once that during the time occupied by the brain stem responses there are responses present in almost the entire brain stem including the auditory nerve. In certain regions, many elements are active in a synchronized way and by plotting neurograms one can determine how well the activity is synchronized.

The degree of synchronization interacts with sharpness of the unit potentials. For instance, the action potentials of myelinated fibers are usually very sharp lasting less than a msec. The potentials resulting from activity of other elements such as dendrites can be much longer lasting.

Spatial orientation is very important because in some parts of the brain the elements may be aligned fairly randomly whereas in other parts they might be very regularly arranged. The aligned cell groups can be folded intricately as in the LSO or simply organized in a plane as in the MSO. An important property of fiber tracts is that the elements within a bundle are all oriented alike.

So, if one thinks about the various potentials talked about in the last few days, such as the brain stem potentials, for example, one notes first that these are fast components; the deflections last about as long as unit potentials of the auditory nerve. Thus it is unlikely that long lasting potentials from cell bodies or dendrites are involved. The best guess at the present time would be that faster events such as synchronized action potentials in oriented elements are the main contributors. For these reasons, most people would tend to suspect fiber tracts such as the trapezoid body or lateral lemniscus as being involved in the brain stem responses. This line of thinking can be traced at least back to Kemp Copee and Robinson. If the "brain stem responses" are not filtered as drastically as most workers do, the sharp sequence of deflections are seen to be riding on some slower components. Thus, during the same time that the fast deflections are occurring, slower activity is also apparently present. These could well be contributions from slower processes such as slow-conducting pathways or more likely activity of cell bodies or processes such as dendrites. In the medial superior olive, for instance, there are elements lined up in a nice simple arrangement in three dimensional space. In fact gross electrodes placed near this nucleus do give large evoked potentials slower than action potentials in the auditory nerve. I was interested in Dr. Terkildson's remarks. He wanted to test responses to low frequencies and was not doing so well with the fast components of the "brain stem responses". He started looking at slower components and did better with those. Recall that the MSO is predominently composed of low-frequency units.

Dr. Starr's report appears to match very well with the brief report of some of the workers from Toronto in that acute lesions involving inferior colliculus do not eliminate the fast brain stem potentials. If the potential contributions from cells in the colliculus are predominently slow component activity, then one might not expect contributions by fiber tracts peripheral to the colliculus to be affected by acute lesions. Perhaps long-term effects might be discernable if some of these tracts degenerate retrogradely.

The question of when one uses brain stem responses and when one uses electrocochleography, all boils down to what information one wants. If one is interested in obtaining an "objective audiogram" where it is relatively clear that the nervous system is intact, any potential can be used so long as it is validated. But if one does not know what is wrong and there is a chance that the central nervous system is not intact, then knowledge of the potentials later than N_1 can become important especially if we know what their origin is.

SYMPOSIUM SUMMARY

SYMPOSIUM SUMMARY: REVIEW AND FORE-VIEW

Hallowell Davis

Central Institute for the Deaf

Thank you for your kind words of introduction but thank you not at all for putting me on the spot in this particular situation. The task of summarizing the symposium is almost an impossible one. It was very nice of you to suggest having the manuscripts submitted to me beforehand so that I could review them, digest them, pick out the particular words of wisdom, and put them in relation to one another.

This worked out about as it usually does. I believe I received about 30 per cent of the manuscripts in St. Louis before leaving, and was presented with another 40 per cent of the manuscripts immediately on arrival in Chicago. That just ruined my Sunday evening.

The upshot of it is that my coverage is spotty and those of you whose manuscripts I did receive may get a little more attention, obviously, then others. This is an excuse for being a little taken by surprise by one or two of the very interesting presentations to which I had to sit and listen with full attention. As a result I am exhausted.

The symposium as a whole in my opinion was admirable. It was a very well-balanced mixture of laboratory research, research into fundamentals and basics, and of clinical problems and consideration of new procedures which are still in development. This bringing together of the experts in the field, who understand the dwellers in the ivory towers, and those who are making use of some of the ideas and techniques that have been developed in the past, is why we need to come together. We need to get acquainted with one another's points of view, and perhaps above all with the different vocabularies so that we can communicate more effectively, one group with another. This is one of the great purposes and accomplishments of symposia like this.

It is good to have also the round tables, with their less formal give-and-take and with questions and answers from the floor. I wish we could have had a little more of that. But somehow the Amtrak syndrome seemed to get the better of us in one or two instances, and things were cut short.

From the kind of interaction that we have been having, I think, develops the clinicians' healthy respect for the laboratory workers, and vice versa. It is essential that we have this.

There is also the recognition of different stages of discussion, "levels of dis-

ISBN 0-12-514960-3

course" I think is the proper phrase for it, of the analyses in the laboratories of the details of certain mechanisms, anatomical relations, and so on; and then the contrasting over-all approach that we make when we start dealing with the practical applications. I am going to quote a little later on to illustrate this point more fully, because I think it is a very important one.

The program started and proceeded in a logical anatomical way, beginning with the ear and working up through the brain stem, and finally coming out the top at the cortex. The material dealing with the cortex you have heard so recently, and it was so well summarized on the clinical side by Dr. Rapin's final remarks, that I am not going to devote much attention to it. We can see there is a gap between the details of the anatomical organization of the fields of the cortex and those of the unit responses. As Dr. Goff pointed out, we still don't know where the vertex potential is generated, and we don't know what its basis really is. Perhaps we can make a guess that it comes from the auditory areas, or auditory fields perhaps I should say, in general. That is a good working hypothesis, but it won't make any difference as far as our empirical use of the vertex potential for clinical testing is concerned.

It is clear that interest in ERA, electric response audiometry, from the cortex is obviously at a low ebb at present. I am delighted that Dr. Salomon is still working with it. We will look forward to his developments of methodology, which I hope he will be able to standardize so that we can really take advantage of them. I saw his manuscript and I hope you will all give it good attention in the final publication. He did not have time to do justice to some of its complexities. Dr. Rapin's point that there still is a place and will be a place from the neurological point of view for cortical testing is valid. One of my predictions for the future is that its stock will go up again.

I had the feeling that the central emphasis in the organization of the program was around electrocochleography and the transtympanic approach; 16 or 18 months ago, when the program was being organized, that certainly was the point of central interest.

These brash interlopers, the brainstem responses, had just shown their heads or at that time, and we had no idea that they would soon rival the electrocochleogram in general interest, particularly in their potentialities for audiology, for getting the complete audiogram, as opposed to the otological potentialities of the electrocochleogram. I believe the electrocochleogram will continue to be the darling of the otologists. It is their private preserve. The ones who can put in that transtympanic electrode are the ones who are chiefly concerned, and most particularly concerned, about the differential diagnoses to which the transtympanic electrocochleogram can contribute.

The particular advantage of the electrocochleogram is the availability of the summating potential. I emphasize the summating potential rather than the cochlear microphonic because I think, as appeared in the discussions on Dr. Dallos's and Dr. Russell's papers, the summating potential and cochlear microphonic are closely related and probably give much the same kind of information. The summating potential is easier to deal with, in my opinion, and I believe both are very closely related to the excitatory mechanisms. So, I will tag both of them as items of future interest, well illuminated by the discussions that we have had here.

When it comes to getting the audiogram, I think the motto of the brain stem audiologists is, "Anything you can do I can do cheaper and safer." I personally am on that side with respect to audiometric studies by frequencies and the functional assessment of the peripheral auditory apparatus.

I do not want to repeat in detail the conclusions that we reached in discussions of round tables and otherwise, but I will simply say that in my opinion this is where a major impact of the discussions has been.

In the section of the program on Tuesday morning dealing with the cochlea there turned up what to me was a surprising item: the cochlear implant. I had not been able to figure out how the cochlear implant turns out to be a part of evoked electrical activity in the auditory nervous system. The implant does not yield an evoked potential; it is an applied potential. But it was nice nevertheless to hear the news about the Bilger study, and I think we were all refreshed by Dr. Black's introduction of a somewhat novel point of view in regard to cost-benefits. That gave us something to think about. I won't say it was a comic relief, but it did reduce the tension arising from our own technical problems.

I suppose the answer is that it was thought, when things were being organized, that the transtympanic electrode might help in the evaluation of candidates for the implant operation. This idea was strongly current in some of our minds at the time the program was put together; but I believe that enthusiasm has subsided, and the thing to test is really whether the person who is deaf can report a sensation of sound when he is stimulated, rather than trying to detect brain stem or cortical responses. The former is cheaper and more to the point.

Dr. Lindsay showed us the pathology of deaf ears, and to me it was rather surprising to learn how many ganglion cells seem to survive in one condition after another. Unless the scala tympani was completely filled with bone it seemed that all cases might, at least in principle, be candidates for the cochlear implant. I don't know what your thoughts might be, Dr. Spoendlin, as to what particular types of cells are surviving in these cases, and what these survivors might contribute to the over-all normal sense of hearing. There is a gap to be closed here, and I hope you will be back again some day and help fill it in.

Speaking of Dr. Spoendlin, he still holds firm to his ratios of distribution of nerve fibers to the inner and outer hair cells: 95 and 5% respectively. As Dr. Dallos would say, it seems to be the inner hair cells that do all the work. This is a very curious situation, and Dr. Spoendlin still stands pat. I was most interested to hear that and think it is extremely important. We have here one of the great zones of uncertainty: what does this innervation ratio mean; what does it imply for the relative importance of inner and outer hair cells; and also what about the efferent nervous system? We heard from Dr. Warr that the efferent nervous system is complicated but well-organized, with the uncrossed and the crossed tracts coming from different sources. And if we look into the evolutionary history of the efferent nervous system, we find that it is strongly represented throughout the entire lateral line-labyrinth-cochlear sensory system.

Incidentally, in the lateral-line organ the function of the efferent system seems to be to reduce the sensitivity of the end-organ when the fish is about to make a movement in the water. The analogy suggests that the olivo-cochlear system goes into action when we get ready to make a noise of our own, that is to speak. Maybe humans have learned to like the sound of their own voices so much that this has become a vestigial system; but seriously I put it to you that the significance of the outer hair cells may be that they are the effector organ for the efferent nerve supply. We should look at nerves and hair cells together to see where they fit into the scheme of things.

Dr. Dallos may have the answer here. He tells us that apparently the outer hair cells in some way sensitize the inner hair cells and give them their extraordinary sensitivity, and incidentally the frequency selectivity, that is revealed by the tuning curves of single auditory units. So, all we have to suppose is that the efferent nerve supply turns off Dallos's sensitizing influence and the picture is complete; if he will only tell us how that sensitization works. This is one of the challenges, one of the paradoxes, that still confronts us in the ear, and it is all tied up with the tip-and-tail story, and how the sharpening of tuning is brought about.

I want to couple the frequency selectivity again with the extraordinary sensitivity of each unit at its best frequency. Dr. Bennett spoke of the sensitivity of the electrical sensory system in certain fish (recall the voltage gradient of a dry cell from New York to Miami), but the absolute sensitivity of the auditory mechanism gets down (as you are all undoubtedly aware) close to the level of the energy of Brownian movement. This seems just too good to be true.

I think these things are all related in some way, and I was hoping that Dr. Bennett would give us some helpful elucidation. But I must say that, not having seen his material beforehand, I was as much confused as most of the rest of you probably were with the "calcium influx" and the "voltage clamps" and other unfamiliar concepts. It is good to know that there are people who are concerned with excitatory mechanisms at the molecular level, and I think that in a relatively short time we will have considerably more enlightenment on the problem of excitation not only by electrical but by mechanical (tactile) stimulation.

The term "calcium influx" raises a thought. I just hope that nobody goes away from here and invents a new treatment for Menière's disease based on eating chalk! All too often a jump is made too quickly from something being mentioned in a particular context and then being put to trial in what turns out to be a ridiculous fashion. This is just a bit of caution.

Seriously, Dr. Bennett gave us some insight into the advances that are being made at the molecular electrochemical level into the problem of electrical excitation and electrogenesis in sense organs, synapses and neurons. The electrical control of the release of chemical transmitter is part of our problem in the organ of Corti. I had hoped that Dr. Bennett would also illuminate the problem of how mechanical deformation initiates the receptor potentials (cochlear microphonic and summating potentials), and how it is that they are so exquisitely sensitive. Unfortunately, his self-regenerating oscillating potentials seem to be too slow and to occur too late in the sequence of activities to be very helpful in this respect. On the other hand, his remarks about spontaneous activity and the adjustment of threshold are very pertinent.

Dr. Smith gave us sound morphological evidence for something we thought we knew all the time, namely that the endolymphatic duct doesn't leak but maintains both the potassium concentration and the electrical polarization of the endolymph of scala media. It is nice to know that it is done in the right way, with the proper conventional types of occluding junctions. A new bit of information is that the stria vascularis seems to be in a sac of its own. Perhaps that will help some of us in our model making.

Turning to the traveling wave. This is something which seems to have been a laboratory curiosity for many years. Dr. Eldredge's film animated the traveling wave for us very helpfully. Visualization of this kind makes the phenomenon more real for us. My point is that we need to think in terms of the traveling wave in order to interpret clinical recordings, both in the electrocochleogram and in the brainstem responses. The traveling wave delay contributes to the latency of the responses. The delay is longer for low frequencies and synchronization is less precise. Such effects turn out to have very considerable clinical significance, as we learned from the round table discussions.

There was one paper that was a breakthrough as far as I am concerned. It was presented by Dr. Russell, and described recording from inner hair cells by intracellular microelectrodes. It is a breakthrough to have these inner hair cells still alive and responding. His final conclusion was both definite and important. As of 1977 we now know that the tip-and-tail tuning pattern exists at the level of the receptor potential; it exists inside the cell; it is not brought about by synaptic action or other neural interactions. This is something I for one had already inferred, not from the silence of anatomists but from their very definite denials that there are any neural connections or synapses between outer and inner hair cells. They have been looking for them for years.

One of my favorite generalizations as a neurophysiologist has been that if you develop a strong physiological inference without anatomical support, an obliging anatomist will supply the support within three years. In this case we have been kept waiting at least 13 years but the physiological inference of neural interaction now collapses. We will take you off the hook, Dr. Spoendlin, and not keep asking about such neural interconnections any longer.

Another impressive point in Dr. Russell's presentation was his emphasis on the large DC component of the receptor potential, with the AC component riding on top of it. This was my basis for an earlier comment that the summating potential is something to watch in the future.

I will now really address the question of the tip and the tail of single-unit tuning curves. The tip remains for me a physiological mystery and paradox. We simply do not have a full understanding of it. But we have it very much with us in our clinical applications and interpretations. The tip is vulnerable to anoxia, to drugs, to various kinds of mistreatment, exposure to noise, -all of the things that we know are not very good for the ear. It is always the tips that are affected first. Whether the tips are really rounded off, as if by the loss of Evans' "second filter", so-called, or whether their thresholds are elevated because of loss of sensitization, as Dr. Dallos has it, these alternatives are still up for grabs, and there may be still other types of explanation still to come. But the clinical problem of recruitment is squarely before us, and we have to do what we can with it on an empirical basis while we wait for further enlightenment.

Perhaps here is a good place for me to introduce a quotation from Dr. Kiang, who talked about the reconstruction of the first whole-nerve action-potential spike from the responses of separate individual units, and the complexities that one encounters in making these reconstructions and inferences. You heard him say it, but this is the way he has it in his written version; and with his permission I will read a paragraph or two:

> "Even such fundamental questions as whether there are two or more populations of sensory cells that have very different response properties; whether the different sensory cells interact; how the hair cells relate to the nerve cells; and whether different nerve cells can influence one another; remain equivocal. While it may be fascinating to speculate on the various theoretical possibilities, the confusion between conjectures and facts in the current literature plagues the beginning student.
>
> "Fortunately, at the auditory-nerve level, one can continue to build a quantitative theory of the gross neural responses in terms of single-unit activity *without completely understanding the mechanisms* that generate such activity. *(Emphasis added)*
>
> "The tuning curves of auditory-nerve fibers are not only determined by cochlear processes but also by all the preceding stages in the external and middle ears, to say nothing of the acoustic system . . . . a variety of complex changes can occur in the tuning curves of the auditory-nerve fibers after insults to the cochlea. Although it is theoretically possible that tests may be developed for the differential diagnosis of various levels of disorders, it may also be that similar electrocochleographic recordings can result from different underlying abnormalities.
>
> "As a general principle, it is probably safest to avoid involved interpretations unless it directly affects treatment or money matters. If surgical intervention is to be considered, if rehabilitation training is to be planned, or if other kinds of tests need to be ordered, then one must proceed on a "best-guess" basis. Gross distinctions in assigning defects to brain or ear can frequently be made with some confidence. Conductive vs sensorineural losses can sometimes be assessed, when other tests are inapplicable. Perhaps the diagnosis of specific conditions

such as Menière's disease or acoustic tumors can also be aided.

"The point is that few of these practical applications require interpretation at a detailed cellular level. The clinician can correlate electrocochleographic recordings and disease entities in a straightforward empirical manner, insisting only that the correlations be validated on their own merits. To couch interpretaions and make recommendations in terms of presumed underlying mechanisms is probably premature and certainly unnecessary."

Thank you, Nelson, for putting things so effectively.

Dr. Kiang told us about his sharply-tuned units in the auditory nerve. We have a rather remarkable convergence between that and information derived by the technique of high-pass masking. Such masking yields "derived responses" which may be called "narrow-band action potentials". Dr. Eldredge's presentation went through the rationale of the masking technique, and Dr. Eggermont gave us a fine demonstration of it as applied to the human electrocochleogram. The correspondence between his curves and the single-unit tuning curves of Dr. Kiang, and also the psychoacoustic tone-on-tone inhibition curves that Dr. Dallos has derived, is really remarkable. It gives us great confidence in the reality of all of these things, and a sound model on which to base the interpretations of the deviations and abnormalities in the electrocochleogram or the brain stem responses that some of us are sure to encounter in practical situations.

Time does not allow me to comment extensively on the papers and the round table discussion of yesterday afternoon. I will, however, remind you by title of the outstanding anatomical presentations by Dr. Kane, dealing with the organization at the cellular level of the primary cochlear nuclei and by Dr. Diamond on the auditory areas of the cerebral cortex. The major lesson for us in each case was the intricate complexity of the neural cell types and their interconnections. It is only on the basis of such anatomical studies that we can make intelligent guesses as to the anatomical sources of the evoked potentials that we observe in the laboratory and in the clinic. Detailed understanding of the neural circuits and their neurological functions is far beyond our reach. Dr. Goff, for example, could describe the scalp-recorded sound-evoked potentials, but for only a few of the waves could he identify a probable source. The best-identified sources were actually *muscles* of the neck or head, activated reflexly by the stimuli. He could not identify the primary response of the auditory cortex. The classical slow cortical "vertex potentials" are a confusing, overlapping array, and Dr. Goff was unable to localize their sources definitely, even with intracranial electrodes. Things may be simpler in the brain stem, where latencies are short and the state of the subject does not complicate the picture, but even here, as Dr. Tsuchitani's presentation reminded us, we face the problem of multiple generators responding simultaneously. Dr. Starr, in the round table, surprised us by evidence that many if not all of the brain stem responses in the "Jewett sequence" may arise from the axonal tracts of white matter (like the auditory nerve) and not from gray matter (as in the cortex).

A moral here was pointed out in discussion by Dr. Davis: "simplistic models of a single ascending pathway and a single auditory area will not suffice; we must learn to think in triplicate." Dr. Kiang agreed in principle but protested that "triplicate" was still far too simple.

The multiplicity of pathways and of types of response in different classes of neurons has a direct bearing on the brain stem response. The various "Jewett waves" are separately identifiable because a group of nerve impulses remains closely synchronized. Transmission times and synaptic delays are remarkably constant, up to and apparently including the inferior colliculus. They are what Dr. Galambos calls the "timekeepers." They are almost certainly the basis of "periodicity pitch" and closely involved in the "lateralization" of a sound source. Their responses are visible precisely because they are good timekeepers. Other pathways carry other temporal patterns of impulses. It is thus possible, if only the timekeepers are impaired, that sounds can be perceived even though no brain stem responses can be identified. This is an important limitation, even though such cases may be rare. The rule is that a positive BSR response of normal form and latency is very strong evidence for an intact peripheral mechanism, but actual hearing may sometimes be better than an absence of or very weak brain stem responses might suggest.

In the round table on brain stem responses Drs. Terkildsen, Osterhammel and Davis agreed that the BSR response best known as "Jewett V" is an excellent indicator for responses to tone pips (filtered clicks) of 1000, 2000 and 4000 Hz but is not so clear at 500 Hz; and furthermore that the later ("middle") responses may be a useful supplement at this lower frequency.

One last reminder to those of you who are just entering the field of auditory evoked potentials. The question of which is "best" among the brain stem responses, the electrocochleogram, the cortical responses, or the middle responses depends on just what your problem is and what your needs are. The same goes for the acoustic stimulus. The unfiltered click is fine for the kind of screening of infants that Dr. Galambos told us about. It is not nearly so good for the derivation of an audiogram. I will repeat my hope that for audiological purposes we can soon standardize on filtered clicks and how to filter them, so that data can be interchanged more freely fron one laboratory and clinic to another. Tone bursts will still have their place. The clear definition of objectives is one of the things that you all have to consider, particularly whether your interest is audiological, otological or neurological; and this will determine the requirements of the equipment that you will install.

INDEX

A B C 8 D 9 E 0 F 1 G 2 H 3 I 4 J 5